Shelter Medicine for Veterinarians and Staff

Shelter Medicine for Veterinarians and Staff

Edited by **Lila Miller, DVM,** and
Stephen Zawistowski, PhD, CAAB

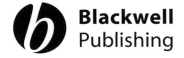
Blackwell
Publishing

LILA MILLER, DVM, is the Senior Director of Animal Sciences and Veterinary Advisor of the American Society for the Prevention of Cruelty to Animals, New York, NY. She has more than 25 years experience working in the field of animal sheltering.

STEPHEN ZAWISTOWSKI, PhD, CAAB, is Senior Vice President and Science Advisor of the American Society for Prevention of Cruelty to Animals. He joined the ASPCA in 1988 as Vice President of Education.

Blackwell Publishing Professional
2121 State Avenue, Ames, Iowa 50014, USA

Orders: 1-800-862-6657
Office: 1-515-292-0140
Fax: 1-515-292-3348
Web site: www.blackwellprofessional.com

Blackwell Publishing Ltd
9600 Garsington Road, Oxford OX4 2DQ, UK
Tel.: +44 (0)1865 776868

Blackwell Publishing Asia
550 Swanston Street, Carlton, Victoria 3053, Australia
Tel.: +61 (0)3 8359 1011

Printed on acid-free paper in the United States of America

First edition, 2004

Library of Congress Cataloging-in-Publication Data
Shelter medicine for veterinarians and staff / edited by Lila Miller and Stephen Zawistowski—1st ed.
p. ; cm.
Includes bibliographical references and index.
ISBN 0-8138-2448-6 (alk. paper)
1. Veterinary medicine. 2. Pets—Diseases.
3. Animal shelters.
[DNLM: 1. Veterinary Medicine—methods.
2. Animal Diseases—diagnosis. 3. Animal Diseases—prevention & control. 4. Animal Welfare.]
I. Miller, Lila. II. Zawistowski, Stephen.
SF745.S46 2004
636.089—dc22
2003023828

The last digit is the print number: 9 8 7 6

Dedication

This book is dedicated to Lloyd Tait, VMD, the ASPCA's first "head of shelter medicine," who was everything one could imagine in a friend and mentor. Irascible, supportive, quixotic, and fiercely dedicated to animal welfare, he laid the early foundation for the formal practice of veterinary medicine in the ASPCA shelters.

Contents

Section 3: Disease Management

Section 4: Shelter and Community Programs

Section 5: Animal Cruelty

Contributors

Leslie D. Appel, DVM
Instructor in Clinical Sciences
Cornell University College of Veterinary
Medicine
Ithaca, New York

Michael Bannasch, BS, RVT
Center for Companion Animal Health
School of Veterinary Medicine
University of California
Davis, California

**Richard Bednarski, DVM, MS,
Diplomate ACVA**
Associate Professor and Hospital Director
Ohio State University College of Veterinary
   Medicine
Columbus, Ohio

Kelley Bollen, MS
Animal Behaviorist
Massachusetts Society for the Prevention of
   Cruelty to Animals (MSPCA)
Springfield, Massachusetts

Linda P. Case, MS
Lecturer, Companion Animal Sciences
Department of Animal Sciences
University of Illinois
Urbana, Illinois

Holly Cheever, DVM
Vice President, New York State Humane
Association (NYSHA)
Voorheesville, New York

Cheryl Diehl
Manager, Wildlife Rehabilitation Center
Wisconsin Humane Society
Milwaukee, Wisconsin

Scott Diehl
Manager, Wildlife Rehabilitation Center
Wisconsin Humane Society
Milwaukee, Wisconsin

Julie Dinnage, DVM
Director of Animal Protection Medicine
MSPCA
South Huntington, Massachusetts

George C. Fahey Jr., PhD
Professor of Animal Sciences and Nutritional
   Sciences
Department of Animal Sciences
University of Illinois
Urbana, Illinois

Janet Foley, DVM, PhD
Assistant Professor
School of Veterinary Medicine, Center for Vector-
   borne Diseases and Department of Medicine and
   Epidemiology
University of California
Davis, California

**Richard B. Ford, DVM, MS, Diplomate ACVIM,
Hon. ACVPM**
Professor of Medicine
North Carolina State University College of
   Veterinary Medicine
Raleigh, North Carolina

Scott M. Giacoppo
Project Coordinator, MSPCA
Metro South Animal Care and Adoption Center
Brockton, Massachusetts

Nicholas Gilman
Vice President of Services
Animal Care and Equipment Services (ACES)
Denver, Colorado

Jill Goldman, PhD
Animal Behavior Fellow
ASPCA
New York, New York

Robert C. Hart, DVM, Diplomate ACVS
Instructor, Orthopedics and Neurosurgery
Cornell University Hospital for Animals
Ithaca, New York

Kate F. Hurley, DVM, MPVM
Director of Maddie's Shelter
    Medicine Program
Center for Companion Animal Health
School of Veterinary Medicine
University of California
Davis, California

Tom Johnson, NCARB
Thomas Johnson Architects
Morton, Pennsylvania

Charlotte A. Lacroix, DVM, Esq.
Priority Veterinary Legal Consultants
Whitehouse Station, New Jersey

Julie Levy, DVM, PhD, Diplomate ACVIM
Assistant Professor, Small Animal
    Medicine
University of Florida College of
    Veterinary Medicine
Gainesville, Florida

Edward A. Leonard, DVM
Retired Special State Police Officer
Slade Veterinary Hospital
Framingham, Massachusetts

Mark Lloyd, DVM
Wildlife Conservation, Management
    and Medicine
Deputy Team Commander, Veterinary
Medical Assistance Team 1
East Setauket, New York

Amy Marder, VMD
Director of Behavior Services
Animal Rescue League of Boston
Boston, Massachusetts

Janet C. Martin, DVM
Director of Veterinary Services
Roger Williams Park Zoo
Providence, Rhode Island

Jörg Mayer, DVM, MS
Clinical Assistant Professor
Head of Exotics Service
Tufts University School of
    Veterinary Medicine
North Grafton, Massachusetts

Lila Miller, DVM
Senior Director and Veterinary Advisor
ASPCA
New York, New York

Julie Morris, MS
Senior Vice President, National Shelter Outreach
SPCA
New York, New York

Gary J. Patronek, VMD, MS, PhD
Associate Professor
Tufts University School of Veterinary Medicine
North Grafton, Massachusetts

Michelle Posage, DVM
New England Veterinary Behavior Associates
Lexington, Massachusetts

Susan M. Prattis, VMD, PhD, Diplomate ACLAM
Assistant Professor of Biology and Schottenstein
Professor of Neuroscience
Yeshiva University
New York, New York

Pamela Reid, PhD, CAAB
Vice President, Animal Behavior Center
American Society for the Prevention of Cruelty to
    Animals (ASPCA)
New York, New York

Robert Reisman, DVM
Coordinator of Abuse Cases
Henry Bergh Memorial Hospital
ASPCA
New York, New York

Janet Scarlett, DVM, MPH, PhD
Associate Professor of Epidemiology
Department of Population Medicine and Diagnostic
    Science
Cornell University College of Veterinary Medicine
Ithaca, New York

Leslie Sinclair, DVM
Shelter Veterinary Services
Columbia, Maryland

Fern Van Sant, DVM
For the Birds, San Jose, California
Maui Animal Rescue and Sanctuary,
    Maui, Hawaii

Bonnie Yoffe-Sharp, DVM
City Veterinarian
Animal Services Division
Palo Alto, California

Stephen Zawistowski, PhD, CAAB
Senior Vice President and Science Advisor
ASPCA
New York, New York

Acknowledgments

This book would not have been possible without the cooperation and support of a great many people. The ASPCA as an organization and our many dear colleagues here have provided a wide range of assistance from important content contributions to a friendly ear. Many of the ideas for the book developed while we worked with three different ASPCA presidents. The late John F. Kullberg, Ed.D., always supported efforts to develop the best possible care for the animals in the shelter incorporating new advances in veterinary medicine and behavioral science during his term as president. Roger A. Caras shared his gift of impatience—why couldn't things get better, faster. Larry Hawk, DVM, was at the helm when the book was started. He provided support for the work flexibility and intellectual freedom so important to a project like this. We now welcome Ed Sayres as president and look forward to seeing the seeds planted here flower under his leadership. Special thanks to Rosemary Rodriquez, without whose valuable assistance, attention to detail, and unflappable personality, this project would have been infinitely more difficult.

Finally, our partners and families have been understanding and supportive of countless weekends, holidays, and vacations spent with file folders, editing pens, and laptops.

Thank you all.

Lila Miller and Stephen Zawistowski

Introduction

On first examination, it might seem surprising that it has taken this long for a book on the practice of veterinary medicine in the shelter environment to appear. After all, both disciplines started with the care of livestock and horses. Over the years, however, they have each followed different paths. Sheltering moved to a primary emphasis on dogs, and to some extent, cats, by 1900. Veterinary medicine did not experience this shift until after WWII. Off and on, shelters and veterinarians were in conflict, sometimes over ideology, sometimes over business practices, and sometimes over what is in the best interest of animals. A variety of social, economic, philosophical, and professional factors have created a new dynamic that both compels and rewards shelters and veterinarians that engage in cooperative ventures. The opportunities are myriad, and the obstacles daunting.

In the past, veterinarians were usually called to give advice without having any understanding of the dynamics that are involved in running a shelter. The call was usually in response to public criticism about conditions in general at the shelter, or in response to a specific disease outbreak. A veterinarian spent a minimum amount of time talking to shelter directors and managers, a hasty shelter visit was arranged, and the options offered were often unworkable or ineffective due to severely limited resources or a failure to understand both the internal and external shelter policies. The experience was deemed an exercise in futility for both parties. Moreover, municipal shelter policies were often aimed at animal control, not animal health and welfare. As long as euthanasia was wielded as the primary weapon against disease and overcrowding, it would seem reasonable that the demand for veterinary expertise was minimal. Any sign of illness, however mild, was often a death sentence for animals.

Today, however, the design of health care programs specifically for animal shelters is a challenge that is being taken up by veterinarians in increasing numbers. The current increase in demand for veterinary services can almost certainly be partially attributed to the rise of the No Kill movement that seeks to end the euthanasia of adoptable animals as a means for population control. It becomes clear to anyone who works at a shelter for any length of time that the longer animals are held, the more likely they are to become ill, whether from direct contact with disease agents or from stress. Most existing health care guidelines for facilities housing multiple small animals were developed for laboratories, catteries, and kennels that operate with an entirely different set of goals and standards. In addition to providing specific disease information and spay/neuter services to address the problem of excess numbers of unwanted animals, veterinarians are now more intimately involved in the management and day-to-day workings of the shelter and are being asked to comment on policies and procedures that were not traditionally seen as part of the veterinarian's domain. Expectations are that the veterinarian can answer questions about shelter design, sanitation protocols, temperament testing, and mass euthanasia—subjects that a typical veterinary education does not begin to address. The issues have become much more complex as standards of care are rising, animal shelters are becoming more professional in their approach to placing animals, and the legal consequences related to zoonosis and other liability issues are increasing.

The prevention of disease in an animal shelter requires a much more comprehensive approach than simply prescribing vaccination and treatment protocols. A review of the veterinary literature seldom reveals any specific data that veterinarians can apply with confidence in shelter settings wherein the predominant population is dogs and cats. Without the benefit of clinical research studies, finding answers to shelter questions poses a real challenge. One of the few published articles specifically about shelter medicine appeared in *Current Veterinary Therapy* more than 10 years ago (Edwards, 1989). A few clinical studies related to shelters have been performed. In 1993, an article appeared in the *Journal of the American Veterinary Medical Association* called "An Idea Whose Time Has Come, Veterinarians in Humane Society Administration" (Patronek, 1993). The AVMA crafted two statements designed to guide veterinarians in their dealings with the humane community as if it were inevitable that there would be misunderstandings, legal and ethical problems, and conflicts of interest. One is an agreement adopted in 1982 by the American Humane association and the AVMA called "A Memorandum of Understanding for Humane Organizations and Veterinarians" (AVMA, 2002). The second is "AVMA Guidelines for Veterinary Associations and Veterinarians Working for Humane Organizations" (AVMA, 2002). The AVMA has adopted numerous other position statements over the years to address programs and concepts that arose from the animal sheltering community—early age neutering, abandoned and feral cat programs, ovariohysterectomy—orchiectomy clinics, dog and cat population control, microchipping, and so on. Lack of awareness of some of the issues concerning shelters and shelter veterinarians has not been a problem.

This textbook was conceived as an aid to the veterinarians and dedicated animal care professionals striving to provide excellent preventive and medical care options in the current existing vacuum of validated clinical research. Unlike many other traditional veterinary textbooks dedicated to one species or one subject that claim to be the only book one will need, the multiplicity of experiences that are encountered in the world of animal sheltering preclude making such a claim. This book should be one of several essential texts in the shelter veterinarian's library. Each section is designed to provide information that will help veterinarians create programs and protocols that meet the specific needs of the shelter and the community. The first section provides an introduction into the world of animal sheltering, discussing the history and operation of animal shelters, the administrative and legal challenges to be met, and a review of the relinquishment data and population statistics that help define pet population issues. The second section on husbandry will give insight into shelter design flaws that must be addressed to help create a healthy physical facility,

and the sanitation protocols that will help maintain a disease-free environment. Brief reviews of care for selected species will be covered with the understanding that in-depth diagnostic protocols and treatment procedures can be found in numerous other veterinary journals and texts. The focus is on temporary care and husbandry issues that are unique to and pertinent for shelters. The lengthy infectious disease management section explains the importance of acquiring and managing data to help minimize disease transmission and provides medical information about canine and feline diseases that are encountered in shelters. The section on shelter and community programs provides information about some subjects that are likely to be encountered by veterinarians working for shelters that are both purely veterinary in nature, such as spay/neuter; some that are less so, such as foster care; and others that are an interesting blend of the veterinary and nonveterinary, such as mass euthanasia protocols, animal handling, feral cat issues and disaster medicine. The final section on animal cruelty gives an insight into how far the profession still has to go to deal with animal cruelty, particularly in developing the field of veterinary forensics and on-site crime scene investigation.

Interest in this specialty area is increasing. The Association of Shelter Veterinarians was formed in 2001. A course in shelter medicine is being taught at Cornell University's Veterinary College, and a shelter residency program is available at the University of California at Davis Veterinary College with more being developed (Auburn is considering one), and an Internet course is being designed for the Veterinary Information Network (VIN). Shelter medicine and community health tracks are being offered at two of the largest veterinary conferences in the country—the North American Veterinary Conference in Orlando and the Western States conference in Las Vegas—and shelter medicine courses are being offered at most of the national and regional animal welfare conferences, including the Shelter Veterinarian's Conference offered at the American Humane annual conference.

The authors who have contributed to this book have been among the first to accept the challenge of defining a new field of practice. It is hoped that this textbook will help begin to establish a body of knowledge and to stimulate further interest in this developing specialty.

REFERENCES

AVMA. 2002. Directory and Resource Manual

Edwards, M.A. 1989. The practice of veterinary medicine in a humane society facility in *Current Veterinary Therapy X,* Kirk and Bonagura, eds. Philadelphia, PA: WB Saunders, 85–90.

Patronek, G. 1993. An idea whose time has come: veterinarians in humane society administration in *Journal of the American Veterinary Medical Association,* Vol.202, 862–864.

Section 1:
Animal Shelters and
Their Functions

INTRODUCTION

When first exposed to the workings of a good-sized, busy animal shelter, people frequently are overwhelmed by the frenetic pace, jargon, and variety of activities. This is not surprising, because animal shelters often fill all of the roles that numerous non-profits and government-operated services provide for the human inhabitants of a community. Homeless shelter, emergency clinic, food bank, police force, and adoption agency for animals often are found under one roof. Section 1 provides a short primer that will help readers to orient themselves in the complicated world of animal sheltering.

Zawistowski and Morris provide a short history of animal shelters in chapter 1, tracing their development from impounds for colonial livestock to modern programs and facilities. Modern efforts to coordinate and harmonize shelter programs and activities will need to overcome a history of independent function and action that dates to the very beginning of animal sheltering. In chapter 2, Scarlett delineates what we know about the pet population issues and how these issues impact animal shelters and their programs. She summarizes the available literature on the numbers of animals entering animal shelters and the reasons for relinquishment, providing a substantive description of the size of the problem. Implementing a successful medical program at an animal shelter is as much about managing people as it is animals. Yoffe-Sharp shares her experiences in the field and makes some recommendations on how to surmount the administrative hurdles of shelter medicine in chapter 3. Working in an animal shelter opens up a new environment of potential legal entanglements for a veterinarian. Lacroix, speaking from the unique perspective of both veterinarian and attorney, provides an introduction to these issues and some guidelines for reducing potential liability in chapter 4.

1

1
The Evolving Animal Shelter

Stephen Zawistowski and Julie Morris

INTRODUCTION

The origins of animal shelters are not so much lost in the mists of time, as they are clouded by the fog of indifference. Animal shelters have long occupied a spot on the periphery of a community's geography and awareness. They have been the place where what we don't want to think about happens to pets we no longer care about. Dramatic changes in the past 20 years have led to new policies and practices at animal shelters, reflecting a change in the expectations of animal shelter performance. These changes draw heavily on the expertise of veterinarians. This chapter traces some of the developments in animal sheltering and their impact on veterinary issues associated with shelters.

FORMATION OF THE FIELD

The Origin of Pounds

Shelters for companion animals arose from the impoundments that were common in colonial towns and villages and that used to contain wandering livestock. Animals captured by the "poundmaster" could later be reclaimed by their owners. Wandering dogs, posing a nuisance and safety risk, would have been picked up and taken to the impound, or "pound." The changing nature of communities, with a growing divide between farms and town, was reflected in a changing role for the poundmasters until their primary focus was not livestock, but dogs, and to a lesser extent, cats. Unlike the livestock, which had value and were generally reclaimed, dogs and cats were often left at the pound. Problems in pound management were compounded by the fact that the poundmasters generally did not receive a salary and depended on the redemption fees paid by individuals reclaiming animals. Owners were either more likely to reclaim livestock, or the poundmasters were able to slaughter or sell unclaimed livestock. Because unclaimed dogs and cats could not be slaughtered as food, limited effort and resources were applied to their death. It was not uncommon for the poundmaster to kill them by clubbing or drowning. Vivid illustrations depict the iron cages filled with dogs that were once lowered into New York City's East River as a way to drown the dogs. Corruption was common. Because owned dogs were easier to catch, and more likely to be reclaimed, a racket developed to kidnap pets and take them to the pound for a bounty. Owners, after they were informed of their lost pet being found at the pound, would hurry to claim their dogs and pay the redemption fees.

Spread of SPCAs and Humane Societies

Henry Bergh, a wealthy New York City philanthropist and diplomat, founded the American Society for the Prevention of Cruelty to Animals (ASPCA) in 1866. Modeled after the Royal SPCA founded in England in 1824, it was the first animal protection organization in the Western Hemisphere. The ASPCA's early focus was on the mistreatment of the many horses that worked to transport people and freight in the city. However, as early as the ASPCA's second annual report (1868), information can be found on correspondence between Henry Bergh and the mayor regarding the treatment of the animals at the pound and the practice of paying bounties for the capture of stray dogs to youth under the age of 18 years (Zawistowski, 1998a).

The ASPCA would soon be joined by sister organizations in Buffalo, New York (1867), and Boston, Philadelphia, and San Francisco (1868). Although the Societies would share many common goals, they were independent organizations that did not operate as branches of a national structure. This independence would come to play a role in the current state of the highly localized nature and management of animal shelter programs. In each case, the formation of these societies was championed by a small group of prominent local citizens. Often, a single individual would be the guiding force within the organization. The Pennsylvania SPCA came about largely through the efforts of Caroline Earle White. At a time when it was unusual for a woman to play such a prominent role, she energized the formation of a society in Philadelphia. When propriety and convention relegated her to a background role with the society she helped bring about, she formed the Women's Branch of the Pennsylvania SPCA in 1869. In 1898, with its own charter and treasury, the Women's Pennsylvania SPCA was recognized, with the removal of "Branch" from its title (Zawistowski, in press). Ninety years later, the society's name would be changed to the Women's Humane Society (see note at the end of this chapter).

Caroline Earle White and the Women's Branch of the Pennsylvania SPCA figure prominently in the development of animal shelters. In 1874, in response to the horrific treatment visited upon the dogs and cats at the Philadelphia pound, the society built and dedicated the City Refuge for Lost and Suffering Animals. It was the first such facility designed and dedicated to the humane treatment of animals, providing medical treatment, placing them into new homes when possible, and when all else failed, providing a quick and painless death. To this end, a steel chamber was developed into which a gas could be introduced to quickly asphyxiate the animals. In New York, while Bergh continued to pressure the city to make reforms at the pound, he steadfastly refused to accept the job for the ASPCA. Bergh was concerned that taking on the job would detract from the society's role as an advocate for animals and would place undue financial strain on the organization. It would not be until 1894, six years after Bergh's death, that the ASPCA would assume management of New York City's animal shelters.

Development of Animal Control

Several developments in other areas of the country would also have an impact on animal sheltering approaches. In 1866, the city of Cleveland, Ohio, introduced the concept of licensing dogs, and in 1877, Dodge City, Kansas, issued the first license tags (Arkow, 1980). License monies eventually would become the primary source of funds for operating animal shelters in many communities. License tags would permit the identification of owned versus unowned dogs. This was particularly important given the general acceptance of allowing owned dogs to run free in some areas.

When the ASPCA did assume the animal control responsibilities for New York City in 1894, the society introduced the concept of full-time salaried staff to carry out the required work. Using dog license monies from a newly enacted state law, these salaried employees were no longer dependent upon the redemption fees collected from pet owners. As a result, they were able to concentrate on the capture of the many unowned dogs that roamed various districts of the city. In 1894, the ASPCA caught and euthanized more dogs and cats than the municipal management had the year before. Given the present social and political climate, it is ironic to note that the organization was *praised* for this enhanced efficiency and public service (Zawistowski et al., 1998). This likely stemmed from two important aspects of the work. First, the use of salaried employees eliminated the racket of kidnapping owned dogs, and second, stray roaming dogs were an important public hazard, and removing them from the streets was indeed a valuable public service. Another important observation was that the ASPCA also handled cats as part of the animal control function. In many areas cats were not handled at that time, and this remains the case in some communities. As cats have been added to the animal sheltering function in various communities, their representation in the sheltered population has tended to increase with their increasing popularity as companion animals. However, at least in New York City, cats have always been the majority of the animals that come into the animal shelters (Zawistowski, et al., 1998).

DEVELOPMENTS IN EUTHANASIA METHODS
Much of the early effort in humane animal sheltering focused on improving the conditions in which dogs and cats lived at the shelter and providing a more humane way of killing those animals that were not reclaimed by owners or not placed into new homes. As indicated, clubbing and drowning were among the most common methods employed. Various gas chambers were developed to provide a

more benign and aesthetically pleasing form of death. The gases used might be derived from specific chemical reactions, or at least in some cases, illuminating gas was used. Until the introduction of electricity for household illumination, gas was piped into homes for this purpose. Derived from coal, it would have asphyxiated animals exposed in a closed environment. Carbon monoxide is still used in a number of animal shelters to euthanize animals. Electricity as a mode of euthanasia for animals was also considered during the time that it was introduced for the execution of human criminals. In one dramatic demonstration, Edison arranged the electrocution of an elephant that had killed one of its keepers during a rampage (*The Commercial Advertiser*, January 5, 1903). The use of rapid decompression chambers was introduced in the 1970s. Eventually, the injection of an overdose of sodium pentobarbital, or other barbiturate, became the most widely accepted form of euthanasia for animals in shelters (Armstrong et al., 2001).

Although it would seem that this aspect of animal sheltering has come to consensus, it is an issue that continues to cause controversy. The American Veterinary Medical Association document on methods for the humane euthanasia of animals generally is accepted as the standard of practice (AVMA Panel on Euthanasia, 2000). However, difficulties associated with the purchase and administration of sodium pentobarbital by shelters without a staff or collaborating veterinarian available and the continuing need for the education of the staff and authorities responsible for shelter function have compromised the universal implementation of euthanasia by injection. Some communities still permit the killing of unwanted dogs and cats with carbon monoxide derived from engine exhaust, gunshots, and other less humane methods.

PET POPULATION ISSUES

Although the question of "how" animals were killed was, and remains, a major theme for developments in animal sheltering since its earliest days, the question of "how many" did not really become an issue until the last third of the twentieth century. The number of mentions of "pet overpopulation" and a concern for the need to euthanize millions of animals across the nation each year is limited until this time. Even the pet care books distributed by humane societies did not emphasize sterilization of

pets as a way to reduce the numbers of unwanted pets (American Humane Education Society, no date; KIND Report, no date; Henley, 1966). Sterilization was seen primarily as a way to cope with inconvenient and unwanted sexual behaviors in pets. Statistics on the numbers of animals received at animal shelters and their subsequent disposition are notoriously rare, and frequently unreliable. Data collected by the ASPCA for a 100-year period from 1894 until 1994 provides a longitudinal view of one specific community, New York City (Zawistowski et al., 1998). The highest recorded total was for 1928 when 85,744 dogs and 217,774 cats were taken in for a total of 303,518 animals. Nearly 95 percent of these animals were euthanized. These numbers remained constant and high during the Depression era. There was a substantial decline during the post World War II period, with 167,712 animals received in 1954. This change is probably associated with the major demographic shift the United States experienced during this era. Many families moved out of cities and into the suburbs. Once there, many acquired pets that they might not have had while living within the confines of smaller city homes and apartments. Coupled with a *laissez-faire* approach to responsible care for their pets was limited attention to the explosive reproductive potential of domesticated companion animals, resulting in a pet population explosion. Regardless of the actual numbers, because these have always been difficult to document, the most salient observation is that the numbers, whatever they were, exceeded the resources required to manage the problem. At the same time, the sense and image of animals was changing. Popular culture helped to change public appreciation of dogs and cats as animals with specific occupations or roles to that of cherished companions (Milekic, 1998). As a result, public tolerance for the caricatured dog pound diminished, resulting in a trend toward greater professionalism in the management of animal shelter functions in many communities (Armstrong, et al., 2001).

NATURE OF SHELTERS

Organization and Function

Communities responded to changing animal shelter needs in a wide variety of ways. In the absence of a national system of oversight or governance, local shelter operations and policies were intimately correlated with community values and economies. Tip O'Neill, former speaker of the United States House of Representatives, who is frequently credited with the statement that, "All politics are local," could have just as easily been describing the condition and operation of animal shelters. Several common approaches did dominate the ways in which animal shelters were operated and funded. Communities with active and effective humane societies or SPCAs often arranged for the society to provide for the animal sheltering needs, similar to the arrangements in Philadelphia and New York City. Funding could come through the collection of dog license fees, redemption fees, fines collected for violations of animal control laws, or other associated service fees. Other communities responded by having an animal shelter operated by a designated municipal agency. This might be the government arm that also provided police protection, sanitation, park maintenance, or health services. A variety of intermediate approaches were also undertaken. An existing humane society that operated an animal shelter might provide contract shelter boarding services for a community, while field services such as capturing strays would be managed through a municipal or government arm. Quite a few larger communities had both a municipally run animal shelter or dog pound and a humane society animal shelter. The level of cooperation between government-operated shelters and humane societies, whether operating a shelter or not, ranged from very close and supportive to tense and critical. The level of tension reflected both the quality of performance at the shelters and the personalities of the individuals involved.

Animal Intake

During this time, a wide variety of activities came under the scope of animal shelter operations. These included services provided within the shelter and those actively projected into the community. At a most basic level, animal shelter functions revolve around the intake, care, and disposition of animals in a community. Animals may arrive at a shelter in a variety of different ways. Two of the most common would be those animals brought in by an owner no longer able, or willing, to provide a home or care or stray animals delivered to the animal shelter. These strays may have been caught by animal shelter or animal control staff or found by members of the public. Another source of animals would be

those seized by law enforcement officials from individuals accused of animal cruelty, abuse, or neglect. Depending on the programs offered, a shelter may also hold animals when caretakers are incapacitated or evicted, fleeing domestic violence, or in other emergency circumstances. In each of these cases, providing care for the animals may be governed by a complex web of laws, documentation of ownership, and court orders, which may in fact contradict one another or act contrary to the best interests of the animals. Shelter managers and veterinarians need to work closely together to coordinate their efforts in these cases.

An increasingly common form of intake is the transfer of animals from another shelter. Dogs or cats will be moved from one location to another where they may have a better chance of placement in a new home. This is especially common for puppies and kittens. In some areas, where spaying and neutering is common, and there is a fairly high level of pet owner responsibility, puppies, small dogs, and kittens may be brought in from other areas for adoption.

ANIMAL CARE

Substantial change has been seen in the level of care provided for animals in a shelter; the many chapters in this volume are a testament to this change. Early shelters or pounds were often designed with large community cages or pens for dogs or cats. Many of the shelters built during the post World War II era were strongly influenced by a rapidly expanding knowledge in veterinary infectious disease medicine and sanitation and incorporated individual housing for all animals to limit the spread of disease in the shelter environment. Modern shelter designs have combined new materials, mechanical equipment, and a better understanding of animal behavior to facilitate maintaining the physical and psychological health of animals. In some cases, dog kennels have been replaced by private apartments that provide more space and a homelike environment. Community housing for cats is becoming common again as well. The length of time that animals may stay in a shelter can vary greatly. Shelters that accept stray animals generally are required to keep them for a minimum number of days to allow an owner to find and reclaim a lost pet. This holding period can range from 2–3 days to 10 or more and depends on community and state law and policy. Other holding periods would be those for animals seized in cruelty cases, animals held after biting someone, and those held when their owners have been arrested or incapacitated.

ANIMAL DISPOSITION

The disposition of animals also has a variety of different options. Euthanasia and placement of dogs and cats in new homes are the two most common. The decision to euthanize can be based on the need to make room for more animals, for humane reasons if the animal is injured or sick, or if the animal is not considered suitable for placement in a new home due to serious behavior problems. Other forms of disposition include returning lost or stray animals to owners who reclaim them or transferring animals to other shelters or various specialty rescue or foster groups. Less common than in the past is releasing dogs and cats to universities or other institutions for research purposes. This practice, known as pound seizure, is in fact prohibited by law in 14 states and by local regulation or policy in many other communities. Native wildlife or uncommon domestic and exotic animals frequently are transferred to other facilities, such as sanctuaries or wildlife rehabilitators.

NATIONAL ORGANIZATIONS

Those who run shelters have not been completely on their own. Both the American Humane Association (AHA) and the Humane Society of the United States (HSUS) provided a variety of support services, guidelines, standards of practice, and training to improve the performance of animal shelters. Phyllis Wright of the HSUS played a significant leadership role, emphasizing that companion animals would benefit most from efforts that combined legislation to provide laws that protect animals, education on the responsible and proper care of animals, and sterilization to reduce the numbers of unwanted animals (Armstrong, et al., 2001). Many current leaders in the animal sheltering field trace their dedication to work in the field to Phyllis Wright. The National Animal Control Association (NACA) was formed to meet the particular needs of the government-operated animal shelter and animal control programs. The Society of Animal Welfare Administrators was formed in 1970, as a way to share information and ideas among the executives who run animal shelters. In 1995, after the ASPCA returned

animal control responsibilities to New York City, the Society also began to offer training and support programs through a National Shelter Outreach department. In addition to training and opportunities for networking, these organizations have also helped to develop benchmarks for animal shelter programs and operations (ASPCA, no date, p. 9).

A NEW PARADIGM?

There have probably always been shelters that accepted animals but did not euthanize to make room for additional animals as needed. These *No Kill* shelters typically played a low profile role in their communities. They were able to receive a limited number of owner-surrendered or relinquished animals and hold them until they were able to place them in new adoptive homes. The past 20 years have seen the development of the *No Kill Movement*. This movement represents the progression in thought from *how* animals were killed, to *how many,* and now to *why*. In a highly controversial and influential essay "In the Name of Mercy," Ed Duvin (1989) took issue with the idea of shelters continuing to facilitate irresponsible pet owners by euthanizing the animals. He argued that if shelters stepped away from this tactic, society would be forced to deal with the problem in a more reasonable and humane fashion.

In a dramatic, and highly publicized endeavor, Richard Avanzino announced that the San Francisco SPCA would give up its animal control contract and work with a city-managed agency to make San Francisco America's first city in which no adoptable pets were euthanized (www.sfspca.org/history). This event in 1989 served as the rallying point for a national movement to promote and support the philosophy that animal shelters should not euthanize unwanted pets as a way of dealing with society's failure to promote and require responsible pet ownership.

A part of this effort has been the recognition that as programs evolve, more and more of the work of animal shelters will need to be proactive and will take place outside the walls of the shelter. Humane groups and animal shelters have offered humane education programs (Zawistowski, 1998b) and other community education programs for more than a century. The key development here has been the evolution of direct animal care programs that go beyond traditional animal control and the capture of strays or dangerous animals. These include off-site adoptions, the use of the Internet to support and promote adoptions, mobile spay/neuter vans, trap-neuter-return programs for feral cats, animal behavior help lines, and dog-training programs. The intent is to expand the shelter's scope of operations beyond its current physical facility and location and to solve problems by preventing them *in situ*. The significance of these efforts, and the importance of veterinary participation, are such that other chapters in this text will address them in some detail.

CONCLUSION

Animal shelters were once thought of as bleak and depressing. Today, innovative shelters are bright and cheerful and offer the comforts of home. Design elements now take advantage of natural sunlight; eliminate bars and cages; create park-like settings; use colorful murals and graphics; provide interactive learning centers, improved air quality, noise abatement, and areas where members of the public can interact with the animals. These changes have helped to change the face and reputation of many animal shelters. These modern shelters offer much more than animal housing. They provide a wide variety of services including humane education, cruelty investigation, behavior help lines for adopters and the public, dog training, off-site adoption centers, spay/neuter services, feral cat programs, and an ever-growing number of community outreach and partnership activities.

The vision of the modern shelter is that shelters are not just for animals; they are for communities. It is the vision that "the best shelter is a humane community," that is revolutionizing the animal shelters in the most profound way.

REFERENCES

The American Humane Education Society, no date. *Dog Care.* Boston, MA: The American Humane Education Society. (Reprinted from the Pennsylvania Society for the Prevention of Cruelty to Animals, Philadelphia, PA.)

The American Veterinary Medical Association. 2001. Report of the AVMA panel on euthanasia. *Journal of the American Veterinary Medical Association*, 218: 669–696.

Arkow, P. 1980. Future trends in animal control. Speech delivered to the Animal Control and Public Health Seminar, Kansas Animal Control Association and Kansas State University, Manhattan, KS, February 29.

Armstrong, M., Tomasello, S., and Hunter, C. 2001. From pets to companion animals. In *The State of the Animals 2001*, D. J. Salem and A. N. Rowan, eds., pp. 77–85. Washington, DC: Humane Society Press.

ASPCA, no date. *ASPCA Keys to a Great Shelter: The ASPCA National Shelter Outreach Guide to Starting and Improving a Humane Organization.*

The Commercial Advertiser, January 5, 1903. Bad elephant killed. Topsy meets quick and painless death at Coney Island.

Duvin, E. 1989. In the name of mercy. *Animalines*. (Reprinted online at www.bestfriends.org/nmhp/pdf/Mercy.pdf.)

Henley, D. (ed.), 1966. ASPCA guide to dog care. New York: Taplinger Publishing Co., Inc.

KIND Report, no date. *Caring for Your Dog.* Washington, DC: KIND, The Humane Society of the United States.

Milekic, S. 1998. Disneyfication. In *Encyclopedia of Animal Rights and Animal Welfare*, M. Bekoff and C. Meaney, eds., pp. 133–134. Westport, CT: Greenwood.

Zawistowski, S. 1998a. The American Society for the Prevention of Cruelty to Animals. In *Encyclopedia of Animal Rights and Animal Welfare*, M. Bekoff and C. Meaney, eds., pp. 9–12. Westport, CT: Greenwood.

Zawistowski, S. 1998b. Humane education movement. In *Encyclopedia of Animal Rights and Animal Welfare*, M. Bekoff and C. Meaney, eds., pp.189–191. Westport, CT: Greenwood.

Zawistowski, S. (in press) The history of SPCAs in America. In *International Animal World Encyclopedia*, Rev. Andrew Linzey, ed. Plymouth, England: Kingsley Media, LTD.

Zawistowski, S., Morris, J., Salman, M. D., and Ruch-Gallie, R. 1998. Population dynamics, overpopulation, and the welfare of companion animals: New insights on old and new data. *Journal of Applied Animal Welfare Science*, 1(*3*): 193–206.

NOTE

The first Humane Society was founded in England in 1774 "...for the recovery of persons apparently drowned." It gained royal status under the patronage of King George III in 1787. Founded by two doctors, the Society also promoted the controversial new technique of resuscitation as a life-saving technique. It is, of course, a long jump from using the term humane to describe a society dedicated to saving drowning humans to its modern application to organizations dedicated to saving animals. The transition apparently happened in the late 1870s and early 1880s in the United States. By that time, humane societies generally were concerned with saving and protecting humans. In 1874, Henry

Bergh, founder of the ASPCA, played an active role in the first successful removal of a child from an abusive home. This led to the formation of the New York Society for the Prevention of Cruelty to Children. Many of the people that Bergh had influenced in the formation of SPCAs across the country took up this new cause as well. However, in many cases, they did not form new organizations. They often merged the saving of animals and children under one roof. Correspondence between Bergh and the leaders of these other SPCAs was at times pointed, as Bergh thought it a mistake to combine the two roles. More often than not, they were combined, and a confusing set of names evolved. In some cases, the two missions were reflected in the ponderous organizational title of Society for the Prevention of Cruelty to Animals and Humane Society. In many cases, the organization eventually truncated its name to the simple title of Humane Society, dropping SPCA all together. When the enforcement of child protection laws was assumed by local governments in most areas around the country, all that might be left to the animal shelter was a name with a curious history and a confusing legacy of organizational titles at the national level.

2

Pet Population Dynamics and Animal Shelter Issues

Janet Scarlett

INTRODUCTION

The word *statistics* is derived from the Latin word *status*, meaning "manner of standing" (Dawson and Trapp, 2001). Early statistics were used to determine Roman residents' assets and to provide the basis for tax assessment (some things never change). Despite their inauspicious beginnings and potentially dry nature, statistics characterize the nature and magnitude of the tragedy of unwanted pets in a manner in which an encounter with one animal or a visit to one shelter cannot do alone. These numbers can lead to insights that enable people to focus on facets of the problem (and the solutions) that can bring about the most benefit. The statistics tell a story of tragedy, progress, hope, and opportunity. Those committed to solving this issue can celebrate the progress already made, the hope that the progress engenders, and the opportunity presented for further progress and the eventual elimination of the problems associated with unwanted animals and their needless deaths.

SOURCES OF DATA

The results of numerous surveys and studies are cited in this chapter. When reading the statistics presented, bear in mind the limitations of the design and conduct of the studies producing the numbers. The perfect survey or observational study will never be conducted. The imperfections do not invalidate the results, only make it incumbent upon the reader to interpret and draw the appropriate inferences. Because results from a few studies are cited frequently in the following review, a brief overview of their strengths and limitations are provided to facil-

itate the reader's understanding and interpretation of the results.

The enumeration of dog and cat populations is not the subject of a national census as is true in people. Estimates of the size of animal populations are derived principally from surveys of samples of American households conducted by various organizations. The most commonly cited figures (that is, from the American Veterinary Medical Association [AVMA], the American Pet Products Manufacturer's Association [APPMA], and the Pet Food Institute [PFI]) are derived from nonrandomly selected household panels that have been assembled to be representative of the U.S. population on certain demographic variables such as income, household size, and so on. The study of household panels results in high response rates, and household characteristics can be characterized readily (Patronek and Rowan, 1995). Studies based on these panels are potentially limited, however, by the often-higher educational and economic status of households willing and able to respond to such surveys. Estimates of pet ownership based on surveys employing random sampling techniques (random digit dialing) (Manning and Rowan, 1992; Teclaw et al. 1992; Patronek et al. 1995) have been approximately 20 lower than those from panels (Patronek and Rowan, 1995). These conflicting results suggest that the panel estimates may be overestimates, which should be borne in mind when reviewing these numbers.

Patronek and Glickman (1994) developed a comprehensive model regarding the dynamics (sources, births, deaths, and movement) of the U.S.-owned dog population using statistics collected from Washington and Iowa in 1991 and a variety of other sources. As acknowledged by the authors, the model is potentially limited by the quality and representativeness of the data upon which it is based and its incorporated assumptions. Despite its limitations, however, this model is the most thoughtful, comprehensive one to date and has produced national estimates, some of which have been replicated subsequently (New, 2001). Unfortunately, because of the dearth of data regarding the large free-roaming cat population and its inter-relationships with owned and sheltered populations, a similar model for cats does not yet exist.

The National Council on Pet Population Study and Policy (NCPPSP) was founded in 1993 to enhance cooperation among national humane and veterinary organizations and to collect data regarding the extent of pet surplus in the United States and the factors contributing to the unacceptably high relinquishment and euthanasia rates of dogs and cats in this country. The Council subsequently funded several studies, three of which are cited in this review. The three studies were titled the *Shelter Statistics Study*, the *Regional Shelter Relinquishment Survey* (RSRS), and the *National Household Survey*.

The *Shelter Statistics Study* was designed to identify all animal shelters in the United States and to collect national data regarding impoundments, euthanasias, adoptions, and redemptions. The study was implemented because no complete list has been collected and maintained by any organization (Rowan, 1991). During the conduct of this study, the reasons for the lack of such a list became clear. Defining a shelter was difficult. Many organizations shelter animals, that is, they identify unowned animals and provide temporary or lifetime care. These include traditional not-for-profit SPCAs and humane societies (some of which provide animal control services), municipally owned facilities, and a growing number of other groups (for example, limited-admission shelters, lifetime sanctuaries, breed and other rescue groups, private individuals, and so on). Not only do these organizations vary widely in size, activities, and lifespan, they also vary in their capability and willingness to provide statistics regarding their operations. This essentially makes the collection and maintenance of a *current* complete national shelter list and national statistics impossible.

The *RSRS* was conducted in 12 full-service animal shelters with animal control responsibilities in four regions of the country (Sacramento County, California; Denver, Larimer, and Weld counties, Colorado; Bergen County, New Jersey and New York City; and Knox and Anderson counties, Tennessee, and Jefferson County, Kentucky) (Salman et al., 1998). The shelters were located in highly urban areas (Denver, New York, and New Jersey), in moderately sized cities (Sacramento) and in semi-rural areas of Colorado, Tennessee, and Kentucky. Data were collected from February 1995 though April 1996. The objectives of this study were to detail owner-reported reasons for relinquishing pets and to identify characteristics of animals surrendered and of their owners over a one-year period. Several publications describe the results of this study (Salman et al., 1998; Salman et al., 2000; New et al., 1999; Scarlett et al., 1999; Kass et al., 2001).

Owners were interviewed personally by trained interviewers using a standardized interview form designed to collect animal characteristics (that is, age, gender, and neuter status), owner characteristics (that is, age, gender, and income level), length of ownership, and original source and cost of the animal. The form allowed for up to five reasons for the relinquishment of an animal(s). The participating shelters were not randomly sampled, but were selected on the basis of their proximity to investigators and interviewers and their willingness to participate. Interviews were collected regarding 3676 surrendered dogs and litters and 1409 cats and litters. Animals impounded for legal reasons or as strays or dead on arrival were excluded.

These study characteristics must be borne in mind as the data are examined. Also, for many analyses, litters were examined separately from individual animals. Although some regional differences were identified, the data generally had high internal consistency, suggesting broad applicability of the results to the shelter community. This, coupled with the consistency with previous investigations and perceptions of leaders in the humane community, suggests that the results are generally valid. Direct application of these results to particular shelters or communities should be made with caution, however, as differences between the sampled shelters and particular shelters and their local circumstances may well exist. Also, because no data were collected from limited-admission shelters or sanctuaries, applicability to these organizations is unknown.

The *National Household Survey* was conducted using a subset of a random sample of 80,000 households in the United States (New et al., 2000). The objectives of this study were 1) to compare the same data collected from people relinquishing animals in the RSRS to that from a sample of U.S. pet-owning households, and 2) to characterize why animals entered and left households, enumerate births and deaths, and estimate the proportions of planned and unplanned litters. The sample included 6899 pet-owning households selected such that approximately half of the sample had a dog or cat leave the household during the previous year. Limitations of this study include possible bias introduced by non-random sampling, over-sampling of households where at least one animal had left during the previous year, and the question of the comparability of the sample of relinquishers to the household sample.

Several other studies have highlighted factors affecting the risk of relinquishment (Patronek et al., 1996a,b; New et al., 2000; Arkow and Dow, 1994; Kidd et al., 1992; Neidhart and Boyd, 2002; Kass and Hart, 1998). The primary limitation of these studies is the lack of random sampling of the shelters studied, the small number of shelters studied, and the consequent questions of generalizability to other areas of the country. Reassuringly, the results have been consistent across these studies, facilitating a more in-depth understanding of the factors contributing to relinquishment and their relative importance.

All studies of the reasons for relinquishment were based on what owners reported. Despite efforts to encourage honest responses, the results of these studies must be evaluated recognizing that false reasons may have been offered to assuage guilt, enhance the likelihood of adoption, and so on.

Summary national estimates relating to pet ownership, dynamics, sheltered animals, and so on masks the wide variability inherent to these statistics. Pet ownership patterns vary by region of the country, urban or rural residence, income levels, and so on (AVMA, 2002); shelter impoundments and euthanasias vary by type of shelter, size of population served, and so on. This inherent variability complicates the estimation of national statistics and

their extrapolation to specific communities and shelters. Also, because most studies did not employ random sampling, confidence intervals and other measures of variability are not presented.

DOG AND CAT POPULATIONS IN THE UNITED STATES

Overall Estimates

Studies of the size and characteristics of pet populations have been conducted by and for a variety of organizations over time. Recently the Pet Food Institute (PFI) released its 2001 figures (Ipsos-NPD, 2001). PFI has sponsored its Pet Incidence Trend Report since 1981, and in 2001 reported 75.6 million cats and 60.2 million dogs in American households. More than a third (34.2 percent) of the approximately 104 million American households owned at least one cat, and 36.9 percent owned at least one dog. Approximately 16 percent of all households owned both species. These data show slight changes in the proportion of households owning dogs and cats since the 1996 PFI survey when 33.4 percent owned cats and 37.6 percent owned dogs. Between 1996 and 2001, a 7.8 percent increase occurred in the number of dogs (up from 55.7 million dogs in 1996), and an 11.2 percent increase occurred in the number of cats (67.9 million cats in 1996), underscoring the rise in multiple-pet households, especially with cats. In 2001 households with cats owned 2.1 cats, whereas households with dogs owned 1.6 dogs.

Data for 2001, published by the American Veterinary Medical Association's Center for Information Management (AVMA, 2002), provided similar estimates for the total owned dogs (61.6 million) and the percentage of households owning dogs (36.1 percent) and somewhat lower estimates of the number of owned cats (70.8 million) and households owning cats (31.6 percent). AVMA estimates of the average number of dogs and cats per household matched those estimated by PFI. Overall, the 2001 AVMA figures suggested that 49.2 percent of cat-owning households owned more than one cat, down somewhat from 1996 when 52 percent of cat-owning households owned multiple cats. As mentioned previously, these estimates may overestimate owned populations by as much as 20 percent.

The figures presented here pertain to owned animals. Because feral dogs no longer constitute a sizeable proportion of the dog population in the United States, these statistics provide reasonable estimates of the total dog population. The data for cats, however, exclude an unknown, but significant, segment of the total feline population. Data from several sources have suggested large numbers of feral or stray cats, at least in some parts of the country. Two California- and one Massachusetts-based study suggested 9–15 percent of households fed cats they did not own (Johnson et al., 1993; Johnson and Lewellen, 1995; Luke 1996). In the California studies, the "fed, but not owned" cats constituted 30–40 percent of all cats enumerated. Alley Cat Allies, a national feral cat advocacy organization, estimated a population of 30–60 million feral and stray cats in the United States (Holton and Manzoor, 1993). Based on these and other data, some authors have estimated that stray and feral cats may account for as many unowned as owned cats in the United States (Patronek and Rowan, 1995). For obvious reasons, precise data are not available, but the not owned, largely unaltered population is an important facet of the pet surplus issue. Because a high proportion of owned cats are neutered (exceeding 75 percent in most surveys) (Manning and Rowan, 1992; New et al., 2000; Patronek et al., 1997), the unowned cat population is undoubtedly the source of many kittens and cats brought to animal shelters each year. Communities searching for solutions to unwanted pets must initiate and maintain programs targeting unowned cats if this major source of cats in shelters is to be controlled or eliminated.

Neutering and Fertility

Relatively high neuter rates among owned dogs (69–73 percent among females and 42–48 percent among males), and the scarcity of puppies in many urban shelters suggest that efforts by humane groups and veterinarians have been successful in lowering canine fertility (New et al., 2000; Patronek et al., 1997; Manning and Rowan, 1992; Teclaw et al., 1992; New, 2001). Patronek and Glickman (1994) estimated that 2.8 percent of dog-owning and 1.1 percent of all households had dogs whelp annually. New et al., (2000) using the National Household Survey data, obtained a similar estimate of 2.6 percent (95 percent C.I.: 2.1–3.1 percent) of U.S dog-owning households had at least one litter born in 1996 (unpublished data). Among these lit-

ters, more than half of the canine litters were unplanned, resulting in approximately 0.55 million unplanned dog litters in 1996. Overall, a crude birth rate of 11.4 puppies per 100 dogs was estimated (New, 2001).

Neuter rates among owned cats consistently exceed those of dogs with approximately 77–80 percent of females and 78–80 percent of males neutered (Manning and Rowan, 1992; New et al., 2000; Patronek et al., 1997). Double the percentage of cat-owning households (95 percent C.I.: 4.5–5.9 percent) reported at least one litter in 1996 as compared to dog-owning households. Two thirds of these litters were unplanned, resulting in approximately 2.1 million unplanned cat litters (New, 2001). The crude birth rate per 100 cats was estimated to be 11.2. While the majority of owned dogs and cats were neutered, 11–16 percent of females (both species) have been reported to have had a litter, many before neutering (Patronek et al., 1997; Johnson et al., 1993; Manning and Rowan, 1992). Reasons given to explain why their animals had given birth before neutering included desire to breed, cost, inconvenience, and accidents, not always in this order of importance (Johnson, 1997; Patronek et al., 1997). The accidents included "she escaped, I didn't think she would go into heat this young," or "I didn't realize that she was in heat." These data suggest that neutering both sheltered and privately owned animals *before* puberty should be a national goal. They also suggest that cost and ease of obtaining neutering services are important.

The high proportion of households owning pets; billion dollar pet expenditures for food, accessories, health care, and other services; and family member status, speak to Americans' adoration and devotion to pets in the latter decades of the twentieth and early twenty-first century. As an indicator of American culture relating to pets, these statistics alone are misleading, however, as the number of animal shelters and the unwanted animals they handle speak to a darker side of Americans' relationship with their pets.

SHELTER DATA: TRAGEDY, PROGRESS, AND HOPE

In the late 1980s and early 1990s, Rowan noted that despite considerable investment in efforts to control pet populations, relatively little had been done to characterize pet surplus and to evaluate the effectiveness of control efforts (Rowan, 1991, 1992; Rowan and Williams, 1987). In 2003, progress has been made, although many questions remain. Precise estimates of the number of dogs and cats entering and being euthanized in shelters in the United States still elude the humane and veterinary communities. Recent efforts to identify all animal shelters and sanctuaries in the United States identified more than 4700 shelters handling at least 100 animals per year (Zawistowski et al., 1998). Attempts to identify every facility sheltering animals were thwarted by a lack of a definition of shelter, the birth of new organizations, changes in animal control officers, changes in the names and locations of shelters, and so on. Therefore, this figure should be regarded as an estimate.

Not surprisingly, in light of the difficulties in identifying shelters and encouraging responsiveness to requests for data, estimates of national impoundment, adoption, and euthanasia rates vary widely. For example, in the early 1990s estimates regarding euthanasia ranged from a low of 5 to 6 million (Patronek and Rowan, 1995) to more than 18 million dogs and cats euthanized annually (Nassar et al., 1992). Using their model, Patronek and Glickman estimated that in 1991, U.S. shelters impounded approximately 4 million dogs and euthanized 2.1 million (53 percent) of them (Patronek and Glickman, 1994). A recent estimate suggests that the number euthanized in 2000 was 4–6 million dogs and cats, representing about 4.5 percent of the owned dog and cat population (Irwin, 2001). Differences among the estimates arise as a result of the differing methodologies and populations surveyed to arrive at the estimates.

Adoption rates of dogs and cats in shelters vary widely as well. They depend on the nature and mission of the organization—limited- or full-admission facilities—and within these categories by size of the community served, resources, and other factors. The lowest published adoption estimates are between 20 and 25 percent for both dogs and cats in some full admission shelters to more than 90 percent in some limited admission facilities (Wenstrup and Dowidchuk, 1999; Zawistowski et al., 1998; Patronek and Glickman, 1994). Shelters are believed to supply their communities with somewhere between 6.3 and 22 percent of all dogs and cats acquired (Patronek and Glickman, 1994; NFO Research, 2000).

Other Statistics

During the past decade, a new statistic, the save rate has been suggested to monitor the progress being made in reducing euthanasias and facilitating comparisons among shelters. This statistic calculates the percentage of animals not euthanized (that is, adopted, redeemed, transferred to breed-rescue, remaining in the shelter, and so on) among all animals entering the shelter (with the exception of those dead on arrival) in a defined time period (for example, month, year). The denominator includes those not euthanized, as well as those euthanized, dying of illness or injury, and escaped from the shelter. The save rate has the advantage of making shelters aware of how well they are doing overall in saving lives, whether that is by reducing euthanasia, reducing disease in their facilities, finding partners in facilitating adoptions, and so on.

Some shelters have reported the proportion of adoptable animals saved. This statistic is limited by the lack of standardized definitions of *adoptable* and *unadoptable*. In a 1999 survey, staff in 186 shelters across the country reported that approximately 39 percent of their impounded animals were unadoptable. When asked for their basis for defining unadoptable, however, 75 percent had no clearly defined criteria (Wenstrup and Dowidchuk, 1999). If shelters employ a moving definition of adoptable (and unadoptable) to attract donations, enhance public image, and so on, then assessments of progress over time and across shelters cannot be made validly.

Trends

Data from national organizations and shelters suggest that, contrary to some reports, the numbers of animals and percentage of owned animals euthanized in shelters has been declining since at least the mid 1970s (Irwin, 2001; Zawistowski et al., 1998). In 1973 the Humane Society of the United States estimated that about 13.5 million dogs and cats were euthanized in shelters (roughly 20 percent of owned animals). In 1991 estimates of 4–5 million (about 5.3 percent of the owned population) underscored the progress made (Rowan, 1991). Over a longer period, the data are equally dramatic. Data from New York City shelters from 1895 to 1994 illustrate the dramatic decline in euthanasias per capita over the last 100 years (Fig. 2.1) (Zawistowski et al., 1998).

Euthanasia per 10,000 Human Population

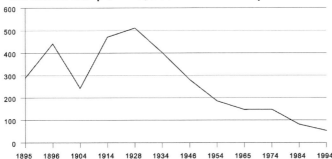

Figure 2.1. ASPCA Animal Control Services. Euthanasia of dogs and cats as a function of the human population of New York City (Zawistowski et al., 1998). Reprinted courtesy of *Journal Applied Animal Welfare Science*, Lawrence Erlebaum Associates (1): 193—206.

The inflow of animals into shelters varies considerably by area of the country and even by shelter within an area. Several sources have suggested that 6–12 percent of the dog population entered shelters in the 1990s (Patronek et al., 1997; Arkow, 1994) and that approximately 50–55 percent of the sheltered dogs were euthanized (representing about 4 percent of the dog population) (Patronek and Glickman, 1994; Wenstrup and Dowidchuk, 1999). Similar figures for cats suggested that 5–8 percent of the estimated owned population entered shelters and that approximately 65–80 percent of those entering were euthanized (Arkow, 1994; Wenstrup and Dowidchuk, 1999). Arkow (1994) estimated that this represents euthanasia of approximately 4–6 percent of the owned cat population.

Age Distribution

The popular use of the terminology, "pet overpopulation," is an unfortunate misnomer. The words imply that successfully reducing canine and feline fertility alone will resolve the euthanasia of millions of adoptable pets. The problem is, not surprisingly, more complex than this terminology suggests. In the RSRS, puppies and kittens accounted for 29 percent and 47 percent, respectively, of animals relinquished to the 12 participating shelters. The age distribution of relinquished animals in this study is presented in Figure 2.2. A survey of 186 shelters nationwide suggested even lower estimates of puppies (13 percent) and kittens (14 percent) entering shelters (Wenstrup and Dowidchuk, 1999). In a growing number of urban shelters, puppies are scarce (Patronek and Glickman, 1994), and potential adopters must adopt an older dog or put their names on puppy waiting lists. The largest age group of dogs and the second largest age group of cats relinquished was 6–24 months of age. These data underscore the importance of investing resources to assist people preferentially to prevent, but alternatively to resolve, issues that lead to relinquishment early in an animal's life and in a new pet-owner relationship. When compared to animals retained in their homes, risk for relinquishment was greatest among puppies and kittens less than 3 months of age (most of whom were in litters), followed by those 3 to 6 months, and those 6 to 24 months of age (New et al., 2000; Patronek et al., 1996a,b). Certainly young animals are not the only age group at risk of relinquishment, but if strong bonds fail to form, weak attachment can also contribute to decisions to relinquish later in the life of the animal.

Owner's Request for Euthanasia

A significant, but often overlooked facet, of relinquishment involves animals surrendered with the owner's request for euthanasia. These animals represented approximately 24 percent and 17 percent of surrendered dogs and cats, respectively (not including litters) in the RSRS (Kass et al., 2001). In contrast to animals relinquished by owners requesting adoption where the median length of ownership was 1–2 years, these animals had been owned a median of 10–11 (cats–dogs) years. Aged or ill dogs and cats accounted for 82 percent of requests for euthanasia, and these animals had a median age of approximately 12 years. Since owners frequently failed to clearly distinguish between illness and old age, these conditions were not examined separately.

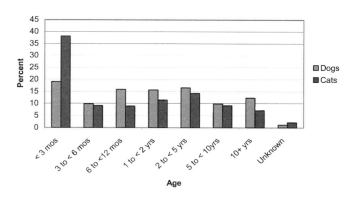

Age Distribution of Relinquished Dogs and Cats in 12 US Animal Shelters in 1995-96

Source: Regional Shelter Relinquishment Survey by National Council on Pet Population Study and Policy (NCPPSP)

Figure 2.2. Age distribution of relinquished dogs and cats in 12 U.S. animal shelters in 1995−96. Reprinted courtesy of *Regional Shelter Relinquishment Survey* by the National Council on Pet Population and Policy (NCPPSP).

Behavioral concerns, most of which were the sole reason cited, accounted for 16 percent and 18 percent of requests for euthanasia for dogs and cats, respectively. Aggression toward people or other animals was by far the most common behavior cited among dog requests for euthanasia. Unlike dogs, inappropriate elimination (38 percent) was the single most common behavioral reason among cats surrendered for euthanasia, followed by aggression to people (28 percent), and biting other animals or people (18 percent). These data remind us that shelters are not only euthanizing young, largely healthy animals, but also providing a service to pet owners often attributed solely to veterinary hospitals. Cost and other factors undoubtedly contribute to the use of this alternate choice for humane euthanasia. The data also strongly suggest that these animals (with the exception of cats with inappropriate elimination) are generally not part of the larger pet surplus crisis and that these animals should be subtracted from the figures cited earlier when the tragedy of pet euthanasia is discussed. They furthermore suggest that generally speaking, euthanasia requests of shelters don't have a trivial basis. Advanced age, illness, and aggressive behaviors, threatening the safety of people or other animals, are reasonable reasons leading many dedicated pet owners to provide a humane death for their animals. Although some of the reasons leading to these requests may

be frivolous or treatable, the vast majority appears not to fall into these categories.

With the growing numbers of shelters instituting temperament testing in order to protect adopters from aggressive and otherwise dangerous dogs, the proportions of animals being euthanized for these reasons must also be discounted from figures relating to the magnitude of unacceptable surrenders and deaths.

REASONS FOR RELINQUISHMENT

Reasons for relinquishment have been presented in various ways, and their interpretation can be colored by the method of presentation. For example, the top 10 individual reasons for relinquishment (and their overall frequency in the surrendered population) reported by relinquishers for dogs and cats from the *RSRS* are listed in Table 2.1. The frequency of the reasons, grouped by similarity to each other, is listed in Table 2.2. Both lists provide somewhat different insights into the issue of relinquishment. For example, looking at the individual reasons obscures the importance of behavioral issues as a cause of dissolution of the human-animal bond, because individual behaviors are not as important as reasons such as moving or cost. When looked at as a group, however, behavior issues were cited as at least one of the reasons for relinquishment in 40 percent of dogs, dwarfing the 7 percent of dogs sur-

Table 2.1. Top 10 individual reasons[a] cited by owners for relinquishing animals[b] to 12 U.S. animal shelters in 1995-96.

	Dogs	%[c]		Cats	%[c]
1.	Moving	7	1.	Too many in house	11
2.	Landlord issues	6	2.	Allergies	8
3.	Cost of pet maintenance	5	3.	Moving	8
4.	No time for pet	4	4.	Cost of pet maintenance	6
5.	Inadequate facilities	4	5.	Landlord issues	6
6.	Too many pets in home	4	6.	No homes for littermates	6
7.	Pet illness(es)	4	7.	House soiling	5
8.	Personal problems	4	8.	Personal problems	4
9.	Biting	3	9.	Pet illness(es)	2
10.	No homes for littermates	3	10.	Inadequate facilities	2

[a] People could cite up to 5 reasons for relinquishment.
[b] Dogs and cats relinquished as strays or for euthanasia due to age or illness were excluded.
[c] Frequency among all animals relinquished.

Table 2.2. Frequency of classes of reasons given at the time of relinquishment of dogs and cats to 12 animal shelters in the United States, 1995-1996.

Reason Class	Dogs[a]		Cats[b]	
	n	%[c]	n	%[c]
Aggression toward people	211	10.3	68	5.0
Aggression to another animal	153	7.5	83	6.1
Nonaggression behavioral problem	603	29.5	283	20.8
Request for euthanasia	362	17.7	157	11.5
Animal's health	167	8.2	78	5.7
Animal characteristics (not behavioral or medical)	91	4.5	25	1.8
Human housing issues	622	30.4	371	27.3
Household animal population	139	6.8	228	16.8
Human health and personal issues	554	27.1	488	35.9
Human preparation or expectation	286	14.0	207	15.2

Source: J Applied Animal Welfare Science (1998) 1:212.
Note. Litters are not included in data.
[a] $n = 2045$.
[b] $n = 1361$.
[c] Percentage of animals with at least one reason in each class. Each animal may have had up to five reasons for relinquishment.

rendered for moving. Moving alone, however, accounted for 7 percent of all surrenders, making it the single most common individual cause cited by owners (New et al., 1999). Similarly, among cats only, house-soiling appears in the top 10 reasons; whereas behavioral issues combined were the second most common cause of relinquishment. The importance of too many cats, the most common individual reason, however, is buried in the fourth most common class of reasons, household animal population. When discussing reasons for relinquishment, the type of data discussed should be clarified. Also, most shelters currently allow people to report only one reason for surrendering an animal. The frequency of multiple reasons (Scarlett et al., 1999; Salman et al., 2000) and the length of owner's deliberation before relinquishment (DiGiacomo et al., 1998) strongly suggest that for many people, it is a combination of reasons that eventually leads to surrender.

Patronek et al. (1996a,b) categorized factors affecting relinquishment into those that were potentially modifiable and those that were not. The following discussion uses their approach.

Potentially Modifiable Factors

Behavior: Behaviors, perceived by owners as unacceptable, were the leading cause of relinquishment of dogs and the second most common group of reasons for cats. In the RSRS, behavior was cited as at least one of the five possible reasons for relinquishment for 40 percent of dogs and 28 percent of cats relinquished. Households surrendering dogs were twice as likely to believe they needed behavioral advice than those not surrendering (Patronek et al., 1996a). Since many owners fail to mention behavioral problems for fear that their disclosure will lead to euthanasia, these figures are probably underestimates. The behaviors most commonly associated with surrender of both dogs and cats were inappropriate elimination, aggressive behaviors to people and other animals, and destructiveness (Table 2.2). The behavioral data excluded litters.

Inappropriate elimination: Despite differences in methodology, dogs and cats urinating inappropriately at least weekly in the home were approximately 2 to 4 and 2 to 6 times more likely, respectively, to be relinquished compared to animals occasionally or never displaying this behavior (New et al., 2000; Patronek et al., 1996a,b). Urinating or defecating inappropriately can be caused by numerous medical and behavioral problems. Medical causes (e.g., cystitis, renal disease, and diabetes mellitus) are well documented and can frequently be treated successfully when diagnosed. Behavioral causes (e.g., separation anxiety, unsuccessful house training, and dirty litter boxes) are also well described, but many veterinarians report less confidence in diagnosing and successfully treating these causes, and owners acknowledge difficulty in finding competent guidance (Patronek and Dodman, 1999).

Common myths and a lack of good information aggravate the problem of inappropriate urinating or defecating in owners' homes. When asked to respond to the statement "It is helpful to rub the dog's nose in its mess when it soils in the house" 31.8 percent of people surrendering dogs believed it was a true statement, and another 11.4 percent were not sure (New et al., 2000). Similarly, despite published data suggesting that cats in multicat households are more likely to urinate outside the litter box compared to cats in single-cat households (Askew, 1996), 35.5 percent of people relinquishing cats were unaware or unsure of this relationship. Since recent growth in cat ownership has been largely due to an increase in number of cats per household, informed adoption counseling and simple measures, such as frequently cleaning litter boxes and providing at least one litter box per cat in households with multiple cats, may help to reduce relinquishments for inappropriate elimination.

Aggressive behaviors: In the National Household Survey, 16 percent of households reported dogs that had growled, snapped or attempted to bite people at least some of the time in the month prior to the interview. In the RSRS, excluding litters, 10.3 percent of dogs were surrendered for displaying these behaviors to people and 7.5 percent were surrendered for displaying these behaviors to other animals (Salman et al., 1998). Of dogs displaying aggression, 69 percent had bitten at least one person. When compared to dogs retained in their homes, surrendered dogs displaying aggression toward people at least weekly or most of the time were at least 1 and a half times more likely to be relinquished compared to dogs lacking signs of aggression (New et al., 2000; Patronek et al., 1996a,b; Kass and Hart, 1998).

A somewhat smaller proportion of relinquished cats were aggressive to people (5.0 percent) and approximately the same percentage (6.1 percent) reportedly were aggressive to other animals. Seventy-one percent of cats displaying aggression to people had bitten a human (Salman et al., 1998). In the National Household Survey, 13.2 percent of owned cats reportedly were aggressive to people at least some of the time, but this was not statistically different from the 12.6 percent of relinquished cats. In contrast, cats with daily aggression to people in another study were four times more likely to be relinquished than cats never exhibiting this behavior (Patronek et al., 1996b).

Destructive behaviors: Chewing, digging, climbing, scratching, and so on were less common than aggression or inappropriate elimination, but important reasons for relinquishment. Dogs damaging property inside or outside the home most of the time were over twice as likely to lose their homes than dogs who did not (New et al., 2000; Patronek et al., 1996a). Inappropriate scratching and other damage daily or most of the time approximately doubled the risk of surrender in cats (New et al., 2000; Patronek et al., 1996b).

Other frequently reported behaviors for dogs included escaping (5.5 percent), disobedience (4.4 percent), and being too active (3.8 percent) in the RSRS. Perceived hyperactivity on a daily basis or most of the time was consistently associated with risks of relinquishment 2–3 times higher than dogs rarely or never exhibiting this behavior (New et al., 2000; Patronek et al., 1996a). Among cats, unfriendliness (1.8 percent), disobedience (1.2 percent), and demanding too much attention and being too active (1.1 percent) were the most frequently reported behaviors besides aggression and inappropriate elimination. Perceived hyperactivity daily or most of the time more than doubled the risk of relinquishment (New et al., 2000). Note: Separation anxiety is also thought to be an important behavioral cause of relinquishment. Since a constellation of behaviors may be associated with separation anxiety (undiagnosed by the owner), this specific diagnosis does not appear in many published studies.

Obedience training: Participation in obedience classes was strongly associated with retention in households; dogs with formal training had approximately one-third the risk of relinquishment of untrained animals (Patronek et al., 1996a).

Veterinary care: Dogs with veterinary care in the previous year were significantly more likely to remain in their homes. Interestingly, receipt of veterinary care for cats in the previous year was not similarly associated with retention (Patronek et al., 1996a,b).

Unrealistic expectations: Unrealistic expectations regarding the role of a new cat in the family and the amount of work associated with a dog was a strong factor (minimally raising the risk four-fold)

influencing relinquishment (Patronek et al., 1996a,b). These data suggest ignorance of feline characteristics, which should be addressed prior to adoption. This interpretation is given further credence by the finding that people who had done some reading about feline behavior had about half the risk of relinquishment compared to those who had not. Interestingly, cats acquired as strays were less likely than those acquired from other sources to be relinquished, suggesting that time spent observing a cat before taking him/her into the home may enhance the likelihood of a lasting relationship. Alternatively, rescuing an animal may enhance a person's bond with the pet.

The effectiveness of adoption counseling has been challenged by data suggesting that dogs acquired from shelters were more likely to be relinquished because the care required exceeded the adopter's expectations. Other studies have estimated that 19–20 percent of dogs adopted from shelters were returned or transferred to another home within 6–12 months (Kidd et al., 1992; Neidhart and Boyd, 2002). The development and evaluation of standardized guidelines regarding adoption counseling for young and adult animals would improve the understanding of the effect of counseling on retention rates in adoptive homes.

Neutering: Spaying and castrating have not only reduced the number of unwanted puppies and kittens but are also associated with reduced risk of relinquishment. Neutered animals had one-half to one-third the risk of surrender compared to sexually intact dogs and cats (New et al., 2000; Patronek, 1996a,b). Presumably, this is a reflection of the reduction in sexually associated behaviors and the inconvenience of unwanted pregnancies.

Decisions to relinquish animal(s) to animal shelters are complex. Often it is a constellation of reasons, including timing, that tips an already precarious balance in favor of removing an animal from the household. When allowed to cite more than one reason for relinquishment, most people surrendering an animal listed more than one. Studies, based on shelter data collecting only one reason for relinquishment, are potentially misleading in that people may report the most socially desirable reason, the one least likely to result in euthanasia, or have other (unknown) motivations for offering the cited reason. Data from several studies suggest that the decision to relinquish is often complex and often not made without thought and considerable guilt (DiGiacomo et al., 1999; Scarlett et al., 1999). It is common to hear shelter staff refer to people surrendering animals as irresponsible. Certainly, there are irresponsible people who surrender, but data suggest that more often ignorance and unfortunate circumstances culminate in relinquishment. This is good news, because it is difficult to rehabilitate irresponsible people, but somewhat easier to educate well-meaning, but uneducated owners or those caught in unfortunate circumstances.

Non-modifiable Factors Associated with Relinquishment

Length of ownership: The length of ownership was a strong determinant for the relinquishment in all studies where it was evaluated. In comparative studies of relinquished to owned animals, both dogs and cats were at highest risk of relinquishment during their first year of ownership. In the National Household Survey in which length of ownership was evaluated within the first year of ownership, the bond between pet and owner was most fragile within the first six months (New et al., 2000). These data underscore the importance of good adoption counseling, nurturing appropriate expectations, and the availability of good advice during the early months of ownership.

Other factors: Low initial cost of animals and mixed breeding were associated with higher risk of surrender (New et al., 2000; Patronek et al., 1996a,b). While purebreds were generally less likely to be abandoned, they were not immune. Thirty percent of relinquished dogs in the RSRS were reportedly purebred, and 7 percent had been purchased for $200 or more.

Widely held beliefs that animals acquired as gifts or from pet stores were less likely to be retained in their homes have been challenged by data suggesting a protective effect (for animals acquired as gifts) or no association with relinquishment (for animals purchased from pet stores) (New et al., 2000; Patronek et al., 1996a,b). Recognizing that gifts, for example, do not result in higher return rates, a growing number of shelters have adoption programs at Christmas that save animals from euthanasia.

Owner characteristics: People with more education and income were generally less likely to relinquish animals, but almost a quarter of people surrendering had annual incomes of $45,000 or more, and more than half had more than a high school education. Although parents frequently acquire pets for their children, families with children were about two times more likely to relinquish their pets compared to those without children (Patronek et al., 1996a). Among adopters from a San Francisco shelter, people returning their pets within six months had a lower mean age and were more often parents, men, or first-time adopters (Kidd et al., 1992). A similar study of adopters from two shelters, an adopt-a-thon and a PETsMART Luv-a-Pet location, found that problems getting along with people or other pets, behavioral issues, running away, allergies, and owner death were the major reasons for pet relinquishment during the first year following adoption (Neidhart and Boyd, 2002).

MEDICAL STATISTICS

Veterinarians who develop population health programs need medical statistics that enable them to monitor disease control and prevention efforts within their facilities. This requires veterinarians to have familiarity with basic health indices, appropriate data collection, and interpretation. Similarly, they must be able to work with databases currently in use in shelters to track disease frequency.

Statistics regarding adoptions, relinquishments, and euthanasias are necessary for fund-raising, planning, prioritizing, evaluating, and so on, but their use must be guided by clear, coherent goals. Fennell (1999) argued that shelters should focus on projects and programs that attract potential adopters to shelters and their animals, rather than to other sources (breeders, pet stores, friends, and so on). She suggested that shelters should concentrate more on a market perspective, looking for every opportunity to attract people to shelter animals, rather than on blaming an irresponsible public. Reviewing the statistics presented here for opportunities to achieve such goals seems highly desirable.

SUMMARY

In the decade since Rowan referred to the statistical black hole that existed with regards to pet population dynamics and euthanasia, progress has been made. Yet, many questions and issues continue to impede progress. Basic definitions still complicate data collection, not the least of which is "what is a shelter?" With the growing advocacy for companion animals by a diverse number of groups, we need a taxonomy of types of groups that handle animals and a census of them.

National statistics are needed by humane organizations for political, fund-raising, educational, and other reasons, but they mask the heterogeneity of situations around the country. The inflow of animals into shelters varies considerably by area of the country and even by shelters within an area. Similarly, the reasons for animals entering, both from animal control and owner-relinquishment, vary, making it incumbent on shelters to understand the animal dynamics in their own communities. Communities need local statistics that enable them to identify, prioritize, and evaluate their programs.

Reasons for animals entering shelters are complex and do not relate to the over-production of puppies and kittens alone. Neutering efforts must continue, but programs assisting people to make wise adoption decisions and supporting the bond between animals and adopters must be developed or strengthened. Although it may seem to staff receiving animals in shelters that most people surrendering animals are irresponsible, much of apparent irresponsibility is due to ignorance, and programs addressing this ignorance (for example, behavior hotlines) offer hope to pet owners and shelters alike. Likewise, facilities and programs (for example, obedience training, agility classes, and dog parks) that encourage well-mannered pets and having fun with pets help foster strong bonds that prevent relinquishments.

Continued breeding of dogs and cats, while at the same time euthanizing millions to control the excess, and the surrender of millions acquired as life-long companions is morally reprehensible. Using statistics to moralize and condemn an irresponsible public, however, is unlikely to change public attitudes and practices. The development of and continued emphasis on new paradigms to attract people to shelters and shelter-animals, rather than acquiring them from friends, pet shops, and breeders, are likely to increase shelters' market-share of animal homes and reduce euthanasias. Similarly, creative approaches to matching pets with appropriate people (for example, pets for seniors) can place animals with characteristics previously believed to condemn them to death.

The future outlook for homeless animals has never been better. The efforts of many groups have decreased unnecessary euthanasias over the past several decades. Increased vitality and dedication to further reducing these numbers in the past 10 years has led to many new programs and brought dramatic changes to the face of animal sheltering. Continued commitment is required to achieve a humane society in which euthanasia is no longer a tool for population control. Veterinarians, whether employed by shelters or working in private practice, have a vital role to play in achieving this goal.

REFERENCES

Arkow, P. (1994) A new look at pet "overpopulation." *Anthrozoos* (7): 202–205.

Arkow, P.S., and Dow, S. (1994) The ties that do not bind: A study of the human-animal bonds that fail. In (R.K. Anderson, B.L. Hart, and L.A. Hart, eds.) *The Pet Connection*. Minneapolis: University of Minnesota Press, 348–354.

Askew, H.R. (1996) *Treatment of behavioral problems in dogs and cats*. Oxford, England: Blackwell Science, 286–287.

AVMA (2002) U.S. *Pet Ownership and Demographics Sourcebook*. Schaumburg, IL: American Veterinary Medical Association; Membership and Field Services.

Dawson, B., and Trapp, R.G. (2001) *Basic and Clinical Biostatistics*. New York: Lange Medical Books/McGraw-Hill, 1.

DiGiacomo, N., Arluke, A., et al. (1999) Surrendering pets to shelters; the relinquishers' perspective. *Anthrozoos* (11): 41–51.

Fennell, L.A. (1999) Beyond overpopulation: a comment on Zawistowski *et al.* and Salman *et al. Journal Applied Animal Welfare Science* (2): 217–228.

Holton, L., and Manzoor, P. (1993) Managing and controlling feral cat populations: Killing the crisis and not the animal. *Veterinary Forum* March: 100–101.

Ipsos-NPD (2001) *Pet Incidence Trend Report*. Washington, DC: Pet Food Institute.

Irwin, P.G. (2001) Overview: the state of animals in 2001. In (D.J. Salem, A.N. Rowan, eds.) *The State of Animals 2001*. Washington, D.C.: Humane Society Press, Humane Society of the United States.

Johnson, K., Lewellen, L., et al. (1993) Santa Clara County's pet population. San Jose, CA: National Pet Alliance.

Johnson, K., and Lewellen, L. (1995) San Diego County: Survey and analysis of the pet population. San Diego, CA: San Diego Cat Fanciers, Inc.

Johnson, K. (1997) Four study comparison. In Proceedings: A critical evaluation of free-roaming/unowned/feral cats in the U.S. Colorado: American Humane Association, Cat Fancier's Association.

Kass, P.H., and Hart, L.A. (1998) An epidemiologic study of determinants of dog and cat relinquishment to animal shelters in Sacramento County, CA. The changing roles of animals in society. 8th International Conference on Human-Animal Interactions, Prague.

Kass, P.H., New, J.C., Jr., et al. (2001) Understanding animal companion surplus in the United States; relinquishment of nonadoptables to animal shelters for euthanasia. *Journal of Applied Animal Welfare Science* 4:237–248.

Kidd, A.H., Kidd, R.M., et al. (1992) Successful and unsuccessful pet adoptions. *Psych Rep* 70:547–561.

Luke, C. (1996) Animal shelter issues. *Journal of the American Veterinary Medical Association* 208:524–527.

Manning, A.M., and Rowan, A.N. (1992) Companion animal demographics and sterilization status: results from a survey in four Massachusetts towns. *Anthrozoos* (5): 192–201.

Nassar, R., Talboy, J., et al. (1992) Animal shelter reporting study 1990. Englewood, CO: American Humane Association.

Neidhart, L., and Boyd, R. (2002) Companion animal adoption study. *Journal of Applied Animal Welfare Science* 5:175–192.

New, J.C., Jr., Salman, M.D., et al. (2000) Characteristics of shelter-relinquished animals and their owners compared with animals and their owners in U.S. pet-owning households. *Journal of Applied Animal Welfare Science* 3:179–201.

New, J.C., Jr., Salman, M.D., et al. (1999) Moving: Characteristics of dogs and cats and those relinquishing them to 12 animal shelters. *Journal of Applied Animal Welfare Science* 2:83–96.

New, J.C., Jr. (2001) Results of a pet-owning household survey: the role of the veterinary profession in keeping pets at home. Presentation: 138th American Veterinary Medical Association Convention, Boston, Mass.

NFO Research, Inc. (2000) National Pet Owners Survey. Scarsdale, NY: American Pet Products Manufacturers Association.

Patronek, G.J., Beck, A.M., et al. (1997) Dynamics of dog and cat populations in a community. *Journal of the American Veterinary Medical Association* 210:637–642.

Patronek, G.J., and Dodman, N.H. (1999) Attitudes, procedures and delivery of behavior services by veterinarians in small animal practices. *Journal of the American Veterinary Medical Association* (215): 1601–1611.

Patronek, G.J., Glickman, L.T., et al. (1996a) Risk factors for relinquishment of dogs to an animal shelter. *Journal of the American Veterinary Medical Association* 209:572–581.

Patronek, G.J., Glickman L.T., et al. (1996b) Risk factors for relinquishment of cats to an animal shelter. *Journal of the American Veterinary Medical Association* 209:582–588.

Patronek, G.J., Glickman, L.T., et al. (1995) Population dynamics and risk of euthanasia for dogs in an animal shelter. *Anthrozoos* (8): 31–43.

Patronek, G.J., and Glickman, L.T. (1994) Development of a model for estimating the size and dynamics of the pet dog population. *Anthrozoos* (7): 25–41.

Patronek, G.J., and Rowan, A.N. (1995) Determining dog and cat numbers and population dynamics: Editorial. *Anthrozoos* (8): 199–205.

Rowan, A.N., and William, J. (1987) The success of companion animal management programs: A review. *Anthrozoos* (1): 110–122.

Rowan, A.N. (1991) What we need to learn from epidemiologic surveys pertaining to pet overpopulation. *Journal of the American Veterinary Medical Association* 198:1233–1236.

Rowan, A.N. (1992) Shelters and pet overpopulation: a statistical black hole. *Anthrozoos* (5): 140–143.

Salman, M.D., Hutchison, J., et al. (2000) Behavioral reasons for relinquishment of dogs and cats to 12 shelters. *Journal of Applied Animal Welfare Science* 3:93–106.

Salman, M.D., New, J.C., Jr., et al. (1998) Human and animal factors related to the relinquishment of dogs and cats in 12 selected animal shelters in the United States. *Journal of Applied Animal Welfare Science* 1:207–226.

Scarlett, J.M., Salman, M.D., et al. (1999) Reasons for relinquishment of companion animals in U.S. animal shelters: Selected health and person issues. *Journal of Applied Animal Welfare Science* (2): 41–57.

Teclaw, R., Mendlein, J., et al. (1992) Characteristics of pet populations and households in the Purdue Comparative Oncology Program catchment area. *Journal of the American Veterinary Medical Association* 201:1725–1729.

Wenstrup, J., and Dowidchuk, A. (1999) Pet overpopulation: Data and measurement issues in shelters. *Journal of Applied Animal Welfare Science* 2:303–319.

Zawistowski, S., Morris, J., et al. (1998) Population dynamics, overpopulation and the welfare of companion animals; new insights on old and new data. *Journal of Applied Animal Welfare Science* 1:193–206.

3
The Administrative Hurdles of Shelter Medicine

Bonnie Yoffe-Sharp

"A pessimist is one who makes difficulties of his opportunities and an optimist is one who makes opportunities of his difficulties."

—Harry S. Truman

INTRODUCTION

Shelter medicine is both an art and a science and can be an incredibly fulfilling career. Caring for those animals that have no one else to care for them, and having the freedom to make decisions about the health and medical care of an animal without having to rely on the owner's consent can be liberating. Many shelter veterinarians agree that not having to deal with the daily idiosyncrasies of clients is a welcome change from private practice.

That is not to say, however, that veterinarians working at or with animal shelters don't have several other sources of stress and frustration. Whether working in a nonprofit humane society, municipal animal control facility, open door or limited admission shelter, most shelter veterinarians have nonmedical, often administrative, hurdles to clear. These hurdles, or challenges, vary from facility to facility and from person to person. Although monetary constraints often seem to be one of the major obstacles that keep shelters from accomplishing their goals, it is the interpersonal conflicts that often lead to the high stress levels that we take home with us.

What are the primary sources of our nonmedical challenges? The list can be endless, but the most common includes the following:

- Staff conflicts
- Employee management
- Boards of Directors
- Government bureaucracy
- The media
- Relationship with local private practitioners

In this chapter, we will take a short look at each of these challenges, as well as the possible approaches to dealing with them.

STAFF CONFLICT AND EMPLOYEE MANAGEMENT

"A healthy attitude is contagious but don't wait to catch it from others. Be a carrier."

—Unknown

Often staff conflict boils down to miscommunication, lack of adequate communication, perception of unfair treatment, and basic personality differences. Open, honest, and clear communication sounds trite and simplistic, however, the reality is that if we practiced communicating this way the quality of our work (and home) lives would dramatically improve.

Effective Communication and Active Listening

It is necessary to customize your communication style based on the other party. Don't assume that you've been understood, just because you've been heard. For example, you may have one staff member who will listen to your instructions for a task or animal treatment to be accomplished, and then performs the task as instructed or asks for clarification if she is unsure of your intent. This gives you the opportunity to give clearer instructions and ensures that the correct action is taken. On the other hand, you may have another staff member who appears as if she is listening to your instructions, and then does something totally different. Or, she may not perform the task at all and act as if she had never been instructed to do so in the first place. These latter scenarios can be extremely frustrating. To help remedy this type of situation, you will need to adjust your communication style with her. When you give her instructions, not only try to be as clear as possible, but also say the same thing at least twice, in two different ways. Then, ask her for acknowledgment that she understands, or have her explain back to you what needs to be done. This can be done in a respectful, nonpatronizing way. The reasons for the employee's poor performance of tasks are moot. You don't need to know if it is a passive-aggressive behavior pattern or if she just doesn't pay attention.

Active listening is critical to effective two-way communication. An enhanced listening ability translates into improved employee relationships that will dramatically improve job performance. We are often so busy with our caseloads that the thought of slowing down to really listen to a staff member's questions or concerns may seem to be a poor use of time. But in the long run, you will need the staff's respect and trust to function effectively. They need to trust that you care enough about them, and the animals, to really hear and understand what they have to say. Use the same technique of asking for clarification if you're not sure you understand what the other person is saying, and repeat back to him/her your understanding of what was said and get confirmation. It's important not to prejudge the message you are receiving. If you've labeled a person as stupid, crazy, unqualified, and so on, then you won't pay attention to what they have to say. Be open to hearing the thoughts and feelings of other people. This is easier said than done; we don't want to believe that an unlikable person has said something worth thinking about.

Working Together

One common area of staff conflict in open-door animal shelters surrounds the important job of "dispositioning" for euthanasia. Choosing which animal is going to live and which one is going to die is tremendously stressful. Similarly, in limited admission shelters, deciding which animals to admit and which to turn away can cause much internal conflict and stress. Every organization will have guidelines, protocols, and certain criteria that they use to help make these often-difficult decisions. It's those cases in the "gray zone" that cause the conflict and bad feelings.

- "Just how old ARE those kittens, and are they really weaned yet?"
- "That dog didn't really growl at the kid, he was just vocalizing to get attention. You just don't like Rottweilers."
- "Last year we put a cat up for adoption that had the exact same kind of medical condition."

The list of such cases is endless. It is critical that there are specific and written criteria specifying what constitutes an adoptable versus a nonadoptable animal. It is also critical to be consistent in the application of such criteria. This does not mean that there aren't multiple factors that contribute to the final decision for any particular animal, such as how overcrowded the shelter is at a particular point in time. It is also difficult to be second-guessed on a medical diagnosis you've made, because it may lead to an animal being determined as unadoptable. Your staff needs to understand and respect your areas of expertise, responsibility, and authority. The flip side, of course, is that you don't make a habit of questioning the dispositioning decisions made outside of your realm of expertise and authority. I like the model of having two people, from different departments, make the disposition decisions on any given day. For one thing, it takes a little bit of the pressure and stress off of each individual by "sharing the (emotional) load," and it instills more trust, and therefore less resistance, from those that would question a particular decision. It also provides a check and balance system. A model I have seen work fairly well is to include one person from the medical team and one person from the shelter department in such decision making.

Positive Reinforcement

When managing employees it is imperative to give positive reinforcement. We all know that when training a new puppy you don't get anywhere by using punishment; you just instill a fear response. Yet, we forget that as humans, we need positive reinforcement too. We not only need to make the staff aware of their mistakes, and how to correct them, but we also must make them aware of when they do things correctly. Compliments for a job well done makes a person's day. A literal, or figurative, pat on the back lets your staff know that you not only are aware of what they actually do, but that you appreciate their efforts. Nothing will improve your working relationships more. And, don't be stingy when it comes to complimenting nondepartmental employees. If someone goes above and beyond, tell him or her and thank them. Also, let their manager know. It will help develop better interdepartmental relations. When a conflict does arise, or you need to lodge a concern about someone else's employee, the pill will be a little less bitter to swallow. A level of trust and respect will already exist, and hopefully your concerns will be heard less defensively.

Fair Play

Last, but not least, be fair. Let's face it, there are some people we just like more than others. There are those individuals that get on our nerves. There are some fellow employees we enjoy, and some we spend time with away from work. But, when at work, everyone must be treated equally. You do not want even the appearance of playing favoritism. This will not only help your relationship with those people with which you don't click, but will keep your at-work relationship with your friends more professional. It is easy to start to take advantage of a friendship if it is not clear that all staff members have the same performance standards.

BOARDS OF DIRECTORS

"I've looked at life from both sides now, from up and down, and still somehow, it's life's illusions I recall . . . ."
— Judy Collins

"If you can't beat them, join them."
— Unknown

I worked for 14 years as a veterinarian for a nonprofit humane society animal shelter. I joined the Board of Directors of that shelter two and a half years later and have been wearing the hat of a board member for the last three years. Therefore, I truly have seen it from both sides. I joined the board because I love the organization and wanted to make positive change.

The Big Picture

From an employee's perspective, it may be hard to understand why boards of directors head nonprofit humane organizations. They may seem to be a group of people who oftentimes have no clue about the day-to-day operations of an animal shelter, and who seem to have no knowledge of, nor interest in, animal issues. Some of their decisions may seem totally uninformed. However, it is important to understand the true function of a board. The main role of the board is to look at the big picture, to develop the direction and mission of the organization, and to work with the executive director to ensure that the organization's general policies and programs reflect that mission. The board's role is not to be involved in the shelter's day-to-day operations. The board is legally responsible for governance of the organization, which includes overseeing finances and ensuring adequate resources for the organization, deciding long-range planning, and reviewing and approving the annual operating budgets.

Big problems can develop if the board and the executive director don't have a strong and cooperative relationship. Staff veterinarians probably have few, if any, direct interactions with the board. The Executive Director (ED) is the staff's interface with the board. If you have a problem with a board's decision that affects your department and ability to provide medical care for the animals, it is the ED that will need to help you make your case. It is never a good idea to go over the head of your ED to the board of directors. (The exception to this rule, of course, is in the case of egregious and/or unlawful behavior, such as sexual harassment, animal cruelty, and so on.)

Here is an example of a board of directors keeping the big picture in mind: Many years ago, while working at a nonprofit humane organization, I started a blood donor program, making canine and feline blood available to local practitioners. (This was back in the days before all the animal blood banks were around.) We only charged the amount it cost us for our time and the materials to collect the blood. It was a great program, and the local vets loved it. We saved animals' lives, and no shelter animals suffered due to the program. About one and a half years after starting the program, the board of directors found out about it and there was an uproar. There was concern that the public would think we were doing animal research or that the animals would be euthanized for their blood, and therefore people would be reluctant to surrender animals to our shelter. My ED understood that no animals were suffering, and in fact many animals were benefiting from the program. But, in the end, she agreed with the board that the possible loss of public support and confidence in the organization outweighed the life-saving benefits of the program.

And in the end, I understood that the community's trust in and support of the organization was more essential and would have a larger impact than the individual animals we helped to save with the donor program. Perhaps the board and ED were practicing population medicine better than I. They had assessed the risk-to-benefit ratio and come to the conclusion that more animals were ultimately served without the program.

Politics

Political issues can be a major problem with a board of directors. There may be hidden, or not so hidden, agendas of certain board members. This can tear a board, and ultimately an organization, apart. If a board is too busy with fighting amongst themselves, there is no time to help build the finances of the organization. This can ultimately affect the bottom line for some of your programs. Unfortunately, as a staff member you will have very little control over these types of problems. Stay out of it as much as you can, and try not to burn any bridges. You never know if you will need the support of the board, or of individual board members, in the future.

GOVERNMENT BUREAUCRACY

> *"Better to light a candle than to curse the darkness."*
> —Chinese Proverb

Working for government has its own set of challenges—the one most prominent being government bureaucracy. A humane organization background can be an asset in helping to run a municipal shelter. This is not the case for many municipal animal control facilities. Some animal control facilities are under the auspices of a police department. That is, the people in authority are not necessarily animal people.

The main problems in this arena concern money (lack of it), bureaucracy (lots of it), and ignorance of animal welfare and sheltering issues. It can be hit or miss as to what priorities of yours are valued. For example, if the Chief of Police is passionate about animals, you're in better shape than if he/she feels that they were "stuck" with having to oversee "the pound." In either case, it behooves you to get to know the people who make the decisions that affect your ability to practice shelter medicine effectively. Make sure they get to know and respect you, and the job you do, not only for the sake of the animals, but also for the animal-owning and animal-loving members of the community. Educate them on important animal issues, and what's in it for them.

For example, at the municipal shelter where I work, I approached our Police Chief with an interest in hosting a daylong course about the link between animal abuse and interpersonal violence. The workshop would be aimed at the constellation of players in violence prevention and in the prosecution of violent offenders, including law enforcement personnel, animal control officers, veterinarians, social workers, educators, and so on. I did not know at the time that our Chief was a member of the county's domestic violence task force. He said that they had never discussed anything about the link in their previous annual conferences. He became very excited and brought the idea up to the task force, which puts on a very large conference annually. Others in the animal welfare field had concurrently expressed an interest in presenting similar material at the conference. The outcome was a 90-minute presentation on the link by two other individuals, including a Humane Officer/Animal Cruelty Investigator and myself, at a very large conference. The task force also decided to host a daylong postinstitute conference the day following the main conference, focusing exclusively on the cycle of violence to people and animals.

It was a lucky coincidence that everything fell into place the way it did. It certainly increased my value in the eyes of the Chief, and improved my ability to approach him with other topics or concerns that I may have in the future. I got more than I could have hoped for in that I was able to address a much larger audience than I had originally anticipated. Also, he has become more sensitized to the issues of animal abuse and its link to interpersonal violence, and is likely to expect more action on the part of his officers when they are presented with cases of possible animal abuse.

THE MEDIA

Shelter veterinarians are most likely to be approached by the media in relation to an animal cruelty or animal hoarder case. These types of cases are big news and spark a lot of public interest. Although these cases provide an opportunity to educate the public about issues of animal cruelty and neglect, one must be careful. People are misquoted, or quoted out of context, all the time. In cruelty cases, there should be one designated media point person for the agency. Refer all inquiries to this person unless that individual asks you to make some statements. Even then, be sure that you know exactly what you plan to say. It is easy to get nervous and forget your main message. You must also take care not to reveal specific details of an ongoing investigation.

When dealing with the media for a less stressful reason, such as an interview about being a shelter vet or an educational piece about geriatric pet care, enjoy yourself. Keep the message clear and in short sound bites. Keep it as simple and nontechnical as possible; otherwise you will lose the interest of your audience or their ability to understand your message.

Here are a few other helpful tips to remember when preparing for a media interview:

- Most reporters want to present accurate information. Assume that he or she is trying to do the best job to write a balanced and honest report, unless proven otherwise.
- The media can serve your agency as a conduit to the community. Remember that the interview is an opportunity to get your information across accurately.
- Be confident and upbeat. Don't forget that you are the expert and you have more control than you think.
- Try to never walk into an interview cold. When a reporter contacts you for an interview, find out what is to be discussed and if need be, promise to call back within 30 minutes. Then, do your homework and hone your message.
- Always return a reporter's phone calls and keep their deadline in mind.
- Assume you are being taped, whether the interview is by phone or in person.
- Be consistent in your message. Say the most important thing first. Prepare two or three main statements and weave them into the interview no matter what. If need be, you can use a bridging technique to get you back to your message. Transitional phrases such as "What's most important for you to know is . . . " work well.
- Be upbeat, enthusiastic, and engaging. Try to smile and be warm and friendly.
- The reporter has the last word, so don't get annoyed or sarcastic with him or her.
- Anticipate questions and give a direct answer to a direct question.
- Avoid the use of the phrase "No comment." Tell the reporter if you cannot discuss certain information, and if possible, why. Admit if you don't know the answer to a question and try to find the answer and get back to the reporter before the deadline.
- Just as in a court testimony, don't say more than necessary. Make your point and then stop. If a reporter pauses, he or she might be hoping that you will fill the void and put your foot in your mouth.
- Don't repeat negative words used in the interviewer's question. For example, if asked, "Don't you feel it was irresponsible of you to euthanize all 20 of the impounded rabbits?" don't say, "I

was not irresponsible." The headline the next day might read, "Dr. Smith denies she was irresponsible."

• Be truthful. It will add to your credibility. Address problems and then move on to your positive message.
• And remember, when dealing with the media, there is no such thing as "off the record."

Another important concept to remember when dealing with the media, whenever possible, is to act rather than wait and then have to react. You want to hit the papers first with a positive spin, rather than have to be defensive and react to someone else's negative spin. For example, in retrospect I could have handled the blood donor program I discussed earlier differently. At the time, there were only a couple of small articles insinuating that animals were being euthanized in order to get blood (totally untrue). If I were to start that program now, I would work with my organization to put out a press release preemptively. In it we would explain how the program worked, and the wonderful life-saving benefits of having fresh whole blood on hand. I would also emphasize that not only owned pets in the community would benefit, but also shelter animals in need of an emergency blood transfusion.

RELATIONSHIP WITH LOCAL PRIVATE PRACTITIONERS

"It's the constant and determined effort that breaks down all resistance and sweeps away all obstacles."
—Claude M. Bristol

Many shelter veterinarians feel as if they are walking a tightrope between their shelters' policies and the opinions of their local private practice colleagues. Some sheltering organizations actually have a predominantly adversarial relationship with their local veterinary community. It is imperative that a healthy and strong relationship be developed and maintained between these two groups for the optimum health of the animals in our communities. Differences aside, both groups have many common goals. So, what can shelter organizations and shelter veterinarians do to improve cooperation, understanding, and their working relationship with local veterinarians? The optimum strategies for forming, or strengthening, positive relationships are unique

to each community. Some things that have worked in the past are discussed in this chapter, however, be creative and use your personal and your organizations' strengths and talents to develop unique approaches to nurture this important relationship.

The following are a couple of guiding principles to keep in mind when establishing or maintaining a healthy and productive relationship:

• The more time an individual gives you, the more invested and loyal they are to you. And "you" can represent either an individual or an organization. This is true for both time and money. Once someone has done something for or given something to your organization, they are more invested in the relationship and are therefore more likely to help or defend you in the future.
• WIIFM or "What's In It For Me?"—Every decision a person makes and every action they take is based on the answer to that underlying question. This doesn't mean we are all incredibly selfish, but that we all have personal motivators. These motivators can run the gamut from personal gain or the need to feel superior to others all the way to altruism or feeling important and needed.

It is important to keep these guiding principles in mind when developing relationships with local practitioners. If you can work together on some small project or come to a consensus on some issue, then you are already beginning to develop an affinity and some rapport. There are many ways to do this. For example, join your local veterinary medical association and attend the meetings. Then, volunteer for office or committee work. This can provide an opportunity to get to know some of the other vets in the community in ways unrelated to your role with the shelter. It is easier to ask somebody for something if they already know you, or at least know who you are. Begin, if possible, by asking for something small. For example, ask if your organization can leave some of your Pet Loss Support Group brochures in their waiting room. In this case, the "what's in it for me" is a new service provided to their clients. It is easy for them to say yes to this because it benefits both the shelter (outreach to people in need of pet loss support) and the practice. With every small "yes" you receive, you are more likely to receive more "yes's" in the future. This is a tried and true technique for sales people.

And let's face it, we are sales people, too. In our case, we are selling our organizations and ourselves.

THE PRINTED WORD: NEWSLETTERS

- Include local veterinarians on your shelter's mailing list for your newsletters. Ask if your shelter can leave extra newsletters in their waiting room.
- Write a "Shelter Notes" column for your local Veterinary Medical Association (VMA) newsletter. Sample topics include your shelter's vaccination protocols, rabies quarantine policies, early-age spay and neuter information, or interesting recent case histories or cruelty cases. The list is endless.
- Ask a local colleague to write a column, either one time or on a regular basis, for your shelter's newsletter. Or, ask different (and appropriate) local vets each time and rotate this responsibility. Sample topics include timely animal health issues (summer time hazards for pets), or an "Ask the Vet" question and answer format.

FACE-TO-FACE INTERACTIONS

People work together more comfortably when they get to know each other. Face-to-face interactions provide opportunities to improve communication, build mutual respect, and develop rapport. They also provide a forum to sound out ideas and work on cooperative programs or projects.

Invite local colleagues to special events hosted by your shelter. Include these people on the organization's mailing list, and consider a personal follow-up call, as appropriate. For example, if your organization has an annual awards event that honors people or animals who have gone above and beyond in helping animals in the community, invite the local veterinarians. Perhaps one of their clients (or patients!) is receiving an award. If the shelter offers classes to the public that may be of interest to their clients or staff, send copies of the flyers or invitations to the local clinics.

Give a speech at your local VMA meeting. It can be a formal lecture on a topic for which you have experience or some expertise. Sample topics include: the veterinarian's role in recognizing and reporting animal abuse, temperament testing of shelter dogs, the role of stress on the incidence of upper respiratory infections in animal shelters, shelter veterinary medicine as herd health, and so on. If you don't feel comfortable doing a formal presentation, give an informal report to the group on the services your shelter offers, or lead a discussion on a community-related animal issue. It is amazing how many local practitioners are unaware of the various services provided and the functions performed by many animal shelters.

Liaison Committees

Establish a liaison committee that consists of a few local VMA members and relevant shelter staff. Your shelter and local veterinary community will dictate the particulars of your program. My experiences with such a committee in the past were very positive and the liaison provided multiple benefits to our organization. I will use my experience as an example of how such a committee can work.

Our committee consisted of four local, and relatively shelter friendly, small animal practitioners. They all happened to be practice owners. Our staff members included myself, our ED, and our Director of Operations. On occasion, other staff members would come to a meeting when necessary. For example, our Spay/Neuter Clinic Manager came to a couple of meetings to discuss a cooperative spay/neuter program. Meetings were held every other month from 6:30 to 8:00 P.M. at the shelter. We sometimes provided soft drinks and a snack.

We used the liaison committee meetings to open up and improve communication with our local veterinary community, to sound out ideas, and to launch new cooperative programs. In the process we came to know and respect one another. The first few meetings were somewhat formal and stiff. In time, they evolved to the point that everyone freely engaged in discussions and heated debates with mutual respect and humor. We became allies, enabling my organization to enlist from local practitioners generous donations of time and expertise for such projects as community outreach vaccination clinics and a spay/neuter referral program.

Topics for discussion included our routine shelter deworming protocols, contents of medical information handouts that went home with the adopters, vaccination policies for wolf hybrids, pet overpopulation legislation, feral cat program protocols, cooperative programs, and very heated debates about declawing cats. I must admit we tended to digress into consulting with each other on interesting and unusual cases. A couple of times I even brought radiographs with me to a meeting in order to get additional opinions. It was not only beneficial for that particular case, but it also helped to build our camaraderie.

At our bimonthly VMA meetings, one of the local practitioners on the liaison committee would give a brief report to the membership. I saw direct benefits as a result of this increased exposure to and knowledge of the shelter and especially of its medical programs. Rather than being criticized by a local veterinarian because some recently adopted kitten came down with an upper respiratory infection, I was more likely to receive a friendly call of concern. I was always happy to receive the information, and I also used the opportunity to not only thank my colleague for the call, but also to solicit ideas on how to decrease this type of problem in a shelter population. This created a "win win win" situation in which I gained new insight on an old problem, we built mutual esteem as professionals, and I was also able to convey all the precautions we were already taking to prevent the spread of infectious disease within the shelter. I often found that local practitioners had underestimated the level of care our patients routinely received.

If there are other animal shelters in your area, you may also consider forming a liaison committee of representatives from each of these organizations to meet on a regular or on an informal basis.

Persuade the Veterinarians to Visit the Shelter

Offer an evening or weekend "behind the scenes" tour of the shelter facilities. You can restrict this to just vets, or also consider inviting them to bring their family members and staff. Providing food increases attendance, especially if you're asking people to come after work. Many people have a negative, preconceived notion of an animal shelter or "pound." I know that I did.

Ask local vets to give a speech or teach a class at the shelter for the public and/or shelter staff. Topics could include geriatric pet care, emergency first aid for pets, how to choose the right companion animal for your family, the importance of vaccinations and routine veterinary care, and so on.

Why, you ask, would a vet want to take time out of his or her busy schedule to prepare and teach a class for your organization? The answers are many and vary from individual to individual. They can include feeling a sense of importance for being asked, the possibility of drawing new potential clients from community members in the audience, and a sense of satisfaction and altruism in giving back to the community.

PROFESSIONAL INPUT

Ask your colleagues for professional advice and help, when needed. People love to be asked; it is a compliment to them as an individual and to their expertise. For example, you can ask for input on shelter health practices such as disinfection, vaccination, or deworming protocols. This does not mean that you are uninformed on such topics; "new and improved" products come out all the time. Before switching your procedures and products, it is helpful to find out the opinions of those people who are using these other products. Be aware of who you are asking certain questions; select colleagues to query carefully. And, don't bother to ask unless you are willing to listen with an open mind. If veterinarians are going to be asked for input, be sure their input will actually be considered, and if not acted upon, that there is clear communication about the reason this occurred. Understandably, vets may be resentful if their advice is asked and then seemingly ignored. Critical evaluation of any information gathered will help you to make informed decisions.

Ask for practical help or advice on selected medical cases from local associates or specialists. If your colleague is going to provide a service for one of your cases, discuss the fees to be paid up front and whether they are to be full price, a reduced fee, "at cost", or pro bono. People feel good about helping, and again, you demonstrate the level of care patients receive at your shelter. I have elicited generous aid via phone consults and during actual office visits and procedures. In the past, I consulted via phone with a local veterinary dermatologist who diagnosed a growth hormone deficiency in a Pomeranian, and with a veterinary ophthalmologist who diagnosed a corneal sequestrum in a cat. Due to these short phone conversations, I was able to make decisions about the adoptability and appropriate treatment for these patients. I've also had shelter animals seen by specialists for free or reduced fees, including the same ophthalmologist diagnosing juvenile cataracts in a dog, a local mixed animal practitioner coming to the shelter to castrate a ram, and a local small animal practitioner who has performed innumerable orthopedic procedures at no charge. All of these generous actions helped to foster our cooperative relationships.

Of course, no good deed should go without appreciation. It is vital to ensure these generous donations of time and expertise are recognized. A thank you note signed by the shelter staff or vet department staff doesn't seem like much, but is highly valued by the recipients. Recognition in the shelter newsletter or on a plaque in the shelter lobby are also nice ways to recognize someone's contribution. Cookies or flowers also work well. A framed picture of the patient with his or her new adopters will usually end up on the wall in the private practitioners' waiting room or office. Everyone wants to be appreciated and people are much more likely to help again in the future if appropriately appreciated in the past.

It is vital that shelter veterinarians establish respect and a good working relationship with their colleagues in private practice. Working together will not only improve the quality of the shelter veterinarian's life (for we all know the adverse effects of stress), it will also improve the quality of life for the animals in their care. We share many common goals, and even if there are philosophical differences on certain issues, shelter veterinarians and private practitioners can certainly work together on those goals that they share. The time and energy invested in developing a strong, cooperative relationship with community veterinarians will bring many rewards. Kirkwood (1999) provides additional advice on how to improve relations with local veterinarians.

CONCLUSION

The practice of veterinary medicine in an animal shelter has its own unique rewards and challenges. The profession as a whole is recognizing the expertise necessary to provide appropriate medical care for the populations of animals cared for in shelters. The vital services animal shelters provide to both the animals and people in our communities also has been increasingly recognized. Shelter veterinarians can be very proud of the roles they play in helping to provide those services. And beyond their specific medical knowledge and skills, they must successfully negotiate the administrative and human sides of shelter medicine. The rewards are priceless.

REFERENCE

Kirkwood, Scott (1999). "A Prescription for Better Veterinary Relations," *Animal Sheltering*. Humane Society of the United States (HSUS). (November-December).

4
Legal Concerns for Shelters and Shelter Veterinarians

Charlotte Lacroix

INTRODUCTION

While veterinarians who work in the animal shelter environment face the same legal issues as general practitioners who provide their services in private practice, some areas of the law are more likely to impact how shelter veterinarians practice veterinary medicine as compared to their general practitioner colleagues.

Shelter veterinarians often are employed by organizations formed for purposes that are generally ancillary to the private practice setting. These purposes include "adopting out" animals to the public, educating owners about the responsibilities of pet ownership, investigating suspected rabies and animal bite cases, handling abandoned animals, providing behavior consultations to new pet owners, investigating animal cruelty cases and instituting animal population control programs, which, in each case, may give rise to challenging legal dilemmas for shelter facilities. What follows are some of the areas more likely to generate legal concerns.

PET ADOPTION

Prior to adopting out animals, shelters and shelter veterinarians should take reasonable measures to ensure that animals put up for adoption are free from zoonotic diseases[1] and behavioral problems, which could potentially result in human injury. Because medicine and animal behavior are imperfect sciences, shelters and their veterinarians cannot guarantee that adopted pets will not pose any danger to their human companions. Although shelters do their best to assess animal personality and adopt out animals that are free of parasitic diseases, shelters should be prepared to share the blame when a child is bitten or loses his sight to ocular larval migrans, which is one possible form of a toxocara or roundworm infection in humans.

For example, in a New Haven case, a child lost his vision due to ocular toxocariasis, and his parents sued the pet shop that had sold them the child's puppy.[2] Although the pet shop ended up settling the case for $1.5 million, if the case had gone to trial the court would likely have addressed the issue of the pet shop's alleged negligence in "failing to deworm the puppy, failing to have any deworming program in place, and failing to keep appropriate records."[3] Although the defendant in this case was a pet shop, the analogy to the animal shelter context is clear. The shelter, like the pet store, must take some responsibility for protecting a naïve public from diagnosable, zoonotic diseases that are common in young and homeless animals.

Another liability issue for shelter veterinarians is assessing the vicious or dangerous nature of an animal before it is adopted out. In a Tennessee case, a woman was killed by her neighbor's two pit bulls that, several months earlier, her city animal shelter had determined were not "vicious."[4] Betty Lou Stidham lived next door to two pit bulls that had on numerous occasions bitten people. When one of these dogs attacked her small dog causing her dog to have a leg amputated, Ms. Stidham filed a "vicious animal complaint" with the city shelter. The shelter then impounded the dogs for evaluation and conducted a "vicious animal hearing." During the hearing, the shelter found that the dogs did not appear to have a "vicious nature" towards humans or animals and thus were not vicious. However, the shelter did classify the dogs as "dangerous" because of their "capability to inflict serious injury,"[5] and thus ordered their owner to repair the fencing around his property and enroll the dogs in obedience classes. The difference between the classifications "vicious" and "dangerous" in this case was that a classification as "vicious" would require that the dogs be impounded, while "dangerous" required only that certain steps be taken by the owner to minimize the dogs' risk to others. Although the shelter followed up with the owner on several occasions and found that he had not followed the order, the shelter did not classify the dogs as vicious or impound them. In a subsequent wrongful death suit against the city animal shelter, the court held that the shelter was negligent in failing to perform its "special duty to . . . protect [Ms. Stidham] from the danger . . . presented by the dogs."[6] The court found that not only was the vicious animal hearing conducted improperly, but also that the city should have impounded the dogs when the dogs' owner disobeyed the shelter's order and did not take them to obedience training. Although this was not a case where the dogs were adopted out from a shelter, the court's ruling is clearly applicable to dogs that are adopted out from shelters; it is thus very important for shelters to properly screen animals before adoption. In addition, it is critical that prospective owners understand that, even though shelters use reasonable efforts to screen animals, no warranty will be given because of the inherent risks in the adoption and ownership of any animal.

Adopting legally defensible policies and screening techniques reduces the risks by ensuring that adopting owners are able and willing to properly care for their new pet (Appendix 4.1).[7] Shelters may also inquire as part of the assessment of prospective owners as to the type of environment to which the recently adopted pet will be exposed. Such inquiries reduce the possibility of pets being returned to the shelter because they did not "fit in" with the family. Examples are a young, large, happy, and rambunctious dog adopted into a family that lives in a highrise apartment or a timid and potentially fearful cat adopted into a house full of active children.

CONFIDENTIALITY OF MEDICAL RECORDS

While veterinarians have a clear ethical obligation to maintain the confidentiality of their clients' and patients' medical records,[8] only a few states (namely Pennsylvania, New York, Georgia, Missouri, Kansas, Texas, and Illinois) have laws, usually in the veterinary practice act, which require veterinarians to maintain client confidentiality. This legal obligation does have exceptions, however, and some states permit veterinarians to reveal confidential information for the purpose of protecting the public health or the health and welfare of the patient. For example, Pennsylvania's act reads, "Veterinarians and their staffs shall protect the personal privacy of clients, unless the veterinarians are required by law to reveal the confidences or it becomes necessary to reveal the confidences to protect the health and welfare of an individual, the animal or others whose health and welfare are endangered."[9]

Shelter veterinarians face a difficult dilemma because, unlike their private practitioner colleagues, many of the animals they treat are strays, either because the owners cannot be located or are unidentifiable. Local and state laws dictate when the ownership of strays or abandoned animals is transferred to shelters, and once shelters are deemed to have ownership rights in the animals they shelter, no duty of confidentiality is owed to the former owner. However, after the animal has been adopted, any medical information generated from the animal's care would remain confidential in those states that impose a legal duty.

Therefore, in this hypothetical example, if Dr. Shelter treated a puppy, "Sammy" for tapeworms after Mrs. Smith adopted the puppy and "Sammy" was later acquired by a second owner, Mr. Jack, then Mr. Jack would not be entitled to the information pertaining to "Sammy's" treatment without Mrs. Smith's authorization. However, if Mr. Jack had been bitten by "Sammy," Dr. Shelter would have to provide "Sammy's" rabies vaccination history if Dr. Shelter is in a state that waives the duty of confidentiality for the purpose of protecting the public health.

The issue of confidentiality arises for shelter veterinarians in several other contexts as well, and it is essential they know what their state laws require. Some states, such as New York, do not permit veterinarians to breach the duty of confidentiality even though such a breach would reunite a lost pet with its original owner. For example, Debbie brings in her new dog, "Fido," to Dr. Can't Tell, whereupon Dr. Can't Tell decides to scan "Fido" for a microchip and finds that "Fido" actually belongs to Julie. In New York, Dr. Can't Tell cannot reveal such "personally identifiable facts, data or information obtained in a professional capacity without the prior consent of the . . . client, except as authorized or required by law."[10] Therefore, if Debbie wants to keep "Fido" and does not want Julie to find out that she has found "Fido", Dr. Can't Tell is not allowed to notify Julie as such would be a breach of confidentiality to his client, Debbie. Such laws are intended to encourage people to obtain veterinary care for animals without penalizing them for doing so by later removing the animal. Unfortunately, the results don't always seem to be fair, and in this case, was contrary to the interests of the original pet owner. This duty also creates a conflict of interest where the shelter veterinarian suspects or knows that clients are abusing their pets. Veterinarians have a duty to their clients to keep this information confidential, but they also have a duty to protect the patient's best interests. For example, a cat is brought to a shelter to be neutered and the veterinarian notices what looks like small burn marks on the cat's paws and chest area. When the client is questioned as to where these marks came from, the client openly admits that he uses a lighter to lightly burn the cat when it scratches the furniture or has accidents in the house. Clearly the client does not realize he is abusing his cat, because when the veterinarian tells him this is not an acceptable way to treat a pet, the client disagrees.

In some states, such as New York, the veterinarian's duty of confidentiality to the client does not permit the reporting of such abuse.[11] However, how can any veterinarian allow this client to continue to burn his cat? There is no clear answer in this situation, and shelter veterinarians must do their best to explain to owners why they should not mistreat, neglect, or abuse their pets. Veterinarians who reasonably believe that pets are in grave danger or harm should consider not allowing the owners to take their pets home and immediately contact their local animal control office or humane organization to report suspected abuse. Under California law, such a contingency is expressly provided for with a provision on confidentiality that says: "Nothing in this section is intended to prevent the sharing of veterinary medical information between veterinarians and peace officers, humane society officers or animal control officers who are acting to protect the welfare of animals."[12] This law clearly seeks a better compromise between the confidentiality of the client and the best interest of the patient. In addition, some states provide veterinarians with immunity from lawsuits when they report animal abuse cases, and veterinarians should check their animal cruelty statutes to determine if such protections are in place.[13]

MALPRACTICE CLAIMS

Generally, shelter veterinarians are subject to the same malpractice claims as private practitioners and must therefore exercise the same standards of care as are expected of reasonably prudent veterinarians under similar circumstances.[14] Examples of specific liabilities that most often concern shelter veterinarians include: the transmission of zoonotic diseases to humans, rabies exposure issues,[15] anesthetic deaths of adopted animals scheduled to be neutered, and human injury due to the adoption of animals with behavioral problems.

Shelters can reduce their risk of liability for most malpractice claims by practicing preventative medicine, communicating with prospective owners, using informed consent forms,[16] controlling the transfer of ownership, and maintaining good clear records on the animals examined and treated at the shelter. Performing spay and neuter surgeries before an animal is adopted out helps prevent shelter liability, should the animal die during surgery. If the animal is owned by the shelter and has not been adopted out to an owner, no owner can sue the shelter for malpractice. Additionally, physical examinations, behavioral evaluations, routine deworming, and diagnostic tests (such as fecal examinations and serological testing), provide information for veterinarians that affects the adoption process. While in an ideal world all of these procedures would be adopted, the variability in resources available to different shelters leads to tremendous variability in the type and number of procedures that are implemented by shelter veterinarians.

SPAY AND NEUTER SURGERY IN THE SHELTER

It is common for shelters to perform spay and neuter operations on shelter-owned animals as well as on pets that have been adopted out to new owners. Some states, however, do not allow shelter veterinarians to spay and neuter client-owned animals. For example, the New York Practice Act, states that "[n]o business corporation, other than a professional service corporation . . . shall be organized for the practice of veterinary medicine," and under this law, the treatment of animals in the shelter is considered to be the practice of veterinary medicine.[17] Because most shelter facilities are nonprofit organizations, such laws were enacted to prohibit nonprofit organizations from competing with for-profit veterinary practices. This means that shelter veterinarians may perform surgeries on animals before they are adopted out to the public, but once these animals have owners, they cannot be brought back to the shelter for treatment, surgery, or any other veterinary care.

Shelter veterinarians should therefore ensure that the laws of their state permit the treatment of client-owned animals before offering veterinary services to newly adopted pets and their owners (Appendix 4.2). In states such as New York that have such "noncompetition" laws, shelters are encouraged to either participate in population control programs by providing low-cost spays and neuters at local veterinary hospitals or to neuter and vaccinate animals before adoption and then charge an adoption fee to cover the cost of these services.

EXPERT WITNESS

Due to their involvement with the admittance and treatment of abused and neglected animals, shelter veterinarians are often asked to provide expert testimony in animal cruelty cases. While veterinarians receive no formal training on how to draft a report, answer interrogatories, or prepare for an appearance in court, serving as an expert witness is an important role that shelter veterinarians should be prepared to assume. Without such experts to assist prosecutors in enforcing animal cruelty statutes, many perpetrators would be acquitted and left free to continue abusing animals.

In addition to the challenges of learning to be an effective expert witness,[18] shelter veterinarians often are concerned with being sued for defaming[19] an individual charged with animal cruelty. Unfortunately these suits do arise, but it should be comforting for veterinarians to know that such allegations are usually very difficult to prove and the *truth* is their best defense! So as not to use personal funds to defend themselves against allegations of defamation, shelter veterinarians should not agree to be experts until they have determined who will pay their legal fees in the event they are sued. Generally,

shelters employing the veterinarians can agree to pay for the veterinarian's defense or insurance can be purchased from a medical malpractice carrier, such as the AVMA-PLIT. Moreover, some states protect veterinarians by forbidding claims brought against the veterinarian on the basis of their involvement in such a case. For example, Florida law states that veterinarians will not be held civilly or criminally liable for "decisions made or services rendered" under the state's cruelty to animals statute. It further clarifies this statement by asserting "[s]uch a veterinarian is, therefore . . . immune from a lawsuit for his or her part in an investigation of cruelty to animals."[20]

While veterinarians should act as experts where they have some experience or knowledge (i.e., regarding poor living conditions for animals deprived of food, water or shelter), it is similarly important that veterinarians not act as experts in areas where they have absolutely no experience. For example, a shelter veterinarian who has spent the last 10 years caring for dogs and cats would not be the ideal person to testify regarding the condition of reptiles and exotic birds found neglected in a pet shop. Although it may be generally recognizable that these animals were in poor condition, it is far too easy for the defense to show that such veterinarian has very little personal experience on which to base an opinion, thus diminishing the credibility of the expert and weakening the case against the pet shop. In such a case, veterinarians with experience, preferably those that have written and spoken on the topic and are well recognized in the industry, are the best expert candidates. Such veterinarians are often employed at universities and large practices and can be located fairly easily. If an exotics expert is not available, it still is essential to get a veterinarian to testify about the animals' condition, as veterinarians are still considered to be the best professionals to comment on the care and treatment of animals.

PERMISSIBLE ACTS OF SHELTER STAFF

Because many shelters are set up as nonprofit organizations and therefore are supported through generous but often limited donations, many are unable to hire "in-house" veterinarians. As a result, many shelters consult or use the services of local private practitioners and have their nonveterinary personnel provide care to the shelter animals.

Private practitioners consulting or working with shelters must consider what forms of care they feel comfortable supervising or delegating to the shelter's nonveterinary staff, while abiding by the guidelines imposed by state law concerning acts that must solely be performed by veterinarians. Generally, these include diagnosing, operating, treating, or prescribing for any animal disease, pain, or other physical conditions.[21]

Private practitioners also must keep in mind those tasks that may be performed by nonveterinarians. The Practice Act of each state governs the types of medically related tasks that may be performed by assistants and the amount of supervision required by veterinarians who are responsible for such individuals' activities. For example, the California Practice Act is very specific and requires certain tasks to be performed under the "direct" (as opposed to "indirect") supervision of a veterinarian. These include performing dental prophylaxis and the administration of anesthesia and various resuscitative procedures.[22] Other duties can be performed with less supervision because they are not considered to be as critical to the life of the animal and therefore only require the veterinarian's "indirect" supervision. These include obtaining x-rays, applying bandages, and administering and applying medications and treatments, including intramuscular, intravenous, and subcutaneous injections.[23] Veterinarians should also keep in mind that some states, such as New York and California, require that technicians performing certain medical procedures be licensed.[24]

When treatments and diagnostics are not clearly set forth in the state's veterinary Practice Act, veterinarians should exercise common sense in determining what nonveterinary staff are qualified to do. And if in doubt, they should contact the Veterinary State Board for guidance. Veterinarians should be aware that they bear the ultimate responsibility for ensuring that staff members perform their duties competently. For example, if a veterinarian sees patients at a shelter one day a week and feels comfortable with the competence of the staff, it may be reasonable to allow the staff to administer fluids to a dehydrated dog or clean and bandage shallow, uncomplicated wounds. Veterinarians should also ensure they are in compliance with state law when allowing nonveterinary shelter employees to perform diagnostic testing on animals put up for adoption. Such diagnostics are important to ensure the animals are free of serious diseases, some of which are zoonotic, including hookworm and ascarid infections, or others such as heartworm disease and feline leukemia.

Another common situation where veterinarians will work with nonveterinary shelter staff is in the context of providing prescription medications to shelters for use on shelter animals. This question also is best answered with common sense. Clearly, by law, veterinarians should not be prescribing medications to shelters for shelter staff to dole out as they see fit.[25] However, with common conditions easily recognizable by shelter staff, shelter veterinarians, after consulting with the staff, often authorize staff members to administer medications. For example, when a cat exhibits the clinical signs of an upper respiratory tract infection, including a runny nose, watery eyes, sneezing, and a low fever, shelter staff will often treat the condition for several days until the veterinarian arrives.

However, even when shelter staff is permitted to treat animals for such common conditions, no medications should be sent home with an adopted animal without the prescription or signature of a licensed veterinarian. Careful consideration must be given to each state's laws, possible negative effects of medications, the abilities and training of the shelter staff, the frequency of veterinary visits, and the accessibility of a veterinarian, before embracing a policy allowing staff to treat animals with medications.

CONTROLLED SUBSTANCES

As one of the main functions of shelters is to euthanize unadoptable animals and few are "no-kill" facilities, shelters use large amounts of euthanasia solution, such as Pentobarbital. The purchase and delivery of these "controlled substances." is regulated by the Drug Enforcement Agency (DEA) (a federal agency formed to guard against the misuse of dangerous substances), and by each state, which have their own laws to regulate the use of these drugs.

Some state laws take into account the fact that euthanasia is an integral part of shelter life, and create unique provisions for the use of controlled substances specifically in shelters as opposed to the private practice setting. Under Florida law, shelter staff, unlike private practice staff, may administer euthanasia solution without direct veterinary supervision.[26] In order to ensure that such lay staff is trained, the law also requires that technicians and employees of animal shelters complete a training program to become certified euthanasia technicians before they can euthanize animals without veterinary supervision.[27]

State laws may also be more flexible regarding the purchase of euthanasia drugs for shelter use. Whereas state laws generally allow only veterinarians to purchase controlled substances, some states permit animal shelters to register as "separate entities," thus qualifying them to purchase euthanasia drugs even without a veterinarian on staff.[28] New York shelter facilities, for example, can apply for a permit from the Department of Health, Bureau of Controlled Substances, which allows them to purchase Beuthanasia solution and ketamine in order to euthanize and tranquilize animals.[29] This is good for shelter veterinarians because they are not held accountable for the ordering, storage, and use of the controlled substances, but rather the shelter's staff is required to take on these responsibilities and keep careful records. When a state requires individual practitioners to order and keep track of the shelter's euthanasia solution, thereby holding veterinarians solely responsible for the use of such drugs, it is essential for veterinarians to implement detailed guidelines for the staff to follow. As mentioned previously, differences exist in the registration and management of controlled substances in the shelter environment in each state, and thus shelter veterinarians should inquire with their state drug enforcement agency or veterinary association to be clear about state procedures.[30]

If an animal shelter is unable to obtain its own DEA license, it is dependent upon veterinarians to purchase controlled substances to be used at the shelter. When a veterinarian decides to leave the shelter, both federal DEA regulations and state law must be followed in order to ensure the proper transfer of controlled substances from one licensed party to another. The veterinarian who purchased these drugs will be held accountable and must take responsibility for them when he or she leaves. If a new veterinarian is already at the shelter (or another responsible party with a DEA license), there should be a clear transfer of the controlled substances to that other party—the departing veterinarian should leave the responsible person with an inventory of all

controlled substances purchased under the departing veterinarian's DEA registration. If there will be a lapse between veterinarians and there is no one else at the shelter with a DEA license, an inventory should be taken when the one veterinarian leaves and again when the new veterinarian arrives, to be certain that all controlled substances are accounted for. In some states, such as New York, it is illegal for a shelter veterinarian to supply a shelter with controlled substances; in such cases, a shelter should obtain its own DEA permit.[31] When the shelter cannot obtain a permit, a shelter veterinarian can agree to provide or "supervise" the treatment of animals with drugs from his own supply, but he cannot store them at the shelter.[32]

Even when careful guidelines are followed, it is possible that some or portions of controlled substances will be lost or stolen; reporting this theft is the responsibility of the licensee who purchased and delivered the drugs. When loss or theft occurs, the licensee must immediately report the theft to the DEA and the local police department or local bureau regulating controlled substances. The report to the DEA must be made on Form DEA-106, Report of Theft or Loss of Controlled Substances, which can be found on their website www.deadiversion.usdoj.gov. An example of a local form would be New York's "Loss of Controlled Substances Report,"[33], which must be filed "promptly" with the Department of Health, Bureau of Controlled Substances, even if the "controlled substances are subsequently recovered, [and] the responsible parties identified or actions taken against them."[34]

RABIES VACCINATION CLINICS

In order to reduce the public health risks associated with rabies, municipalities frequently host "Rabies Clinics" that provide low-cost vaccinations to the cats and dogs owned by members of the community. Such clinics are held at shelter facilities or public places such as fire stations and large parking lots. Shelter veterinarians and private practitioners often donate their time and administer vaccines to what is frequently a large number of dogs and cats.

Though there are a number of liability issues that arise in this context, there are certain requirements that are standard in most state laws regarding vaccination clinics. First, while it is impossible to do a complete physical examination on each of these patients, most states (such as New York) require that the administering veterinarian perform physical exams to determine whether the pets are sufficiently healthy to tolerate the vaccinations.[35] Additionally, owners must complete an information sheet before seeing the doctor, with such requisite information as their name, address, phone number, pet's name, age, species, sex, color, breed, and weight (Appendix 4.3). Thereafter, the veterinarian must fill in the rabies certificate for each patient, including the date of vaccination and the expiration date of the vaccine. Generally this is sufficient information, which, with the help of an assistant and a little advance planning, should not be too burdensome for veterinarians. Some states such as Florida require that the rabies vaccine manufacturer, the vaccine lot and expiration date, and the type and brand of vaccine be noted on the certificate, but even this information can be printed on the rabies certificate in advance.[36]

A significant constraint on the veterinarian's time is the signature requirement for the rabies certificate. Some states (such as Florida), have specifically stated that a signature stamp is acceptable,[37] while others (such as New York), do not address the issue of whether an actual signature is required or whether a signature stamp is sufficient. It is probably safe to assume that a signature stamp is acceptable, even if the certificate is stamped by someone other than the administering veterinarian, so long as, like most other permissible acts of nonveterinarians, it is done under the "direct supervision" of the veterinarian. This would mean that the veterinarian's assistant sits at a table in the same room or one adjoining the room where the vaccinations are being given, applying the signature stamp as each patient emerges from the vaccination area. However, the administering veterinarian should inquire with their state board of examiners whether the signature stamp is an acceptable substitute for an actual signature.

Time constraints in rabies clinics make it virtually impossible to get a thorough medical history on every dog and cat that comes in and, even with such a history, veterinarians cannot predict with any degree of certainty which dogs will suffer side effects from the vaccine. However rare such side effects may be, in order to reduce the risk of liability for administering veterinarians, it is essential that owners be warned of the potential side effects

and what to do if they occur. Then, if a serious side effect does arise, veterinarians are less likely to be held liable because they properly warned owners of such a possibility and instructed them to see a veterinarian at the first sign of a reaction.

Some states have limited the liability by adopting laws that provide immunity for veterinarians working in the rabies clinic setting so that if injury or death to the animal does occur, the veterinarian is not held responsible.[38] However, these provisions are not universal and do not protect veterinarians in cases of gross negligence or willful misconduct, or where the veterinarian's behavior falls below the standards generally practiced by other veterinarians in like circumstances.[39] For this reason, it is best for veterinarians to prepare owners for the possible side effects. One way of minimizing the drain on the veterinarian's time is to distribute a short list of side effects that clients should look for in the first 24–48 hours after the vaccination. This list should differentiate between common side effects and those that need a veterinarian's attention, and possibly include the phone number of a local veterinary emergency practice. To further protect the veterinarian, owners may be required to sign a waiver of liability, confirming their understanding that there is no guarantee against serious side effects from the vaccine, and that they are waiving the right to sue the administering veterinarian if such side effects occur (Appendix 4.2).

Unfortunately, liability from the vaccine itself is not the only risk to the shelter veterinarian involved in such clinics. Accidents can and do occur during the clinic, such as a client falling in the waiting area, a pet escaping and/or biting another pet or owner, or a pet slipping away from the veterinarian and escaping from the facility. Accidents are virtually inevitable, especially in a small area filled with several people and their animals. However, there are several ways that administering veterinarians can protect themselves and limit their liability for such accidents. First, veterinarians should request that the municipality sponsoring the free clinic obtain public liability insurance for such accidents. Veterinarians also can ask that the municipality agree to indemnify them for damages and legal fees that they may incur as a result of a judgment from a lawsuit.

Another option is to have pet owners sign waivers releasing veterinarians from liabilities stemming from accidents occurring at the clinic, which is similar to the waiver signed by the pet owner concerning the vaccination itself. In fact, both releases can be included on the same form. This waiver says that the owner will hold Dr. Q and the ABC Animal Shelter or Municipality harmless from any act or any failure to act that results in injury to the owner or pet. Furthermore, a form stating that the owner releases the veterinarian from liability for both the possible side effects of the vaccine as well as for any accidents that may occur during the clinic visitation, will go a long way towards removing clinic experience anxiety (Appendix 4.2).

RABIES OBSERVATION PERIOD/ QUARANTINE

Rabies is clearly an important public health issue in animal shelters, where most animals come in with no history, and shelters must determine whether each animal presents a public health risk. It is the responsibility of the shelter and its veterinarians to protect the public by quarantining any animal suspected of having been exposed to rabies. State and local laws regulate the treatment of animals suspected of having been exposed to rabies, and designate how long the animal must remain under observation or in quarantine. These laws will generally also set out the procedures to follow if the animal has bitten a human or another animal, or if it dies while in quarantine.

By and large, these laws state that if the exposed animal has a current rabies vaccination, the animal must be observed for any rabies symptoms for at least 10 days.[40] If the exposed animal has not been vaccinated or the vaccination has expired, the quarantine can last up to six months in an approved veterinary facility or locked enclosure, and if at any point the animal shows symptoms of rabies it must be euthanized. The shelter veterinarian is responsible for observing the quarantined animal for any changes in its behavior or health, and this responsibility should not be delegated to shelter staff. The animal's owner is responsible for the isolation expenses as well as the cost of any necessary veterinary treatment during the observation or quarantine period.[41] If an animal is suspected of having rabies and no owner is located after the requisite holding period in the shelter, the animal should be euthanized and the head sent to the state laboratory for rabies testing. In addition to state law, the Rabies Compendium published yearly by the *Journal of the American Veterinary Medical Association* (JAVMA) is an excellent resource regarding rabies issues.[42]

LIABILITY FOR EUTHANASIA

Most shelters cannot find homes for all the animals that they admit and are therefore permitted by state law to euthanize unadopted animals, including pets that have been lost by their owners. These laws have been necessary to keep shelters functioning as they experience a large influx of animals and need to maintain a continuous supply of cages. Before such animals can be euthanized, the laws of most states require that animals be held for a given waiting period to allow sufficient time for owners to locate their pets. This period, ranging anywhere from four to eight days, is often long enough for pets that can be identified, either by a collar, tattoo, or microchip, to be reunited with their owners.

However, the situation does occasionally arise when pets are euthanized before their owners locate them at the shelters. While such situations leave owners without their beloved pets and are very difficult for both the owners and shelter personnel, the shelters are generally not liable to the owners, so long as the animals were held for the requisite number of days. Some state statutes clearly protect shelters and their veterinarians by specifically prohibiting the imposition of civil or criminal liability on veterinarians in such cases. For example, regarding cats, Maine law states that "A veterinarian, a humane agent, an animal control officer or an animal shelter, including a person employed by an animal shelter, is not civilly liable to the owner of a cat for the loss of that cat resulting from actions taken in compliance with this section."[43] Colorado law applies this immunity to all pets, stating that for any animal held for the minimum holding period, the shelter and its employees "shall be immune from liability in a civil action brought by the owner of a pet animal for the shelter's disposition of a pet animal."[44]

Otherwise, when an animal is euthanized before the holding period is up and the owner comes in within the prescribed period to find the animal already gone, a negligence claim may arise. Especially in today's litigious climate, where the loss of a pet can invoke damages for loss of consortium and infliction of emotional distress, euthanizing an animal before the holding period has expired must be avoided. Shelters can implement policies to minimize such risks by requiring their staff and veterinarians to check several times that an animal has been at the shelter for the requisite time period, before performing any euthanasia. This does not mean doing an exhaustive history on where, how, and by whom the dog was brought in, but rather it entails the use of reasonable measures such as checking the date that the animal arrived and having those who actually euthanize the animals initial next to the date the animal was admitted to ensure they, too, have double-checked the holding period.

A recent Illinois case illustrates that lawsuits against shelters for wrongly euthanizing pets are not theoretical but actually present a real risk.[45] In this 2001 case, a woman who had lost her cat, Bosco, had attempted for several weeks to locate him by advertising in the local newspaper and having her friend visit the shelter weekly. Though the shelter held the cat for the requisite seven days as required by local law, the cat was labeled unadoptable because of scarring and therefore was kept in an area inaccessible to the public. On the eighth day, the owner learned that her cat had been taken to the shelter, but the cat was euthanized several hours before she arrived. When asked how this could have happened, a shelter employee callously replied that they didn't have time to check newspaper ads and that the pet's "time was up." The owner sued the shelter, claiming that the shelter breached a duty to her to exercise reasonable care to prevent the loss of her pet, and that the shelter had misrepresented itself by saying that it would make "every effort" to find the owners of lost pets. Clearly, the shelter was careless in euthanizing a pet whose owner had been actively looking for him, but the court dismissed the case, stating that the behavior was not "extreme and outrageous" enough for the shelter to be found guilty.[46]

While the shelter was not found to be negligent in this situation, the bad publicity and harm to the shelter's public image was likely quite damaging. Given that most shelters' budgets depend heavily on donations, it behooves shelter personnel to adopt and follow policies that reduce the incidence of such tragedies and the lawsuits that follow.

WILDLIFE

Though the majority of animals that shelter veterinarians encounter are domestic companion animals, such as, dogs, cats, rabbits, and ferrets, occasions arise when they are faced with greater challenges, namely the treatment and care of wildlife. As the boundaries between human living space and animal habitats continue to diminish, humans are more likely to come into contact with wildlife and invariably these animals will find their way to shelters. Commonly, people will injure or find injured animals and bring them to animal shelters for treatment, instead of wildlife rehabilitation facilities that are either nonexistent or difficult to find in communities.

Wildlife rehabilitators are scattered throughout the United States and can be found by contacting the Wildlife Commission of the state in which the shelter is located, as well as through certain organizations such as the National Wildlife Rehabilitator's Association. However, because these facilities are scarce and often unknown to the public, shelter veterinarians will frequently admit injured wild animals into shelter facilities. State law regulates the treatment of wildlife, and in most states, anyone attempting to rehabilitate wildlife must have a wildlife rehabilitator's permit.[47] While it is not difficult for most veterinarians to obtain such permits, it often is unnecessary, as a majority of states allow veterinarians to provide emergency treatment to wildlife, provided that the wildlife are transferred to rehabilitation as soon as possible.

Shelter veterinarians should be aware that because migratory birds readily cross state lines, they are treated differently from wildlife and are regulated by the federal government and not state wildlife commissions. Similar to state laws created for wildlife, federal law allows veterinarians to handle injured birds, triage and stabilize them, so long as the birds are transferred within 48 hours to federal permit holders who are authorized to rehabilitate migratory birds. In treating migratory birds, shelter veterinarians should exercise caution before euthanizing such birds unless it is clear that the bird is in severe pain and there exists no hope of rehabilitation. Faced with a bird that must be euthanized, shelter veterinarians should attempt to contact a licensed bird rehabilitator to get their input on the situation. For this reason, it makes sense for most shelters to have clearly posted the names and numbers of the licensed rehabilitators that are located in their state in addition to the contact information for the state's wildlife rehabilitators.

CONCLUSION

Shelter veterinarians have a unique relationship with the animals they treat and the owners that adopt these animals, and therefore they frequently are faced with legal dilemmas that they may not otherwise encounter as private practitioners. There are, of course, many other legal issues that challenge shelters and shelter veterinarians on a daily basis, but this chapter is meant to guide shelter veterinarians in combination with their own common sense and caution; clearly, there is not one answer that will apply to all situations. Additionally, this chapter should not serve as legal advice, and shelter veterinarians should seek the direction of their state veterinary board as well as legal counsel, as needed, to determine the appropriate course of action in any particular situation.

The author is very grateful for the invaluable research and contributions she received from Michelle Winn, Esq., without whose assistance this chapter would not have been possible.

NOTES

1. Wilson, James F. et al. January 1996 "Zoonotic parasitic diseases: A legal and medical update." *Veterinary Forum*, pp. 40–46.
2. *Id.*
3. *Id.*
4. *Chase v. City of Memphis*, 1998 Tenn. LEXIS 435.
5. *Id.*
6. *Id.*
7. Wilson, J. F., and Lacroix, C.A. 1995 *Legal Consent Forms for Veterinary Practices*. (Yardley: Priority Press Ltd.).
8. Principles of Veterinary Medical Ethics of The American Veterinary Medical Association, Principle VII. Medical Records (1999 Revision).
9. Pennsylvania Code, Rules of Professional Conduct for Veterinarians 49 Pa. Code § 31.21, Principle 7 (http://www.pacode.com/secure/search.asp).
10. New York Rules of the Board of Regents, Part 29, Unprofessional Conduct, NY Reg 29.1 (b) (8) (http://www.op.nysed.gov/part29.htm#29.6).
11. *Id.*
12. California Business and Professions Code § 4857 (2001) (http://www.leginfo.ca.gov/).
13. Florida Statutes § 828.12(3) (2001) (http://www.leg.state.fl.us/).
14. Wilson, James F. 1990 *Professional Liability, Law and Ethics of the Veterinary Profession* (Yardley: Priority Press Ltd.), pp. 131–174.
15. "Public veterinary medicine: Public health, Compendium of Animal Rabies Prevention and Control, 2000." *Journal of the American Veterinary Medical Association* 216, no. 3 (February 1, 2000): 338–343.
16. Wilson, J. F., and Lacroix, C.A. 1995 *Legal Consent Forms For Veterinary Practices*. (Yardley: Priority Press Ltd.).
17. New York State Consolidated Laws, Education Law, Title 8, Article 135 § 6706 (http://www.op.nysed.gov/title8.htm).
18. Wilson, James F. *The Veterinarian as an Expert Witness, Law and Ethics of the Veterinary Profession* (Yardley: Priority Press Ltd., 1990), pp. 284–293.
19. Wilson, James F. *Libel and Slander, Law and Ethics of the Veterinary Profession*. (Yardley: Priority Press Ltd., 1990), pp. 166–170.
20. Florida Statute § 828.12(3) (2001).
21. California Business and Professions Code § 4826 (b), (c), (d) (2001); New York Consolidated Laws, Education Law, Title 8, Article 135 § 6701.
22. Pennsylvania Code, 49 Pa. Code § 31.31 (a) (1).
23. Pennsylvania Code, 49 Pa. Code § 31.31 (a) (2).
24. New York State Consolidated Laws, Education Law, Title 8, Article 135 §6709, 6711; California Business and Professions Code § 4832-4842 (2001).
25. California Business and Professions Code § 4826 (b) (2001); NY State Consolidated Laws § 6701.
26. Florida Statute § 828.058(4) (a) (2001).
27. *Id.*
28. Wilson, James F. *Law and Ethics of the Veterinary Profession* (Yardley: Priority Press Ltd., 1990), pp. 264–268.
29. NYCRR Title 10, Article 33, Public Health Law, § 80.134(d) (w3.health.state.ny.us/dbspace/NYCRR10.nsf/).
30. *Id.*
31. *New York State Veterinary News/NYS,* November 1998, page 9.
32. *Id.*
33. NYCRR Title 10, Article 33, Public Health Law § 80.20.
34. *Id.*
35. New York Regulations, Veterinary Standards of Practice, NY Reg § 638.620.
36. Florida Statute § 828.30 (2001).
37. Florida Statute § 828.30 (2001).
38. Maine Revised Statutes, Title 7, Part 9, Chapter 720, § 39.17 (2001) (janus.state.me.us/legis/statutes/7/title7sec3917).

39. Texas Health and Safety Code § 826.047, (www.capitol.state.tx.us/); Pennsylvania Code § 455.9a(a).

40. Pennsylvania Code, 7 Pa. Code § 16.22 (a) (1,2).

41. See note xviii; New York State Sanitary Code, Chapter 10, Part 2, Section 2.14 (http// www.health.state.ny.us/nysdoh/sancode.htm).

42. *JAVMA* 218, no. 1, (January 2001): pp. 26–31.

43. *Maine Revised Statutes, Title 7, Part 9, Chapter 720* § 3919-A (5) (2001).

44. Colorado Statute, Title 35, Agriculture, § 35-80-106.3 (2001).

45. *Clinite v. The Anti-Cruelty Society*, 312 Ill. App. 3d 8 (2000).

46. *Id.*

47. Pennsylvania Code, 58 Pa. Code §147.302; New York State Consolidated Laws, Environmental Conservation Law §11-0919.

Appendix 4.1

"Insert Shelter Name" PET ADOPTION AGREEMENT

Adopter Information:

Name:_____   Employer: _____

Address:_____   Employer's address: _____

_____   _____

Phone:_____   Phone: _____

I hereby acknowledge receiving from the **"Insert Shelter Name"** a:

1) Dog; Cat; Puppy; Kitten (Circle appropriate) named _____

2) Age: _____ (as estimated by "Insert Shelter Name" staff)

3) Breed: _____ Color: _____ Weight: _____

4) Microchip ID #: _____

5) Male; Female; Male-neutered; Female-spayed (Circle appropriate)

6) Vaccination History:_____

7) Deforming History:_____

I AGREE: (Please initial each statement)

Appendix 4.1 (*continues*)

_____ 1.   To provide proper and adequate food, water, housing, exercise, grooming, and humane treatment at all times.

_____ 2.   To provide veterinary care in the form of annual vaccinations, preventive heartworm medications as appropriate, and such veterinary medical care as is necessary to prevent and/or treat accidents and illnesses.

_____ 3.   To obey local licensing and animal confinement laws.

_____ 4.   To keep this animal as a pet and companion animal only, and not to use it for any other purpose.

_____ 5.   Not to sell, give away or use this animal for experimental purposes, allow it to engage in dog fighting or train it or have it trained to attack other persons or animals.

I **ACKNOWLEDGE** that: (Please initial each statement)

_____ 1.   I have been informed that all animals can from time to time carry and transmit diseases, some of which affect people, including bacteria, viruses, parasites, and fungal diseases (i.e., ringworm) and that these diseases may be undetectable in what appears to be a healthy animal at the time of adoption.

_____ 2.   I am aware that pets may exhibit normal but potentially undesirable behaviors including, but not limited to, aggression, house soiling, biting, scratching (people, furniture, and woodwork), barking, digging, mounting people's legs, urine marking (dogs), urine spraying (cats) and that these normal behavior patterns may be difficult to manage. No one at   **"Insert Shelter Name"** has told me that this pet will **not** engage in any of these behavior patterns.

_____ 3.   **"Insert Shelter Name"** is not responsible for any damage which the animal may inflict on another person, my property or the property of another and no attempt will be made by me to hold the **"Insert Shelter Name"** responsible for such damage.

Appendix 4.1   (*continues*)

_____   4.   I am aware that it usually costs between $250.00 and $750.00 per year to feed, house, train and provide veterinary care for a pet and that I am financially able to meet these expenses for my adoptive pet.

_____   5.   I accept the animal as it is at the time of adoption and understand that the **"Insert Shelter Name"** is not responsible for any medical conditions not readily detected or detectable prior to or at the time of this adoption or discovered after such adoption.

_____   6.   I acknowledge that I have read this agreement and hereby release the **"Insert Shelter Name"** from any present or future liability associated with my adoption of this animal.

I agree to adopt the above mentioned animal as of _____ (date).

_____   _____

Signature of Adopter   Date

---

1. All forms in these appendixes are courtesy of Wilson, J. F., DVM, JD, and Lacroix, C. A., DVM, JD. 2001. *Legal Consent Forms for Veterinary Practices*, Priority Press, Ltd.

Appendix 4.2

<u>**Spay and Neuter Certificate**</u>

Authorization for Anesthesia and/or Surgery [3]

Client's Name _____ Pet's Name _____

Anesthetic and surgical procedure(s) to be performed:

_____

_____

I, the undersigned owner or agent of the owner of the pet identified above, certify that **I am** _____ **I am**

not _____ (check one) eighteen years of age or over and authorize the veterinarian(s) at (shelter name) to

perform the above procedure(s). I understand that some risks always exist with anesthesia and/or surgery

and that I am encouraged to discuss any concerns I have about those risks with the attending veterinarian

before the procedure(s) is/are initiated. My signature on this form indicates that any questions I have

regarding the following issues have been answered to my satisfaction:

- The reasonable medical and/or surgical treatment options for my pet

- Sufficient details of the procedures to understand what will be performed

- How fully my pet will recover and how long it will take

- The most common and serious complications

Appendix 4.2 (*continues*)

- The length and type of follow-up care and home restraint required

- The estimate of the fees for all services

- Any necessary payment arrangements

While I accept that all procedures will be performed to the best of the abilities of the staff at this hospital, I understand that no guarantee or warranty has been made regarding the results that may be achieved. I agree to pay a deposit of _____% of the estimated fees, assume financial responsibility for the remaining fees, and provide payment via cash, credit card, or check at the time my pet is discharged from the hospital. Should unexpected life-saving emergency care be required and the hospital staff is unable to reach me, the staff **has** _____ **does not have** _____ (check one) my permission to provide such treatment and I agree to pay for such services.

I have read and fully understand the terms and conditions set forth above.

_____   _____

Signature of Owner or Agent   Date

(or) Signature of Parent or Legal Guardian (if owner/agent less than 18 years of age)

Phone number(s) at which owner or agent can be reached today and/or tomorrow:_____

---

1. All forms in these appendixes are courtesy of Wilson, J. F., DVM, JD, and Lacroix, C. A., DVM, JD. 2001. *Legal Consent Forms for Veterinary Practices*, Priority Press, Ltd.

Appendix 4.3

Vaccination Certificate

1. I, _____, give permission for my pet(s) to be vaccinated at this clinic and acknowledge that such vaccinations do not constitute complete pet health care. (*It is essential that my pet receive a yearly physical examination.*)

2. I also state that my pet(s) have no sign of disease, are not allergic to vaccines, and are not pregnant.

3. I understand that vaccinations may cause unexpected reactions in pets. I also agree to accept all risks of vaccination and personally accept both legal and financial responsibility for all charges incurred as a result of all such risks. I also accept that it is my responsibility to seek emergency care as needed or directed.

Owner name:_____

                  Last   First

Street Address:_____

           City   State   Zip

Home Phone No.:(___)_____Work Phone No.:(___)_____

Appendix 4.3 (*continues*)

Signature of Owner:_____Date:_____

Animal's Name:_____M / F: Neutered/Spay

Breed:_____Color:_____ Age_____

_____

To be Completed by Shelter Staff

Rabies Vaccine

Vaccine Manufacturer:_____Vaccine Serial No.:_____

Vaccination Tag No.:_____ Vaccination Expiration Date:_____

(signature)_____

(Name of Veterinarian)

---

1. All forms in these appendixes are courtesy of Wilson, J. F., DVM, JD, and Lacroix, C. A., DVM, JD. 2001. *Legal Consent Forms for Veterinary Practices*, Priority Press, Ltd.

Section 2:
Husbandry

INTRODUCTION

Shelter veterinarians often find that some of the most challenging demands that are placed upon them are not always medical. While basic medical information is readily accessible from a variety of sources, answers to husbandry questions are less readily obtained, especially when being applied to the unique shelter environment.

Solutions to disease transmission problems often rest in preventative measures and changes in shelter design and sanitation procedures, rather than changing vaccination or treatment protocols. Veterinary knowledge is essential to avoid the useless waste of resources to combat disease. Chapter 5 by Johnson on shelter design will help veterinarians be an effective part of a management team that examines the shelter environment in an attempt to identify and remedy physical facility problems that may contribute to disease spread. In Chapter 6, Gilman describes the concepts and implementation of a sound sanitation program. A thorough understanding of disease and the methods that will prevent and disrupt their transmission is one of the most invaluable contributions that veterinarians can make to

maintain a healthy shelter population. The role of good nutrition in maintaining a healthy population is covered by Case and Fahey in chapter 7. This frequently neglected component of a good health care program is often relegated to purchasing departments and managers who have little, if any background in feeding stressed animals with special needs.

The last few chapters in this section are devoted to the special care concerns for various animal species that find their way into shelters. Although the ultimate goal of shelters is to rehome or release animals as quickly as possible, many shelters are housing animals for prolonged periods, giving rise to more concern about the quality standards of care. Every species could not be covered here, and most of the information provides only basic guidelines for handling animals upon their arrival at the shelter, and how to deal with immediate and short-term health care and management concerns. Relationships with species specialists and wildlife rehabilitators should be developed in advance for assistance in dealing with complex medical problems and disease outbreaks in unfamiliar species when they occur.

5

The Animal Shelter Building: Design and Maintenance of a Healthy and Efficient Facility

Tom Johnson

INTRODUCTION

Very few animal shelters operate in an effective and efficient building environment. Unfortunately, this also includes many new facilities that suffer from the lack of maintenance of relatively new equipment, and that were often built by inexperienced consultants or contractors providing little design relief other than "new" finishes. Older facilities range from the progressively deteriorating to badly deteriorated. Complicating the advancing building age and general systems degeneration could be many changes in the mission for which the building was originally created. The older shelters, which were basically created as "dog pounds", did not provide for cats. Animal health was seldom considered as a pound's responsibility. Few "pounds" were built that maintained an environment necessary to sustain the health and safety of the staff and the animals, and little was done other than meet the public animal control's ordinance requirements for a mandatory holding period and subsequent "disposal."

Today's staff medical professional may be working in the old "physical plant" of one of these antiquated facilities in conditions that need to be changed to meet the needs of a healthy, safe, animal-holding environment. With your professional training you can be a key team member in the improvement of all physical conditions in the shelter.

The following are medical parallels to consider:

1. Health maintenance—Doing preventative building maintenance
2. Triage—Recognizing the building's symptoms and planning the appropriate treatment
3. Rehabilitation—Identifying the building's systemic problem(s) and helping to plan for renovations and/or additions.

Begin with the "physical exam." Every building needs a complete and thorough examination, and few are receiving them. Every building needs a tailored program of "health" maintenance, and few are receiving it. Every building needs to be understood for what it can do and what it can't; few are.

The responsibility is a great one, considering that the successful implementation of the "exam," the "rehabilitation"; and the application of "prevention" will directly affect the conditions in which the staff will work and will determine the public's opinion of the facility. Will it be an accessible, safe, and healthy environment where the building provides for the security, health, and comfort of the staff and the shelter animals? Working in some degree of substandard conditions is an unfortunate and almost universal characteristic in most animal shelters. However, it shouldn't be. Understanding that your medical evaluation and diagnostic process is very similar to the way an architect manages a design process can make you a key contributor to the successful rehabilitation of a "sick" building.

Every building had its "mission" and was designed to meet the particular "program" that created the design at that particular time. A typical suburban veterinary clinic is not an animal shelter any more than a suburban branch bank is a hardware store. The design process doesn't start with the things that a building "won't do", it starts with the program of things that the building is intended "to do". Each component of the "things" that must be done becomes a part of the design. The administrative office should be very different from the medical treatment room. The feline initial holding room should be very different from the feline adoption space. The Animal Control Officers' holding kennels should be very different from the public adoption kennels. When rooms, finishes, equipment, and materials are victims of unintended uses and exposures, problems almost always occur.

How can the medical professional in the shelter environment best contribute to reducing or eliminating problems? Consider the problems that "plague" most shelters, and consider how you can actively contribute to preventive treatment for the facility. Because contagious diseases always require a vehicle of transmission, the facility "examination" needs to begin at that point. Look for virus "safe harbors". Find shelter climatic circumstances that contribute to disease transmission, and identify environmental conditions that nurture bacterial development. Then, you can participate in the team effort to decide on the selected "rehabilitation" and recommend the appropriate "treatment" for these conditions.

LIMITING DISEASE TRANSMISSION

If there's the possibility of an infectious animal population, the only "treatment" that will prevent any disease transmission is true isolation. Unfortunately, few facilities have a space that is physically and environmentally separate from the rest of the shelter. This area of isolation must be totally outside the building's occupied space envelope; it must have an outside-only entrance; its heating and ventilation must be completely separate. Careful atten-

tion must be paid to any potential disease transmission by the staff, the tools that are used in the room, movement of dirty bowls, and so forth from the area. How can an isolation area be effectively monitored by staff when it's so far away from the normal work zone? Consider the problems; then consider the alternative solutions. A room "outside" the building can be built physically "inside" the structure but still allow exterior-access only and include all necessary cleaning and feeding provisions. If a wall of this isolation room could be adjacent to an interior building corridor, a large fixed glass window would then allow staff to continually monitor the space. A "three-way" switch, for the light in the room, located in this corridor lets shelter staff turn on the isolation room lights without having to leave the building and then enter the isolated room. Think completely through the details and all procedures needed. This is only an example of diagnosing the core of the problem and considering alternative treatments. Consult with the other members of your specialty team and then "prescribe" the appropriate process to achieve a successful end for your particular environment and problem.

Because the canine population typically exhibits problems limited to a few common diseases, your study of the "treatment" of the building should reasonably focus initially on those diseases. What reasonably can be done to reduce the occurrence of infectious tracheobronchitis, canine distemper, and canine parvovirus? In the feline community, you would consider the respiratory infections, while also considering the implications of the more insidious diseases and their effects on an adopted animal and the adopter. Because prevention is the best treatment, we need to focus our attention on how best to prevent the transmission of diseases between sheltered animals, between animals and staff, and between the staff with equipment, materials, and finishes that are uncompromising in their ability to maintain antiseptic conditions.

Disease management can also be addressed through careful planning of traffic patterns through the shelter building. The flow of people, equipment, and air should always progress from areas of highest health to those areas of less healthy or questionable-status animals. Healthy animals available for adoption should be readily accessible for viewing by the public, without needing to pass through other shelter areas. Stray animals of questionable health status should be in a separate area and staff or the public should not be allowed to go directly from this area to the adoption area to prevent the possible spread of disease. In the same way, movement from disease isolation areas to areas where strays or adoption animals are housed should be controlled or prevented.

EVALUATING NEEDS

Consider the total shelter as the problem. What are the symptoms of a "sick" shelter? What can be done about it? Let's first consider existing buildings and then the planning for, and the understanding of, the options that can be applied successfully in new facilities. The building is the "patient". Be systematic in your examination and your triage of all the spaces in the building. Start by making a summary list of all the spaces in the building. Note how the spaces "feel"; Are they comfortable, how do they smell? Does a room feel humid or does is feel too dry? Does the room have floor drains? Do they look dry and dirty? Is the lighting adequate? Look at the wall and floor surfaces; is there deterioration, cracking, or open joints (especially between the walls and the floor), is the base of wall material peeling away? What is the floor made of? Are there open joints and is there cracking? Do the floors in the treatment spaces look like they can really be cleaned? Considering the use of the space will enable you to make critical decisions on the appropriate "treatment." Painted drywall construction is usually acceptable with traditional "office type finishes" but *never* in animal holding areas. Walls must be washable and only epoxy-painted surfaces or other totally impervious materials should be used in animal spaces. Cabinetry must be commercial grade without the delaminating of the plastic surfaces or joints. There should be no failing hinges on doors and drawers, and cabinets should be made of a base material that withstands the continuous moisture they will be exposed to in continual cleaning. When you look around a room that is used for animal care, is there anything that shows rust? Are there any wooden surfaces? Are there cracks between floors and walls that can't be cleaned? Any hidden surfaces under old drains? Record all the "symptoms," as they will be the foundation of your "diagnosis" for appropriate "treatment".

How old is your building? Have individual areas outgrown their intended use? Have needs changed and have rooms been forced to accommodate them? A usual example is finding cat-holding spaces that have been forced into old buildings intended to function only as dog pounds. Has the building had an effective and adequately funded program of planned maintenance? Did experienced specialists design it specifically as a shelter, or was it more "home grown"? Review the condition of all spaces, the floors, walls, hardware, ceilings, lighting, windows, doors, and all built-in equipment. Look for deterioration, rust, cracks, and lack of maintenance. Record them all as problematic conditions.

SEARCHING FOR THE "QUICK FIX"

In the wild west the patent medicine salesman had the cure for everything. In the shelter environment, many vendors and sales promotions may offer you a "quick fix" for your shelter problems. Just like the wild west, most of the offerings are temporary, are basically very remedial, and are usually marginally successful at best. The vendor will be long gone, and so will be your money, before you realize you've "been had." There are very few quick fixes in the animal sheltering environment.

SURFACES

Floors

Most shelter floors are concrete. Many have had something applied to the concrete surface, but there are only a few materials that may successfully be applied to this concrete for a successful finished surface if the bare concrete is not acceptable. To paint a concrete floor is never an option. Realizing that concrete floors are not impervious, something must be done to it to create the necessary waterproof and cleanable finish. New or old, your concrete is probably cracked, because it's the nature of the material to crack and shrink on poorly prepared substrates and often even in the normal curing process. These cracks must be filled. If you are working on bare concrete, some "treatment" options were probably made when the material was originally cast. Now, with proper cleaning, drying, and surface preparation, there are more "treatments" reasonably available. This successful surfacing of concrete can usually only be accomplished with one of several epoxy flooring systems (not paint) or with a specialty group of materials that harden and seal the exposed concrete surface. If you have diagnosed one problem as deteriorated concrete surfaces and you are in a facility that can't vacate a total space for an extended period of time for cleaning, drying, and surface preparation, do not consider the application of any remedial surfacing material. It will not be successful. Your only "treatment" is keeping the surface, cracks, and voids really clean until you can replace this portion of your facility.

Because being able to maintain durability and to effectively clean all surfaces is a companion requirement in a new facility, bare concrete should be finished only by the specialty group of products specifically designed to create an impervious, long-lasting, and very hard surface. If aesthetics dictate a more "finished" appearance, the choice of materials becomes more limited and the cost of the material increases dramatically: this stuff is not cheap! The best of these systems are the poured epoxy systems, which provide excellent surfacing, an integral curb at the wall, fill most cracks, and are very costly. Other 100 percent solids epoxy options are available from some reputable manufacturers but need careful and thorough evaluation. Sheet vinyl, with heat-welded seams and a chemically welded vinyl base, is a less costly and often an acceptable alternative, but only when the concrete floor can be determined to be a dry material. Someone may suggest commercial vinyl tile squares and, while they may be an alternative in the administrative area, they are not in animal care areas. Each square has a crack between it and the next tile. The only way to fill these cracks is with heavy periodic waxing and polishing. At the meeting of the floor and the wall, usually a vinyl strip is glued to the wall and butts the floor: Another open joint exists there that cannot be filled. If that joint is at the top of the base, against the wall, there is an open seam that water may penetrate during cleaning and it will not dry or drain.

If you can vacate a total space, the resurfacing of deteriorated concrete floors is a possibility. Do your research and consider only tested materials that have worked well for others. Do not rely on the advice of salespeople or local vendors. You need a specialist to guide you through all the alternatives as you select the appropriate material. Then, all surfaces must be clean, dry, and properly prepared before applying the selected finish. This is absolutely gospel for both new and renovated surfaces, and there are no compromises or alternatives. Reflect that "clean" is relatively easy for shelter staff personnel: They're good at "clean", but "dry" is something else. The specialist will perform tests on the floor to determine when it is acceptably dry. Preparation of the concrete usually requires acid etching, grinding, shot-blasting, and/or patching before a system of 100 percent solids epoxies can be properly applied. Systems vary widely; some require several layers of skilled application, and others are more parochial. Again, do not paint concrete floors.

Walls

The walls of animal-holding areas in most shelters are usually built of concrete blocks and are probably coated with one of the many epoxy-type paints, in just as many different chemical compounds, that have been available for several decades. Frequently, the concrete blocks weren't properly prepared for the surface material, the paint didn't really fill all the cavities in the surface, and many start deteriorating almost immediately after curing. There are likely broken edges and holes in the existing concrete blocks. The painted surface may have been improperly applied, leaving air holes that have filled with dirt and other small debris particles, giving bacteria and viruses a possible "safe harbor." In and around these concrete block walls, you may find other locations of severe deterioration. Metal doors and frames may be severely rusted; windows may have deteriorated frames. You may find patches, holes, and other long forgotten parts of some additions, renovations, or other questionable conditions in areas that were repainted with some material that was not compatible with the original finish. If your facility has these symptoms, accurately locate them and then find the cause. Then, you can prepare a plan to treat the problem. The rusted doors and frames were probably not galvanized, and oxidation in the high humidity environment was impossible to prevent. The treatment is difficult, but possible. First, the rusted frames must be surgically removed from the wall by an experienced contractor. Then, a "retrofit" galvanized hollow-metal frame can be installed with a new hollow-metal galvanized door, but experience suggests the selection of materials that absolutely will not rust is a better alternative. Aluminum store-front materials work well and are economical. If the wall surfaces need repainting, the same criteria apply as to resurfacing floors: They must be clean, dry, and prepared for the selected surfacing material. The preparation again will require the consultation of a specialist. Many materials have different preparation system requirements. All manufacturers publish very detailed procedures and usually have local field representatives that will visit the facility and make detailed recommendations for the specific location for use in the final installation with the local contractor. Don't compromise their recommendations because this is the only way to insure satisfactory and effective results.

Ceilings

Ceilings can reveal symptoms that are strong diagnostic tools. Hopefully your ceilings are "suspended acoustic systems", that is, they are the typical rectangular panels set in a suspended grid frame. There's a wealth of diagnostic information hiding up there. Get a very bright light, climb up on a ladder, remove a portion of the ceiling, and investigate the hidden area up in the cavity above. Is it dirty? Where is the insulation? Is there evidence that the ductwork and equipment have been tampered with? Have additions of TV cable, computer wiring, and so forth, destroyed a portion of the hidden walls or insulation? Below the ceiling, are the air grills in the ceiling dirty? Are the lighting fixtures clean? Are they making loud buzzing sounds? All of these are symptoms of neglect and deterioration, and they need to be attention items in a good preventive maintenance plan.

What makes an effective shelter ceiling? If it's a high humidity space, which is usually the case in areas without the recommended frequent total air change, do not use any components that could rust, and only use ceiling panels that will resist moisture. Suspended ceiling grids are available with aluminum and plastic components only and they work very well. The aluminum system is very satisfactory and less expensive than the plastic alternatives. Considering that in an animal-holding space, and most particularly a kennel, the ceiling is about the only area where there is some potential for sound mitigation; don't waste this opportunity. With concrete floors, concrete block walls, and all other surfaces adjacent being hard and reflective, the space above you must perform any acoustic treatment. Higher is better and angles, in the ceiling plane which provide more surface area, are better than flat horizontal surfaces.

ENVIRONMENT

Sound

Sound is a form of energy and, as with any form of energy, it can be changed but not eliminated. When a dog barks, the sound energy strikes all available surfaces in a line-of-sight direction. A small portion of this energy is transmitted through the material; some hopefully is absorbed, but most is reflected to strike another surface with similar results. Effective modulation might be an intermediate acoustic plane in a sound-proof room, where angled surfaces give the opportunity for more acoustic surface area with reduced reflectivity. The higher wall surfaces, above the height of the top of the doors, are also acoustic treatment opportunities and should be used effectively. Soft panels that can be hung in the space are often marketed as solutions, however, they offer minimal sound mitigation, require cleaning, and block lighting. They are relatively expensive for the minimal mitigation effect they achieve. When considering an acoustic modulating surface reflect on the fact that all acoustic materials are rated by their NRC (noise reduction coefficient, which is the arithmetic average of the absorption coefficients at 250, 500, 1000, and 2000 Hz). This represents the frequency of sound that may be expected in a normal administrative environment. Because a dog's bark is between 250 and 4000 Hz (a very wide range), we can only consider the NRC as a general guide for material selection in animal care facilities. Pick a product with a high NCR, but study its density and moisture resistance as well, because the dirty, sagging, ceiling tile is usually the result of a budget material that was inappropriately selected.

Some ceiling systems offer perforated plates backed with very effective sound reduction materials. Some are very resistant to surface damage, some are extremely good sound reducers but are very light and easily damaged, and the costs vary accordingly. Do not lose the only sound absorption opportunity by only allowing hard surfaces for the ceilings, and continuously consider that the only way that sound can be managed is by either *insulation* or *isolation*. Pick an appropriate one that will work in your shelter building.

Lighting

In the animal-holding area, where are the existing light fixtures? Do they effectively light the animals or were they installed to light the path of people travel? Do they offer switching alternatives so that a bright space, without shadows, is available to the morning cleaning crew, but a lower level of lighting is available during the hours when the public is in the spaces? Lighting fixtures are relatively easy to move, so do not discount this opportunity. If they are fluorescent, consider the color rendition of the selected tube. Typical fluorescent tubes are available in standard "warm" and "cool" white. The warm emphasizes the red side of the color spectrum; the cool emphasizes the blue. Also available are tubes that come very close to "natural" coloration. Consider the location and tell your maintenance team to have all three types available. Install the natural color in the triage, exam rooms, and any other spaces that need natural light. Study the color scheme of the building, and then consider which side of the color spectrum would best enhance that color scheme. Sometimes it's tempting to mix the tubes in a fixture; resist the impulse. It's not very effective.

Contemporary lighting fixtures rarely use incandescent bulbs. Common in the past, these bulbs delivered much of their energy in the form of heat and not light. If you have a ceiling with small circular holes and an incandescent bulb up in a can, suggest replacing them with the new generation of compact fluorescent lamps. They'll last longer, they are much more energy efficient, and they create very little heat energy. Also, there will be appreciable savings in operational costs. Dramatic lighting effects are also available with many low-voltage lighting systems. Most of these utilize a version of the MR-16 lamp that was originally designed for 35mm slide projectors. Because of the very low voltage, these systems are easy to wire, and lamping is available in a variety of brightness levels and beam widths. Remember that the 12v transformer they use must be hidden somewhere; it can usually be above a ceiling or behind an access panel. Local fire and other codes demand usually lighted exit signs. Even the selection of an exit fixture with a low-voltage lamp can be a large long-term financial savings because these fixtures are always on and will, over time, consume a large amount of power.

Ventilation

The successful system, properly designed for an animal-holding facility, will provide at a minimum 10 air changes per hour in all animal spaces and effectively manage humidity levels. Be aware that there is a big difference between air "changes" and air "exchanges". Most commercial air systems only exchange most of the air in a building over and over, sharing air in all the spaces. These systems provide the vehicle for the transmission of many shelter diseases. If the air in your facility is recirculated by a typical commercial system, no "quick fix" exists to solve the problem. Consult a heating and ventilation specialist who can properly direct the selection of changes to your system, if possible, or to discuss the options available for new equipment.

You must consider the very critical role of filtering in the effective heating and ventilating (HVAC) system. In a typical commercial system, filters are usually located adjacent to the air-handling equipment to protect this portion of the equipment from the exchanged air that will be carrying contaminates from the building. The normal commercial installation provides minimal filter protection, because this is not often a major concern in the typical office or commercial environment. This is not so in an animal sheltering facility, where the air is heavily loaded with large and small particulates. While inexpensive systems are available that will provide 100 percent fresh supply air and discharge 100 percent of the exhaust air, they seldom include any engineered energy recovery modules. These systems end up being extremely expensive to operate, and the filtering of all air in animal spaces is still required to protect the equipment. If you have or are considering a replacement ventilation system that will operate with the recommended minimum of 10 true air "changes" an hour, have air conditioning, and provide heated air, you must consider adding modules that will provide heat exchange between supply and exhaust air. These "energy recovery units" transfer the heat/cooling energy from the 100 percent exhausted air to the 100 percent fresh incoming air with up to approximately 80 percent efficiency. No system can operate at a reasonable cost without these energy recovery units. Available in several configurations, they are usually a plate-type or a wheel-type system with four duct connections in the shape of an X, with the energy recovery plate or wheel at the center. When operating, exhaust air enters one corner of the X, passes through the wheel or wiping the plates, and transferring the heat or cooling energy to the incoming air that "wipes" the other side of the plate as it rotates into the path of the wheel for a similar exchange. These efficient modules will usually totally recover their initial costs in about three years. Consult with an HVAC specialist, not the local air conditioning salesperson, when considering such a system as regional climatic conditions affect the selection of the proper type of system.

Specialty filters are required to remove large-, small-, and micron-sized airborne contaminate particles in the building air stream. There are also other specialty filters available for other applications that include the removal of objectionable odors. Unfortunately, in an animal holding-environment, without several filtering locations, by the time the return air has reached the filters adjacent to the air-handling equipment, it has already severely contaminated the air distribution duct system. We need to first filter our returning (exhausting) air at the source (i.e., directly behind the return air grills in the animal holding spaces). Look around the rooms that hold animals in your facility. Are all the grills located only in the ceiling? Are some located close to floor level? Which are the dirtiest grills? Hold a piece of letter-type paper across the face of the grill. Is the air being pulled (the return air) or is it being pushed (the supply air)? How strong is the force of the flow? If the grill is a supply air grill (we'll continue to call it a grill, but it's called a diffuser in the industry if it's supplying air) and there is evidence of streaking dirt around it, it is probably only an indication of the wiping effect of the air flow and not dirty supply air. The return air grill will be different. Remove the grill and shine a flashlight into the ductwork. How dirty is it? Ask your HVAC contractor if a washable filter can be installed behind the grill and if the grill can be modified for relatively easy removal in order to access this washable filter. This is a very effective "treatment" application.

For example, in one project that we designed, the existing cat-holding room was to have air conditioning added to the existing heated air supply ducting. When the contractor inspected the existing ductwork above the ceiling, he reported to me that the job would be easier than he had originally thought, because the existing ductwork was already insulated. Surprised, I climbed into the ceiling space to check this ductwork. What the contractor had found was not commercial insulation but 20 years of accumulated cat hair!

Vendors are often anxious to sell high-efficiency particulate accumulators (HEPA) filtering, however, as a single stand-alone unit, it is relatively inexpensive, marginally effective, and requires the frequent replacement of expensive filters. Understand that these expensive filters are truly functioning at 100 percent efficiency the instant they are turned on. As they filter airborne contaminates, both large and small, they become progressively blocked until they relatively quickly reduce the air flow to the point that they become part of the problem instead of the solution. HEPA filtering does have its place, however, as a component of some central systems, but it is not a stand-alone piece of equipment. In such a central system, first a washable filter should be located just behind the return air grills in all the animal-holding spaces. These filters remove the gross contaminates, hair, and other large particles in the air stream. Next in the ducted air return system is a second filter location, which typically includes pleated fine polyester filters, often located adjacent to or in the air-handling equipment. These relatively inexpensive filters remove the smaller particles that pass through the initial washable filters. Following these filters are a series of high-efficiency filters that remove all but the micron-sized contaminates. This progressively sized air filtering may finally include HEPA filtering. All of this initial filtering is necessary, because the HEPA module is so efficient (removing particles from 99.97 percent to better than 99.99995 percent) that, unless well protected by gross filtering, they will collect all passing contaminates, and will easily and quickly clog. Being uncleanable, these very expensive modules must be then replaced.

Another option is the substitution of the HEPA filtering module with a component of ultra-violet (UV) radiation. UV units will not clog and will not degrade until the light source needs to be replaced. These light sources, when properly designed and located, effectively neutralize all virus and other small organic particulates; it's a component worth considering.

Ozone generation is also marketed as a defense mechanism in your air supply system. Unfortunately, this is a dangerous and potentially harmful alternative. The Environmental Protection Agency (EPA) has issued many warnings about the toxic effects of ozone, but vendors are still trying to sell these units to the uninformed. Ozone is an oxygen molecule with an errant additional atom of oxygen loosely attached. This atom can re-attach to other substances and alter the chemical makeup of that substance affecting its smell and other characteristics. Unfortunately, it can also attach to the respiratory system of staff members, as well as the animals' systems, complicating any existing chronic respiratory diseases. In addition, the invasion of this severe irritant can also compromise the individual's ability to fight other respiratory infections. As a potential hazard to shelter staff, as well as to the shelter animals, do not consider ozone generators anywhere in your shelter's HVAC system.

ANIMAL HOUSING

Canine

Canine holding options range from stacked cages to "real life" rooms and everything between. In the 1970s, the Humane Society of the United States (HSUS) published their landmark guide to shelter planning. It brought into focus "indoor-only" dog kenneling, which was relatively revolutionary in the days of the traditional inside-outside kennel. The basic idea was a back-to-back rectangular concrete block kennel space with a guillotine door in the rear wall to allow animal passage from one side to the other inside a kennel. Kennel drainage was an open floor drain located in one corner of each kennel. The gated fronts were swinging or sliding chain-link fence.

Kenneling problems occurred in the management of these kennels because the plan's success depended on only one side of the back-to-back kennel being used for a single animal. This gave the morning cleaning crew the opportunity to move the animal from one side the other, clean the dirty kennel, and maintain the animal without having to remove it from its kenneling location. In most of these locations, however, kennel crowding almost always lead to both sides of the kennel being used for animal holding, creating the need to remove the animal from the kennel for morning cleaning. Some other shelters opted to just wash down the kennel with the animal remaining in the space. A recent evolution of the inside-only concept provides an alternative kenneling design with alternative cleaning/holding possibilities. This adaptation sacrifices no holding kennels for cleaning, while retaining the ability to clean without removing the animal from the dedicated kennel.

Kennel materials range from the traditional painted concrete block to space-age plastic panels and proprietary systems. Local fence contractors are quick to provide seemingly budget installations that almost always quickly show their unsuitability. Always use specialty materials in the kennel area and relegate the local fence contractor to building the exterior exercise run enclosures.

Kennel drainage has also evolved from the open floor drain that quickly showed its unsuitability with accidents involving broken legs and some small animals lost into the sewerage piping system. The "open pipe" was an attempt to provide an alternative that did not require the picking up of feces, theorizing that with a pressure washing system, they could be washed into the open sewer. It didn't work well and most shelters have covered all drains and, if they didn't eliminate the pressure washer when it first broke, have dramatically "throttled-down" the pressure in the systems so that "aero-socialization" in the cleaning process didn't continue to transfer vaporized contaminates throughout the kennel space. This design also required that the plumbing "rough-in", performed very early in the construction process, be very accurate to locate these drains to be precisely in the corner of kennels that were not yet built. The chance for error was great and too often they were not properly placed, thus resulting in drains under walls or in other unworkable portions of the floors. Unless local construction codes dictate otherwise, floor drains now are almost always located in the open area of the front or rear of the kennel space, allowing easier construction locating, providing sloped floor construction to the drain, and then covering the drain with stainless-steel strainers on easily cleaned plastic piping.

The new generation of trench drains offer very workable alternatives to the traditional floor drain. Most kennel cleaning involves the use of squeegees to dry kennel surfaces, and they are difficult to steer into a floor drain. A trench drain, with a plastic or stainless steel grate, located immediately in front of the kennel gate provides easy squeegee movement to the drain, does not allow the draining transfer of sewage from kennel to kennel, and is easy to clean.

Regardless of the chosen system, the location of the drain must not allow open sewers, or the surface drainage of urine and washing of feces from kennel to kennel. The side walls of the kennel should be solid and high enough so the animals can't see each other or come into nose-to-nose contact. Most kennel component manufacturers also provide secure options for food and water bowls rather than allowing them to rattle around the kennel. Plan the kennel to provide space for chosen amenities such as resting benches, blankets, and toys. Some shelters are fortunate to have a variety of sizes for kenneling needs; others do not. In larger kennels, the opportunity to provide animals with companions has shown that they may adjust more quickly, be quieter, and present more normal behavior characteristics. Progressive training, as an animal "graduates" from holding kennels to adoption kennels, can reinforce the positive expectations of a potential adopter.

Feline

In the HSUS publication, mentioned previously, cat holding was suggested in wall-mounted stainless steel cages arranged in two ranks, with the bottom units about 18 inches above the floor, and the upper rank on top of the lower one. It was and still is a good plan, but for years shelters have continued to try to maximize the stacking of cat-holding cages, often trying configurations up to four rows high. Experience has shown that cages mounted very low were difficult to maintain and very awkward for public viewing. Cages above the two ranks were too high for maintenance, and cats were unable to be seen by most people. Shelters that installed these high units inevitably used them only for very expensive storage or they just sit empty.

Feline holding has evolved, allowing for many alternatives. Cat colony rooms and cages with connecting port holes, utilizing various levels, and the addition of transparent surfaces give the cats a welcome relief from the traditional stainless steel cage. Effective space planning allow cats to see general shelter activity, but protects them with specialty ventilation systems and provides shields from the public's poking fingers. Cat colony rooms are built to allow grouping of felines in a "family" environment, typically maintaining the "family" group without the introduction of any new animals until the entire population has been adopted or the last remaining cats are moved to other locations. If you are in an older shelter and are considering the use of a space not specifically designed as a colony room, exercise the diagnostic process to evaluate the space. Consider the existing surfaces: Can they be cleaned? Will the ventilation system provide the necessary air changes in the space? Are there accessible filters located behind accessible return air grills? Is the lighting compatible with the intended use? If these considerations can be satisfied, the space may be acceptable for a colony use. If not, you must then provide renovations that will satisfy the need and not compromise the program requirements.

Other Animals

The modern animal shelter may receive a wide variety of animals other than dogs and cats. Depending on the regional location and function of a particular shelter, the design may need to provide space for small mammals, birds, wildlife, or livestock. Some of the other chapters in this text will provide specific details on the types of housing required for these species. All of the previously discussed concerns about surfaces that are easy to clean will still apply. Several additional modifications will also be important to include. Small animals and birds will often require humidity and temperatures that are different from the balance of the facility. Separate controls may be needed for these rooms. In addition, it is helpful to provide electrical power strips part way up the walls because many small animals and reptiles will require heating pads and lights. Because these animals will often be kept in cages on tables or shelves, placing the electrical outlets 42 inches above floor level will eliminate the need to crawl under or behind the cages to plug in equipment.

REDUCING STRESS

The responsibility of all shelter personnel is the maintenance of the health, safety, welfare, and accessibility of the animals, the staff, and the public. This mission accountability must weigh in when deciding on the uncompromised final diagnosis and appropriate "treatment" for the facility. Often neglected, but a very important component of overall health, is the management of stress. Because the impact of stress is a staff issue as well as an animal consideration, the "building triage" must consider the factors that will reduce or increase stress for both the animal and human population. Whether renovating or designing a new facility, if the public and the staff functions can be positively separated one major stress contributing factor can be eliminated. The public has its zones of adoption, education, and related activities, and they do not need to become part of the problem as the staff routinely carries out daily activities.

For a shelter animal, there is almost nothing warm, friendly, or familiar about the space in which the animals must be housed. Consequently, a degree of stress is almost unavoidable in all shelter animals. The shelter has many different holding environments, however, they are often in the same room. The focused evaluation of all cages and kennels will assist the staff in making a guided selection of the best location for the different animals. Most animal behaviorists have noted that if an animal does not arrive at the shelter with a behavior problem, the chances are pretty good that it will acquire one or more while it is there. An example is in a typical kennel room where the first kennel is immediately adjacent to the typical closed solid entry door. If a stressed barker is located in this most stimulating location, the kennel will be constantly under barking siege. If a quieter animal is located here, the surprise factor that would normally stimulate barking may be reduced.

Every animal received in the sheltering environment will be subject to some degree of stress. This will affect the animal's health, behavioral characteristics, and the ability to effectively predict the animal's adoptability. Stress reduction, for the animals, can be affected by taking advantage of all the opportunities available to positively change the holding environment. Almost all dogs bark. Barking is loud and irritating, and when one dog barks, probably more will communicate in response. What can be done to reduce this cacophony? Kennels that face kennels contribute to increased barking. Animals placed face to face will "talk" more spontaneously than animals that cannot make eye contact. We've already noted what can realistically be done to "treat" a space acoustically, but effective early kennel planning can create even more dramatic changes. Because dogs are pack animals, they often

do better together when some kennel opportunities offer enough space for selected animals to be companioned. Then, with a planned program of basic obedience training and appropriate pre-adoption evaluation, the animal will be more well-adjusted, will more often display normal behavior characteristics, and will be quieter than animals in a single kennel. These animals will then be excellent adoption candidates. Planning for larger kennels (real-life or dog rooms) in renovations, additions, and/or new construction is usually the choice, however, because modifying the existing typical small individual kennel area is usually difficult and expensive.

While most issues of health maintenance for the animal population can probably be accomplished with extensive medical treatment, the alternative involving prevention as the best treatment may be most effective and efficient. Good space planning can effectively change the holding options and provide a health maintenance alternative for many shelter animals. While the dog that's just been surrendered with a continuous record of periodic veterinary health maintenance probably may be quickly placed in an adoption environment, the "road hard" stray will need isolated holding options. The cat that has outlived its little old lady companion is also probably a candidate for adoption. The feral cat brought in by the ACO requires a very different holding option. An appropriate location is one that is separate, quiet, and offers positive isolation from other shelter animals.

SPACE PLANNING

The subtleties of space planning must have high priority in the design process of all renovation and new building projects because they will contribute greatly to the delivery of a facility that provides an effective and efficient working environment. Some examples would include a plan for doors that provide for visual as well as environmental separation only where it is necessary. The door from a staff corridor to a kennel provides separation to usually isolate portions of the HVAC system and also to attempt to acoustically provide some isolation of internal noise. Visual separation is not necessary and even not desirable: It's usually there because it wasn't considered in the original planning process. An aluminum store front door, with a large glass area leading to a kennel, will provide acoustical separation, will not rust, and gives a staff member an advance visual check before entering a kennel. Is the light switch placed adjacent to this kennel door? Usually they are adjacent to the knob side of the door immediately on the inside of the room. Why? Because that's where they've always been. If, instead, the switch was placed on the outside of the door, a staff member could turn on the lights before entering the room. It's a subtle difference, but one that may be important when the big psychotic pit-bull, that broke through the kennel gate during the night, is waiting inside the kennel door to greet the first morning staff member into the room.

In space planning, the tendency is to attempt to put different activities in different rooms. Why? If it's an activity that needs an individual space (i.e., an exam room or an office that has full-time use and needs security), plan accordingly. Many other activities, however, will work better, part time, in large central spaces. Food prep is space demanding and requires generous movement to and from animal holding spaces, but it is concentrated in relatively short periods of the day. Washing and drying bowls, litter pans, and so on, is a similar activity. The laundry accumulates piles of dirty towels and blankets needing space for folding and storage. Local storage needs to supply the food preparation area, the stocking of carts for cleaning, and be a repository for inventory materials. All these activities may use the same aggregate space effectively when it is well planned.

Movement through the shelter can be a relatively easy or a stressful experience. Corridors are the building's "streets" and "intersections," and locations of high activity need special treatment. The "sight-lines" along these "streets" should avoid surprise intersections where accidents may frequently occur. Careful planning of the new or renovated facility will treat these "streets" much like a city, with a few wide "super-highways" and only limited access "roads." In effective space planning, all corridors and other nondedicated spaces make up the building's "grossing factor." Less space in the "streets" means more opportunity to add used dedicated spaces for the same total building area.

Consider the many opportunities needed to provide specific spaces for behavior modification. The characteristics of unacceptable behavior are well documented, and many training programs are available for staff, volunteers, and the adopting public.

The need for socialization of all dogs is well established, and while some dogs arrive ready for adoption, most are not. Many studies show that behavior problems are one of the most common reasons that an animal is surrendered to a shelter (Salman, et al., 1998). Taking advantage of all socialization opportunities is difficult to incorporate into many aspects of shelter life, but very necessary. The San Francisco SPCA has prepared "dog apartments" in their canine adoption setting. These rooms are complete with upholstered furniture and items of domestic decorations (i.e., tables, lamps, rugs, and so on), and usually include a playing TV. The potential adopter sees an animal in a domestic setting and is somewhat reassured that maybe this animal will fit into their home setting as well. While few shelters can afford the space, the furniture, and the time necessary to manage such a setting, alternatives are available.

Staff offices are ideal socialization opportunities. If these offices are provided with Dutch doors, the maintenance of staff duties and interference with animal socialization is minimized. Few special construction measures need to be taken because, even if the spaces are carpeted, they are usually small. Furthermore, if carpet replacement is periodically necessary, it is not expensive. Choose a tightly woven, level-loop material that is easily cleaned. Carpet tiles provide for easy replacement of portions of the carpet, and are available with antimicrobial modules at reasonable costs. Get-acquainted rooms need to be used by staff and volunteers for more than the few minutes of getting acquainted with potential adopters. These rooms are animal spaces and surfaces should be provided that can be easily and effectively cleaned but do not have a kennel atmosphere. Use rugs that can be washed, throws over a soft chair or loveseat, and windows looking to quiet activities. These items give an animal an opportunity to experience the alternative to the kennel, and these breaks from kennel life are much more effective with a staff or volunteer companion. In the daily routine, provide large exterior exercise enclosures. These should be built of concrete or other cleanable surfaces. In this environment, a selected group of dogs can be given the opportunity for exercise, socialization, and behavior evaluation with a skilled staff member. The better spaces are also relatively secluded and do not offer the general public casual visual exposure.

CONCLUSION

The "diagnosis" of the building, just as the animal, must also assign a degree of risk to the conclusion. Treatments are then assigned that are appropriate to these risk factors. Many shelters have conducted a thorough evaluation of their existing conditions. Through this evaluation, the shelters have reached the conclusion that only dramatic renovations or a new building would relieve their compounding problems and prepare them to adequately serve the health, safety, and accessibility requirements of the community that they serve. Then, the decision whether to try and renovate or to build new must be faced. Renovations may seem to be the more attractive option until carefully studied. Must the facility remain in full operation during the work? Is this reasonable? Is it possible? Is everyone aware that renovations are often more expensive than new construction? Now is the time to see the "specialist". Rely on the advice of these professionals before making a renovation decision.

Few sheltering operations are prepared for the new or renovation project, which might be normal to the commercial building market. Establish a building committee with members that have a business and/or construction background. Keep the committee small, with no more than three or four members. Then, interview several professional design candidates and select members based on experience, references, and trust. All successful construction projects are carefully planned and executed only by this type of team effort.

The selection of all shelter "treatments" must be made after considering the broad range of circumstances that may be experienced: Remember, "alternatives" not "compromises" because the selection decision on most shelter materials and equipment is permanent and not easily changed or renovated.

All shelters should proactively anticipate and prepare for problems, because the reaction to a crisis, when it occurs, is usually unsuccessful, inefficient, and very demanding of the staff. The shelter cannot prevent problems. It must provide the appropriate systems, space, and the appropriate staff actions to manage the "treatment" of them. With no one, easy "fix", the medical staff member is as professionally prepared with the ability to direct the "treatment" as anyone. A plan for all anticipated problems will provide the shelter with the ability to handle crisis intervention in all but the most unusual of situations.

REFERENCE

Salman, M. D., New, J. G., Scarlett, J. M., Kass, P. H., Ruch-Gallie, R. and Hetts, S. (1998) Human and animal factors related to the relinquishment of dogs and cats in 12 selected animal shelters in the United States. *Journal of Applied Animal Welfare Science* 13: 207–226.

6
Sanitation in the Animal Shelter

Nicholas Gilman

INTRODUCTION

There is an increasing effort on the part of animal shelters in the United States to keep animals for longer periods of time. This may in part be due to a stabilization of the number of incoming animals and an increase in the number of acceptable homes. It may be influenced by the trends established by "no-kill" shelters and by the incorporation of increasingly progressive adoption programs. It may have something to do with greater visibility of local animal shelters to their communities over the past few years. In any case, animals are staying longer in animal shelters.

This trend toward providing longer-term refuge for dogs and cats forces the shelters to give greater consideration to maintaining the health of the animals under their care. After all, keeping animals healthy in a shelter environment is difficult to manage for even short durations. To do so with a large shelter population and for longer time periods requires a strong health care program. One of the key elements of that program includes effective cleaning and disinfection regimens.

While it is expected that all animal shelters clean and disinfect their facilities on a regular basis, the advent of animal sanctuaries, shelters that focus solely on adoption programs, and humane organizations that choose to rehabilitate sick animals (as opposed to euthanasia) means that disinfection programs must be aggressive, well-executed, and take advantage of the best disinfectants, cleaning tools and techniques. Keeping animals with different health profiles in close proximity forces shelter administrators to accept nothing but the most strin-

gent protocols in the cleaning regimen if the organization expects to keep diseases at bay. While there are modern and effective disinfectants and cleaning tools, it is the animal care staff's attention to detail that will make a critical difference in the health of the shelter animals. In addition to staff awareness of principles of disease transmission and cleaning practices, volunteers and the public must also be made aware of the role they have to play in maintaining a healthy shelter environment.

For the purposes of this chapter, the four levels of cleaning an animal shelter will be as follows:

1. Physical Cleaning—This process is the removal of gross wastes and organic materials from the environment. Physical cleaning will not, in itself, kill pathogens but will remove some of the medium in which contagions can grow.
2. Sanitation—This process is the killing or removal of "the number of bacterial contaminants to a safe level" (Greene, 1998). Sanitation is usually accomplished through an application of a chemical, but it does not achieve the same level of kill as disinfection.
3. Disinfection—This process will kill most of the contaminants in a given area. With the exception of bacterial spores, disinfection will kill all the pathogens that can cause the onset of disease. However, it should be noted that true disinfection rarely is achieved in the animal shelter environment.
4. Sterilization—This process is the killing of all life forms at all levels, including bacterial spores. It is typically achieved through chemical or ther-

mal means. With the exception of surgical instruments put through an autoclave cycle, true sterilization does not occur at an animal shelter.

Although animal shelters have staff who are prepared to work hard and perhaps to a high level of attention to detail, and in spite of modern disinfectants, most shelters achieve little more than good cleaning or mild sanitation on a daily basis in their animal care areas. For example, most disinfectants used by animal care facilities require 10 minutes of contact time to achieve disinfection. However, the general practice in cat care rooms is to spray a disinfectant into a cage and to wipe the surface clean almost immediately. It is arguable whether this has any chemical effect whatsoever, much less to achieve true disinfection. The reality of shelter work is that attendants often do not have the time to allow disinfectant to sit for the full 10 minutes. Yet in the face of a disease outbreak, this overlooked step may be the critical one that was key to helping prevent or control the spread of the disease.

In dog runs, on the other hand, the disinfectant is often left on the kennel floors for the recommended 10 minutes. However, a shelter's flooring surfaces are often in poor condition or are porous, and thus retain organic matter that can harbor disease organisms. These conditions, which are common to shelters, will severely compromise the effectiveness of disinfectants. Again, we can assume that cleaning or sanitation has taken place, but it would be rare for true disinfection to take place in an animal shelter. This, by no means, should discourage the practice of using disinfectants to achieve cleaning or sanitization levels. The goal of the shelter staff should be to seek true disinfection through the utilization of techniques, chemicals and equipment that are appropriate for each shelter's unique set of circumstances.

Resource allocation is important in designing a sanitation protocol that will address the condition of the shelter, budget, labor force, characteristics of the shelter animal population and diseases commonly encountered in the shelter and surrounding areas. Even if such practices fail to achieve true disinfection, pathogens are reduced and the facility does not suffer from repellent odors.

Odors are more than a deterrent to good public relations. While the source of many odors may be microbial and not viral, the presence of odors indicates the presence of a medium in which noxious organisms and contagions can grow. Covering up the odor with masking sprays is not a solution. It should be generally accepted by the cleaning staff that odors are indicative of an unhealthy environment.

The importance of good physical cleaning of the shelter cannot be stressed enough. It is essential for maintaining a healthy and sanitary environment. A facility cannot be disinfected without being properly cleaned first due to the inability of most disinfectants to penetrate and kill disease organisms in organic debris. In addition, some of the organisms that cause serious health problems in shelter animals are highly resistant to disinfection, so their physical removal is critical to ensure the best possible opportunity for minimizing disease contamination and spread. Among some of the most resistant disease organisms are parvovirus, calici virus, ringworm spores, coccidia, and other protozoans. Without proper cleaning and disinfection, some of these contaminants can survive in the environment for months to even years.

THE ANIMAL SHELTER ENVIRONMENT

Unfortunately, not all animal shelters are designed to be easily cleaned. The materials, floors, drains, and air-handling systems should be designed to move contagions out of the environment as quickly as possible and to make cleaning uncomplicated, but this is not always the case. Furthermore, shelters that have dirt, grass, and gravel runs should be aware that these surfaces cannot be effectively disinfected. There are cleaning techniques that animal care attendants can use even in poorly designed shelters to keep disease rates down.

Creating a Healthier Shelter Environment

Some form of cleaning and disinfection must occur on a daily basis. If shelter staff time allows, twice daily cleaning and disinfection is preferable for shelters that are experiencing regular disease outbreaks or for shelters that have a very high turnover of animals. Animal care facilities that have stable and healthy populations and relatively low animal turnover rates, such as some sanctuaries, may decide to clean but not to disinfect quite as often to reduce stress levels from moving cats unnecessarily every day. There is no formula to determine the best system; most shelters will make the determination through trial and error.

According to Greene, hands are one of the most common animate means of fomite transmission of disease (Greene, 1998). Install hand sanitizers in all animal areas and encourage staff, visitors and volunteers to use them after handling each animal to minimize fomite disease transmission. Ensure that the contents of the hand sanitizers are effective against the types of contagions of concern. The Center for Disease Control (CDC) has a report on hand washing that includes information about hand sanitizers (www.cdc.gov). They can be very effective when hand washing is not practical or feasible. Place signs to politely inform the public and to remind the staff to use hand sanitizers after contact with each animal.

To further control fomite disease transmission, footbaths should be used whenever disease outbreaks occur. If the shelter regularly has disease problems, footbaths should be used on a regular basis. These footbaths should be changed in accordance to how often that room is accessed and the product being used. For example, bleach breaks down fairly rapidly in water, so bleach footbaths must be changed at least once a day. Instructions for use of Roccal® include daily changes and whenever the footbath solution appears soiled (www.cdfa.ca.gov). In addition, the efficacy of the disinfectant will be compromised if the surface area is too broad.

When removing an animal from its cage for any reason, even if the animal appears healthy, they should be returned to the same cage whenever possible to minimize disease spread. This is especially important when considering diseases that are resistant to disinfection such as parvo and ringworm. This practice will also reduce errors in cage cards not following the animal to its new quarters. Whenever temporary transport cages are used to house animals while cleaning their cages, they should be assigned to that animal for the duration of their stay when possible and disinfected after each use. If cardboard carriers are used, the animal may be sent home in that carrier, it can be used for a nonanimal purpose, or it should be discarded.

Remember that any and all surfaces that an animal comes into contact with are subject to cleaning and disinfection. This includes humane traps, transport cages, squeeze cages, restraint poles, medical instruments, muzzles, rope leads, collars, scales, exam tables, anesthesia equipment, and so on.

Staff charged with the cleaning of several animal housing areas should begin their work in the healthiest rooms and work towards quarters housing known contagious animals. In doing so, there is less chance of fomite disease transmission. Puppy and kitten areas should be cleaned and disinfected first, as they are most susceptible to diseases. The use of disposable aprons is recommended when several areas must be cleaned during a disease outbreak. In extreme situations, it may be necessary to remove and launder clothing before going into the areas with the most disease susceptible animals. Clothing, bedding, rags, and other reusable cloth materials should be laundered with soap and bleach in water temperatures above 160°F for 25 minutes to kill most infectious agents (Greene, 1998).

Disposable litter boxes and food dishes should be utilized if possible. If disposable litter boxes are not used, substitutes should be found for the more common plastic litter boxes that become scratched and damaged over time and are more difficult to properly disinfect. Fecal material containing corona and parvovirus, giardia cysts, coccidia, and a host of other disease organisms that are spread through the fecal oral route could easily be spread through contact with a dirty litter box.

Infestation of insects and rodents in the shelter can cause disease outbreaks, odors and, in rare cases, potential bite trauma. In order to keep rodents and insects from being attracted to an animal care area, remove all animal waste as soon as possible, remove all animal feed from floors, and keep a tight lid on feed bins and trash receptacles. Consider the use of a commercial rodent/insect control program, but be aware of potential dangers of poisons on shelter animals. If in doubt, contact the ASPCA Animal Poison Control Center (888-426-4435 [there is a charge for the telephone call] or www.appc.aspca.org) for information regarding product safety for use around animals.

One strong consideration for the shelter staff is strategies that keep the animal care areas as dry as possible. A wet environment is one in which contagions can more easily grow. In addition, odors that the public find objectionable are often aggravated by a wet or moist kennel area. Finally, dogs that are wet are not only sources of odor, but are compromised in their ability to stay warm. This, in turn, may contribute to an increase in disease rates.

In order to keep the shelter as dry as possible, consider the following:

1. Squeegee standing fluids into drains. Do not allow a floor to simply air dry as this will allow moisture to evaporate into the kennel environment. This, in turn, will contribute to dank, musty odors.
2. Whenever the animal care areas are wet, turn up the air-exchange rate and increase the airflow in the wet areas. Air exchange rates should be 10 times an hour or higher during this time.
3. The use of mops is discouraged for the general cleaning of animal care areas as they tend to harbor odors and may be a prime vector for the spread of disease. If used, however, do not allow damp mop heads to remain in the animal care areas. Remove them to a separate area to dry. Empty and disinfect mop buckets as soon as mopping is finished.
4. Do not spray or mop areas with plain water unless it is followed by the application of disinfectant. Emphasize to the cleaning staff that a freshly mopped or hosed-down floor is only a medium for the growth of contagions unless it is followed by the application of disinfectant.
5. Repair leaking sinks, pipes, and hoses as soon as possible.

Controlling Air Flow to Minimize Disease

Adequate ventilation is essential to help maintain the health of populations of animals in enclosed spaces. Although it may seem that air handling and filtration is part of shelter design or building maintenance, because it has a profound effect on the health of the animals, veterinarians should be aware of the limitations of and problems with the ventilation system. By adjusting the rate of airflow (15 times per hour or more), the temperature, and the humidity, the animal care staff will be able to complement a good disinfection program. The HVAC (heating, ventilation and air-conditioning) system designed for a shelter should allow for adjustments depending upon the season, the disease rate, the

weather, and other factors that can influence the health of the animals.

For example, the animal care staff should be able to regulate the air-handling system in three ways: temperature, air exchange rate, and ratio of recirculated air versus fresh air.

Monitoring Temperature

The Animal Welfare Act standards permit ambient temperatures in facilities housing dogs and cats to go as high as 85°F or as low as 45°F for no longer than four hours (Animal Welfare Act, http://www.nal.usda.gov/awic/index.html). However, shelters that are tempted to use these standards should be aware that these minimums were not developed for, nor do they apply to, animal shelters. These extremes of temperature contribute to increasing stress levels and should be avoided. The temperature in animal care areas should be kept at a reasonable level for the animals, staff, and public, typically, 68°F to 75°F. Areas that are used as recovery rooms for surgical patients or treatment areas should be monitored to avoid extreme temperature fluctuations as this also contributes to stress. However, remember that if the cages or runs are near the floor that the temperature may be a few degrees colder at that level than five or six feet above floor level. Also different rooms in different areas of the building may be at a different temperature so the entire building should be checked to make certain all the animals are comfortable. Therefore, when selecting a temperature for an animal care room, consider which animals are there (e.g., post-op recovery, puppies, sick animals) and which building area will best suit their needs if different areas typically reach different temperatures.

Monitoring Air Exchange

By exhausting air from an animal care room and bringing in fresh or filtered (recycled) air, one achieves air exchange. The rate of exchange should be about 15 times an hour. This rate is predicated by the air volume that the fans in the air-handling system are able to move. The dangers of a low air exchange rate are a potential increase in disease transmission (as animals have a greater chance of breathing in the contagions exhaled by sick animals), an increase in odors, and a longer time for the room to dry after the cleaning and disinfection process. Inlet vents should be near the ceiling to bring in fresh or filtered air, and outlets should be near the floor to properly recirculate the air to where disease organisms are generally found (Greene, 1998).

Controlling the Recirculation Ratio

Animal care staff should be able to control to what degree the incoming air is recycled versus fresh air. The advantage of recycled air is lower utility bills: Recycled air is already the temperature selected for a given room. Recycled air can also be filtered with the following filters to reduce contagions, particulates, and odors:

- Ultra-violet light (for reducing air-borne diseases, especially in cat care rooms)
- Charcoal (for odor control only)
- Electro-static (disease and particulate control)
- Negative ion (disease control)
- HEPA (High Efficiency Particulate Accumulator, for disease and particulate control)

The advantage that fresh air has over recycled air is that it brings in air that has not been exposed to animals and, presumably, contagions. However, a 100-percent fresh air system would be expensive, as all of the incoming air would have to be heated or cooled to the desired room temperature.

Most systems include a combination of recycled and fresh air. Animal care staff should be able to control the proportion of recycled to fresh air based on the needs of the animals and the agency. For example, if there were an outbreak of air-borne disease in the facility, the staff would be well advised to increase the amount of fresh air and reduce the recycled air. On the other hand, if the shelter population were relatively healthy, using recycled air would help keep utility bills down.

One aspect of both air handling and general cleaning and disinfection that is typically overlooked is the regular and thorough cleaning of air ducts and registers. Too often, these items are not cleaned on a regular basis and become a dangerous breeding ground for contagions. Just as with cages or surgical instruments, the grates covering the air ducts and registers should be removed and thoroughly cleaned and disinfected. In critical areas such as isolation, quarantine, and clinical areas, the cleaning and disinfection of air duct grates should be done weekly. If there is a disease outbreak, all

grates should be cleaned and disinfected more often than normal. Changing of the air filters should also be increased during times of disease outbreak.

Some considerations for controlling air in the shelter are as follows:

1. Keep the fans and air circulation system on until the facility is dry.
2. Cats should not be exposed to temperatures that cause them to pant for long periods. Panting may indicate unacceptable stress levels. If necessary, mechanically cool the air. If possible, keep temperatures below 80°F for animal housing areas.
3. High humidity levels can allow mold spores to grow and is in general a good breeding ground for contagions. If your HVAC system allows it, adjust it to remove as much humidity as possible.
4. As noted previously, some HVAC systems allow for adjustments in the ratio of fresh air to recycled air. Adjust this ratio to fit the needs of the animals. Ensure that recycled air is never exhausted from the isolation or quarantine areas to the adoption wards.
5. Some shelters take advantage of automatic "air fresheners" that periodically spray a scented aerosol from a wall-mounted unit. The problem with such units is that they mask odors of which animal care staff should be aware. The best use of such units is to have them in operation during the hours when open to the public. Otherwise, simply masking odors makes it difficult to catch unpleasant, but important, odors–such as the distinctive odor of an ear infection or bloody diarrhea.

SANITIZING CAT CAGES

Maintaining the health of the cat population within an animal shelter is a commonly voiced concern for many shelter administrators. Although feline upper respiratory diseases can be spread through airborne contamination, cats isolated to their own cages are infected by sick cats housed in the same room primarily through fomite contamination. Aerosol transmission is not the most prominent way respiratory viruses are spread (Gaskell and Dawson, 1998). Sneeze droplets may travel a distance up to 4 to 5 feet (Greene, 1998), but freshly aerosolized particles with microbes greater than 5μm in diameter rarely remain airborne for more than one minute (Greene, 1998, p. 673). Instead, fomite transmission is probably the most common way diseases are spread in shelters. The most common animate fomites are hands, while clothing, litter boxes, water bowls, toys, and medical or cleaning equipment is only a partial list of inanimate fomites. A good disinfection regimen is not enough for keeping cats healthy in a shelter environment; a preventative health program that includes constant disease surveillance, vaccinations and deworming, prompt isolation of sick cats in a separate area (not just an area in a room with healthy animals), and quarantine areas for cats that still need time to manifest symptoms of incubating diseases is also necessary.

Daily Cleaning Steps for Cat Care Areas

Although individuals may develop their own styles of cleaning, some basic steps need to be followed, in order, for effective cleaning:

1. Turn up ceiling fans and air circulation as high as possible. This will circulate air and cause faster drying. However, during times of disease outbreak, do not use the ceiling fans. In such times, fans only serve to potentially spread the disease.
2. Relocate the cat to a suitable location (see the following section).
3. Remove all bowls, toys, newspaper, cage liners, litter pans, and so on, and either throw away (if disposable) or empty and wash if not disposable. All nondisposable litter boxes, water bowls, food dishes, and so on, should be disinfected daily and whenever a new animal is placed in a cage.
4. Launder all bedding and clothes in bleach, hot water, and soap.
5. Sweep out the cage with a brush or hand broom.
6. Scrape out the soiled areas with a nonabrasive scouring pad.
7. If possible, use hot water and soap and/or detergent to thoroughly clean cage and cage gates. Physical cleaning must be completed thoroughly in order for the chemical disinfection process to work properly. The entire cage must be cleaned including sides, doors, front, bars, and so on. The temptation to just clean the floor should be avoided.
8. Spray cage with appropriate disinfectant (see section on disinfectants), including cage floor, walls, ceiling, and doors.
9. Leave disinfectant on for as long as possible (10 minutes to achieve disinfection). If rinsing is called for by the manufacturer's instructions, be sure to do so thoroughly. Wipe out and dry cage with paper towels. Do not re-use paper towels on the next cage. If using rags to wipe out cages, change rags for each cage. Ensure all surfaces have been wiped clean of disinfectant, as many disinfectants can be irritating to the sensitive skin and paws of cats. Thorough rinsing will also get rid of any odors from the disinfectant that may be an irritant to the eyes and mucus membranes. Place clean cage liner, bowls, and litter pan in cage to complete the process.

Tools:
- Hand-held sprayer
- Paper towels
- Nylon spatula or nonabrasive scraper
- Hand-held brush

Placing Cats during Cleaning Process

With the one exception perhaps being handling fractious feral cats, it is not acceptable to leave a cat in its cage during cleaning and disinfecting. Therefore, the animal care staff must be familiar with some of the techniques used to complete the cage cleaning process, while keeping the cats safe from direct exposure to the disinfectants. According to the American Humane Association's Shelter Operations School (American Humane, 2001), there are a number of ways to keep cats clear of the cleaning process. Each has its own distinct advantages and disadvantages:

1. The Pass-the-Cat Method—In this method, one cage in each cat room is left empty and clean at all times. The daily cleaning process begins by moving a cat (typically a cat in an adjoining cage) to the empty cage. The now-empty cage can now be worked on. When clean, a new cat can be placed in this cage while its old cage is sanitized. In this manner, the animal care attendant can continue around the room, always having a place for a new cat. The disadvantages to this system is that every cat gets moved to a new cage in every cleaning session; while the cages have been sanitized, the cats are nevertheless exposed to an environment only recently occupied by another, perhaps sick, cat. In addition, there is a danger that cage cards will not be moved along with the cat. On the whole, this

method works best in rooms where the cat population is known to be healthy, such as an adoption room.

2. The Summer Home Method—The summer home method relies on each cat having its own, typically adjacent, temporary cage in which to be put while its regular cage is cleaned. This type of system is best used when the caging in the room has been designed for such a system. For example, there are caging systems in which a large cat cage has a much smaller cage immediately above or below it expressly for the temporary placement of the cat. The advantages are that no cat will be exposed to any but its own cage(s). The disadvantages are that for each cat there must be a corresponding empty cage, and most shelters do not have the luxury of always having that many empty cages.

3. The Cat-in-the-Box Method—This method puts the cat into an airline-type crate or cat carrier for the duration of the cleaning process. Unless the carrier can be assigned to the same cat throughout its stay, the disadvantages are that each carrier must be sanitized between cats. Disposable cardboard carriers could be used, then discarded or used for transporting animals other than cats (assuming that other animals may not pick up cat diseases as readily as other cats). This system is best used only when there is no other option is simply available for the animal care staff; it uses up valuable time and resources.

4. The Hold-the-Cat Method—This system uses a second person to hold the cat while the cage is cleaned. The strong advantages of such a system is that the person holding the cat can take its temperature, inspect the animal for physical ailments, socialize with it, and so on. Although it will not prevent fomite transmission, this may be the most professional method of those listed here; the ability to record a cat's temperature on a daily basis allows animal care staff to get a jump on incubating diseases and to remove cats with elevated temperatures before sneezing–and therefore, transmission–sets in. In other words, while this labor-intensive method requires two people, it satisfies much more than the cleaning process. It collects data about the cat that will help to reduce the spread of disease in the facility. It is best used in quarantine and adoption areas where early detection of diseases is impor-

tant, and works only with cats that are easily handled.

5. The Dry Cleaning Method—The dry cleaning method keeps the cat in the cage being cleaned. Instead of applying disinfectant, the cage is simply straightened up, bowls removed and cleaned, and litter pan sifted or replaced. The logic to such a method is that because no cat is moved into any environment other than its own, that disinfection is not necessary. This system works best when the shelter is critically shorthanded or when the completion of cleaning in a short amount of time is important. The disadvantages lie in unkempt cages (it's difficult to clean and straighten around the cat) and in less odor control.

None of these methods is perfect. However, it is possible to take maximum advantage of these methods by applying them in different parts of the shelter. For example, the pass-the-cat method works well in the adoption areas, while the two-person method works best in quarantine areas. The summer home method can work well in the isolation and clinic areas. The dry cleaning method works best when shelters are shorthanded and in places where appearance is less critical and where the cat population in that room is healthy. Each shelter can apply different methods as they see fit. In all cases, the critical issue of keeping cats from direct contact with disinfectants is acknowledged.

SANITIZING DOG HOUSING

The cleaning process for dogs in a shelter environment can be both a disease preventative and a disease vector. Some of the most virulent diseases that affect canines are borne by fecal matter. In many cases, the transmission of fecal matter from one kennel run to another by the animal care attendant allows for contamination to take place. The soles of the attendant's shoes, the hose that is dragged into and out of each run, the inappropriate placement of trench drains, and especially the "pooper scooper," become the vector by which feces migrates from dog to dog. Therefore, it is again the attention to detail that will, in large part, determine the spread of viral diseases such as parvo and corona, which are both viruses that are spread by contact with infected feces. A strong sanitization program for the dog care areas will, assuming that attention is paid to detail, reduce contagions and odors. As with cats and other animals, it is important that the facility allow for the segregation of healthy animals from sick ones if the spread of disease is to be kept to a minimum.

Daily Cleaning Steps for Dog Care Areas

Effective cleaning of canine areas requires the following steps, in the order listed:

1. Increase the airflow into the dog care areas. If possible, increase the ratio of fresh air to recycled air. One hundred percent fresh air should be used when possible.
2. Move dogs out of the area to be sanitized. If the dogs are in the runs, move them all to one side. Dog "runs" are defined as being comprised of two dog pens that are separated by a guillotine-type door that can be operated by an animal care attendant from the outside of the run. (These are excellent for housing aggressive animals because it minimizes handling them.) If the dogs are in cages or pens, move them individually out of the area to be cleaned. Dog "pens" are defined as areas in which the animal has enough room to establish a sleeping area and a soiling area. Dog "cages" are large enough to accept a dog but not to allow for separate sleeping and soiling. Do not apply chemical disinfectants where an animal can come into direct contact with it.
3. Remove all toys, blankets, bowls, resting platforms or mats, and any other objects not attached to the enclosure. Launder, clean, disinfect, or dispose of the objects as appropriate.
4. Launder all bedding and clothes in bleach, hot water, and soap.
5. Scoop up fecal matter and dispose of it properly. Do not use a spray of water to flush fecal matter down the drain. By spraying water at organic matter, it can splash into other areas. Always use a scoop to pick up and remove fecal matter. Care should be taken to keep the migration of fecal matter to a minimum in the scooping process. Physical cleaning must be completed thoroughly in order for the chemical disinfection process to work properly.
6. Spray enclosure with water to rinse away urine, hair, feed, remaining fecal matter, and so forth. The optimal water temperature to kill most organisms is 82°C or 180°F (Greene, 1998).

Always start rinsing at the top of the enclosure. This allows the draining water to gently rinse away the organic matter without splashing it. Use a scrub brush to remove any stubborn soiled areas. Rinse all surfaces thoroughly, including the bottoms of the attached dog beds.

7. Spray the enclosure with the appropriate disinfectant. Ensure that the proper dilution ratio is used. Apply disinfectant with a hand-held proportionator or a system that supplies working-strength disinfectant prediluted through a hose. Do not apply disinfectant by throwing a bucket of working strength solution onto the floor. The entire cage must be cleaned, including its sides, doors, front, bars, and so on. The temptation to just clean the floor should be avoided.
8. Allow the disinfectant to sit on the surface for as long as the manufacturer recommends, or at least 10 minutes. Rinse if appropriate.
9. Squeegee the standing disinfectant away.
10. Return clean water and feed bowls, toys, blankets, and so on.
11. When the surface of the kennel floor is dry, allow the dog to return to its run, cage, or pen.

Tools

- High quality hose
- Hand-held, gardening-type, hose-end sprayer
- Hand-held proportionator
- Scrub brush
- Fecal scoop
- Squeegee
- Bucket lined with garbage bag for feces

Cleaning Kennel Aisles

The use of mops in most animal care areas is not recommended. Mopping dirty floors simply tends to move the contaminants around in an increasingly septic "soup." Additionally, mops are a major source of odor wherever they are housed as they are rarely cleaned and disinfected themselves. Instead, consider scrubbing floors with a hard bristle brush and a working strength disinfectant. Rinse with fresh disinfectant and remove the standing liquid with a squeegee. Administrative space and other nonanimal care areas may be cleaned with mops and pails.

If dogs are placed in a communal holding area while their individual cages are cleaned, staff should be aware that this is a source of contamination and disease spread. As a regular course of business, this may be unavoidable, but should be re-evaluated whenever there is a disease outbreak.

DISINFECTANTS

While it is possible for an animal care facility to try to prevent the spread of disease by rinsing, scrubbing, scooping, and closely monitoring the conditions of the animals, it is not possible to kill contagions–and therefore sanitize, disinfect, or sterilize–unless chemical or thermal methods are used. Because thermal cleaning is not always practical in animal shelters, chemical disinfection is the remaining choice for routine purposes. In all cases, however, physical cleaning **must** precede disinfection in order to be effective. Even the most modern disinfectants cannot work effectively in the presence of organic matter. Although some products combine detergent and disinfectant actions in one bottle, taking each step separately is more likely to be effective. If the staff does not allow the disinfectant to sit for 10 minutes, by cleaning effectively they will have at least reduced the particle load. If the two steps are combined into one and poorly performed, neither cleaning nor disinfection will have been achieved.

Methods

Some shelters use steam cleaners as a daily cleaning procedure or in response to a disease outbreak. Steam heat is a type of thermal cleaning, and is the most effective means of achieving sterility. When all else fails, it will kill coccidia and Toxoplasmosis cysts (Greene, 1998). As a practical matter, thermal or steam cleaning seems to work better for small, specific applications such as the sterilization of surgical tools or for a specific stainless steel cage. The reasons commonly cited for not using steam cleaners for daily disinfection include the following:

• Steam cleaning (at a disinfection level) requires more staff time than that of chemical disinfection. In order for steam to kill pathogens at a disinfection level, the steam must be directed at a given spot for at least a few seconds. In contrast, chemicals can be applied to a broad area in those same few seconds. The chemical can then be simply left to complete the disinfection. Steam must

be applied by an attendant until disinfection is achieved.
• Steam increases the amount of water introduced into the shelter, contributing to a wet and/or humid environment.
• Steam is better suited for spot disinfection than for large surface areas.
• The entire area should be evacuated for effective steam disinfecting rather than just removing animals from individual cages. However, there may not be another empty space in the shelter to place several animals at once while waiting until the area is dry.

In cases of intractable disease outbreaks, steam cleaning utilizing a heavy-duty commercial-grade machine remains one of the most effective means of disinfecting a facility, especially if depopulation and other methods have already been attempted.

The advantages to modern chemical disinfectants and the techniques and tools used to apply them are as follows:

1. Easily purchased and delivered in bulk
2. Consistent performance if manufacturers' directions are followed
3. Easily applied to surfaces with only a few specialized tools
4. Quick-acting (10-minute surface time)
5. Broad effectiveness against bacteria, viruses, and microbes
6. Relatively inexpensive at working strength

The following are the disadvantages of disinfectants used in animal shelters:

1. May be harmful to skin and nasal tissues for both humans and animals.
2. Tend not to work well at temperatures below 50°F.
3. Can be corrosive to metals.
4. May or may not be effective against non-enveloped.
5. Requires OSHA (Occupational Safety and Health Administration) compliance.
6. May not work well in the presence of organic materials.

Although there are many different types of disinfectants used in hospitals and for industrial purposes, there are only two types of disinfectants in common use in animal shelters today. Sodium hypochlorite (bleach) and quaternary ammonium compounds are in use in the vast majority of animal shelters in the United States. Although phenol-based disinfectants were common in shelters in years past, its toxic properties, especially to cats makes it contraindicated for animal care purposes. Calcium hypochlorite, though more commonly used as a swimming pool cleaner, also may be used as a shelter disinfectant, although its use as such is still limited. Iodine-based disinfectants have also been tried in shelters, but are now no longer in common use. There are, in fact, much more effective disinfectants available to kill pathogens of all types, but their application, cost, availability, or composition make them impractical as animal shelter disinfectants. (For a more comprehensive discussion of disinfectants, see Greene's discussion on "Environmental Factors in Infectious Disease" in *Infectious Diseases of the Dog and Cat,* 1998.)

Chemical Disinfectants

For almost all of the animal shelters in the United States, the common choices of disinfectants for routine sanitizing are sodium hypochlorite and quaternary ammonium compounds. However, while most animal shelters tend to use one or the other disinfectant, or opt for a rotation of the two disinfectants, there seems to be a long list of concerns that shelters have expressed over the relative pros and cons of each. Whichever product is selected, shelter staff should wear gloves, protective eyewear, and boots when applying chemicals, and they should follow all appropriate OSHA and common sense safety precautions.

SODIUM HYPOCHLORITE
Sodium hypochlorite (or bleach) used at a dilution ratio of 1:32 is an effective disinfectant against most of the pathogens that affect animals in shelters. It is easy to procure, relatively inexpensive, and is straightforward to apply. However, due to its corrosive properties, it tends to cause metal fixtures in animals shelters to rust, is less effective in the presence of organic material, tends to irritate nasal tissues of cats if not properly diluted, and can cause sores if exposed to skin. The most commonly cited reason for the use of bleach in animal shelters is that it is known to kill parvovirus.

The following are recommendations for using sodium hypochlorite:

• Follow all manufacturer recommendations for storage and application and observe the information on the material safety data sheet (MSDS). In addition, follow all OSHA recommendations about the use and handling of bleach.
• Apply bleach through a proportionating unit (either a hand-held system or part of a system built into the facility) at a dilution ratio of 1:32. Do not apply by splashing on surfaces with a bucket. When dealing with an outbreak of feline ringworm, use bleach at a dilution ratio of 1:10. In such a circumstance, use special care to thoroughly rinse and dry the cage before returning the cat to its cage
• Allow solution to sit on the surface for at least 10 minutes.
• Rinse surface with water to reduce likelihood of chemical burns.
• Squeegee away leftover liquid.
• Keep sodium hypochlorite containers, both concentrate and working strength, stoppered when not drawing liquid. Open bleach containers present both a hazard and the likelihood that the strength of the mixture will be reduced though escaping gas.
• Store sodium hypochlorite in a well-ventilated area away from metal electronic circuit boxes or other metallic fixtures. Protect it from light and prepare fresh daily.
• Do not mix bleach with anything but water. Mixing with other chemical such as ammonia can release fumes that are harmful to both animals and people.

QUATERNARY AMMONIUM COMPOUNDS
Quaternary ammonium (commonly known as "quats", brand names Roccal®, Spectrasol®, Parvo-sol™, A33) compounds are the subject of some controversy over whether they do, or do not, kill nonenveloped (such as parvo). Federal government testing has certified some quats to be an effective agent against parvo in the most recent of testing protocols, yet many in the general veterinary community remains unconvinced. Textbook references, conference presentations on shelter medicine, and a number of recent studies have indicated that quaternary ammonium compounds are not effective

against certain viruses (Greene, 1998; Eleraky Pot-gieter, and Kennedy, 2002; Kennedy, Mellon, Cald-well, et al., 1995). Parvo is the virus of most concern due to its resistance to disinfection, its ability to survive for long periods in the environment, and its deadly effects on shelter animals in particular. However, because of quaternary ammonium's other strengths (e.g., less corrosive and more effective at killing Giardia cysts) many U.S. shelters continue to use quats for disinfection. Nevertheless, in the event of an outbreak of viral infections in the shelter, it is recommended that a known virucidal such as sodium hypochlorite be used for disinfection until the outbreak is controlled.

Quats can come in different dilution ratios including 1:32, 1:64, 1:128, and 1:256. The best overall ratio for shelter use may be 1:64 as more concentrated ratios will not have the strong odor-control agents. Most quats have no, or very little, caustic properties that will cause rusting or corrosion of metal gates, cages, and fittings in the shelter. However, just as with other disinfectants, they must be used according to the material safety data (MSDS) sheet.

Final Recommendations for the Use of Chemical Disinfectants

The ultimate choice of a shelter disinfectant is made more difficult because of the confusing and contra-dictory information–both scientific and anec-dotal–about the efficacy of commonly available disinfectants. Shelters are encouraged to use what works best for them. No scientific test exactly replicates real-life conditions. Some shelters achieve excellent results using quats while scorning bleach, while many other health care professionals are of the strong opinion that bleach is the best product to use when diluted and applied properly. Ultimately, a disinfectant must work for the shelter in which it is to be used. Shelter administrators are also encouraged to gather as much data as they can from their animal care technicians on how well they perceive the disinfectant to work. Much of their opinions will be corrupted by whether or not they like the smell of the disinfectant, how easy it is to dispense or to dilute, and so forth. However, these impressions also should carry weight, as the more the technicians like the disinfectant and are convinced of its efficacy, the more they will enthusiastically and faithfully use the product. The technicians can also

provide anecdotal information on how healthy the animals seem to be under the effect of different disinfectants.

In order to introduce a more scientific approach to what has typically been an informal and anec-dotal process, shelter veterinarians are encouraged to do the following:

- Maintain complete records on disease outbreaks, including the type of disease and date of manifestations of the symptoms.
- Record the results, if measurable, of the disinfectant action on the disease with which is being dealt.
- Direct the response of the cleaning staff in times of disease outbreak. This may include mandating the switch from quaternary ammonium compounds to sodium hypochlorites when parvovirus outbreaks occur.
- Cleaning protocols and practice may be two different things. A cleaning staff sometimes develops "shortcuts" that to them seem harmless, but which result in an increase in disease transmission. Monitor the staff periodically to ensure compliance with the established cleaning and disinfection protocols.

Finally, each shelter might employ several disinfectants for use at different times or in different places. Because quaternary ammoniums are good at controlling odors, they might be used prior to opening in the morning. They would also be the best choice if giardia cysts were detected in shelter animal stools. Sodium hypochlorite might be used following an outbreak of a nonenveloped virus or in areas where corrosion or odor-control are not vital. Another method might be to rotate the products on a daily or weekly basis. What remains important, however, is that such decisions are made not on personal whims or on cost-control alone, but on how the disinfectant controls disease and odor.

CONCLUSION

Veterinarians play a key part in providing guidance to the shelter when designing an effective sanitation program. When disease outbreaks occur, the sanitation protocol should be carefully scrutinized and changed if necessary to reflect the properties of the causative disease agent and to break or control its modes of transmission. There is no one method of cleaning and disinfecting that will work all the time for every shelter in every situation. Management must be prepared to tailor their methods to utilize their resources to their best advantage. Attention should also be paid to the development of newer, more effective disinfectants that are being made available. Two products that should be watched for are the alcides and potassium peroxymonosulfate. Alcides are a new form of sodium hypochlorite that are reportedly less corrosive to metal, work better in the presence of organic materials, and have a broad spectrum of activity and low toxicity. The solution is effective for 14 days. It is more expensive than bleach and less readily available. Potassium peroxymonosulfate (Virkon S®, Trifectant) is another newer disinfectant that has been reported found to be virucidal (Eleraky, Potgieter, and Kennedy, 2002), fungicidal, and bactericidal, less irritating to mucus membranes, less corrosive to metal than bleach, and less likely to be inactivated by organic material. It has instructions for use on carpets, which would give it a definite advantage over bleach when disinfecting households. Effective cleaning and disinfecting are essential to minimize disease transmission under all circumstances, but if the shelter is unable to implement a strong veteri-nary health care program, has a poor ventilation system, or is unable to effectively isolate all sick animals from healthy ones, proper sanitation becomes even more critical. Finally, a clean facility is a more pleasant place for both the staff and visi-tors.

REFERENCES

American Humane Shelter Operations Guides, 2001. American Humane Association, Englewood, CO.

Animal Welfare Act, http://www.nal.usda.gov/awic/index.html, Title 9, Chapter 1, Part 3, Subpart A, Sections 3.2 and 3.3.

Eleraky, N. Z., Potgieter, L. N. D., and Kennedy, M. May/June 2002. Virucidal efficacy of four new dis-infectants. *Journal of the American Animal Hospital Association* 38:231–234.

Gaskell, R., and Dawson, S. 1998. Feline Respiratory Disease in *Infectious Diseases of the Dog and Cat* edited by Craig E. Greene, WB Saunders, Philadel-phia, PA.

Greene, C. E., ed. 1998. Environmental Factors in Infectious Disease. *Infectious Diseases of the Dog and Cat*. Philadelphia, PA: W.B Saunders.

Kennedy, M. A., Mellon, V. S., Caldwell, G., et al. 1995. Virucidal efficacy of the newer quaternary ammonium compounds. *Journal of the American Animal Hospital Association* 31: 254–258.

7

Nutritional Challenges for Shelter Animals

Linda P. Case and George C. Fahey, Jr.

INTRODUCTION

Along with proper health care and clean housing, the nutritional needs and feeding of shelter animals is an important component of shelter care. Proper nutrition is frequently overlooked because of the mistaken notion that the nutrition of animals being held for short periods is inconsequential to either the individual animal or the overall well being of all the shelter animals. Poor nutrition, especially in animals whose health is already compromised may contribute to increased disease susceptibility and disease spread. Shelters typically receive dogs and cats of various ages, reproductive status, and health and body conditions. Many shelters have established foster programs and are responsible for the care and feeding of neonatal puppies and kittens, as well as gestating and lactating females. Animals in conditions of severe malnourishment through morbidly obese will also be shelter residents. This chapter provides information regarding the basic nutritional needs of dogs and cats, the selection of the appropriate foods, and feeding management for all stages of life and body conditions. Specific information that will aid shelter staff and veterinarians in the care and feeding of shelter dogs and cats also is included. Feeding options in the shelter require balancing the nutritional and medical needs of the animals, and the financial and staffing resources available for implementation. The decision-making process should include the expertise of veterinarians and other qualified staff and consultants to ensure that all animals are receiving the proper amount and quality of nutrients based on species, age, and medical condition. Because edu-

cation is an important role of shelters in communities, the final portion of this chapter provides basic feeding management tips for educating new adopters regarding the proper feeding of their animal companion.

DIETARY REQUIREMENTS OF DOGS AND CATS: SIMILARITIES AND DIFFERENCES

Important Nutrient Requirement References for Dogs and Cats

The pivotal references supplying information about the nutrients needed by dogs and cats are the National Research Council (NRC) publications (NRC, 1985 for dogs; NRC, 1986 for cats). These publications summarize current information regarding canine and feline nutrient requirements, how they were determined, and the factors affecting them. Many advancements in companion animal nutrition occurred in the 14- to 15-year period since these documents were first published. Therefore, in 2003, a new NRC text titled *Nutrient Requirements of Dogs and Cats* was published. In this volume, an updated evaluation of the nutrient requirements of each species is presented along with information dealing with their digestive physiology, food intake and factors affecting intake, feeding management, physical activity and its effects on nutrient requirements, diet formulation and feed processing, and unique food constituents (those having nutritive value and those added to diets for reasons other than providing nutritive value). This volume is much more comprehensive than any of the previously published NRC documents dealing with dog and cat nutrition, and will serve as a valuable reference for all persons interested in companion animal science including those involved with shelter animals.

Another excellent source of information on nutrients important to dogs and cats is the Association of American Feed Control Officials (AAFCO) publication (AAFCO, 2002). Canine and feline nutrition expert subcommittees were named by the AAFCO Pet Food Committee and charged with establishing practical nutrient profiles for dog and cat foods based on commonly used ingredients. These established profiles are the "AAFCO Dog Food Nutrient Profiles" and the "AAFCO Cat Food Nutrient Profiles" as the terms are applied in AAFCO pet food regulations referring to nutritional adequacy. The profiles were designed to establish practical minimum and maximum nutrient concentrations for dog and cats foods formulated from nonpurified ingredients that are commonly included in dog and cat foods. The AAFCO subcommittees built the profiles starting with the NRC requirements with modifications based on the known effects of ingredients and processing and the potential for lower digestibility of some ingredients. Recommendations on nutrient source are made based on findings of low bioavailability. The AAFCO Dog and Cat Food Nutrient Profiles and the AAFCO Feeding Protocols are the only AAFCO-recognized methods for substantiating the nutritional adequacy of "complete and balanced" pet foods. Minimum, and some maximum, nutrient concentrations were established in these Profiles for maintenance, growth, and reproduction (gestation/lactation). Maximum nutrient concentrations also were established for nutrients for which the potential for overuse or toxicosis was a concern.

When specific issues related to nutrient requirements of dogs and cats emerge, shelter personnel are referred to the previously cited publications for authoritative information on the topic. They are readily available from the locations listed in the References section of this chapter.

Nutritional Idiosyncrasies of the Cat

Both the dog and the cat belong to the class, Mammalia and the order, Carnivora. However, the dog belongs to the Canoidea super family and the cat to the Feloidea super family (Case et al., 2000). The cat is a strict carnivore, whereas the dog is an omnivore. Thus, it would be expected that nutrient requirements and nutritional management programs pertaining to each species would be different. The nutritional idiosyncrasies of the cat may be divided into those that are of practical importance and those of academic interest. The former category includes requirements for higher concentrations of dietary protein, for the amino acid, taurine, for arachidonic acid, and for preformed Vitamin A. The latter category includes unique features of glucose and energy metabolism by the cat, its sensitivity to arginine deficiency, and the inability of the cat to convert tryptophan to niacin (Case et al., 2000). As a strict carnivore, the cat cannot obtain all of its essential nutrients from plants and, therefore, requires consumption of animal products to meet certain nutrient requirements. This is important; some caretakers (and shelter staff) believe (incorrectly) that cats may be fed similarly to dogs. The nutritional idiosyncrasies of the cat result in more stringent dietary requirements than those of the dog. Shelter personnel responsible for feeding kittens and cats need to be aware of the unique features of cats and ensure that they are provided with diets that have been specifically formulated for cats. Both NRC and AAFCO consider the uniqueness of the cat when publishing requirement and nutrient profile recommendations, respectively. Likewise, pet food manufacturers prepare diets for cats that account for their unique nutritional needs.

Feeding Approaches (Dog versus Cat)

Early feeding experiences can influence dietary choices made by dogs and cats. Exposure to specific dietary flavors and textures early in life can enhance preferences later in life. Kuo (1967) showed that puppies fed a single, uniquely flavored diet for six months would not eat novel foods, whereas puppies fed a mixed diet would eat any new food presented to them. Cats who become accustomed to one particular flavor will often not accept foods with different flavors whereas if the diet is varied, they seldom select only one type of diet or one particular flavor. The palatability and novelty of a particular food, as well as hunger intensity and presence of stress, are important factors affecting the acceptance and choice of particular foods at particular times.

Dogs should be offered fresh food at least once daily. Most adult dogs are capable of consuming their daily energy needs in a single meal. However, growing dogs and gestating/lactating bitches usually require at least two meals per day. Multiple daily feedings are preferable in shelter settings because they help alleviate boredom, facilitate staff interactions with animals, and reduce the risk of gastric dilatation/volvulus in susceptible breeds. On the other hand, free-choice feeding may result in excess consumption and weight gain in some animals (especially dogs), and can increase the risk of developmental bone disease in growing large and giant breed dogs (NRC, 2003).

Texture and moisture content of the food are important considerations when feeding cats (NRC, 2003). Many cats will select a moist diet (meat or canned food) over a dry pelleted or expanded diet. However, some cats that have been fed a dry commercial diet for long periods will select this type of diet. Unique features of cat feeding behavior include the lack of stimulation of food intake by sugar, the negative effects of short-chain fatty acids (alone or in the triglyceride form) on food intake, and the aversion by the cat to bitter tastes. Cats prefer small meals provided frequently throughout the day and night. Dry food offered free choice is the most practical means of feeding. Fresh food should be offered daily to prevent spoilage that would hinder normal consumption. Cats who are malnourished, stressed, or underweight may benefit from free-choice feeding with dry food, plus one or two additional small meals of canned food.

LIFE STAGE NUTRITION

Shelters are responsible for housing and feeding companion animals that can range significantly in size, body condition, health, and age. An appreciation of the energy and nutrient needs of companion animals during different life stages is important for their optimal care and feeding.

Feeding Adult Dogs and Cats

Adult dogs and cats that are not reproducing are said to be in a state of maintenance. This category includes the majority of animal companions found in the United States today. In shelter settings, many owner-relinquished pets are young or middle-aged adults, and may range from severely malnourished

to morbidly obese. A primary nutritional goal for feeding these animals is to attain (or maintain) optimal body condition and weight, and to promote health and longevity. If at all possible, adult dogs and cats at shelters should be fed a high-quality food that has been formulated for either maintenance or all life stages, and has been proven to be nutritionally adequate through AAFCO feeding trials. Dogs are best maintained feeding 2–3 portion-controlled meals each day. Either canned or dry food or a combination of the two can be fed. The choice between dry or canned needs to consider the factors of cost, convenience, and palatability, among other things. Today, there are a wide variety of both types of food available, and feeding a poor quality dry food, while certainly convenient and cost effective, may not be in the best interests of the animal's health. Similarly, feeding canned foods can be the best choice of food for stressed animals, those not eating well, or have dental problems that preclude a dry diet. Poor quality foods, regardless of type, can cause diarrhea or loose stools and compromise the health of the dog. Animals who are underweight or who have stopped eating may benefit from feeding a canned diet during the first few days of their stay. For adults who are overweight, daily food intake should be monitored for the first few days, and the amount of food that is offered should be gradually reduced to achieve a moderate rate of weight loss. Because even overweight animals will stop eating in response to stress, it is recommended that food intake be monitored for several days without restricting intake. Once the dog or cat is eating reliably, the amount that is fed can be adjusted. This is especially important for overweight adult cats that are at increased risk of developing hepatic lipidosis if they refuse to eat for an extended period.

Neonates

It is not uncommon for shelters to receive entire litters of newborn kittens and puppies, with or without the mother. In normal circumstances, preweaning mortality estimates for puppies and kittens have been estimated to be as high as 40 percent, with the vast majority of deaths occurring during the neonatal period (Hoskins, 1995). In shelter settings, mortality rates may be even higher. Proper nutritional support during this time period is critical for preventing neonatal illness and mortality. One of the first concerns with neonates at shelters is whether or not they received colostrum during the first 48 hours of life. In dogs and cats, the major proportion of passive immunity is acquired via colostrum, and so neonates who have not received colostrum will be immunologically compromised. In addition to its immunological benefits, colostrum provides essential nutritional benefits and contributes significantly to the postnatal circulating blood volume (Lepine, 1997). Because the period during which the newborn's gastrointestinal tract is permeable to the intact immunoglobulins of colostrum is very short (~ 48 hours), it is vitally important that newborns receive adequate colostrum as soon after birth as possible.

Healthy puppies and kittens born to a well-nourished mother require only their mother's milk until they are about four weeks of age. However, in shelter settings, supplementing neonates with commercial milk replacer is often necessary if the mother is underweight or in poor health. When puppies and kittens are four weeks old, semisolid food should be introduced, as the mother's milk is no longer nutritionally adequate to support normal development after this age. A commercial food made specifically for weaning puppies or kittens can be used, or a thick gruel can be made by mixing a small amount of warm water with commercial puppy or kitten food. Cow's milk should never be used to make the gruel because it has higher lactose content than bitch's and queen's milk and may cause diarrhea. Similarly, puppies and kittens should not be fed a homemade "weaning formula" unless the formula has been shown to simulate the nutrient profile of natural bitch's or queen's milk.

The semisolid food should be provided in a shallow dish, and puppies and kittens should be allowed access to fresh food several times per day. The food should be removed after 15 to 20 minutes. By five weeks of age, most puppies and kittens are readily consuming semisolid food, and by six weeks of age, they are able to chew and consume dry food. Nutritional weaning is usually complete by six weeks of age, although many bitches and queens will continue to allow their young to nurse until they are eight weeks or even older. Weaning studies indicate that puppies will continue to suckle at seven weeks of age even when offered free access to solid food (Malm and Jensen, 1996). The psychological and emotional benefits of suckling may be as important as the nutritional benefits in puppies that are older than five weeks of age. For this reason, complete weaning (behavioral weaning) should not be instituted until puppies and kittens are at least seven to eight weeks of age.

Orphans

An orphan is any young animal that does not have access to the milk or care of the mother. Circumstances that may render young puppies and kittens orphans at animal shelters or in foster homes include the death of the dam, an inability to locate or capture the mother, or illness or malnourishment of the mother. Orphaned animals must be kept in a warm, draft-free, and clean environment. The best possible nutrition for newborn animals comes from their dam, so foster mothering is the best solution for orphaned newborns. Shelters with active foster care programs may be capable of "doubling up" litters to allow natural fostering. This is usually more practical in cats than in dogs because of the seasonal breeding cycle of the domestic cat. When cross-fostering is used, it is imperative that all foster mothers are prescreened for infectious diseases and that sanitation protocols are strictly followed to prevent cross-contamination among newborns (see Chapter 21 on foster care). When a foster mother of the same species is not available, nutrition must be provided through a well-formulated milk replacer. The milk replacer nourishes the puppies and kittens for the first few weeks of life, until their digestive and metabolic functions develop to the point at which solid food can be introduced. A number of commercially produced canine and feline milk replacers are available. Most of these products are composed of cow's milk that has been modified to closely match the nutrient profiles of bitch's and queen's milk (Lepine et al., 1998; Kelley et al., 1998). Compared with cow's milk, the milk from bitches and queens contains a larger proportion of calories from fat and protein and a lower proportion from lactose. Evaporated cow's milk is occasionally recommended for raising orphans because it has a level of protein, fat, calcium, and phosphorus that is similar to bitch's milk. However, the lactose content of evaporated milk is still much too high, and for this reason it should not be used.

During the first few weeks, the food intake of neonatal puppies and kittens is largely limited by stomach volume. A general rule of thumb is to limit each feeding for newborn puppies to 10 to 20 milliliters of milk. Newborn kittens are able to handle approximately one third to one half of this amount. The concentration of the formula is extremely important. The milk replacer should be prepared exactly according to directions, and new formula should be prepared daily. If the concentration of the formula is too low (diluted formula), more feedings per day will be necessary to meet the neonate's needs. In this case, the intake of excess fluid can adversely affect water balance and may stress the immature kidneys. Conversely, if the energy density of the formula is too high, severe digestive upsets and diarrhea may occur. Orphans should be weighed daily to ensure that they are receiving enough nourishment to support normal weight increases. General rules of thumb during the first three weeks of life are increases of 10 percent Body Weight (BW)/day for puppies and 10–15 g/day for kittens (Daristotle et al., 2002).

If the concentration of the formula is correct, neonates that are bottle-fed are able to self-regulate their formula intake. Feeding orphans four to five times per day is usually practical, with feedings spaced at even time intervals. This schedule is often reasonable for human caretakers, and it also allows the neonates to obtain their needed hours of uninterrupted sleep. Orphans can be fed either with a small animal-nursing bottle or through a stomach tube. When bottle-fed, orphans will usually reject the bottle when their stomachs are full. However, the correct volume of formula should still be estimated and measured for each feeding. Because neonates who are tube-fed cannot self-regulate intake, formula volume must always be carefully measured to avoid over- or under-feeding.

Growth (Adolescence to Adult)

Kittens and puppies are usually fully weaned by the time they are seven to nine weeks old. Shelters receive recently weaned kittens and puppies (often entire litters), and also accept a substantial proportion of adolescents (especially dogs). Proper feeding and nutrition are essential during the first six to 12 months because dogs and cats are rapidly growing and developing. In dogs, the rate of growth and the age that they reach maturity is dependent upon breed and adult size. Large and giant breeds attain mature size when they are between 12 and 18

months of age, while small and toy breeds reach adult size at a younger age, usually between seven and 12 months (Allard et al., 1988).

The enormous amount of growth and development that occurs during a relatively short period of time translates to high-energy requirements in growing dogs and cats. From weaning until about six months of age, the energy needs of growing puppies are approximately twice those of an adult dog of the same weight. After six months of age, energy requirements begin to decrease as the rate of growth declines. A general guideline suggests that a young dog's energy intake should be approximately two times maintenance until 40 percent of adult weight has been reached. At this point, intake should be decreased to approximately 1.6 times maintenance, and further decreased to 1.2 times maintenance when the dog has reached 80 percent of adult size (Daristotle et al., 2002). Energy requirements for growing cats are estimated to be 200 to 250 kcal/kg BW for the month after weaning, and slowly decline to 90 to 100 kcal/kg by adolescence (six to nine months). Active adult cats require about 60 to 70 kcal/kg BW (Case et al., 2000).

The type of food that is fed is an important consideration for growing dogs and cats living in shelters. Because growing animals need to consume higher food quantities, the diet's digestibility and energy density are important considerations. Puppies and kittens have less digestive capacity, smaller mouths, and smaller and fewer teeth than adults. As a result, they are limited in the amount of food that can be consumed and digested in a single meal. If the diet is poorly digestible or has low energy and nutrient density, a larger quantity must be consumed. In this situation, the limits of the stomach may be reached before adequate nutrients and energy have been consumed. Excess consumption of food also can cause intermittent diarrhea, which is often exacerbated by the stress of a kennel environment. The long-term result can be compromised growth and impaired muscle and skeletal development. Therefore, young animals in shelters ultimately benefit from eating high quality commercial pet foods rather than the more economical generic or private label brands.

If at all possible, growing dogs and cats in shelters should be fed high quality commercial foods that are guaranteed to be nutritionally adequate for growth or for all stages of life, proven by the use of AAFCO feeding trials. They should be fed amounts of food that will support normal muscle and skeletal development and a typical rate of growth for their species and size. Although it may be tempting to over-feed shelter animals (especially puppies and kittens who are underweight), feeding growing dogs and cats to attain a "plump" body condition should be avoided. Providing too many calories early in life can lead to increased numbers of fat cells and may predispose the animal to obesity later in life. In addition, it is known that feeding dogs, especially large and giant breeds, for rapid growth is incompatible with normal skeletal development and can contribute to the development of a number of skeletal disorders (Lepine, 1998).

While some shelters may find it easier and possibly less costly to simply feed an adult maintenance food rather than a growth diet to young animals, adult maintenance foods (for both dogs and cats) are not specifically formulated for growth and their nutrients are not balanced with energy to meet the needs of growing animals. For example, because a growing puppy requires up to twice the amount of energy per day as an adult of the same weight, a puppy will need to consume a larger volume of an adult food to meet energy needs. This may result in the inadvertent consumption of excess amounts of other nutrients (such as calcium). If very large volumes of food are fed to meet the puppy's energy needs, this also can lead to digestive upsets, gastric discomfort, or diarrhea. It is therefore best to feed highly digestible growth diets in which the nutrient content has been thoroughly evaluated, and which has an energy and nutrient density formulated to meet the requirements of growing dogs and cats. Puppies and kittens under six months of age should be fed premeasured food three to four times a day.

Pregnant and Lactating Females

Pregnancy and lactation are periods of high physiological stress for female dogs and cats. Increased energy and nutrients are needed for fetal growth during gestation and for milk production during lactation. Because many of the pregnant dogs and cats who arrive at animal shelters are malnourished and in poor health, providing optimal nutrition to them attains an even greater importance. Pregnant queens and bitches should be fed highly digestible, nutrient-dense foods because this type of food is capable of supplying the extra energy and nutrients need during reproduction without necessitating excess volume consumption. The amount of food provided should be gradually increased, starting during the second (cats) or sixth (dogs) week of gestation and continued until parturition. At the end of gestation, the female should be receiving approximately 25 to 50 percent more food than her normal maintenance needs. Because most cats adapt well to free-choice feeding, this is often the best way to provide the pregnant queen with adequate nutrition during pregnancy. Free-choice feeding also is appropriate for underweight dogs or dogs not eating well. In all cases, weight gain should be monitored closely to prevent excessive weight gain during pregnancy.

After parturition, the mother should be provided with fresh water and food. Most females will begin eating within 24 hours of giving birth. If necessary, the mother's appetite can be stimulated by moistening her food with warm water or switching to canned food. This also ensures that adequate fluid is consumed, which is essential for normal milk production. During lactation, energy and water are the two nutrients of greatest concern. Ample energy intake allows sufficient milk production and prevents drastic weight loss from occurring. Adequate water intake is necessary for the production of a sufficient volume of milk. The nutritional demands of lactation are influenced by the mother's nutritional status and weight at the time of birth and the size of her litter. Females who have large litters or who are malnourished are at greatest risk for excessive weight loss. In these cases, supplemental feeding of puppies or kittens with milk replacer can help to offset the mother's energy loss, especially during peak lactation.

Depending on the size of the litter, female dogs and cats require up to two to three times normal maintenance energy needs during lactation. A general guideline is to feed one and one half times maintenance during the first week of lactation, two times maintenance during the second week, and two and one half to three times maintenance during the third to fourth week of lactation. Many mothers do best if simply allowed free access to their food throughout this period. After the fourth week, the amount of mother's milk that is consumed by the puppies and kittens will decrease as their solid food intake gradually increases. This will translate into a gradual reduction in milk production and reduced energy needs of the mother. By the time that the kittens and puppies are of weaning age, the dam's food consumption should be less than 50 percent above her normal maintenance needs.

Special Concerns for Older Animals

Improvements in the control of infectious diseases and in the nutrition of dogs and cats have resulted in a gradual increase in the average life span of companion animals. Unfortunately, shelters also experience this trend and receive older and geriatric animals that may require extra care and attention in terms of optimal feeding and nutrition. A primary physiological change that occurs with aging in most animals, and which directly affects nutrition and feeding, is a decline in resting metabolic rate. This is caused by a natural age-associated decrease in lean body tissue and by the voluntary reduction in activity. Together, these changes may result in a 20 to 40 percent decline in daily energy requirements. While this decline appears to be consistent among dogs, the aging cat has been shown to be rather unique. Unlike dogs, as cats age, lean body mass does not decrease appreciably, and cats vary enormously in age-related changes in voluntary activity. As a result, many older cats do not show the expected age-associated reduction in their daily energy requirement. In addition to reduced energy needs, older animals are subject to increased incidence of disease and stress and are, therefore, especially vulnerable in a shelter environment.

Older animals may have reduced abilities to efficiently digest and absorb dietary nutrients. Again, there are some differences between dogs and cats. While older dogs that are otherwise healthy usually show no change in their ability to efficiently digest and utilize dietary nutrients, the digestive efficiency of cats declines slightly in cats with age, and the nutrient that is most affected is dietary fat (Anantharaman-Barr et al., 1991). Older cats seem to easily compensate for this decreased digestive efficiency by slightly increasing the amount of food that they consume. If cats are meal-fed, however, it is important that shelter personnel consider that older cats (but not older dogs) may actually need slightly more food each day than young adult cats of the same weight. Finally, the presence of chronic disease can present an additional nutritional challenge to shelters caring for geriatric animals. This is especially important when assessing pet health.

Health problems that are more common in older animals than in young adults include chronic renal disease, diabetes mellitus, constipation, and neoplastic disease (cancer). Dietary changes often can be helpful in relieving symptoms or slowing the progression of some of these diseases.

Caloric intake and body weight should be carefully monitored in older animals in shelters to ensure adequate intake of calories and nutrients. Commercial pet foods marketed for geriatric dogs and cats tend to fall into one of two categories: those that contain slightly reduced fat content and a decreased caloric density (compared with a maintenance food), and those that are calorie- and nutrient-dense and are formulated for older animals who are experiencing a loss of body weight or a chronic disease. Appropriate senior diets should be selected by shelter staff, based upon an individual animal's energy needs, health, and weight status. In all cases, foods for older animals should contain high quality ingredients, especially highly digestible protein.

SELECTION OF FOODS BY SHELTER MANAGEMENT

Types of Food Available

Commercial dog and cat foods generally fall into three major categories: dry, canned, and semimoist. Dry-expanded pet foods are dominant in the pet food marketplace. They contain between 10 and 12 percent moisture, a feature important for proper shelf life, and are formulated using many categories of ingredients. Dry dog foods are marketed as meals, pellets, kibbles, or extruded products, but the majority of dry cat foods are processed by extrusion cooking. Cats have fewer premolars and molars than dogs, so food particles must be produced in a size and shape suitable for incising rather than grinding. Extrusion processing is well suited for accomplishing this. Most of the dry pet food sold today is extrusion processed, which means that most of its starch has been gelatinized. This cooking process greatly improves starch digestion (NRC, 2003).

Semimoist pet foods contain between 25 and 35 percent moisture. They are prepared similarly to dry-expanded foods. Shelf-life stability is obtained by controlling water activity, which may be predicted and controlled through the use of humectants added to the food. These foods contain many of the same ingredients as dry-expanded foods, but they often contain meat or meat byproduct slurries that are incorporated prior to or during extrusion. Semi-moist cat foods often contain a variety of ingredients to include meats, animal byproduct meals, fish products, grains, soy products, fats and oils, and vitamin and mineral supplements. Semimoist dog foods are prepared using similar ingredients but often are shaped into a size convenient for feeding or packaged to simulate meat chunks. All semimoist foods must be packaged in low moisture diffusion packaging to prevent moisture loss and changes in water activity (NRC, 2003).

A third category of extrusion-processed pet food is soft-expanded food. These products are similar to semimoist in that they often contain a relatively high level of meat byproducts and often have higher levels of fats than dry-expanded foods. Ingredients used are more like those found in semimoist foods and include humectants to control water activity. Moisture concentrations range from 27 to 32 percent.

Baked pet foods are prepared in various stylized shapes (e.g., bones) to attract buyers. They are produced using traditional means of dough formation, shape cutting or stamping, and oven baking. They contain over 50 percent cereal flours and have limited capacity to incorporate wet meat byproducts or slurries, and thus contain only three to six percent crude fat. Most baked products marketed today are dog biscuits and treats.

Many of the same ingredients are used in canned pet foods as are used in their dry-expanded and semimoist counterparts. Canned pet foods contain 74 to 78 percent moisture and, thus, have much higher concentrations of fresh or frozen meat, poultry, or fish. A meat-based formula may contain from 25 to 75 percent meat or meat byproducts. Foods with the higher concentrations of meat are generally designated as "dinners". Many canned pet foods may contain a significant concentration of textured vegetable protein (soy or wheat gluten) that is essentially a meat analog and has a structure that mimics the appearance of meat. These products have all but replaced earlier fortified "all meat" formulas because of reduced formula costs and, more importantly, because of improved nutrient profiles possible with meat/texturized vegetable protein combinations. While designed to be fed alone as a complete and balanced diet, canned foods are commonly used as supplements to improve acceptability of dry foods (NRC, 2003).

Homemade diets are popular with a small sector of the pet owner population. If a homemade diet is used, it is critical that the diet is formulated to be complete and balanced for either dogs or cats. In most cases, homemade recipes have not been thoroughly tested for nutritional adequacy. Conversely, homemade diets can provide adequate nutrition to dogs and cats, provided that a properly formulated recipe is used, the correct ingredients are included, and the recipe is strictly adhered to on a long-term basis (Case et al., 2000). In recent years, raw diets have become popular and are the basis of much discussion on the part of pet professionals. The pros and cons of feeding these types of diets are presented in the Proceedings of Petfood Forum 2000 (Brown, 2000; Grieshop, 2000).

Therapeutic, or veterinary, diets are available to veterinarians and pet caretakers. They are distinguished from pet foods formulated for healthy animals by their mode of sale and the manner in which they are labeled. Specifically, veterinary diets are sold only through veterinary clinics and are labeled for use only under the direction of a veterinarian (Case et al., 2000).

Finally, snacks and treats are becoming increasingly popular with pet caretakers. Although they are not required to be nutritionally complete, a significant number are formulated to be complete and balanced, and some carry the same nutritional label claims as dog and cats foods (Case et al., 2000). Treats and biscuits are often offered to the pet by the caretaker as a means of demonstrating affection for the animal, for reinforcing desired behaviors, at times of arrival and departure, as a means of providing a sense of variety in the pet's diet, and as an aid to proper dental health (Case et al., 2000).

Brands of Food Available

Brands of commercial pet food may be classified into four general categories—generic, private label, popular, and premium. Generic pet foods are those that do not carry a brand name. They may be produced and marketed locally or regionally, and minimizing the cost of production is a primary consideration of manufacturers of these products. Inexpensive, low quality ingredients often are used in these diets, and the foods are rarely subjected to thorough animal feeding tests. Generic foods are usually lower in palatability and digestibility than other brands of food available, and so are not suitable for many animals in shelters. Overall, generic foods represent the least expensive and typically the poorest quality of pet foods commercially available (Case et al., 2000). Private label pet foods are products that carry the house name of the grocery store chain or other store in which they are sold. From a quality perspective, they are similar to generic brands.

Popular brands include foods that are marketed nationally or regionally and sold in grocery store chains. They are usually quite palatable and are produced using variable formulations (i.e., ingredients in a particular brand may vary from batch to batch, depending on ingredient availability and the cost to the manufacturer). This type of formulation system sometimes results in variable product quality and digestibility, and may cause gastrointestinal upset in some dogs and cats.

Premium pet foods include high quality ingredients and are prepared using fixed formulations (i.e., ingredients will not change regardless of ingredient availability or market price). Different premium products are produced for dogs and cats at different stages of life or with different lifestyles. Most manufacturers of these foods validate their label claims through AAFCO feeding studies. These foods are the most costly of the four available brands but, because these products are more digestible and nutrient dense, smaller amounts may need to be fed to meet an animal's nutrient requirements (Case et al., 2000).

Food Quality

The quality or nutritive value of commercial pet foods may be assessed using laboratory-based and/or animal feeding tests. All foods should be tested for nutrient composition. At the bare minimum, the proximate components should be assayed. These components include dry matter, ash, crude protein, crude fiber, ether extract, and nitrogen-free extract. The crude fiber analysis is of little value as it drastically underestimates the percentage fiber in an ingredient or diet, and should be replaced with a better assessment of fiber concentration such as total dietary fiber (TDF) analysis. In order to capture all of the lipid content present in pet diets, an acid hydrolysis should be done on the sample before it is subjected to ether extraction. Nitrogen-

free extract theoretically represents the digestible carbohydrate concentration of the sample and is calculated as the sum of the concentrations of crude protein, crude fiber, and ether extract subtracted from 100 percent. A better means of obtaining the carbohydrate content of the food is to actually analyze for its carbohydrate constituents (e.g., starch, total dietary fiber, total nonstructural carbohydrates, oligosaccharides, and so on). It is also wise to analyze for the micronutrient content (i.e., vitamins and minerals) of the food.

Food stability directly affects food quality. It is important that the food has a shelf life of at least one year, and to accomplish that, antioxidants, either natural or synthetic, need to be a part of the diet. Ideally, foods should be tested for stability using assays such as the peroxide value or free fatty acid analysis. Stability tests are sometimes conducted under accelerated storage conditions in which the food is placed in an artificial environment where humidity, temperature, and other criteria can be varied. The stored product then is compared to a fresh product in regards to nutrient content, appearance, and palatability. In addition to problems that may occur with fats, vitamins are particularly susceptible to degradation at high temperatures and humidity (Irlbeck, 1996). All pet foods should be stored in a dry, cool area. Because canned food is sterile and hermetically sealed, little effort is needed for it to retain its wholesomeness and nutritive value. In general, if shelter personnel are concerned about the odor, color, or texture of the food, they should always discard it and replace with fresh food. Expired food should not be fed because the loss of antioxidant and preservative protection can lead to rancidity, loss of palatability, and loss of nutrients.

Other laboratory measurements that may relate to the nutritive value of pet foods include measures of texture, density, size, and shape. All of these factors may affect "mouth feel," which may be more important to cats than dogs (Irlbeck, 1996). This is especially important for shelter animals that may reduce intake or become anorexic in response to stress.

Usually the very first animal test performed on a new food is for purposes of determining palatability. This characteristic of a complete diet is important because shelter staff may tend to purchase food on the basis of its palatability and the quality of the stool excreted by the animal fed that food. Good palatability is not necessarily associated with complete and balanced diets that meet all nutrient requirements of dogs and cats, but most foods with these attributes are highly palatable. Details of the protocol for palatability testing are outlined in Irlbeck (1996).

AAFCO (2002) defines feeding protocols that will determine whether a food is suitable for dogs and cats at maintenance, for growth, and for sustaining pregnancy and lactation. A protocol for determining metabolizable energy (ME) also is outlined in the AAFCO (2002) manual. Many of the foods sold today will have been tested using these protocols.

Other animal tests that can be conducted to determine food quality, but which are not required from a regulatory standpoint, include nutrient digestibility and nutrient metabolism determinations. Data collected from these types of experiments provide information about the bioavailability of selected nutrients, data that are sorely lacking in the entire animal nutrition arena. Much more bioavailability data are needed for the many ingredients that make up dog and cat food. Having such information would allow "precision nutrition" principles to dictate formulation of companion animal diets.

Food Assessment and Selection

Selecting foods for shelter dogs and cats is a difficult assignment. The buyer should be confident that the food purchased is balanced and will meet the physiological requirements of shelter animals. In addition, appropriate foods that meet the needs of shelter dogs and cats in different physiological states and health must be purchased. This selection process was aided by the AAFCO (1987) ruling that the label of a dog or cat food (excluding treats or snacks) should bear a statement of nutritional adequacy or purpose for the food. The four categories listed under that statement include: 1) food which meets or exceeds the requirements of one or more recognized physiological states for nutritional adequacy, including gestation, lactation, growth, maintenance, and which are complete for all life states; 2) food which is not a complete diet, but has a nutritional or dietary claim; 3) those products that should be fed under the supervision of a veterinarian; and 4) foods designed for supplemental or intermittent feeding. The buyer of the food needs to

be confident that it meets AAFCO standards as a complete diet. And if it does, it will be clearly marked on the label (Irlbeck, 1996).

Dogs and cats who have stopped eating due to stress or who are ill may need to be fed a highly palatable and nutrient-dense food to encourage adequate consumption (NRC, 2003). If a new food is introduced, the diet should be changed very gradually, substituting an increasing proportion of the former diet with the new diet over a four- to seven-day period. Inadequate intake of nutrients can affect both immunocompetence and tissue repair (for those animals where surgery has been required). In the case of anorexia or where surgery may limit voluntary food consumption, use of a complete and balanced liquid or gel-type diet that can be delivered by feeding tube may be necessary.

FEEDING MANAGEMENT

Assessing Body Condition in Dogs and Cats

The ultimate goal when feeding shelter animals is to feed all dogs and cats to maintain or attain an ideal body weight and condition. Because many shelter animals arrive in a debilitated state, weight increase is often a primary goal. Conversely, owner-relinquished animals may arrive at the shelter in overweight or obese conditions. Initial intake evaluations always should include an objective assessment of body condition and weight. Shelter staff can use body condition scoring systems that are designed to objectively score the canine and feline body condition. Several systems are available that involve ranking body composition based upon visual assessment and palpation. The most common systems in use are from Purina (www.purina.com) and Tufts University (www.vetgate.ac.uk). The Tufts system, more commonly referred to as Tufts Animal Care and Condition (TACC) score is used more widely in cruelty cases to standardize descriptions of body condition.

In general, dogs and cats that are too thin will have easily palpable ribs, with little or no overlying fat layer. In dogs, the tail base may be prominent, and the overhead profile of the dog will appear as an exaggerated hourglass. Dogs and cats that are at their ideal body weight should have an hourglass shape when viewed from above, with an easily observed waist behind the ribs. If the animal has a heavy coat, the waist can still be easily palpated beneath the coat. In contrast, an overweight dog or cat will have a moderate to heavy layer of fat over-lying the ribs. In obese animals, the ribs may be difficult to feel. The profile will show only a slight hourglass shape, and in very overweight dogs and cats, there is no waist at all. Thickening around the tail base (where the tail meets the body) is common in overweight dogs, while cats typically develop a pendulous abdomen as a result of fat accumulation in intra-abdominal sites.

Determining How Much to Feed

Food intake in all animals is governed principally by energy requirements. When cats and dogs are successfully fed free-choice meals, the underlying control over the amount of food that is consumed is primarily the animal's need for energy. Commercial pet foods that are sold for particular life stages or activity levels are formulated to provide the proper amount of essential nutrients when a quantity is fed that meets the animal's energy requirement. Balancing energy density with nutrient content ensures that when caloric needs are met, the needs for all other essential nutrients will be met by the same quantity of food. It is for this reason that shelters are best served to attempt to procure high-quality commercial foods that have been formulated for different life stages and feed these appropriately, as opposed to attempting to feed using a "one food fits all" approach.

A number of factors affects an individual animal's energy requirement. These factors include age, body condition, activity level, temperament, and the animal's reaction to the shelter environment. Feeding recommendations are provided as guidelines on pet food bags and should be considered to be a starting point when calculating how much to feed. The amount of food can then be adjusted up or down to meet an individual animal's needs. In general, dogs that are highly stressed in a shelter environment and react with hyperactivity will require more than recommended amounts. In contrast, cats that are housed in cages, and animals that become depressed in response to the shelter environment, will have reduced energy needs.

Although shelters often receive a wide variety of donated food, switching the brand or type of food that is fed to an individual animal is not recommended. A solution to the donated food issue is to assign a particular brand of food to a particular animal once his or her body condition and life stage has been assessed. The same food should be fed to the animal for the duration of his/her stay. Most dogs and cats are best maintained on a consistent diet of a balanced pet food. Changing the diet frequently can result in a refusal to eat or in gastrointestinal tract upsets. Animals are especially susceptible when they are stressed. If it is inevitable that a dog or cat's diet must be changed while at the shelter, the new food should be introduced slowly by mixing it in increasing amounts with the animal's original food over a period of four days.

Feeding for Weight Control

Just as is the case for humans, maintenance of "ideal" body weight results in optimal health and body function of dogs and cats. But, for a variety of reasons, weight control is a serious problem in a portion of the pet population. Obesity, defined as a body weight more than 15 to 20 percent above normal, is the most common nutritional disorder of companion animals in the United States, with the majority of the problem occurring in middle age (Case et al., 2000). The incidence of obesity appears to be increasing in both dogs and cats and may be attributed to factors such as sedentary lifestyle and provision of highly palatable and energy-dense foods. While many stray dogs at shelters are underweight and malnourished, a substantial proportion of owner-relinquished dogs and cats are overweight or obese at the time of relinquishment.

The short-term goal of the treatment of obesity is to reduce body fat stores. For a period of time, the dog or cat must be in negative energy balance. This is accomplished by restricting dietary intake, stimulating total energy expenditure, or by a combination of the two. Fasting as an approach to weight loss is never advisable for dogs or cats. The long-term goal of treatment is for the pet to attain the ideal body weight and maintain this weight for the remainder of life.

Dogs and cats that are 15 percent or more above their ideal body weight should be placed on a weight loss program. For animals that are at the shelter for several weeks or months, a goal of one to two percent loss per week is recommended (Case et al., 2000). From the dietary perspective, the most important component of a weight loss program is caloric restriction (60 to 70 percent of maintenance energy requirements). This amount of caloric restriction will allow most dogs and cats to lose one to two percent of body weight per week. Because of the cat's higher protein requirement and its inability to adapt to restricted protein feeding, providing sufficient dietary protein is very important. Overweight animals in shelters should always be meal fed using premeasured portions, even if a commercially prepared weight reduction diet is fed. This allows strict monitoring of the total food intake and removes the opportunity for the animal to spontaneously increase intake of a reduced energy food (Case et al., 2000). Once the target weight has been reached, the daily volume of food can be slowly increased until an amount that maintains ideal body weight is provided.

Commercial pet foods formulated for adult maintenance contain adequate amounts of nutrients to meet the needs of an animal at normal weight consuming adequate calories. If the volume of the maintenance diet is reduced too drastically in order to limit calories, nutrient deficiencies may develop. Commercially prepared foods with reduced energy densities are formulated to contain adequate concentrations of nutrients while supplying fewer calories. Dogs and cats that are just slightly overweight benefit from feeding slightly reduced portions of a normal maintenance diet. However, in cases of moderate to severe obesity, a change of diet is recommended. Reduced calorie diets are either low in fat and high in digestible complex carbohydrate or high in dietary fiber. Some high fiber weight reduction diets also have a reduced concentration of fat, while others contain concentrations of fats similar to or greater than those found in maintenance diets, and so may be more palatable. High fiber diets are not always suitable for shelter environments, however, because they cause increased defecation frequency and stool volume.

Feeding during Periods of Stress

Individual dogs and cats react differently to stress. For some dogs, a kennel environment is highly stimulating and they react with hyperactive excitation, barking, fence running, and in some cases, fence fighting. Other dogs react with depression and may lie quietly for hours, severely reducing their activity. Conversely, stressed cats either will typically become very quiet and reserved or will

attempt to flee whenever they are approached or handled. If cats are housed in cages, their opportunities for movement are severely restricted, and this will affect both the level of stress and their energy needs. Many dogs and cats react to shelter environments by either eating sporadically or by refusing to eat altogether. This is especially common in cats, and is of special concern in adult cats that are overweight as they are at increased risk for idiopathic hepatic lipidosis (Dimski and Taboada, 1995).

In general, canned foods, and dry foods to which warm water has been added, are highly palatable to dogs and cats. Simply adding some water to the dry food may entice some dogs (less commonly, cats) to begin to eat. Similarly, because eating is a socially facilitated behavior in dogs, the presence of other dogs may either intimidate a dog enough to inhibit eating, or may motivate a dog to eat. Providing a nervous dog with a quiet place to eat, or housing him with a companion can entice some dogs to begin to eat. For cats, providing several different flavors of canned food can be used to attempt a reluctant cat to begin eating. This may be especially important to try with owner-relinquished cats because individuals who have been fed a single type or flavor of food for several years will often refuse to consume any other type of food. Cats whose ability to smell is compromised by upper respiratory infections may be encouraged to eat by providing foods that have a strong aroma or adding tuna or sardine juice to their diet, for example. Finally, selecting a food that is highly digestible and energy dense is recommended for stressed animals and is also appropriate for underweight or malnourished animals. These foods are highly palatable and so have a greater likelihood of inducing the animal to eat, and they also deliver more energy and nutrients in a small volume of food. Several "recovery diets" formulated for ill, recovering, or starved animals are available through veterinarians and are well-suited for highly stressed animals who are refusing to eat or who are consuming very little food (Daristotle et al., 2002). These foods are also suitable for refeeding underweight or neglected animals that need to gain weight and body condition. As with ill animals, underweight animals should be fed numerous small meals, several times per day to allow gradual and consistent weight gain.

EDUCATING ADOPTERS ABOUT NUTRITION AND FEEDING

Client education is an important function of animal shelters today, and most include staff and trained volunteers who act as adoption counselors to facilitate successful dog and cat adoptions. This staff typically provides information about health care, behavior, and training for dogs and cats. Nutrition and feeding are equally important topics to discuss with new adopters. Topics that may be important include the type of food to feed (commercial versus homemade), feeding table scraps and human foods, and deciding on the type of feeding regimen to use.

Feeding Dogs versus Cats

Dogs are omnivores who thrive when fed a mixture of animal and plant products. In contrast, cats are carnivores that require certain nutrients found only in animal tissues. Because dogs and cats have differing nutritional needs, only foods that have been specifically formulated and marketed for the respective species should be fed. Most importantly, cats should not be allowed to simply "eat the dog's food", as the long-term consumption of an adult maintenance dog food may result in deficiencies in taurine, protein, and several other essential nutrients.

Selecting a Food

Today, the majority of most companion animal guardians in the United States feed on commercially produced pet foods. These foods are available in several forms (canned, dry, or semimoist) and are formulated and marketed for different stages of life and activity levels. In addition, pet foods vary significantly in both quality and cost. An optimal pet food is one that provides all of the essential nutrients in their proper amounts and proportions. The food must be palatable and acceptable enough to ensure long-term consumption. It should also be properly prepared and preserved to ensure safety and health. Selecting a food that matches a pet's age, size, and lifestyle is the best way to provide optimal nutrition and maintain proper body condition and weight. Some caretakers prefer to feed homemade diets. A homemade pet food also can provide adequate nutrition, if the recipe is properly formulated to provide complete and balanced nutrition for dogs or cats. Specifically, the diet must have

been thoroughly tested at some point for nutrient content and availability. Unfortunately, most of the homemade recipes that are available have not been properly tested and so are often not recommended for use.

Feeding Table Scraps and Human Foods

Many guardians add human foods and table scraps to their pet's diet because they enjoy giving their animal companion something extra or because they believe that the supplement is necessary for their pet's health. Providing a special food is a way of showing affection and love, and is usually harmless if kept to moderation. However, it is important to realize that the nutritional needs of dogs and cats are somewhat different than those of humans. Regardless, most human foods pose a danger to animal health only if they make up a high proportion of the pet's diet.

It is a common belief that cats "need" to be fed milk. While it is true that almost all cats enjoy the taste of milk, they do not need to have milk or any other dairy product in their diet. Although milk is an excellent source of calcium, protein, phosphorus, and several vitamins, the consumption of high amounts of dairy products by cats (or dogs) can cause digestive upsets and diarrhea. This occurs because the lactose that is present in milk requires the intestinal enzyme, lactase, for digestion. As in most mammals, lactase activity decreases as dogs and cats reach maturity. This change results in lactose maldigestion. Undigested lactose travels to the large intestine where it is fermented by bacteria, resulting in the production of gas, loose stools, and possibly diarrhea. While some companion animals continue to tolerate dairy products as adults, others do not. Most can enjoy an occasional bowl of milk but overall, the practice of feeding dairy products should be limited. Other "human foods" to avoid or limit carefully include high-fat table scraps, chocolate, raw meat or fish, raw egg whites, and onions.

Feeding Regimens (Free-Choice versus Meal Feeding)

The method of feeding that is used with companion animals often depends upon the caretaker's daily schedule and the pet's life stage and lifestyle. Meal feeding involves providing premeasured amounts of food for a limited period, several times per day.

Free-choice feeding (also called *ad libitum* feeding) involves providing a continual supply of food and allowing the pet to self-regulate the amount consumed each day. In general, meal feeding with controlled portion sizes is the preferred method of feeding for the majority of dogs and for many cats. This approach allows caretakers to carefully monitor their animal's food intake and nutritional health.

Portion-controlled feeding is always recommended for growing dogs, and a minimum of two meals per day should be provided. Some large and giant breeds of dogs may benefit from three or more feedings per day as a precaution again the development of gastric dilatation volvulus (bloat). A distinct advantage of portion-controlled feeding is that the caretaker can control the dog or cat's food consumption and will immediately observe any changes in food intake or eating behavior, which are often the first signs of illness. In most households, the animal companion is fed one meal in the morning and a second meal in the early evening. The dog or cat's response to feeding and its body condition are the best guides to use when adjusting the volume of food that is provided each meal.

Free-choice feeding involves having a bowl of food available to the dog or cat at all times and allowing the pet to self-regulate energy intake. Dry pet food is most suitable for this feeding regimen because expanded foods do not spoil as quickly as canned products. Free-choice feeding is probably preferred by cats because they are, by nature, nibblers who prefer to consume small meals. Cats who are fed free choice typically eat numerous small meals throughout the day and night. Free-choice feeding is a distinct advantage for pets that do not readily eat enough to meet their energy needs when meal-fed. In contrast, a free-choice regimen is not a good method for animals that have a tendency to over-consume and gain weight. Compared with meal feeding, free-choice feeding requires the least amount of work and involvement on the part of the pet's caretaker. Free-choice feeding can be beneficial in multiple cat households because it usually allows all cats to get enough to eat. Conversely, it is often contraindicated in multiple dog households due to food-guarding behaviors that may develop among dogs.

CONCLUSIONS

Feeding shelter dogs and cats to achieve or maintain optimal health is challenging, given the wide range in ages, body condition, and health of the animals who are housed in shelters. These factors must all be considered when selecting the appropriate foods for shelter dogs and cats, and when determining the correct method and amount to feed. Ultimately, just as with pets in homes, providing diets that are formulated for specific life stages, and which are palatable, digestible, and contain highly available nutrients is the best approach to feeding shelter animals. In addition, educating new adopters regarding the proper feeding practices for their new animal companion is an important role of shelter staff, as optimal feeding positively impacts the animal throughout his/her life in their new home.

REFERENCES

Association of American Feed Control Officials (AAFCO). 1987. *Official Publication*. Charleston, WV: Association of American Feed Control Officials.

Association of American Feed Control Officials (AAFCO). 2002. *Official Publication*. Oxford, IN: Association of American Feed Control Officials.

Allard, R. L., Douglass, G. M., et al. 1988. The effects of breed and sex on dog growth. *Companion Animal Practice*, 2:9–12.

Anantharaman-Barr, H. G., Gicquello, P., et al. 1991. The effect of age on the digestibility of macronutrients and energy in cats. *Proceedings of the British Small Animal Veterinary Association Congress*. Birmingham, AL. Abstract #164.

Brown, S. 2000. Raw: Pro's. *Proceedings of the Petfood Forum 2000*. Mt. Morris, IL: Watt Publishing Co., pp. 34–41.

Case, L. P., Carey, D. P., et al. 2000. *Canine and Feline Nutrition: A Resource for Companion Animal Professionals*. 2nd ed. St. Louis: Mosby Inc.

Daristotle, L., Tetrick, M. A., et al. 2002. *Current Concepts in Clinical Nutrition for Dogs and Cats*. Philadelphia, PA: Harcourt Health Communications, p. 264.

Dimski, D. S., and Taboada, J. 1995. Feline idiopathic hepatic lipidosis. *Veterinary Clinics of North America, Small Animal Practice* 25:357–373.

Grieshop, C. M. 2000. Raw: Con's. *Proceedings of the Petfood Forum 2000*. Mt. Morris, IL: Watt Publishing Co., pp. 42–50.

Hoskins, J. D. 1995. Puppy and kitten losses. *Veterinary Pediatrics: Dogs and Cats from Birth to Six Months*. Philadelphia, PA: WB Saunders, pp. 51–55.

Irlbeck, N. A. 1996. *Nutrition and Care of Companion Animals*. Dubuque, IA: Kendall/Hunt Publishing Co.

Kelley, R. L., Lepine, A. J., et al. 1998. Effect of milk composition on growth and body composition of puppies (Abstr). *FASEB (Federation of American Societies for Experimental Biology) Proceedings*, 12: A837.

Kuo, Z. Y. 1967. *The Dynamics of Behaviour Development*: An Epigenetic View. New York: Random House.

Lepine, A. 1997. Nutrition of the neonatal puppy. *Proceedings of the North American Veterinary Conference*, pp. 27–29.

Lepine, A. J. 1998. Nutritional influences on skeletal growth of the large-breed puppy. *Proceedings of the North American Veterinary Conference*, pp. 15–18.

Lepine, A. J., Kelley, R. L., et al. 1998. Effect of feline milk replacers on growth and body composition of nursing kittens. (Abstr). *Proceedings of the ACVIM (American College of Veterinary Internal Medicine) Forum*, p. 737.

Malm, K., and Jensen, P. 1996. Weaning in dogs: Within and between litter variation in milk and solid food intake. *Applied Animal Behavior Science* 49: 223–235.

National Research Council. 1985. *Nutrient Requirements of Dogs*. Washington, DC: National Academy Press.

National Research Council. 1986. *Nutrient Requirements of Cats*. Washington, DC: National Academy Press.

National Research Council. 2003. *Nutrient Requirements of Dogs and Cats*. Washington, DC: National Academy Press.

8
Dog and Cat Care in the Animal Shelter

Lila Miller

INTRODUCTION

Veterinary education traditionally has been divided into two areas of interest—large and small animal practice. This general division has persisted despite the development of several specialty areas, such as laboratory or exotic animal medicine, or estimates that the volume of veterinary information doubles approximately every 10 years. The significance of this distinction for shelter veterinarians lies in the different approaches to handling disease. Traditional large animal practice involves herd health management of sizeable numbers of agricultural animals. Final decisions about the delivery of health care services are determined primarily by the economic value of the animals. The shift in focus at many veterinary colleges to small companion animal medicine has led to an emphasis on the delivery of individualized treatment protocols that have no relationship to the actual economic value of the animal, which often is viewed as a member of the family. One of the main dilemmas for veterinarians working for and with animal shelters is to find a means of manipulating principles of herd health management to deliver high-quality health care to individual dogs and cats housed together in relatively confined areas in which disease outbreaks are fairly inevitable. Disease outbreaks in laboratory animal colonies, large animal herds, or agricultural herds usually are handled by culling and euthanizing sick, in-contact, and exposed animals, closing the herd to newcomers until the outbreak is over, and repopulating with animals that have tested negative for the disease. The herd is managed as a group. These traditional methods of disease eradi-

cation and control in animal herds are generally not acceptable for use in many of today's modern open-admission animal shelters. The health care approach on paper may emphasize the minimization and/or elimination of disease transmission, but in practice, the goal often is obscured as attempts are made to treat each animal individually as if it were not part of the herd. So, while euthanizing clinically ill animals may be acceptable, the emotional bond that most humans feel for dogs and cats makes it extremely difficult to authorize the euthanasia of apparently healthy puppies and kittens, who have merely been exposed to or have come in contact with an infectious disease agent. The fact that many shelter diseases such as upper respiratory infections (URIs) and ringworm, for example, are typically not life-threatening to the individual animal makes the task even more difficult. The veterinarian's argument that keeping exposed and sick animals in the shelter jeopardizes the health of current and future populations often falls on the deaf ears of untrained professionals who are frequently in final, decision-making positions and who are influenced heavily by public opinion. The search goes on, therefore, for effective disease management strategies to use in animal shelters. Because there have been precious few clinical studies or scientific research on disease patterns in shelter animals, veterinarians are forced to rely heavily on instinct, clinical impressions, networking, informal trials, extrapolation from other data, and anecdotal information to design new health care systems for shelters that may be holding small animal "herds" for long periods of time regardless of their negative health status. Questions are being asked for which no answers currently exist.

An effective, comprehensive shelter disease control program requires more than a list of vaccinations and veterinary procedures. The program must consider the importance of several key but seemingly unrelated medical and nonmedical factors and integrate them into the final plan. Some of these factors include consideration of the number and types of animals received, the different modes of disease transmission, shelter design, sanitation measures, stress levels, and staff and volunteer training. Additional attention must be paid to the role of the public in transmitting disease, a factor with which most other veterinary facilities do not have to contend. Detailed information about specific infectious diseases, data management, sanitation, shelter design, foster care, spay/neuter, and euthanasia programs that are pertinent to disease management will be found elsewhere in this text. There will be some overlap and repetition, but this chapter explores relationships between these key elements to help veterinarians working for and with a shelter design an effective disease management plan based on current medical knowledge, which reflects a realistic goal of minimizing disease transmission. No one single plan will ever suit all shelters because of the different communities they serve and the varying circumstances (that is, budget and mission) under which they operate. However, the goal of every shelter should be to provide 1) a clean, comfortable, and sanitary environment in which stress is minimized; 2) a husbandry program that focuses on proper diet, exercise, behavioral enrichment, and maintenance of comfortable environmental conditions; 3) foster care for sick and debilitated animals that are adoptable; 4) a health care program that addresses the needs of the animals while making optimal use of the available resources; 5) ongoing staff and volunteer training and development; and 6) humane euthanasia when appropriate according to shelter policy and the needs of the community and animals.

THE SHELTER

In order for veterinarians to work effectively with shelters, they should understand the various roles or functions they may be asked to serve, and the mission and philosophy of the shelter. Many communities have more than one shelter, and a satisfactory relationship can be forged when the appropriate shelter is found whose needs match the level of service the veterinarian feels comfortable providing.

The Role of the Veterinarian

Veterinarians provide health care service to shelters in a variety of ways. These services are offered through a variety of contractual arrangements, ranging from fees for staff services to *pro bono*. In some cases, the role of the veterinarian may be advisory only, usually in response to a disease outbreak, health care, or public relations crisis. Shelters may often solicit the opinion of more than one veterinarian. Many nonveterinarians working in animal shelters have an extensive background in animal husbandry, veterinary medicine, and allied subjects, so the veterinarian may often find nonveterinary opinions also being solicited. Without a good understanding of the mission and operation of the shelter, all parties often are frustrated by this relationship when conflicting opinions are offered.

Shelters often seek out veterinarians to join their boards of directors or advisory boards. The role of the board varies according to each individual shelter, but the general role is to set overall policy guidelines and raise funds. This not only lends the shelter a certain degree of legitimacy but also provides much needed links to the private veterinary community. The degree of active participation in program development varies widely from shelter to shelter. (See chapter 3.)

Many veterinarians provide on-call service to the shelter specifically to render medical care to injured or sick animals that must be held. They may also provide periodic service to the shelter by providing examinations, rabies vaccinations, Department of Health inspections, and so on. Some veterinarians enter into agreements that allow the shelter to purchase euthanasia solution and other controlled substances on their license. (Veterinarians should refer to chapter 4 for information on legal issues and check with the State Board or veterinary practice act in their state and with their liability insurance before entering into these agreements.)

Veterinarians are finding employment at shelters to be an increasingly attractive career option as shelters focus less on euthanasia and more on preventative health care and treatment programs. Many work part-time only, providing medical and surgical services (predominantly spay/neuter) on a fixed or flexible schedule. Others work full-time, fulfilling medical and/or administrative functions. Some shelters operate hospitals that are open to the public in addition to providing health care to the shelter animals. Playing an administrative role at the shelter allows for the more effective implementation of policy decisions, but also opens the door for other management headaches and frustration. (Chapter 3 on administrative hurdles deals with some of these concerns.)

Many veterinarians are intimately involved in all aspects of shelter operations, not just the medical ones. They are designing and implementing training programs for staff and volunteers; performing behavior evaluations and helping develop adoptability guidelines; consulting on plans for designing or retrofitting shelters; designing sanitation, behavioral enrichment, foster care, feral cat management, and euthanasia programs; providing protocols for humanely trapping animals and chemical capture; participating in bite prevention, media events, and other humane education projects; working with investigators on cruelty investigations, and so on. The demands placed upon shelter veterinarians certainly require knowledge and skills that far exceed what is acquired via formal training at the veterinary college.

Mission and Philosophy of the Shelter

Understanding the mission of the shelter is critical to designing an effective health care program. There are many different types of shelters, and no one is exactly sure how many there are or how many animals pass through their doors. (See chapter 2 for information on population statistics.) They tend to be classified as municipal, private, "open admission," or "no kill" (limited admission). There are also animal sanctuaries, breed, and animal rescue groups.

Municipal, open admission animal shelters are often primarily concerned with animal control. They do not turn animals away. They can range from being marginally funded by the city and managed by the police department with minimal standards of care, to being well funded with the highest standards of care developed by animal care profes-

sionals. In some cases, a Society for the Prevention of Cruelty to Animals (SPCA) or humane society may accept the contract for animal control and receive municipal as well as private funding. Animal shelter funding is often limited, whether it is private or municipal, restricting the implementation of optimal health care protocols. Local laws tied to municipal funding may also have an impact on the implementation of animal welfare oriented policies, such as limiting the ability of the shelter to screen potential adopters for their suitability.

Some private shelters are run by the local SPCA or the local humane society with no municipal funding. They may be limited or open admission. Although they are also bound by the legal restrictions imposed by local and state government, their internal policies will affect many of the decisions the veterinarian must make, especially in the face of disease outbreaks and overcrowding.

Private, no-kill shelters represent a growing trend in animal sheltering. Their internal policies generally state that they will not euthanize "adoptable" animals, thus eliminating the use of euthanasia to control overcrowding or manage disease outbreaks. They maintain the right to refuse to admit animals when they run out of space, thus effectively eliminating them from performing municipal animal control functions. Adoptability is defined by each agency and may be affected by many factors, including their financial ability to treat disease, ability to isolate sick animals, expertise of the staff in performing behavior evaluations and treatments, and so on. (A well-behaved puppy with parvo is only unadoptable if the shelter cannot treat it, whether the treatment is performed off-site, in-house, or through foster care. Some shelters impose age restrictions on adoptable animals, and others do not, based on their resources and willingness of the public to accept them.)

No-kill shelters may keep animals for several months to years before they are placed. They have been partly responsible for the increased demand for on-site veterinary services. Edinboro (1999) showed that the longer cats stay in shelters, the more likely they are to contract disease. Puppies that contracted parvovirus in a study on pediatric neutering (Howe et al., 2001) were being housed in a long-term facility. Although the *No Kill Movement* has received enormous attention from the media as cities and states strive to reduce the number of animals they euthanize, many shelters still euthanize to prevent overcrowding and manage disease outbreaks, and few, if any no-kill shelters never euthanize animals. Because the term no-kill can be inflammatory and misleading, and many of these shelters are able to reduce their euthanasia numbers by limiting their admissions, they will from this point hereon be referred to as "limited admission" shelters.

Although consideration of the philosophy and policies of the shelter is critical to designing health care programs, a high-quality shelter is defined by more than its health care plan. The benchmarks of a good shelter include 1) reasoned placement of animals into responsible homes; 2) convenient hours; 3) well maintained, cheerful, and bright appearance; 4) polite, well-informed, and helpful staff; 5) a policy of mandatory neutering; 6) information about proper pet care and responsible ownership, animal behavior, and so on; 7) stress reduction and behavioral enrichment programs; 8) clean, dry, and safe environment for the animals; 9) community outreach; and 10) comprehensive health care program that both treats animals and provides preventative health care (ASPCA). Veterinarians have an important role to play in helping the shelter meet and maintain the standards that will make it an outstanding facility.

OBSTACLES TO CONTROLLING DISEASE TRANSMISSION

Maintaining a disease-free shelter can be difficult for many reasons. The limitations that are inherent in animal sheltering operations must be understood so that realistic goals may be set. Animal lives may be lost unnecessarily, and staff morale often plummets if definitive measures are not put in place to deal with disease outbreaks when they occur. It should be remembered that even research laboratories, breeding colonies, animal hospitals, catteries, and kennels all have occasional disease outbreaks, despite the facts that they can control the influx of animals and do not have to deal with a constant influx of visitors or management policies that are not always designed with the prevention of disease transmission as a primary objective. Furthermore, they seldom face the budgetary restrictions or scrutiny of the media and volunteers that must be factored into decision making. An understanding of

all the factors relating to disease transmission and an analysis of the strengths and weaknesses of the shelter is critical for designing a program that overcomes its weak points and emphasizes and capitalizes on its strong ones. Some shelter programs in marginal facilities have minimal disease problems because they have a well-trained staff to implement an excellent sanitation and health care program, and programs in new so-called state-of–the-art facilities suffer from chronic problems because of overconfidence in technology, lack of staff training, poor design, and inadequate sanitation programs. A health care program built upon vaccination, deworming, and disease testing, no matter how excellent, can seldom, if ever, overcome poor sanitation procedures, lack of staff training, and overcrowding.

Some of the reasons why disease transmission is so difficult to control are found in Table 8.1. Limited resources are only one part of the problem. Other factors are discussed in this chapter and the other chapters listed in Table 8.1.

Disease Transmission

A traditional veterinary education provides access to detailed information about disease pathogenesis, diagnostic and treatment protocols, and so on, and that information need not be duplicated in this text. However, there are several characteristics about diseases and their modes of transmission that are of special interest to shelter veterinarians because of their impact on the health of the general population, and they will be described briefly in the following sections.

VARIETY OF WAYS DISEASES ARE SPREAD

A discussion of some of the most important infectious diseases that affect dogs and cats in shelters is found in chapter 16. At one time, it was believed that the spread of disease in shelters could be virtually eliminated if animals were housed individually rather than in group or communal housing. That has not proven to be the case. Two of the most common feline diseases found in shelters, dermatophytosis (ringworm) and upper respiratory infections, are also spread by aerosolization and indirect contact via animate and inanimate objects, also known as fomites. Hands are one of the most common fomites, but the list includes clothing, medical equipment (including anesthesia machines, stetho-

Table 8.1. Obstacles to Maintaining a Disease-Free Environment

Problem	Chapter(s)
Multiple means of disease transmission	8, 16
Incubation periods, carrier states, viral shedding, and so on	8, 16
Resistance to disinfection, long survival rates in the environment	6, 8, 16
Mandatory shelter holding periods	8
Poor sanitation methods	6, 8
Poor shelter design—inadequate space, poor ventilation	5, 6, 8
Overcrowding	8
Constant influx of new animals with unknown medical backgrounds	8
Inadequate staffing	8
Lack of training	8
Poor data collection and data management	15
Poorly designed veterinary health care program	8, 15, 16, 17, 18
Ambiguous shelter mission, vague operational policies	3
Poor or disorganized management	3
No stress management plan	8, 19
Limited resources	8

scopes, and so on), water bowls, litter boxes, ropes, muzzles, and even pens and pencils. So although the ability to physically separate animals from each other is vitally important, it will not be effective as a singular means of disease control. One must consider all the ways disease organisms are shed—that is in feces, urine, saliva, ocular and nasal discharges, and other body excretions and secretions—and the fact that they may also remain on the hair coat of infected and recovered animals indefinitely. One must consider vector transmission via rodents, ticks, flies, fleas, mosquitoes, and so on. Veterinarians may be tempted to design programs that focus on bolstering the individual animal's immune system through improved nutrition, vaccinations, deworming, and treatment, but those efforts are destined to fail if disrupting these modes of disease transmission are not also addressed. This means the

veterinarian must also pay attention to details like the location and maintenance of air vents, sanitation, pest and vermin control, safe food storage, laundering guidelines for disinfecting uniforms and bedding, and so on.

RESISTANCE TO DISINFECTION

Another critical factor to consider is the length of time some disease organisms persist in the environment and their resistance to disinfection. Two diseases that can be devastating to shelter animals are parvo, which is highly infectious and can have a high mortality rate in puppies, and ringworm, which is self-limiting and zoonotic. What they both have in common is their ability to survive in the environment for months (to years) and their uncommon resistance to routine disinfection. Disinfecting carpets and air vents contaminated with ringworm spores can be nearly impossible, and because dirt, grass, and gravel cannot be chemically disinfected, play areas and runs contaminated with parvovirus may be off limits to susceptible animals for prolonged periods of time, unless the surface materials are replaced. The situation is complicated by some conflicting information about the efficacy of various disinfectants. Despite the fact that some of the newer quaternary ammonium products are labeled to inactivate parvovirus, some studies have shown this to not be the case (Kennedy, 1995; Eleraky et al., 2002). It has been shown, however, that sodium hypochlorite (common household bleach) and potassium peroxymonosulfate (Trifectant®) are virucidal (parvocidal) and fungicidal at proper dilutions (Eleraky et al., 2002). Effective disease management requires accurate diagnoses so that effective sanitation methods may be employed. A discussion of sanitation procedures can be found in chapter 6.

INCUBATION PERIODS, CARRIER STATES AND VIRUS SHEDDING

Detailed knowledge about incubation periods, viral shedding, and carrier states of diseases is essential when setting appropriate time lines for quarantine and isolation periods, providing recommendations for adoption guidelines, and for the accurate interpretation of tests. No infallible method is available to shelters to hasten the detection of disease in animals during the incubation period. Physical examinations and disease tests are often inconclusive.

Ten-to-fourteen day quarantines are the option many shelters use to detect disease before an animal is adopted. It is always distressing when homes are found for apparently healthy animals only to have them turn up at the local veterinarian's office or back at the shelter a few days later due to an infectious disease. Not only is it a heartbreaking situation for everyone involved, it also can damage the reputation of the shelter and alienate the adopter from returning to the shelter. Some community veterinarians will criticize the shelter for having poor health standards. One downside to quarantines, however, is that at least one study has shown a 5 percent increased risk of cats developing URI for each additional day spent at the shelter (Edinboro, 1999).

The inapparent carrier state of many diseases complicates their detection. (See chapter 16 for more information on infectious diseases.) *Microsporum canis* fungal spores have been isolated from the hair coats of normal dogs and cats (Moriello et al., 1991). After this zoonotic disease is endemic in the environment, routine toothbrush culturing may not distinguish between true infection and the transient carriage of spores (Moriello et al., 1994). Approximately 80 percent of cats that have recovered from herpes virus infections will become carriers that may be viremic for life; they will shed virus in their oronasal and conjunctival secretions spontaneously or intermittently with stress, typically one week after the stressful incident and lasting up to three weeks after the stress. Viral shedding cannot be detected in latent carriers. Cats infected with calici virus may be lifelong carriers or eventually rid themselves of the virus, but until they do, they may shed virus continuously. Vaccination does not prevent the carrier state (Gaskell and Dawson, 1998). This fact has enormous implications for shelters that treat upper respiratory infections and house cats in groups. The safest disease prevention strategy appears to be to house recovered cats in individual cages, yet the group housing option should not be summarily dismissed because preliminary anecdotal information from shelters indicates that reduced stress levels may offset the impact of increased direct contact as a mode of disease transmission.

Viral shedding is a concern in both naturally infected and vaccinated animals. Puppies infected by parvovirus will shed virus on day three post-infection, before clinical disease symptoms are observed. They can shed virus in their feces for 12 to 14 days after infection (Hoskins, 1998; Carmichael, 1997; Sherdig, 1994) and carry the virus on their hair for months; therefore puppies that have recovered from parvovirus infections should be bathed and housed individually for at least two weeks post clinical recovery. Vaccination will also induce viral shedding that is infectious and that will cause false positives on parvo fecal antigen tests anywhere starting from three to 7 days post vaccination (www.vetmed.ucdavis.edu/CCAH/Prog-ShelterMed/Parvo). False negatives may be obtained early in the course of the disease if the dog is not shedding antigen, or late in the course of the disease, especially if the dog is immune competent and producing antigen binding antibodies. Viral shedding periods should always be considered when housing, disease testing, and offering shelter animals for adoption. Animals who may be shedding virus should not be adopted to households with susceptible puppies and kittens without counseling about the risks, advising physically separate housing for a period encompassing the anticipated period of viral shedding, and making certain that other pets at home are current on their vaccinations and immune competent.

CROSS SPECIES INFECTIVITY OF DISEASES

A strategy that was often used by shelters dealing with disease outbreaks was to place the dogs in the cat room and vice versa, on the theory that most infectious disease agents were species specific. However, this is not always the case, and animals in shelters are more likely to contract otherwise rarely occurring cross infections because additional stresses have compromised their immune systems. The 2a and 2b strains of parvovirus in dogs have been found in cats suffering from clinical signs of panleukopenia, which is normally caused by a different strain of parvovirus (Mochizuki et al., 1996). Bordetella bronchiseptica, one of the disease agents involved in the canine infectious tracheobronchitis (kennel cough) respiratory syndrome has now been implicated as a possible primary pathogen in clinical upper respiratory disease in cats, primarily kittens. (It has been reported, at least anecdotally, that some shelters have experienced a reduction in URI when using the intranasal Bordetella vaccine in their cats.)

Bordetella can also cause disease in rabbits, guinea pigs, and other small mammals. *Sarcoptes scabiei,* which is typically a canine parasite that causes scabies, may infect cats, rabbits, and other animals, including humans, and *Notoedres cati,* the causative agent of head mange in cats may also opportunistically infect dogs, rabbits, other animals, and humans. The predominant cause of ringworm in cats, *Microsporum canis,* can also infect dogs, rabbits, humans, and other animals. Because fomite transmission is such an important mode of disease spread, staff must use extra care when cleaning both dog and cat rooms and when handling other small mammals and rabbits.

Proper Shelter Design

Many shelters are housed in facilities that provide a breeding ground for disease. Scrupulous sanitation techniques must be used to overcome problems like poor ventilation, cracked and porous floors, and inadequate space. Shelter design and sanitation are covered in detail in chapters 5 and 6. Some of the key points for veterinarians and health care staff to consider when creating health care programs and shelter policies include traffic flow patterns, isolation areas, and ventilation. Many policy decisions actually will be determined by the design of the shelter. Resource allocation to increase the treatment of infectious disease must include a sufficient number of physically separate isolation areas to house animals until they are clinically recovered and viral shedding has ceased. Euthanasia decisions often have to be implemented based on the lack of isolation space to treat rather than the severity of the disease being treated. URI and ringworm are non-life-threatening diseases under ordinary circumstances, but have become two very deadly shelter diseases partially for this reason.

Traffic Patterns

The flow of traffic in shelters should progress from the rooms with the healthiest and most disease-susceptible animals (puppies and kittens) first to the unadoptable and diseased animals last. They should preferably be located as far away from each other as physically possible. This is particularly important in shelters that have chronic disease problems. While placing less adoptable adult animals at the front of the shelter to encourage their selection before visitors arrive at the puppy room may be a good mar-

keting strategy, it jeopardizes the health of the puppies. Visitors who wish to see the puppy room at the end of their trip to the shelter should be discouraged from doing so on the same day unless hand sanitizers, footbaths, and disposable aprons are available for their use. Staff who clean multiple rooms should start at the healthiest areas first and end at the isolation and euthanasia rooms to prevent fomite transmission.

Isolation Areas

Effective isolation procedures require placing sick animals in physically separate rooms, not at opposite ends of the same room housing healthy animals. Cat cages that face each other should be at least four to five feet apart because that is the distance that disease droplets can be propelled by a sneeze (Greene, 1998, p. 673). Treatment of animals should occur in the isolation areas, and when isolation areas are full, no further treatments should be initiated until other appropriate isolation areas can be created. Once diseased animals are housed inappropriately with healthy animals, even temporarily, the potential for disease spread increases greatly. In an ideal situation, serious, active ringworm and URI cases would be kept in separate isolation areas, and other areas would be designated for mildly infected or recovering animals. Limited admission shelters that house FeLV and FIV cats long-term must also consider their isolation options, ideally housing FeLV positive cats separately from FIV positive cats. Despite the fact that neither virus lives long outside the host's body and transmission requires prolonged close contact through mutual grooming, shared bowls and litter boxes, or bites, it is prudent to observe strict isolation and sanitation measures. Some shelters even house these animals in separate buildings.

Staff who work in the isolation area should wear protective garments dedicated for use in that area only, including disposable aprons, gloves, foot covers, and so on. There should also be footbaths located at the door. Separate drainage and ventilation would be ideal, and drugs and other medical and cleaning equipment would be used in that room only. Traffic in and out of the room should be restricted to essential personnel only. The public should be directed to this room last when searching for lost animals unless it is fairly certain that the animal being sought is in that room.

OTHER DESIGN CONSIDERATIONS

Debilitated and stressed animals with noninfectious disease should be housed separately in a special care room. Very young and orphan animals should be placed in foster care (see chapter 21), as their care needs are extensive, and the shelter environment is usually too harsh for these animals to survive. This room should be equipped with special equipment such as heat lamps, blankets, towels, medications, and so on. It may be necessary to keep this room warmer than other animal areas. It should be quiet and have minimal foot traffic. All staff who work in this area should receive additional training to meet the special needs of these animals.

In addition to an isolation room for infectious disease, there should be several other distinct separate rooms that provide for separation by age, health, adoption, and legal status. Adoption areas should hold healthy, currently adoptable animals only. A separate adoption area for puppies and kittens should be provided so that young susceptible animals will not be exposed to disease from healthy, immunocompetent adults. If the decision is made to permit the adoption of animals with mild upper respiratory diseases, they should be housed separately. (However, many shelters accept the argument that if 1) URI is an inevitability, 2) many animals are carriers who are probably shedding virus anyway, and 3) the other cats are either immune competent or not, then housing mildly infected cats with healthy ones doesn't increase the risk factor to an unacceptable level, especially if insufficient isolation areas exist and the only alternative is euthanasia. Shelters that elect to follow this path should monitor disease levels and change policies when and if disease levels rise.)

Many shelters provide a quarantine area for observation of animals when they first arrive. (Animals with symptoms of infectious disease should be placed in isolation, not quarantine.) A 14-day quarantine is recommended to cover the incubation period of most infectious diseases, but this is not feasible for many shelters, especially if they intake large numbers of animals or have a rapid turnover. However, quarantines are strongly recommended 1) for animals that appear to be in questionable health; 2) during periods of disease outbreaks; 3) for animals entering from foster care, other shelters, or other regions where disease incidence may be high or unknown; 4) for animals that will be placed in

communal housing; 5) for animals entering limited admission shelters. Animals should be moved immediately as soon as the quarantine period is over or disease symptoms appear, and prompt decisions should be made about their care. If healthy, they should be placed in adoptions. If sick, they should be moved to isolation for treatment, adopted out (with appropriate counseling), placed in foster care, or euthanized. Data are inconclusive as to whether or not animals in quarantine should be permitted to be adopted or held until the quarantine is up. Since the Edinboro study (1999) concluded that the longer cats remain in the shelter the more likely they are to become ill, it would seem reasonable to release apparently healthy adoptable animals at any point during the quarantine period with proper adoption and medical counseling. To accommodate this policy, it would make sense to vaccinate and deworm adoptable animals in quarantine.

The examination room should be separate from the euthanasia room, and each should have enough space for their respective tasks to be performed; a sink, appropriate lighting and equipment, cabinetry, a safe to store the equipment, drugs appropriate to the purpose, and so on. Equipment should not be carried from room to room to discourage disease transmission via fomites. Nor should animals be euthanized in the exam room because of the high rate of contamination, the durability of many disease agents, and the amount of time it takes to properly disinfect the room. The euthanasia room should be cleaned and disinfected rigorously and be located as far away from areas housing healthy animals as possible and close to the area designated for body disposal. (See chapter 24.)

The designation of other shelter areas will depend upon the mission of the shelter. Some shelters must accept animals regardless of the circumstances surrounding their relinquishment. Shelters that are involved in long-term holding for legal reasons pertaining to animal control should have a separate area for these animals. Shelters that receive large numbers of exotic animals (that is, reptiles, birds, small mammals, rabbits, wildlife, and so on) should create separate space to meet their special environmental and behavioral requirements. Other areas should be designated for segregating animals by their 1) age—under 3 months of age, 3–6 months of age, 6 months to a year, seniors over 8 years of age; 2) health status—very sick, mildly sick, recovered, and so on—or infectious versus noninfectious; 3) legal status—owned or stray, currently adoptable, waiting for the legal holding period to be up before eligible for adoption or euthanasia, and so on. The more areas in the shelter, the more opportunities to isolate animals and thus minimize disease spread via direct contact.

VENTILATION

The importance of good ventilation cannot be overemphasized, nor can its limitations be ignored. Dogs housed in indoor-outdoor runs in California still suffer from kennel cough despite the constant access to fresh air. The ventilation system should always be evaluated when investigating a disease outbreak. When evaluating the system, it is important to visit all the animal areas and ensure that the environment in each area is appropriate for the animals' needs—that is, exotics, puppies and kittens, recovery areas, and so on. Ventilation ducts should be located optimally for directing the air flow appropriately within the room and then air flow patterns throughout the building should go from healthy areas to disease areas last. Chapter 5 discusses HEPA filtration, ozone generators, and other equipment frequently used to augment ventilation systems.

Stress

Programs for stress reduction are an essential component of a comprehensive health care program. Stress is defined as "the sum of the biological reactions to any adverse stimulus, physical, mental or emotional, internal or external, that tends to disturb the homeostasis of an organism. Should these reactions be inappropriate they may lead to disease states" (Blood and Studdert, 1988). Animals that enter a shelter are either already stressed or undergo stress, which compromises immunocompetency and renders them more susceptible to disease caused a) by the opportunistic organisms that they may already be harboring, b) by indirect contact via fomites or aerosolization, or c) by direct contact with other sick individuals. Stress adversely affects immune competent as well as debilitated animals. Cats that are carriers of herpes virus will show clinical signs of disease and shed virus when stressed at any point during their stay in the shelter.

Stress reduces an animal's ability to respond to vaccination (Greene, 1998, p. 725) Some shelter veterinarians have suggested that it is better to wait a few days for stress levels to decline in order to produce a more effective response to vaccination. One study (Hennessy, 1997) that indicated stress-related cortisol levels are elevated for the first three days of a dog's stay in the shelter would support the theory that vaccinating a dog on the fourth day after arrival might stimulate a more effective immune response than vaccinating on arrival. Again, no conclusive data exist to support or refute this strategy.

Many diseases are directly stress related. Some examples of canine diseases are parvo, kennel cough, Giardiasis, and Coccidiosis; stress-related feline diseases include upper respiratory infections, Giardia, Coccidia, and FIP. Some physical responses to stress include inappetance, depression, vomiting, diarrhea, self-induced mutilation, aggression, and drooling. The fact that it is extremely difficult to distinguish real clinical symptoms from those induced by stress poses a real problem for shelters.

TYPES OF STRESS

Stress can be physical, emotional, or environmental. Not all shelter stressors can be controlled. Animals that are malnourished, pregnant, lactating, or injured are stressed and at higher risk for contracting disease or further debilitation. These states of physical stress should be addressed as soon as possible for the health and well being of all the animals in the shelter, regardless of the length of time they will be in residence. They should be placed in quiet areas with less foot traffic, and their extra needs should be met with nutritional supplementation, medical care, special housing, extra warmth, careful handling, and so on.

Every animal that enters a shelter for the first time is subject to emotional stress. Stress occurs when the animal encounters unfamiliar surroundings, new human and animal companions, changes in routine, diet and exercise, new noises and odors, and so on. Pain, fear, excitement, boredom, and depression may precipitate behavioral problems in the form of stereotypies (such as spinning or leaping up and down in repetitive motion), withdrawal or aggression, excessive barking, excessive grooming, cessation of normal grooming habits, and so on. (See chapter 19.) The impact of stress on owned animals might be more dramatic because of the drastic disruption of the routine in their lives that strays do not have. Although no formal studies were ever conducted, it appeared to ASPCA staff that owned animals contracted disease at a higher rate than the strays despite the fact that they had often been vaccinated and dewormed before entering the shelter. Speculation was that this might have been attributable to their higher stress levels. (Shelter strays who have survived exposure to myriad diseases may also have greater natural immunity. An opposing theory is that free-roaming strays actually undergo greater stress due to their sudden enforced confinement.)

Environmental stresses are the one type of stress that every shelter has the ability to control to some degree. One of these stresses is overcrowding, which is a major contributing factor to disease spread. Overcrowding occurs when limited admissions shelters do not close their doors to new arrivals or euthanize to create space, and in open admissions shelters as a result of the influx of large numbers of animals and legal holding periods during which they cannot be euthanized or adopted. Budget cuts that reduce operating hours and staffing, well-intentioned local ordinances, neuter before adoption policies that result in longer holding periods, and the sudden arrival of large numbers of animals brought in by local authorities also contribute to overcrowding. Overcrowding should be viewed as a serious problem to be avoided whenever possible, and should be managed efficiently to minimize its negative impact on the shelter residents. Because systems of isolation and segregation of animals inevitably break down as a result of overcrowding, stress levels rise, and more disease transmission via direct contact occurs. Allowing overcrowding to continue indefinitely almost always results in more disease, more animal deaths, and eventually more euthanasia.

Temperature, humidity, and ventilation should always be maintained at appropriate levels to increase the comfort of each animal and, thus, minimize stress. Animals that are hypothermic, hyperthermic, or subjected to drafts or wide fluctuations in temperature and humidity are more susceptible to illness. In general, if humans are comfortable, dogs and cats will be also. Different conditions will have to be provided for exotic animals. Excessive noise (see chapters 5 and 19), lack of sleep, and failure to accommodate diurnal habits of dogs and cats can also increase stress levels.

METHODS OF MINIMIZING STRESS

Whenever overcrowding occurs and animals must be doubled up, following some guidelines can help minimize stress. These guidelines include keeping housemates and litters together (although different litters should not be mixed together) and segregating animals by age (less than 3 months, 3–6 months of age, 6 months to 7 years, and 8 years and over), size, sexual status, and temperament. Male dogs should not be housed together, even if they are neutered, unless they can be carefully monitored for fighting. Aggressive animals or "bullies" that don't necessarily fight but intimidate should also be housed alone. Animals showing very mild symptoms of illness may be housed together since they are already exposed and infected, but seriously ill animals should always be housed separately and treated or euthanized for humane reasons. Pregnant, nursing, and injured animals should always be housed alone. Nursing animals with puppies and kittens greater than four weeks of age should be given the opportunity to spend some time away from their offspring.

Difficult management decisions must be made to control overcrowding as quickly as possible, including closing the doors to new arrivals, transferring animals to other shelters or animal facilities, using foster and volunteer care to remove animals from the building (see chapter 21), and euthanasia. Shelters that suffer from chronic overcrowding should reassess their situations and seek larger spaces, reduce their intake, or change their policies.

Noise by both other animals and staff should be kept to a minimum. In some shelters, soft music has been used to calm both the staff and the animals. At least one study showed classical music to be the most soothing (Wells, Graham, and Hepper, 2002). Dogs that are constantly barking can present a tremendous source of stress to cats (not to mention staff and other animals, including other dogs), and efforts should be made to calm them by providing enrichment or removing them from situations that may provoke excessive barking, such as placement by the door where high traffic serves to arouse them. Behavioral enrichment is discussed in chapter 19.

Environmental temperatures should be kept as constant as possible. Humidity levels should be comfortable, and the temperature in rooms housing healthy dogs and cats should be 65–75°F (www.

hsus2.org/international/library/operate.html). Some states regulate animal shelters. Heat should be provided when the ambient temperature drops below 50°F for more than four hours according to Colorado statute (www.ag.state.co.us), but New Jersey statutes require heat at temperatures below 55°F (www.awfnj.org/regulations.html). According to statute, cooling should be provided at temperatures greater than 85°F in New Jersey and 90°F in Colorado. (The Animal Welfare Act has minimum standards of care for dogs and cats that restrict exposing them to temperatures greater than 85°F or below 40°F for more than four hours. These guidelines were not developed with shelters in mind, and these extremes in temperature should be avoided (http://www.aphis.usda.gov/ac/9CFR99.html). See chapter 26 for more information on this subject.

Drafts, odors, and moisture condensation from high humidity should be minimized, and fresh air should be provided by windows, doors, vents, and exhaust fans. Open windows should have screens to prevent the entry of insects and other unwanted animals and pests, and the exit of escaped, at-large shelter animals. If animals are housed outdoors, they must have access to protection from wind, rain, snow, excessive heat, sunlight, cold, predators, malicious acts from humans, and so on. Additional bedding should be provided for animals housed outdoors in temperatures below 40°F. In general, exclusive outdoor housing of shelter animals should be discouraged.

In keeping with providing a healthy environment for shelter animals, smoking should not be permitted in the shelter. In addition to the health hazards for humans, a link has been shown between secondhand smoke and the development of bronchial asthma and lymphoma in cats (Bertone et al., 2002) and nasal tumors in certain breeds of dogs (Reif et al., 1998).

The stress created from the daily performance of routine procedures such as moving animals from cages for cleaning, grooming, and feeding, walking, or taking them to the veterinarian's office can be minimized by setting up a schedule and assigning staff to work the same rooms so that they can develop a relationship with the animals. Staff should be advised to take a few extra minutes to complete a task if animals are frightened or distressed. Safe and efficient handling techniques should be an important part of any training program

for all shelter staff and volunteers. Overhandling should be avoided if it causes stress.

Shelters are implementing behavioral enrichment programs to break the monotony of the average shelter dog's existence. Boredom and enforced long-term confinement can lead to other problems like self-mutilation or food and cage guarding. Toys, frequent dog walks, agility programs, and play time are some of the enrichment programs in place at many shelters. Toys should be evaluated to make certain they are safe. In general, toys should not be shared even if they are disinfected first. Disposable toys are best. Behavior problems can be extremely detrimental to an animal's chances of successful placement in a new home. Chapter 2 discusses relinquishment data, and chapter 19 has more information on behavior enrichment.

Lack of sleep is a source of stress to diurnal animals, which is frequently overlooked. The lights and music should be turned off at night. Table 8.2 is a summary of some methods of reducing stress.

HUSBANDRY

Nutrition

It is well known that good nutrition is essential to combat stress and promote good health, yet decisions about feeding animals in shelters are often made casually, based on cost or acceptance of food donations. Chapter 7 provides detailed information about dog and cat nutrition. In short, the highest quality, nutritionally complete and balanced food that is obtainable should be fed. Food should be wholesome, fresh, and stored securely so that ver-

Table 8.2. Methods of Minimizing Stress

Avoid overcrowding.
Provide the best nutrition affordable, tailored to meet individual needs.
Maintain stable and comfortable environmental conditions.
Minimize noise.
Establish routines for feeding, cleaning, play time, and so on.
Avoid overhandling and over stimulation.
Provide toys and other behavioral enrichment.
Provide exercise.
Turn lights and music off at night.
Provide soft music.

min and pests do not have access to it. Donated food should be accepted with caution, and the use of generic or expired food should be avoided. Most shelters will need supplies of both dry and canned food in addition to milk replacers for orphan animals, recovery diets, and other specialty foods to meet the special needs of a diverse shelter population. Food intake should be adjusted when weight loss, obesity, or chronic diarrhea occurs. Obesity can become a serious problem in animals held long-term in shelters. Inappetance should be investigated by switching foods to help distinguish between a true clinical health problem and a finicky appetite.

Controlled feeding trials should be designed to test new foods for palatability and quality before accepting large donations or switching brands of food. Poor quality diets that require feeding larger quantities to meet energy requirements, cause diarrhea, or create eating disorders are poor bargains. Shelters that have long-term residents who are accustomed to one brand of food should change diets gradually to avoid diarrhea and other digestive upset.

Fresh water should be readily available at all times. Some shelters withhold water from animals that play with, sit in, destroy, or overturn their water bowls or to prevent excessive urination, but this practice should be discouraged unless a medical reason exists.

Sanitation

Chapter 6 discusses sanitation methods in detail. It is critical for all staff and volunteers to understand the role of fomite transmission of disease in the shelter and how failure to control it may be a major contributing factor to the shelter's inability to prevent or end a disease outbreak. An in-depth review of sanitation protocols should be conducted as one of the first steps whenever a disease outbreak occurs to make certain that animal enclosures are being properly cleaned and disinfected. This is often more valuable than changing vaccination protocols or other veterinary procedures. See Table 8.3 for a brief review of sanitation procedures and Table 8.4 for methods of reducing fomite transmission of disease. In short, cages and animal enclosures should be cleaned and disinfected at least once daily, between different occupants and as frequently as necessary to ensure that the animal is kept in clean, dry, and comfortable quarters and that odors are

minimized. In the case of stable colonies of group-housed cats, the enclosures should be cleaned at least twice a day, but disinfected less frequently (once or twice a week if no new residents are introduced until all the cats have been adopted) to avoid the stress of moving all the cats out each day. There is no way of knowing if this strategy will be successful without implementing it, but the cleaning protocol must be followed stringently.

Staff should be aware of the limitations of sanitation. Dirt and gravel cannot be chemically disinfected, and at least 12 inches must be replaced to render it safe again if contaminated with parvovirus, which otherwise can survive in the environment for months (personal communication with Dr. Janet Foley). Carpets may require professional steam-cleaning to reach temperatures that are high enough

Table 8.3. Review of Sanitation Procedures

Establish diagnosis and determine etiology.
Identify appropriate disinfectant.
Observe staff cleaning procedures—removal of all materials and organic debris from cage, use of proper water temperature and detergent, cleaning entire cage, and so on.
Verify proper usage of disinfectant—proper mixing and application, sufficient surface contact time, and rinsing.
Remove animals from cage and make certain that they are not wet during cleaning process.
Increase frequency of cleaning, especially if using a single product that combines a detergent and disinfectant.
Review methods of minimizing fomite transmission (see Table 8.4).
Install hand sanitizers and foot baths.
Avoid high-pressure hosing and common drainage.
Use disposable rags and paper towels—avoid sponges and mops in animal areas.
Vacuum, clean, and disinfect vents, check and/or replace filters.
Ensure workers cleaning multiple areas start in healthiest areas first and progress toward disease areas.
Make certain that staff utilize safety equipment when cleaning—eye goggles, masks, and gloves.
Disinfect transport cages and communal animal holding areas.

Table 8.4. Methods of Reducing Fomite Transmission

Wash hands frequently, wear gloves and disposable aprons.

Use disposables as much as possible—litter boxes, food trays, toys, aprons, gloves, shoe covers, muzzles, temporary holding boxes, and so on.

Post signs to warn visitors about animal handling precautions.

Return animals to same cage after cleaning.

Make certain communal animal areas and transport cages are disinfected after each use.

Disinfect all equipment—stethoscopes, anesthesia machines (hoses), ropes, muzzles, and so on.

Launder clothes, towels, blankets, uniforms, and so on in hot water, soap, and bleach.

Assign cleaning equipment to one room.

Clean and disinfect water bowls daily and between different animals' use.

Use nonporous, disinfectable materials—avoid wood and carpet.

---

to reduce the disease particle load, but this does not ensure disinfection. Staff should be observed cleaning and disinfecting during a disease outbreak to ensure compliance with policy; verbal assurances should not be accepted.

Housing

GENERAL CONSIDERATIONS

Housing options for dogs and cats in animal shelters have changed over the years. At one time, colony kennels were commonly used for both species. Animal segregation consisted of separating cats from dogs and males from females. Cats were separated by gender, and dogs were separated according to the day of the week they entered the shelter. Tuesday's kennel might be filled to overcrowding, but Wednesday's kennel might be virtually empty. At the end of the holding period, a few animals were selected for adoption, and the others were euthanized. This management tool facilitated searches for lost animals and lessened the chance that animals were mistakenly euthanized before their holding period was over. Disease transmission was of minimal concern because sick animals were euthanized. Veterinarians were consulted about animal housing when standards of care issues were

raised, along with concerns about disease transmission. Housing animals individually became the goal of most progressive animal shelters. Some shelters still use communal housing routinely because of facility restrictions, so it is almost ironic that many shelters are switching to group housing to create a more natural environment, reduce stress, and increase adoptability. Whatever housing options are selected, they should be maintained in proper condition. They should be safe, with no sharp, rusty or jagged edges, constructed of nonporous, durable materials, and easily cleaned, disinfected, and dried. Drains that are located within the enclosure should be covered with grates with small openings that will prevent injuries to legs, paws, or nails.

Most species should be housed separately, and intact females separated from males. Rabbits and other small mammals should be housed separately from dogs and cats because barking and being close predators is stressful for prey animals. There are also concerns about disease spread due to species cross infectivity. Dog enclosures should be rendered escapeproof if cats are housed in them; small cats and kittens can squeeze out between widely spaced bars or ill-fitting doors. Animals should not be placed in the top level of three-tiered cage systems if the cages can't be cleaned easily, and if the animals cannot be easily and safely reached by staff or seen by the public.

DOGS

Guidelines or recommendations for housing dogs, including minimum space requirements, vary widely. Table 8.5 summarizes some space recommendations for both dog and cat housing. Dogs may be housed in cages, runs, enclosures (pens), or kennels. Most shelters will need a variety of types of housing to accommodate different breeds and temperaments and to fulfill the mission of the shelter. At least a few of the enclosures should be designed to withstand destruction from strong or active dogs that are either bored or determined to escape. (Shelters that house pit bulls or other large, dangerous dogs should pay particular attention to this concern, as pit bulls have been known to escape and break into cages to kill other dogs. See chapter 30.) Walls that are a minimum of four feet high (and higher) may be necessary to prevent dogs from visual or direct contact with other. Smaller cages may be

Table 8.5. Housing: Comparison of Minimum Space Recommendations for Primary Enclosures

Source	Dogs		Cats	
	Floor space	Height	Floor space	Height
Colorado Statute Title 35 Agriculture, Article 42.5–101, Animal Shelters and Pounds	Mathematical square of the sum of length of dog in inches,[a] add 6 inches, divide by 144 and multiply by 2—minimum is 6 sq. ft., maximum is 24 sq. ft.	1½ times the height of the dog at the shoulder or minimum of 18 in. and maximum of 48 in.	Weight / Size[b]: <2lbs → 2.5 sq. ft; 2–5 lbs. → 3 sq. ft; 6–10 lbs → 4 sq ft; 10–20 lbs → 5 sq ft	Minimum is 21 in.
New Jersey Statute N.J.A.C 8.23A-1.6(a), 7b, and 8.23A-1.99(g)	Mathematical square of the length of the dog in inches, plus 6 inches, expressed in square feet (sq. ft.)	N/A	Minimum of 7 cubic feet (if kept over 15 days)	N/A
Humane Society of the United States	Cages: Weight: >50 lbs; 36–50 lbs; 10–35 lbs. Kennels[b]: 4 ft by 6 ft. Runs[b]: 4 ft by 8 ft.	Size[b]: 24 sq. ft.; 20 sq. ft.; 12 sq. ft.	Minimum of 9 sq. ft	N/A
Animal Welfare Act[c]	"Must allow space for each animal to express all species-typical postures, social adjustments, behaviors, and movements. For example, animals must be able to lie down with limbs extended in a normal manner without obstruction from enclosure sides or having to extend feet through feeder doors or bars."			

[a] Length in inches measured from tip of nose to base of tail
[b] Minimum size
[c] Rules are minimum guidelines and do not apply to animal shelters as law.
Animal Welfare Act: http://www.aphis.usda.gov/ac/9CFR99.html

acceptable for small dogs and treatment areas, isolation, and recovery rooms, where the stay may be short or where restriction of excessive movement is desirable, while large dogs will be more comfortable in runs or kennels. Dangerous dogs are best housed in runs divided by a guillotine door to minimize handling when cleaning. Pregnant or nursing bitches should be given extra space and always housed individually with extra bedding. Shelters that hold animals long-term will need larger cages and enclosures and more space devoted to play and exercise areas. Dogs that are housed in cages that meet only minimum space requirements should be given opportunities for exercise daily, especially if they are being held for long periods of time. (New Jersey and Colorado statutes for housing dogs in shelters require that they receive at least 20 minutes of daily exercise.)

In general, shelters with disease problems should house dogs individually unless they are less than four months of age or from the same litter or household. Individually housed animals may benefit from play time with other compatible dogs to reduce stress (see chapter 19). If a reasoned decision is made to group house unrelated dogs as a means of providing behavioral enrichment, cage mates should first be quarantined, vaccinated, tested for endoparasites, treated according to the test results, and/or prophylactically dewormed, neutered, and evaluated for behavioral compatibility. When dogs are group housed, Colorado state guidelines require each additional dog be given one-half the minimum space required (www.ag.state.co.us), whereas HSUS recommends that each dog should have a minimum of 4 feet by 4 feet of floor space (www. hsus2.org/international/library/operate.html). Dogs should be provided with mats, resting boards, blankets, towels, or other bedding in their enclosures, especially if they have short, thin hair coats and/or are being held long-term or are sick or injured. These materials should be inspected daily and removed if the dog is destructive. Some dogs will even destroy metal water bowls or copper tubing from automatic watering systems, so the entire enclosure and its contents should be inspected regularly when cleaned (Fig. 8.1).

Tethering is not an acceptable or alternative means of confining animals in an animal shelter. Although the Animal Welfare Act standards do not apply to animal shelters and are minimal guidelines

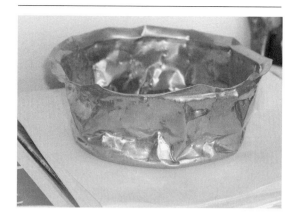

Figure 8.1. Water bowl destroyed by a pit bull. Photo credit Lila Miller.

only, they also prohibit tethering as a means of confining dogs and cats.

Cats

Cats may also be housed individually or as a group. Group housing for behavioral enrichment is probably more common for cats than dogs. Shelters that group house should also have single cages for animals that must be individually housed—that is, for isolation, recovery, quarantine, nursing, pregnant, injured, and feral cats or cats that are aggressive or simply don't like other cats. See Table 8.5 for space recommendations for cages. To minimize disease transmission, some shelters use cages with Plexiglas® fronts so animals may be seen but not touched by the public unless supervised by staff. Some of these cat cages or condo units have hidden litter box areas and separate air exchange systems for each cage. Despite these high-tech systems that prevent or limit disease transmission, some cats still exhibit signs of URI, especially if they are herpes or calici virus carriers.

Cages should have litter boxes (preferably disposable, with clumping litter), elevated resting perches or shelves, scratching posts, and toys. Bedding should also be provided, even if the cat prefers to sit and sleep in its litter box. Cage items should be disposable or disinfectable (Fig. 8.2).

Group housing for cats is increasing in popularity despite concerns about potential increased disease transmission. Thus far, at least anecdotally, shelters that group house cats have not reported an

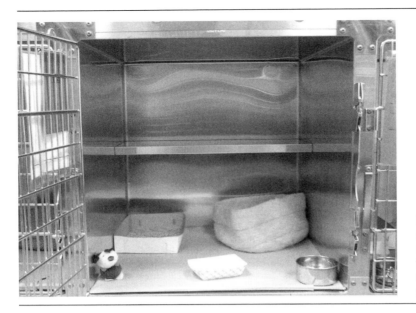

Figure 8.2. Stainless steel cat cage. Notice disposable litter and food tray, bed, toy, and resting shelf inside cage. Photo credit Lila Miller.

increase in upper respiratory infections, ringworm, or stress-induced illness. Table 8.6 contains two space recommendations for group housing. Table 8.7 contains guidelines to follow for group housing cats. Chapter 19 has more recommendations about group housing considerations. In general, cats should be observed for behavior compatibility and removed if they should hide constantly, are overly aggressive, refuse to eat, overeat, and so on. The guidelines in Tables 8.6 and 8.7 are recommendations only. Many experts recommend that households with multiple cats provide at least one litter box per cat, plus one to ensure that there are no problems. This rule of thumb doesn't appear to be necessary in shelters, but litter boxes should be added or cats removed if fecal material appears constantly outside the box. Group housed cats in particular should be given a physical exam on a regular basis, and their weight should be monitored, as

they are less likely to be observed as closely as cats housed individually, and free-choice feeding may lead to obesity.

VETERINARY HEALTH CARE PROGRAM

A typical comprehensive health care program should incorporate, or at the very least consider, the following elements: thorough physical examination of animals; vaccinations (chapter 17); disease testing (chapter 18); development of realistic and practical treatment protocols utilizing data management (chapters 15 and 16); rounds; foster care (chapter 21); and euthanasia (chapter 24). Other programs may include spay/neuter programs for both the shelter and community animals (chapter 22) or trap-neuter release programs to manage feral cats (chapter 23). Community outreach projects may include special programs such as vaccination clinics and mobile medical vans.

Table 8.6. Group Housing Space Recommendations for Cats

Source	Floor space recommendation
HSUS (www.hsus.org)	Maximum 15 adult or 20 kittens in a 10 ft by 15 ft. room
Colorado statute Title 35	Minimum of 10 sq. ft. per cat over 4 months of age
Agriculture Article 42.5–101	Minimum of 7.5 sq. ft. per cat over 6 weeks of age
	Requires solid resting surfaces that cat can fit under
	Maximum of 25 cats

Table 8.7. Guidelines for Group Housing Cats

Quarantine for 7–14 days.

Segregate intact males from females or neuter all cats first.

Segregate by age groups—ideally <3 months, 3–6 months, 6 months–8 years, and senior cats.

Vaccinate with core vaccines—FVRCP and rabies in accordance with shelter policy.

Deworm prophylactically with broad spectrum anthelmintics.

Perform fecal and deworm in accordance with results.

Toothbrush culture for ringworm in high incidence areas.

Test for FIV and FeLV.

Behavior test for compatibility with other cats.

Provide one litter pan per 3–4 cats, clean and disinfect daily, and monitor usage. (Increase number if cats soil outside box.)

Clean and disinfect enclosure daily if constantly introducing new animals.

Provide multiple feeding stations.

Monitor cats closely for signs of infectious disease—sneezing and diarrhea.

Physical Examination

Physical examinations should be performed on animals as soon as they arrive at the shelter. Without the benefit of medical histories and clinical laboratory data, establishment of a definitive diagnosis or prognosis for future health is not always possible. The physical examination takes on additional importance in shelter animals.

A separate area in the shelter should exist where entering animals are held temporarily until these triage examinations can be performed, whether by the veterinarian or other designated, trained animal care staff. The primary reason for this urgency is to identify animals with injuries needing immediate medical attention and to separate those with infectious disease symptoms before they have contact with the general population. Routinely placing them in quarantine without examining them first may jeopardize the health of the other animals in quarantine. Facilities without a quarantine will need to decide where to place the animals according to their legal and health status. Stray animals admitted to shelters with animal control responsibilities must be held in accordance with legal holding periods for lost and found, generally 5–7 days. Healthy adoptable strays should be separated from unadoptable ones. Animals relinquished by their owners, brought in by the authorities, or under a legal hold should be processed as soon as possible in accordance with the conditions of their agreements.

All animals that are accepted by the shelter, including owner relinquishments, should be checked for identification tags, licenses, and tattoos (ears, abdomen, and inguinal region are primary sites) and scanned for a microchip. They should be accurately identified by breed, age, sexual status, all colors and distinguishing characteristics (ears cropped, eye color, tail, and so on) to aid the lost and found department. Tables 27.1 and 27.2 provide guidelines for estimating the age of dogs and cats by their dental pattern. Medical staff should take the time to verify that each animal has an identification band and that any accompanying paperwork matches the animal. Verification of the animal's identity as soon as possible may avert future tragedy.

Animal care staff should be given an examination checklist for the physical examination. The examination should be as methodical and thorough as the animal will permit. See appendix 18.1 for a sample health checklist. A medical record should be prepared and maintained for each animal in the shelter, including a history when available, vaccinations, deworming, diagnosis, and all other pertinent observations. Table 8.8 contains normal values, along with other physiologic information. (On days when the ambient temperature is very high or the animal is excited, the temperature, heart, and respiratory rates may be elevated.) All staff should be trained to recognize infectious disease signs and instructed to report them to the veterinarian or other management staff authorized to move animals as soon as possible. The common signs to train staff to observe for include sneezing, coughing, ocular and nasal discharges, and diarrhea. Other signs may include anorexia, vomiting, depression, and so on. Dangerous or feral animals that cannot be given an immediate hands-on physical examination should be examined visually for signs of infectious disease. Shelter policies may vary as to when the exam must take place, whether on arrival or a few days later when the animal is calm. Decisions must be made quickly as to whether to tranquilize dangerous animals that must be held, if their medical conditions

Table 8.8. Dog and Cat Physiologic Values

Parameter	Dogs	Cats
Temperature[a]—Fahrenheit	99.5–102.5	100.5–102.5
Respiratory rate[a]—breaths/minute	10–30	24–42
Pulse rate[a]—beats/minute	60–180	140–220
Estrous cycle	Seasonally monoestrous	Seasonally polyestrous
Age of puberty for males	6–9 months[b]	9–12 months[c]
Age of puberty for female	6–9 months[b]	4–12 months[c]
Gestation period	56–72 days[b]	63–65 days[c]
Miscellaneous	Spontaneous ovulator	Induced ovulator

[a]Kirk, R., and Bistner, S. *Handbook of Veterinary Procedures and Emergency Treatment* 7th edition. 2000. Philadelphia: W.B. Saunders.

[b]Case, L. 1999. *The Dog.* Ames, IA: Iowa State University Press

[c]ASPCA. 1999. *Complete Guide to Cats.* Jim Richards Chronicle Books

permit it and there are no legal restrictions, in order to safely place an identification band, examine, vaccinate, and render other necessary medical care. Some shelters may require vaccination, disease testing, deworming, and so on upon completion of the initial physical examination if the animal is deemed adoptable, while others may decide to wait a few days for stress levels to decline or for the animal to be adopted first. See chapter 17 for more information on vaccinations.

If veterinarians are not required to examine every animal, guidelines should be developed for when the veterinarian must be called. This "must see" list will vary from shelter to shelter, partially dependent upon the credentialing and expertise of the staff and should include all animals that are accepted for placement, animals with serious injuries or diseases that require treatment, cases on special holds, and animals with a questionable health problem. A licensed veterinarian should always examine animals under rabies observation. In rabies endemic areas, special attention must be paid to wounds on stray animals that may have been caused by animal bites, as these animals may be considered as "rabies exposed" (see the sections on rabies later in this chapter and in chapter 16).

ANIMAL PLACEMENT PROGRAM

The selection of animals to enter the animal placement program will rely heavily, but not entirely, upon the results of the physical examination and behavior evaluation. (See chapter 19.) Adoption

animals should be vaccinated, routinely dewormed prophylactically and specifically for parasites found on fecal examinations.

It is strongly recommended that shelters microchip all animals before their release from the shelter. Most animals can be microchipped; the manufacturer's directions should be followed for proper procedure and site selection. Some private practitioners also microchip, and both the AVMA and some states have declared microchipping to be the practice of veterinary medicine, but others have created a special exemption for shelter staff. Microchip companies offer free scanners to shelters, and the development of a universal scanner that can read all microchips has made microchipping more acceptable. (Adopters pay a fee if they want to continue registration with the microchip companies.) Some municipalities require that dangerous dogs be microchipped so that they may be positively identified in case of future incidents.

Vaccination and disease testing may be performed before adoption or at the actual point of adoption, although most shelters try to vaccinate animals that will be held as soon as possible after arrival at the shelter. Some shelters import animals from other regions of the country and in some cases, even the world, when their population numbers are low. Veterinarians should familiarize themselves with the common disease problems of that region in order to institute proper quarantine, parasite and disease testing protocols to ensure the health of the adopter, the animal, and the other shelter residents.

Adoptability guidelines vary widely from shelter to shelter, community to community, and season to season. Despite the development of written guidelines, decisions may rely heavily on emotion rather than sound medical judgments, which can be a real source of frustration for veterinary professionals. Shelters may euthanize kittens with mild disease symptoms to prevent overcrowding during kitten season and treat them aggressively when there is a shortage, so reasonable exceptions should be built into guidelines. Some shelters find it easy to place animals with physical handicaps such as three legs, or one eye, but other shelters do not have the necessary resources for properly evaluating their medical needs and marketing them. Some shelters have age restrictions, although more older animals are now being placed than previously. Some communities and shelter internal policies may ban placing certain breeds considered dangerous, such as pit bulls. Some shelters place animals regardless of their medical and behavioral problems as long as the adopter assumes all liability, and others may be so strict as to continually have empty cages. Decisions to place animals with zoonotic diseases should be considered carefully. Animals with roundworms should be treated and readily adopted out with written advice on follow up deworming, but more care should be given when adopting out animals with Giardia, especially if a household member is immunocompromised (see chapter 16.) Verbal and written guidelines should be provided to adopters for both wellness care and management of animals with special health and disease concerns. Shelters should consult with legal counsel for advice on developing guidelines for counseling immunocompromised individuals who adopt shelter animals. Information on zoonosis and pet ownership for immunocompromised individuals is available from the Center for Disease Control (www.cdc.gov) and the American Veterinary Medical Association (www.avma.org). A brochure on this subject may be obtained directly from Tuskegee University (Tuskegee University).

Veterinarians will often be asked to estimate the size a puppy will attain at adulthood. No hard and fast guidelines exist for making these estimates, and staff are cautioned about misleading adopters with seemingly factual information. If staff feel compelled to make a guess, one rule of thumb that has most commonly been used is that puppies will reach 50 percent of their adult size by four months of age and 75 percent of their adult size by six months of age. Toy breeds are closer to their adult size at a younger age, whereas giant breeds are farther away.

Advice is often sought for potential adopters who will be bringing animals into home environments previously inhabited by animals with contagious disease. It was common practice to advise adopters to wait for prolonged periods of time if the cases involved parvo, ringworm, feline leukemia, feline infectious peritonitis, and other resistant organisms that persist in the environment for long periods of time or cause fatal disease. To be a truly effective measure, adopters in some cases would have to wait for several months to a year before the organism no longer posed any threat. Potential adopters should instead be advised to 1) discard all bedding, litter boxes, dishes, utensils, leashes, collars, toys, and so on; 2) disinfect with bleach diluted 1:32, allowing surface contact for 10 minutes before rinsing; 3) professionally steam-clean carpets and other fabric surfaces to help reduce the disease particle load; 4) select an adult animal that is more immune competent; and 5) make certain the new pet is healthy and has been properly vaccinated and dewormed. In the case of diseases caused by organisms that do not persist in the environment like corona, FeLV or FIV, it would be good practice to clean and disinfect as a rule, but waiting periods are not necessary. (Personal communication with Dr. Janet Foley, March 2003.)

Most shelters require adoption animals to be neutered either before adoption or through contractual or other low cost agreements with local private practitioners. They should be thoroughly evaluated before surgery. Although minor health problems do not preclude surgery being performed, they must be addressed through appropriate pre- and post-operative care (see chapter 23 on spay/neuter programs) to avoid problems.

Rounds

After animals are triaged and placed in their new quarters, rounds should be conducted at least once a day to continually monitor and reassess health. Animals should be observed for their posture, gait, demeanor, and signs of infectious disease. The cage should be checked for uneaten food, blood, vomit, diarrhea, telltale droplets on the front of the cage from sneezing, and so on. The primary responsibility for rounds should rest with the veterinarian, but all staff should be held accountable for reporting disease symptoms as soon as they are noticed. (In some cases, shelter workers have been known to withhold information about diseased animals to prevent their euthanasia.) Animal wards should have a bulletin board for staff to post important observations that the veterinarian may see immediately upon entering the ward. Animals that are being adopted should be given another complete physical examination before their release to their new owners rather than relying on observations gathered during rounds to assess health. Animals that have been in the shelter long-term should receive a hands-on physical examination at least weekly, including being weighed.

Treatment Protocols

Vaccinations, prophylactic deworming, and routine disease testing should be performed in accordance with the medical guidelines provided elsewhere in this and other clinical texts and in accordance with shelter policy. They will be discussed briefly here. Vaccination decisions are affected by many variables, as are decisions as to when, who, or whether to test for FeLV, FIV, heartworms, or parvo, but all animals held in the shelter and/or placed for adoption should be prophylactically dewormed with a broad spectrum anthelmintic in accordance with the CDC guidelines (www.cdc.gov or see chapter 16) to both promote animal health and prevent visceral larval migrans from ascarid infections.

VACCINATIONS

The role of vaccinations in shelter health programs is poorly understood. Unrealistic expectations exist for vaccines that do not prevent infection but merely reduce the severity of clinical disease in the individual animal. Some of the factors to consider when recommending a vaccination protocol are described in chapter 17; some common obstacles to successful immunization are summarized in Table 8.9. Despite the obstacles, vaccines are considered an integral part of most health care programs, and the clinical impression of veterinarians who worked in shelters before the widespread use of vaccines is that they are very useful in minimizing overall dis-

Table 8.9. Obstacles to Successful Immunization in the Shelter Environment

Maternal antibody interference

Lag time between vaccination and successful immune response may be 2–7 days or more

Unpredictable to negative effect in unidentifiable animals incubating disease

Stress delays or impairs response

Killed vaccines require boosters in 2–4 weeks to be effective

Modified live vaccines may induce viral shedding, cause illness in debilitated animals

Intranasal vaccines cause faster immune response but may produce mild clinical symptoms, more difficult to administer

Less than 100 percent efficacy

Vaccines lessen disease severity, do not prevent infection

ease. A clinical trial of intranasal and subcutaneous vaccines to prevent upper respiratory infection (URI) in cats (Edinboro et al., 1999) yielded some interesting results that would appear to confirm this impression. In this study of 90 apparently healthy cats that were admitted to a shelter, cats with no history of vaccination were 18 times more likely to develop URI, and each additional day at the shelter increased the likelihood of developing URI by 5 percent. Purebred cats were four times more likely to develop URI, and the use of a bivalent intranasal vaccine (calici and herpes) in addition to the subcutaneous vaccination (panleukopenia, herpes, and calici) resulted in a 76 percent reduction in the overall risk of developing URI. Shelters that make reasoned decisions not to vaccinate should be aware that they will probably be heavily criticized and accused of negligence by the public and other veterinary professionals if a disease outbreak occurs.

Low-cost vaccination clinics are the subject of much controversy. Some communities promote rabies vaccination clinics because of public health concerns but draw the line at other routine vaccinations being offered because of opposition from local veterinarians who argue that many people who use these services are not low income. Some of the medical arguments include failure to perform a physical examination before vaccinating, failure to keep adequate medical records, and inability to provide timely boosters or follow-up care for vaccine reactions. Yet vaccination clinics serve a useful purpose that parallels the human health care model for preventative health care, and they are being offered at both remote locations and in urban centers. Veterinarians who choose to participate in these programs should follow the minimum guidelines provided in Table 8.10 and refer to chapter 4.

DISEASE TESTING

Each shelter must examine its mission and resources to determine whether disease testing is a necessary part of the health care program. The results of disease tests in the shelter must be interpreted carefully to avoid errors, especially ones that lead to medically unjustified euthanasia. In most cases, no animal should be diagnosed with an infectious disease based on the results of a single test without corroborating physical symptoms or adjunctive clinical laboratory testing. This is particularly true for FeLV and FIV testing. Although the Association of Feline Practitioners recommends routine testing of all cats, these guidelines were

Table 8.10. Guidelines for Participation in a Vaccination Clinic

Check liability insurance for coverage.
Ensure adequate administrative staffing to prepare records and control crowds.
Ensure adequate technical staffing for handling animals, drawing up vaccines, and so on.
Ensure appropriate medical waste disposal is available.
Ensure availability of both restraint equipment and emergency drugs.
Provide for proper vaccine storage (refrigeration) if at an off-site location.
Perform a mini physical examination on each animal.
Provide vaccination certificates, tags, and written guidelines for follow-up boosters and watch for signs of vaccine reactions.
Keep records.
Maintain control of signature stamps.
Ensure that appropriate inventory is available—correct vaccines, syringes and needles, cotton, alcohol, peroxide, and so on.
Ensure that follow-up care information is available.

developed for pet cats and may not be applicable to all shelters. It is more important (and practical) for shelters that hold cats long-term or that use group housing to test for these diseases on admission than for shelters with a rapid turnover or that house cats in individual cages. Neither virus persists in the environment, and transmission requires prolonged close contact or bites, so disease outbreaks do not typically occur in shelters, especially if they house animals in separate cages. Therefore, it may be more appropriate for some shelters to test animals after they have been selected for adoption to avoid the expense of testing animals that may later be euthanized. Queens and members of litters should be tested individually, and FIV tests in animals under six months should be repeated due to transient positives caused by maternal antibodies. Additional information may be found in chapters 16 and 18, and at www.aafp.com.

Shelters that choose to test for parvo using fecal antigen tests should be familiar with the concerns viral shedding patterns pose for test interpretation. (Also see the section in this chapter on viral shedding and chapters 16 and 18.) Testing apparently healthy cats for Feline Infectious Peritonitis (FIP) is not recommended because of the pathogenesis of the disease and the fact that current tests are not specific for the disease. Heartworm testing may be conducted in areas where the disease is commonly encountered, but it is not generally recommended for routine testing of all dogs. However, it is advisable to test animals that may be in the shelter on a long-term legal hold before using medications that cause adverse effects in heartworm-positive animals and for adopted animals in cases in which the shelter would be unwilling or unable to treat heartworm-positive animals. Cats may be placed on heartworm prevention without disease testing first in areas where the incidence of heartworm disease is high.

SELECTION OF TREATMENT PROTOCOLS

It is beyond the scope of this book to offer specific treatment protocols for medical conditions. This information changes rapidly and is easily found in other clinical texts. However, the criteria used for the selection of treatment protocols in shelters is often very different from the criteria used in private practice. Treatment decisions are affected by the number of animals being treated, the total number of animals in the shelter, adoptability and temperament of the animals to be treated, the experience level of the staff to render treatment, cost, prognosis, board of directors' or community policy, and so on. Although drugs that require multiple doses during the day may be more effective, drugs with once-a-day dosing are more likely to be part of the treatment protocol, especially if multiple animals must be treated, because treatment compliance by staff will be higher. Ease of dosing is another consideration, and selection of drugs that can be compounded into liquids or injectable drugs may be preferable to pilling, especially for cats. Ophthalmic solutions may be preferable to ointments because of easier application. Intranasal vaccination may not be effective because of the difficulty in properly administering the vaccine to uncooperative patients rather than because of inherent problems with the vaccine. Although considered extra-label drug use, weekly doses of Ivermectin may be the drug of choice over other approved earmite treatments that require daily dosing or extensive handling of the patient. Drug treatments in shelters also go in cycles, based on the ease of availability, cost, and convention rather than effectiveness. Amoxicillin and Clavamox were the drugs of choice to treat upper respiratory infections in cats for years, but doxycycline now seems to be more effective, especially if *Mycoplasma* is implicated.

Treatment decisions will also be affected by the availability of animals. Relatively minor problems may go untreated as the decision is made to euthanize instead. In shelters that are overrun with kittens during kitten season, it is not unusual to euthanize animals with fleas and ear mites.

Antibiotic use should be considered carefully when dispensing medication for conditions that typically do not require treatment. The 2001 AVMA Guidelines for Judicious Therapeutic Use of Antimicrobials in Cats states that "antimicrobial therapy is not indicated in feline viral upper respiratory (feline herpesvirus and calicivirus) infections not complicated by secondary bacterial infection" (AVMA, 2002 p. 84). In private homes, mild cases of upper respiratory disease in dogs and cats go untreated, and symptoms eventually resolve on their own. In the shelter, however, there is greater concern about secondary bacterial infection because the conditions in the shelter environment and compromised health status of many shelter animals increases their risk. Failure to treat mild upper res-

piratory infections often elicits criticism if the animal's condition worsens.

Flea and tick treatment options are too numerous to describe here, consisting of topical sprays, powders, dips, flea and tick collars, pills, topical drops applied to the skin, veterinary prescription products, over-the-counter products, and so on. New growth regulators reduce or eliminate the need for environmental decontamination of the home but should not be relied on to prevent contamination of the shelter environment. The broad-spectrum spot-on products that are labeled to control intestinal parasites should not be used in place of a primary deworming product. The use of permethrin spot-on flea products for dogs should be avoided in the shelter because of their toxicity to cats. Check with the ASPCA Poison Control Center (www.appc.aspca.org or 888-426-4435, for which there may be a charge) whenever uncertain about the use of new insecticides or other products to treat animals and/or the environment.

Treatment of infectious diseases should be undertaken in the shelter only if viable isolation areas are available. Once those areas are filled, ongoing cases should be reassessed before placing new cases into unsuitable isolation areas. Animals that are nonresponsive after several days of therapy, continue to run high fevers, refuse to eat, continue to be dehydrated, are deeply depressed, or generally have a poor prognosis should be considered for euthanasia to reduce the risk of disease spread to the other animals in the shelter. Decisions to treat highly infectious diseases with high morbidity and/or high mortality rates risk the health of present and future shelter residents if the disease agents are highly resistant to disinfection or prolonged intensive care therapy is required. Time estimates for recovery and entry into the placement program must also take into account viral shedding periods and the time required for debilitated animals to exhibit sufficient health to be deemed adoptable. Animals that have recovered from infectious diseases like parvo or giardia should be bathed to remove the residual disease load that may survive on their hair and serve to infect other animals. Zoonotic diseases like ringworm that are not life-threatening to either the animals or humans can still present liability issues and bad publicity that threaten the credibility of the entire health care program.

Veterinarians should be proactive in providing

adequate analgesia for animals who are suffering from traumatic injuries, wounds, burns, or other clearly painful conditions. The assumption should be made that if the condition would be painful to humans, it will be painful to animals despite the lack of clear behavioral indicators of pain. Chapter 27 discusses pain assessment and recommends an analgesic protocol. See Appendix 8.3 for a list of pain medications. Shelters that must hold animals with traumatic and painful injuries that do not have hospitals, clinics, or arrangements for care with local private veterinarians should consult their regional regulations for guidelines for euthanizing animals for humane reasons (EHR). Every effort should be made to contact an owner, guardian, or caretaker before EHR is performed. Some municipalities may require a licensed veterinarian's authorization, and others may delegate the authority to shelter managers or two reasonable, concerned members of the public. In New York State, the statute reads "Any agent or officer of the ASPCA or of any society duly incorporated for that purpose or any police officer, may lawfully and humanely destroy or cause to be destroyed any animal found abandoned and not properly cared for, or any lost, strayed homeless or unwanted animal, if upon examination a licensed veterinarian surgeon shall certify, in writing, or if two reputable citizens called by him to view the same in his presence find that the animal is so maimed, diseased or infirm so as to be unfit for any useful purpose" (New York Agriculture and Markets Law).

It may be helpful to try to promulgate some broadly written guidelines for the veterinarian to use when making EHR decisions. For example, a shelter that can provide adequate nursing care for an animal that suffers from treatable hind limb paralysis is justified holding that animal for 3–5 days, especially if it appears to be owned, but if the shelter staff cannot properly evaluate the animal, express the bladder, provide a comfortable cage environment or appropriate drug therapy or nursing care, they should consider euthanasia for humane reasons or move the animal to a hospital. Animals that are dyspneic, in irreversible shock, have extensive traumatic injuries or burns, or are showing profound, irreversible neurological deficits usually can be justifiably euthanized for humane reasons as long as the proper guidelines are followed, including consideration of rabies regulations. The medical record should contain a detailed description of any animal whose condition warrants EHR, and it never hurts to have corroborating signatures from other experienced shelter staff.

Care for Long-Term Holding Cases

Shelters that cannot turn animals away must often hold animals for long periods of time. Owned animals end up in shelters for a variety of reasons in addition to voluntary relinquishment; the owner may have been arrested, evicted, homeless, in the hospital, fleeing a domestic violence situation, and so on. Animals that may have been deliberately abandoned at a veterinary hospital or when the owner moved away or is deceased often end up at the shelter. Animals that have bitten a person or been bitten by another animal may be held for rabies observation at the shelter. If the shelter does not have legal custody of the animals, the liability associated with care of these owned animals is often high, so it is even more critical to observe strict sanitation procedures and ensure the continued health of these animals. Medical record keeping is vitally important in these cases, especially if they are cruelty or animal abuse cases. (See chapter 27.)

Long-term shelter residents should be given a complete physical examination, weighed, vaccinated, and dewormed. A previous medical history should be obtained whenever possible. Young animals should be given booster vaccinations and rewormed at appropriate intervals. They should be weighed weekly, and medical records should reflect any ongoing medical treatment or changes in the animal's condition. Dogs should be walked and given the opportunity to exercise under safe and secure conditions. It may be necessary to obtain prior permission from the owner, court, or other legal guardian to administer medical care to animals that have not been legally relinquished to the shelter. Inability to obtain permission can present a serious dilemma, especially in the case of animal hoarding cases where multiple, poorly socialized, and diseased animals may need care, or if serious non-neurological medical problems develop in animals being held for rabies observation. In many cases, the court or shelter's attorney may need to be consulted before treatment can be rendered in non-emergency situations. This information should be obtained as soon as special cases arrive at the shelter.

RABIES

Animals that are under observation for rabies present a special case. As of 2003, dogs, cats, and ferrets that have bitten someone must be held for 10 days for observation; vaccinated dogs, cats, and ferrets that have been exposed to rabies must be revaccinated and held for 45 days; unvaccinated animals must be euthanized or held for six months and vaccinated one month before release. (Consult the *Compendium of Animal Rabies Prevention and Control*, which can be found at www.avma.org or through the Department of Health for the current complete regulation.) Despite the fact that many of the animals that end up in rabies quarantine are friendly, they should be kept in strict isolation, handled minimally and by experienced staff, always returned to the same cage after cleaning, and housed in secure enclosures in rooms located away from heavily trafficked general public areas. Signs about their status should be posted on their cage. They should be exercised in escape-proof areas if they can be safely handled. The Department (or Board) of Health should be consulted when animals being held for rabies observation become ill. In most cases, stray animals can be euthanized for humane reasons with permission of the department and the head submitted for testing. If the animal is owned and the owner wishes to reclaim the animal after the observation period, both the Department of Health and the owner should be notified to determine the appropriate course of action. In areas where rabies is endemic or a source of unusual concern or where concern exists about other zoonotic or reportable diseases, a daily sign-in book should be maintained so that if an exposure occurs, a log will exist with the names of all the visitors to the shelter during the period of concern.

Unless a veterinarian is well-grounded in behavior, requests to assess the temperament of a dangerous dog should be referred to a veterinary or certified applied animal behaviorist, dog trainer, or other qualified individual. A thorough physical examination should also be performed to establish that the incident was not the result of disease, abuse, or pain. Some physical examinations have revealed painful ear infections, rubber bands or ligatures placed on extremities or genitalia, other evidence of sexual assault (objects inserted in rectum or vagina), or other animal abuse (Munro, 2001) that may have precipitated a bite.

MANAGEMENT OF DISEASE OUTBREAKS AND ZOONOSIS

These subjects are covered in chapters 15, 16, and 18. Summaries are provided in appendixes 8.1 and 8.2

CONCLUSION

Many questions about the practice of shelter medicine have no conclusive answers. It can be quite frustrating to offer professional advice without the benefit of clinical studies or research to guide one's answers. Conflicting recommendations may be offered based on reasonable but different interpretations of the same sets of data. More often than not, decisions must be made without any data at all. Much of shelter practice is not just about medicine and forces veterinarians to reach beyond the information gleaned from a traditional veterinary education. Veterinarians are urged to seek out and consult with other experts in their respective fields for help and to encourage research into methods of sheltering animals that meet the needs of both animals and society.

REFERENCES

Animal Welfare Act: http://www.aphis.usda.gov/ac/9CFR99.html Title 9, Chapter 1, Part 3, Subpart A Sections 3.2 and 3.3

ASPCA (no date). Keys to A Great Shelter. New York, NY: ASPCA.

Blood, D.C., and Studdert, V., 1988. *Baillière's Comprehensive Veterinary Dictionary* London, UK: Baillière-Tindall.

Bertone, E., Snyder, L., et al., 2002 (August 1). Environmental tobacco smoke and risk of malignant lymphoma in pet cats. *American Journal of Epidemiology* 156:268–273.

Carmichael, L., 1997. Parvoviral Infection—Dogs in the Five Minute Veterinary Consult—Dogs and Cats (Larry Tilley and Francis W.K. Smith, Jr., eds.). Baltimore, MD: Williams and Wilkins, 910–911.

Colorado Statute Title 35 Agriculture, Article 42.5-101 Animal Shelters and Pounds (www.ag.state.co.us).

Eleraky, N.K., et al., 2002. Virucidal efficacy of four new disinfectants *Journal of the American Animal Hospital Association*; 38: 231–234

Edinboro, C.H., Janowitz, L.K., et al., 1999. A clinical trial of intranasal and subcutaneous vaccines to prevent upper respiratory infection in cats at an animal shelter *Feline Practice*; 27:7–11, 13.

Foley, J., April 2003. Personal communication, University of California at Davis Veterinary College.

Gaskell, R., and Dawson, S., 1998. Feline respiratory diseases in *Infectious Diseases of the Dog and Cat* (Craig E. Greene, ed.). Philadelphia, PA: WB Saunders, 97–106.

Greene, C. Immunoprophylaxis and immunotherapy in *Infectious Diseases of the Dog and Cat* (Craig E. Greene, ed.). Philadelphia, PA: WB Saunders, 717–750.

Greene, C. Environmental factors in infectious disease in *Infectious Diseases of the Dog and Cat* (Craig E. Greene, ed.). Philadelphia, PA: WB Saunders, 673A–683.

Hennessy, M.B., Davis, H.N., et al., 1997. Plasma cortisol levels of dogs at a county animal shelter *Physiological Behaviour,* 21:295–297.

Hoskins, J., 1998. Canine viral enteritis in *Infectious Diseases of the Dog and Cat* (Craig E. Greene, ed.). Philadelphia, PA: WB Saunders, 40–44.

Howe, L., and Slater, M. et al. January 15, 2001. Long-term outcome of gonadectomy performed at an early age or traditional age in dogs *Journal of the American Veterinary Medical Association* 218, (2): 217–221.

Kennedy, M.A., Mellon, V.S., et al., 1995. Virucidal efficacy of the newer quaternary ammonium compounds *Journal of the American Animal Hospital Association;* 31:254–258.

Maddie's Shelter Medicine Program (www.vetmed.ucdavis.edu/CCAH/Prog-ShelterMed/Parvo).

Mochizuki, M., Horiuchi, M., et al., 1996. Isolation of canine Parvovirus from a cat manifesting clinical signs of feline panleukopenia *Journal of Clinical Microbiology* 34:2101–2105.

Moriello, K.A., DeBoer, D.J., 1991. Fungal flora of the hair coats of cats with and without dermatophytosis *J Med Vet Mycology* 29:285–292.

Moriello, K.A., Kunkle, G.A., DeBoer, D.J., 1994. Isolation of dermatophytes from the hair coats of stray cats from selected animal shelters in two different geographic regions in the United States *Veterinary Dermatology* 5:57–62.

Munro, H.M.C. and Thrusfield, M.V., 2001. Battered Pets: sexual abuse *Journal of Small Animal Practice* 42: 333–337

New York State Agriculture and Markets Law Article 26, Section 374.

Reif, J.S., Brun, C., et al., March 1, 1998. Cancer of the nasal cavity and paranasal sinuses and exposure to environmental tobacco smoke in pet dogs *American Journal of Epidemiology* 147:(5) 488–92.

Sherdig, R., 1994. Intestinal viruses in *Saunders Manual of Small Animal Practice* (Stephen Birchard and Robert Sherdig, eds.). Philadelphia PA: WB Saunders 110–113.

Tuskegee University Brochure entitled HIV/AIDS & Pet Ownership. Tuskegee University School of Veterinary Medicine, Tuskegee AL 36088.

Wells, D.L., Graham, L., et al., 2002. The influence of auditory stimulation on the behaviour of dogs housed in a rescue shelter *Animal Welfare* 11, 385–393.

Appendix 8.1
Management Strategies to Prevent and Control Zoonosis

Create written policies regarding handling animals with zoonotic diseases.

Instruct staff to always wash hands frequently, especially after handling animals or feces.

Confirm the diagnosis and initiate prompt treatment if appropriate.

House sick animals in isolation and limit human contact.

Post signs on cage to advise about the condition.

Wear protective garments when handling animals or cleaning cages and animal enclosures—gloves, masks, gowns, and so on.

Educate staff about zoonotic conditions that occur in asymptomatic animals—Salmonella, Campylobacter, Dermatophytosis, and so on.

Stress importance of pest and vermin control to reduce vector-borne disease transmission.

Contact appropriate authorities promptly for reportable diseases.

Store human food separately from biologics, test samples, and so on.

Prepare animal food in separate areas from human food.

Provide staff with a lunchroom to avoid eating in animal areas.

Provide staff with pre-exposure rabies prophylaxis vaccinations.

Review and enforce sanitation procedures.

Store animal feeds securely to prevent vermin contamination.

Avoid self treatment of wounds acquired in the shelter—seek professional medical care.

Notify physicians you work with animals when unusual disease problems occur.

Appendix 8.2
Summary of Disease Management Protocols

Identify all affected animals (currently ill and exposed) and isolate them immediately.

Trace the arrival and movements of affected animals in the shelter to identify all other previously exposed animals—place in isolation.

Make an accurate diagnosis and determine whether treatment is appropriate—if yes, initiate immediately or place in foster care; if no, remove or euthanize.

Restrict the movement of animals, staff, and equipment throughout the building.

Initiate or strengthen quarantine procedures.

Identify appropriate disinfectant and instruct staff in its proper usage.

Review sanitation protocols on paper and in person—initiate tougher controls—install hand sanitizers, provide foot baths, mandate the use of gloves, and so on.

Inspect shelter, paying particular attention to ventilation system.

Perform rounds more frequently.

Review health care program—would vaccinations, disease testing help?

Determine when it is time to depopulate—cases are increasing, isolation is full, animals are showing no response to treatment, and so on.

Disinfect and shut down disease-infected areas for periods of time related to infectivity of disease organisms.

Appendix 8.3
Pain Management Drugs and Protocols

Opioid Drugs for Treating Pain in Dogs and Cats

Drug	Dog dosage mg/kg (IV, IM, SC)	Cat dosage mg/kg (IV, IM, SC)	Duration of action (hrs)	Comments	DEA schedule
Morphine	0.2–1	0.2–0.3	2–4	Histamine release possible with large IV bolus dose; CRI[*]:0.1–0.3 mg/kg/hr; Epidurally[#]: 0.1 mg/kg preservative-free product	II
Hydromorphone	0.1–0.2	0.1–0.2	2–4		II
Oxymorphone	0.05–0.1	0.05–0.1	2–4		II
Fentanyl	.004–.008	.002–.004	<1 hr	CRI[*]: 1–4 ug/kg/hr	II
Fentanyl Transdermal Patch	25 µg/kg/hr-small dog; 50 medium dog; 75 large dog; 100 giant breed	25 µg/kg/hr size	3–4 days	Takes 12 hr (cat) and 18 hr (dog) to reach therapeutic concentrations	
Meperidine	2–5	2–5	0.5–1	Histamine release possible after IV	II
Butorphanol	0.1–0.5	0.1–0.4	< 1 hr dog; Up to 2 hr cat		IV
Buprenorphine	0.005–0.02	0.005–0.01	6–8	Useful orally in cats BID–TID; Epidurally[#]: 5 µg/kg	V
Pentazocine	2–3	2–3	Up to 2 hr	Higher doses provide up to 2 hr	IV

[*] Constant Rate Infusion; Usually preceded by a bolus dose to rapidly achieve therapeutic plasma concentration
[#] Duration of action up to 24 hrs with morphine and buprenorphine

Appendix 8.3 *(continues)*

Other Sedative and Anesthetic Drugs for Treating Pain in Dogs and Cats

Drug	Dog Dosage	Cat Dosage	Duration of action (hrs)	Comments	DEA schedule
Ketamine	CRI: 2–10 µg/kg/min	CRI: 2–10 µg/kg/min	Duration of infusion	Subanesthetic dose; useful as analgesic adjunct when given with other analgesics	III
Xylazine	0.1–0. 2 mg/kg	0.1–0.2 mg/kg	< 1 hr	Sedation accompanies analgesia; not recommended if cardiovascular compromise present	—
Medetomidine	2–10 µg/kg	10–20 µg/kg	1–2 hr	Sedation accompanies analgesia; not recommended if cardiovascular compromise present	—

Nonsteroidal Anti-inflammatory Drugs for Treating Pain in Dogs and Cats

Drug	Dog dosage mg/kg	Cat dosage mg/kg
Aspirin	10–22 p.o. BID	10 p.o. q 48 hrs.
Carprofen	2 p.o., SC, BID or 4 SC, p.o.–SID	4 one time only
Deracoxib	3–4 p.o. SID for up to 7 days	Not recommended
Etodolac	10–15 SID	Not recommended
Katoprofen	2 SC, p.o. initially followed by 1 daily	2 SC, p.o. initially followed by 1 daily for 5 days
Meloxicam	0.2 SC, p.o. initially followed by 0.1 daily for 2–3 days	0.2 SC, p.o. initially followed by 0.1 daily for 2–3 days
Naproxen	1.2–2.2 p.o.q 1–2 days	Not recommended
Tepoxalin	10–20 p.o. 1st day 10 p.o. sid subsequent days	Not recommended

Appendix 8.3   *(continues)*

Local Anesthetic Drugs

Drug	Duration of action (hrs.)	Constant rate infusion	Nerve block or local infiltration*	Epidural
Lidocaine	1	40–60 µg/kg/min	1–2 mg/kg	4.0 mg/kg
Bupivacaine	2–4	—	1–2 mg/kg	1–2 mg/kg
Ropivacaine	2–4	—	1–2 mg/kg	1–2 mg/kg

*Includes Maxillary and Mandibular nerve blocks; nerve blocks for onychectomy; splash blocks and incisional line blocks

Sample Pain Treatment Protocols*

Example	Drug(s)	Comments
Ovariohysterectomy and castration	Opioid and/or alpha 2 agonist as part of preanesthetic regimen; Opioid and NSAID immediately postsurgically; NSAID continued for 3 days post surgery	Any opioid listed in previous table is acceptable as long as attention is given to dosing interval.
Fractures and severe soft tissue trauma#	Systemic Opioid; Epidural Opioid for rear limb fractures; Fentanyl Patch; Constant rate infusion of opioid plus lidocaine plus ketamine	Maximum analgesia needed. Combinations involving several categories are most useful for more severe degrees of trauma
Arthritis	NSAID	Use only with normal liver and kidney function

*Refer to Drug Tables for choice of specific drugs and dosing regimens
*Pain treatment protocols depend on drug availability and the availability of qualified personnel to administer controlled drugs.
#Trauma* of increasing magnitude requires relatively high doses and combination therapy using more than one category of drug

The source for all the tables in this appendix is Richard M. Bednarski, DVM, Diplomate ACVA, College of Veterinary Medicine, The Ohio State University.

9

Small Mammal Care in the Animal Shelter

Susan M. Prattis

INTRODUCTION

Small mammals are becoming popular as pets and scholarly subjects, offering many advantages to individual owners and/or educational communities; an additional bonus is that educational and research institutions increasingly are developing adoption programs for animals within specific experimental or educational criteria. Among the most commonly encountered species are mice, *Mus musculus;* rats, *Rattus norvegicus;* hamsters, including the Golden Syrian hamster, *Mesocricetus auratus,* the Chinese hamster *Cricetulus griseus,* and the dwarf hamster, *Phodopus sungorus;* gerbils, *Meriones unguiculatus;* guinea pigs, *Cavia porcellus*, including both Abyssian and Peruvian strains; Chinchilla, *Chinchilla laniger;* and exotic marsupials such as the sugar glider, *Petaurus brevicups*, African hedgehog, *Atalerix albiventris*, and the larger European hedgehog, *Erinaceus europaeus.*

In most instances, these smaller mammals are quiet, intelligent, and docile animals that when handled frequently and appropriately can become quite tame and affectionate, live a short to moderately long lifespan, are infected with relatively few diseases of zoonotic concern to humans, and provide many hours of interest and enjoyment. Rodent species have especially been used extensively in comparative medicine research settings due to cross-species physiological and genetic similarities in normative biology and disease pathogenesis mechanisms. In these settings, small mammals that serve as spontaneous animal models—surgically induced models or most frequently, genetically induced rodent models of normative biology and disease—typically are observed closely by scientists involved in their development and are housed under the professional care of laboratory animal veterinarians, laboratory animal technologists, and research animal caretakers. More recently, veterinarians in humane organization practice have begun to encounter these pets as outpatients or in a shelter setting along with traditional small animal and other exotic species, where there may be more questions arising about care for them in this arena.

The goal of this review chapter is to provide information to serve as a basis for providing quality care for small mammals and marsupials in the shelter, to consider facility and disease management in caring for these animal populations, and for using regulatory standards by individual veterinarians in animal husbandry and care in their individual shelter environments.

CLINICAL EXAMINATION AND EVALUATION

Prior to individual handling, small mammals should be initially evaluated for overall appearance at rest in their home cage environment, and their owners should be questioned closely about their pet's normative appearance, behavior, activity level, and medical/surgical history. (See Table 9.1, Small Mammal and Marsupial Normative Biology.) Healthy small mammals are active (frequently most apparent during nocturnal time periods) and exhibit all normal behavioral patterns such as grooming, burrowing, jumping, ambulation, and exploratory behavior following the introduction of novel stimuli and enrichment devices or after cage husbandry changes. Healthy small mammals also have normal food and water intake and excretion, with sleek fur, clear bright eyes, and no apparent abnormal ocular, nasal, or urogenital discharges or peripheral or dermatological masses.

Table 9.1. Small Mammal and Marsupial Normative Biology[a–e]

Species	Body Weight	RR	HR	Temp.	Gestation
	Grams	breaths/min	beats/min	C°	Days
Mice	20–40	60–220	325–780	36.0–37.0	19–21
Rats	250–520	70–115	50–450	36.5–37.5	21–23
Gerbils	55–100	90	360	37–38.5	24–26
Hamsters	85–150	35–135	250–500	37–38	15–16
Guinea Pigs	700–1200	42–104	200–300	37.2–9.5	59–62
Chinchilla	400–800	40–80	200–350	36.1–38.0	105–108
Sugar Gliders	95–160	16–40	200–3000	34.6–36.8	15–17
Afr. Hedge.	250–600	N/A	N/A	34.0–37.0	32–36
Eur. Hedge	400–1200	N/A	N/A	34.0–37.0	N/A

[a] Antinoff, N. Small mammal critical care *Veterinary Clinics of North America: Exotic Animal Practice* 1998; 1(1): 153–175.

[b] Harkness, J.E. 1994. Small rodents *Veterinary Clinics of North America: Small Animal Practice*; 24(1): 89–102.

[c] Harkness, J.E., and Wagner, J.W. 1995. *Clinical Procedures, Biology and Medicine of Rodents and Rabbits*; 44–95.

[d] Pye, G.W., and Carpenter, J.W. A Guide to Medicine and Surgery in Sugar Gliders www.hilltopanimal-hospital.com/sugarglider.htm.

[e] African Hedgehogs www.lpzoo.com/tour/factsheet/mammals/hedgego.html.

In contrast, a "sick rodent" appearance is customarily one in which fur is unkempt and ruffled (rats and mice) or matted (chinchilla, gerbil, and hamster), accompanied by a hunched appearance, closed and/or sunken eyes, nasal or ocular discharge that may be pigmented and found on forelimb paws, and a change in respiratory pattern and general activity in comparison to unaffected animals (Harkness and Wagner, 1995; Wagner and Farrar, 1987; Harkness, 1994). Sick sugar gliders have a similar appearance, with their head held low and ears flattened (MacPherson, 1997). This appearance, termed *sickness behavior*, is thought to be due in part to the effects of elevated cytokine expression in key neuroimmunological pathways (Konsmal, Parnet, and Dantzer, 2002). Sugar gliders are susceptible to bacterial and fungal systemic diseases, and so lethargy, matted fur, inappetance, diarrhea, vocalization, convulsions, and local or generalized swellings are indicative of a potential problem; in some instances, sudden death may be the only indication of acute disease (Salmonellosis, Toxoplasmosis) (Lightfoot, 2000; Pye and Carpenter, 2002).

Hedgehogs are especially susceptible to skin parasitic disease, to tumors, and to some bacterial infections (Lightfoot, 2000; Lightfoot, 1999; MacPherson, 1997). Parasitized animals may exhibit pruritis, quill loss, "moving quills," seborrhea, crusting, and other similar signs; those experiencing systemic disease will present with inappetance, depression, swelling, diarrhea, and other general signs of disease.

Rodent and small marsupial physical examinations are enhanced by the use of a quiet area, the provision of enhanced light, and gentle handling by the examiner; when stressed, rodents and other small mammals will communicate using ultrasonic vocalizations (Blom et al., 1995) that are potentially upsetting to other colony members or cage mates, making them subsequently more difficult to handle. It is helpful to have the following materials and equipment available prior to examination (Harkness, 1994; Antinoff, 1998): towels, plastic rodent restrainers; a penlight; rongeurs or dental burr to trim overgrown incisors or molars; a small (postal) scale with a restraint basket; a heat source, such as a circulating water pad, fluid pack, or a dry rice pack that may be microwaved for 1–2 minutes prior to use; cellophane tape and glass slides to assess pinworm ova and skin scrapings; fungal or other culture media; microhematological tubes (Microtainer, Becton Dickson, *Fisher Scientific*) and heparinized micropipette collection tubes; 1-ml and 3-ml syringes with 22–27 gauge needles; fine hair clippers or a depilatory cream; small to microsurgical instruments, surgical glue, and metal surgical clips; and parenteral fluids, antimicrobial preparations, and analgesic/anesthetic drugs as needed. Recently, a rodent health assessment applications package using Palm devices and local area network intranet has become available, which will allow computerized health and assessment screening of rodent populations (Hampshire, 2001). The program uses a weight composite distress paradigm chiefly characterized by weight loss as a means of identifying animals that might be at risk for metabolic or behavioral abnormalities or clinical disease (Hampshire, 2001). This type of package and equipment might be very useful for animal health triage and enhanced rodent welfare in shelters carrying large small mammal populations, or those with variable staffing responsibility for animal health evaluation without accompanying intensive animal care training in the husbandry, management and diseases of these species (Hampshire, 2001; Hampshire, 2001; *ILAR [Institute for Laboratory Animal Research] Guide for the Care and Use of Laboratory Animals*, 1998).

Many rodents and exotic mammals will defecate and/or urinate (rats and mice), ball up (hedgehogs) or vocalize audibly (sugar gliders) initially when picked up, but this tendency may decrease in animals that are handled routinely. Mice may be cupped in hand, picked up using a gentle grip by the base of the tail and placed on a cage top, hand, or arm for further examination, or by lightly applying pressure against their back while firmly grasping the skin over the neck, shoulders, and back; this grip is the most secure one and allows closer examination of the animal with better manipulation of limbs and digits, abdominal palpation, gender determination, and drug administration while preventing bite injury to the examiner. Male and female weanling mice are similar in size; however, a greater anogenital distance exists in male mice

(1.5–2 times larger than female), and their testes can be detected through the skin. It is best to determine gender composition of a litter by picking up the mice, lifting their tails, and comparing them directly (Harkness and Wagner, 1995). In addition, male mice have a larger genital papillae than do female mice, and female mice exhibit prominent nipples by nine days of age (Harkness and Wagner, 1995). Mice reach sexual maturity by 21 days of age, with first estrous occurring at 28–40 days of age (Harkness and Wagner, 1995). Females exhibit a four-to-five day estrous cycle with a period of nocturnal behavioral estrous lasting 12 hours in duration (Harkness and Wagner, 1995).

Rats should be picked up using a gentle grip of the base of the tail and subsequent placement on a surface or cage lid; alternatively, they may be grasped gently around the thorax with thumb and forefingers held under the animal's mandible and chin, with support provided to the rat's hindquarters. Large retractable testes are apparent in weanling and adult rats and are completely descended by 20–50 days (when they drop down from the inguinal canal), and nipples are prominent in females by 8–15 days of age. As in the mouse, rats exhibit differences in anogenital distance with males having a longer distance than do females (Harkness and Wagner, 1995). Rats are polyestrous, cycling every four to five days with a nocturnal estrous behavioral period of 12 hours in length.

Guinea pigs may also be picked up by scooping them against the body while supporting the hind limbs; however, chinchillas prefer to be scooped up and held close to the body, with their head tucked underneath the arm (Lightfoot, 1999). Male guinea pigs are distinguished by their larger size, smaller nipples, and scrotal pouches containing large testes (Harkness and Wagner, 1995). As is the case in the dog, there is a penile baculum (*os penis*) in the guinea pig (Harkness and Wagner, 1995). Female guinea pigs have a Y-shaped genital anal opening, a closed vaginal membrane and a bicornuate uterus. Male guinea pigs reach puberty by eight weeks of age and females by five to six weeks of age (Harkness and Wagner, 1995). Guinea pigs exhibit a 15–17 day estrous period, with a 24–48 hour behavioral estrous. Gestation is 58–60 days in length.

Hamsters have large amounts of excessive skin and cheek pouches that necessitate a firm grasp, using the dorsal approach noted previously for mice; to do otherwise may result in bites from the hamster. Common pet species include the golden hamster and the Siberian hamster; both species exhibit equally feisty temperaments. Siberan hamsters are smaller, although males can be differentiated by their larger size; males and females reach maturity at 150 days and 90–130 days, respectively (Harkness and Wagner, 1995). Gestation is 18 days in length; both males and females may be housed in groups.

Gerbils, characteristically curious rodents, will readily approach a hand that is placed into their cage; they should be lifted gently by the base of their tail and placed onto a surface. There is a very pronounced difference in anogenital distance between male and female gerbils, with female distance being extremely short (5 mm) compared to the male (10 mm). In addition, male gerbils have a very large scrotal sac, a dark scrotum, and in adults, a large, midventral androgen–responsive scent marking gland (Harkness and Wagner, 1995). Both genders exhibit a pronounced genital papillae (Harkness and Wagner, 1995).

Chinchilla are similar to guinea pigs in overall biology but are less weighty and reactive animals than are other rodents. Gender determination in chinchilla is determined by the presence of a penis cranial to the rectum in males of any age, and, visible testes in adult animals. Female chinchilla are much smaller than are the male chinchilla and also exhibit vaginal membrane closure prior to estrous, breeding, and parturition (Lightfoot, 1999).

One common phenomenon exhibited by chinchilla, gerbils, and to a lesser extent, rats, is that of fur slip or tail slip, in which the application of excessive pressure to the end of the tail will result in slippage of skin and fur (rats and gerbils) or epilation of fur (chinchilla) and release of the rodent; this reaction is a prey species adaptation meant to facilitate escape from predator species and can be avoided with gentle handling as noted previously (Lightfoot, 1999).

African, European, or Asian Hedgehogs have become popular as pets and are relatively tame as young animals but become increasingly more difficult to handle as they approach adulthood (Lightfoot, 1999; Lightfoot, 2000). Examination is impeded by their characteristic behavioral pattern of curling into a ball with extruding noninjurious

spines, and inhalant isoflurane anesthesia is recommended to facilitate full physical examination if this behavior occurs (Lightfoot, 1999). Gender determination in hedgehogs is slightly different than in rodents. Male hedgehogs are larger than females (up to 600 gm body weight), have a small prepuce, and have a penis that is located very far forward of the anus; there is no scrotal sac (Lightfoot, 1999). However, testicles can be palpated in the subcutaneous skin in anesthetized animals (Lightfoot, 1999).

Sugar gliders, marsupials so termed because of the presence of a ptargium between the lateral aspect of the front leg and the tarsus, which enables gliding (MacPherson, 1997), are a social species and should be housed in paired or group housing (Lightfoot, 1999; MacPherson, 1997). Although active in dim light in the presence of an owner, it is difficult for an unfamiliar person to examine sugar gliders while fully awake. An initial examination should consist of a prolonged discussion with the owner, if possible, or with the handler during which activity level and external physical indices can be observed. A more in-depth examination may require inhalant isoflurane anesthesia for full clinical assessment and manipulation (Lightfoot, 1999). Sugar gliders reach a weight of 100–150 grams as adults.

Young sugar gliders (*joeys*) are sexually dimorphic: males exhibit a scrotum, a wart–like area on the ventral abdomen, and females have a furless midventral longitudinal slit area that is the site of the pouch (MacPherson, 1997). The scrotum in adult male gliders is covered with fur, and there are prominent diamond-shaped bald spots on the forehead and chest, which are scent marking glands; scent and urine marking is used by sugar gliders to identify territory and family or group members (MacPherson, 1997). Adult female sugar gliders have a pouch, which is used following parturition for further development of young sugar gliders.

Male and female sugar gliders have a cloacal aperture, which serves the combined purposes of reproduction, urinary, and alimentary tract excretion (MacPherson, 1997). In adult male sugar gliders, penile extrusion will occur from this cavity (MacPherson, 1997). Sugar gliders reach sexual maturity at five months and breed year round; females undergo a 29-day estrous period. Gestation is 16 days in duration; after parturition, immature young (eyelids and ears fused) migrate to the pouch, take the nipple in their mouths, and proceed to nurse (MacPherson, 1997). The nipple increases in size to allow for continual nursing without the requirement of strong suckling muscles to allow the joey to remain attached to the dam. When they emerge from the pouch approximately eight weeks later, their eyes remain shut for an additional seven to ten days; emergence occurs in stages, with limbs and the tail preceding total emergence from the pouch (MacPherson, 1997). After joeys have arrived, male and female sugar gliders share equally in raising their young (MacPherson, 1997).

PHYSICAL EXAMINATION AND DISEASE ASSESSMENT

When examining small mammals it is important to evaluate systemic organ systems in parallel to those of larger animals (Lightfoot, 1999; Lightfoot, 2000; Wagner and Farra, 1994; Quesenberry, 1994). Physical examination should consist of palpation and auscultation of the thorax and abdomen and palpation of appendicular skeletal structures. Assessment of hydration status, which is crucial in small rodents and marsupials as they can become rapidly dehydrated and expire, uses similar indices to those found in larger animals, e.g., skin elasticity and turgor, ocular distension, and mucosal observation and/or refill time responses. Anogenital sites should be examined for gender determination as well as for dermatitis, diarrhea, or fecal staining, fecal impaction, and physiological or pathological vaginal/preprutial discharge or swelling. Some species are prone to disease conditions resulting in abdominal swelling (for example, cystic ovaries in guinea pigs, hepatic lipidosis and hepatic adenocarcinoma in hedgehogs, and neoplasia in all small mammals; similarly, firm hepatosplenic or renal palpation may be detected in amyloidosis–affected hamsters) (Harkness, 1994; Lightfoot, 1999, Lightfoot, 2000; Quesenberry, 1994; Wagner and Farrar, 1994).

Skin is the largest organ system and is the site of numerous parasitic, fungal, and primary and secondary disease manifestations in small mammals (Ellis and Mori, 2001; Harkness, 1994; Wagner and Farrar, 1994; Lightfoot, 1999; Lightfoot, 2000). Barberism, or barbering, is a behavioral grooming phenomena in which an individual(s) removes hair from selected haircoat areas (while underlying skin remains completely normal) of another individual of the same species during periods in which domi-

nance hierarchies are established, or shifted. Some similarities in clinical syndromes have been described across species due to barberism in chinchillas, mice, hamsters, and gerbils. The lesion distribution in barbering differs among the species, with hair loss on shoulders, flanks, sides, and paws in chinchillas or the base of the tail and head in gerbils, and whiskers, head, shoulders, back, and tail-base in mice and hamsters (Ellis and Mori, 2001). The pathogenesis of this behavioral phenomenon has not been definitively identified but has included husbandry, nutritional, heritable, metabolic, endocrinological, and potential fungal factors (Ellis and Mori, 2001). In all species treatment includes the removal of the aggressive or dominant individual and in chinchilla, the adjustment of room temperature and relative humidity levels to 16–21 degrees Centigrade (60–70 degrees Fahrenheit), and 40–60 percent RH, along with additional roughage, increased dust bath exposure (one part Fuller's earth and nine parts silver sand), and toys to enrich the environment (Ellis and Mori, 2001). Behavioral modification has been suggested for use especially in chinchilla, including fluoxetine hydrochloride (Prozac, Dista Products, Indianapolis, IN) at a recommended dosage of 5–10 mg/kg per os (Ellis and Mori, 2001).

Other common causes of alopecia considered as differential diagnoses must be excluded, including parasitism, fungal and bacterial skin infections, and various environmental, behavioral or physiological conditions contributing to fur loss (Ellis and Mori, 2001; Harkness, 1994; Quesenberry, 1994). Chief among them is rodent ectoparasitism, including rodent fleas Xenopsylla, Leptosylla, and Nosopsylla spp., which serve as vectors for Yersinia pestis and Ricettsia typhus and an intermediate host for Hymenolepsis spp. tapeworm infections in humans and other species (Ellis and Mori, 2001). Mites and lice can be quite common in wild mice but less frequently observed in other rodents (Ellis and Mori, 2001; Harkness and Wagner, 1995). Parasitic species observed include Demodex auratis; Liponyssoides sanguineus in chinchilla and gerbil; Myobia musculi, Mycoptes musculinus, Radafordia affinis, and Psoregates simplex in mice; Radfordia ensifera and Notoedres muris in rats; and Liponyssus bacoti (a zoonotic agent and vector for murine typhus, tularemia, Q fever, and plague) in rats and mice (Ellis and Mori, 2001). Polyplax serrata, the only louse infecting mice, is a vector for Encephal-itozoon cuniculi, Eperythrozoon coccoides, and Haembartonella muris, all of which may affect other animal species that might be encountered in a shelter housing environment (Ellis and Mori, 2001).

Guinea pigs are susceptible to Trixacaris cariae (see below); Sarcoptes mures and Notoedres spp mites may rarely infect guinea pigs. Chirodiscoides caviae fur mites are distinct in that they are typically detected in mating pairs (Ellis and Mori, 2001; Harkness and Wagner, 1995). Guinea pigs are also susceptible to lice such as Gyropus ovalis and Gliricola porcelli, Trimenopen jenningsi and Tri-menopen hispidum nosocomial infections have also been described in guinea pigs (Ellis and Mori, 2001). Trixacaris caviae is a common sarcoptic mite in guinea pigs that should be treated aggressively with ivermectin and environmental decontamina-tion when detected to avoid fatalities (Ellis and Mori, 2001). D. criceti and aurati have been re-ported in hamsters as have Notoedres notoedres and N. cati, and Liponyssus bacoti; unlike other rodent species, L. bacoti is a transient parasite in hamsters, and so treatment is directed at frequent cage changes in lieu of antiparasitic medication (Ellis and Mori, 2001).

Hedgehog species are very susceptible to ec-toparasitic agents such as Caparinia tripilis, a psoroptid mite that is large enough to be detected visually, Sarcoptes and Notoedres spp. in European and New Zealand hedgehogs; Chorioptes spp. in African pygmy hedgehogs; and the hedgehog flea (Archaeopsylla erinacei). At present time no lice species have been reported in association with hedgehog species (Ellis and Mori, 2001). Sugar gliders are susceptible to ectoparasitic species sim-ilar to those described in rodents and may be treated accordingly (Ellis and Mori, 2001).

Ear pinna necrosis has been noted in some mouse strains and in chinchilla; the pathogenesis has been identified as otitis media, frostbite, and acariasis. In addition, chinchillas and mice will exhibit intra-species aggressions resulting in bite wound injuries to the outer pinna, and in chinchilla, ear he-matomas. These lesions are treated in a similar fashion to other traditional species, including de-bridement as needed with the use of antiseptics such as betadine or chlorhexidine-based products. Lancing and draining the hematoma with a surgical

suture support layer with topical antibiotics as noted are also indicated (Ellis and Mori, 2001).

Oral examination is difficult in many species due to the narrow orifice, decreased range of motion, and excess folds and tissues within the oropharyn-gal cavity. Sedation or anesthesia induced by par-enteral drug administration (Wagner and Farrar, 1994; Adamcak and Otten, 2000; Antinoff, 1998; Johnson–Delaney, 2000) followed by use of intense focal lighting, an otoscope with a short cone attach-ment, and either 1) a curved pediatric nasal specu-lum or pediatric laryngoscope (Lightfoot, 1999), 2) a larnygoscope with a no. 0 Wisconsin blade, or 3) a straight Miller no. 0 neonatal blade to displace the tongue will assist in visualizing incisor and molar teeth (Quesenberry, 1994). Those that cannot be vi-sualized can also be assessed by inserting a cot-ton–tipped applicator into the oropharynx to iden-tify points and sharp edges caused by uneven dental wear that can then be removed using bone rongeurs or a rotating dental drill (Lightfoot, 1999; Quesen-berry, 1994).

Incisor (rodents, sugar gliders) or incisor and mo-lar malocclusion can result in buccal laceration or tongue entrapment in guinea pigs and chinchilla. It is a major underlying cause of morbidity in small mammals and is exhibited as inappetance or anorexia, drooling and food dropping, weight loss and chronic malnutrition due to protein and caloric deficiencies, infertility, alopecia, mucosal lacera-tion with secondary bacterial infection, and in-creased susceptibility to other secondary infections (Harkness, 1994; Wagner and Farrar, 1994; Light-foot, 1999; Lightfoot, 2000; Quesenberry, 1994). Hedgehogs do not have open rooted dentition and rarely experience malocclusion (Lightfoot, 1999). However, they are susceptible to gingivitis, peri-odontal disease, and oral neoplasia and should be examined closely as they age for these diseases (Lightfoot, 1999). This species has also been impli-cated as a carrier of viral stomatitis (foot and mouth disease) with broad implications for importation regulations and disease exposure patterns (Light-foot, 1999).

Ocular disease has been noted in hedgehogs and chinchilla as a sequela of trauma toward their slightly protruding eyes, and in mice and rats fol-lowing infection (Pasturella pneumotropica in mice, Sialodacryoadenitis virus in rats), overt exposure to continuous and/or high ambient light levels in susceptible strains, and as an iatrogenic consequence of ocular bleeding from the posterior venous sinus in the back of the orbit (Small, 1994). Topical administration of antibiotics and analgesics/topical anesthetics to mitigate corneal ulceration or laceration are indicated as in traditional small animal species. It is worth noting that ocular bleeding is no longer considered to be a humane methodology when performed without first placing rodents under anesthesia (ILAR, 1998). Proptosis of the globe has been reported in rodents and hedgehogs; as long as a functional papillary response is present, an acute proptosis can be replaced with gentle pressure following application of DMSO or Dextrose, two agents that aid in decreasing traumatic swelling after the event (Antinoff, 1998). In the event of chronic proptosis, surgical anesthesia followed by an eye enucleation procedure is indicated.

DISEASE SURVEILLANCE AND PREVENTION

In most instances, small mammals relinquished to shelters are turned in with their cages. If the cages are appropriate, most shelters will keep them in their individual cages, thus minimizing the risk of disease spread through isolation. In some cases, however, there will be ongoing and continual introduction of new animals into open small mammal and marsupial housing colonies. The occasion may also arise wherein several animals are brought to the shelter as a result of a cruelty investigation, and they may have to be held for long periods of time. Most rodent infectious diseases especially are subclinical in nature, and incoming populations may appear superficially to be healthy. If shelters have large rodent populations, rapid turnover, mixing of incoming rodent species, or intrusion of wild rodents into existing facilities, institution of a disease surveillance program (Dillehay et al., 1990; Thigpen, J.E., 1989; Otto and Talwani, 2001) would be appropriate. Use of principles of sanitation and disease prevention in all species housing rooms is particularly applicable and important in this setting. It might be useful to evaluate index cases using serology and histopathological examination.

Some diseases are transmissible between species. Examples include Bordetella bronchiseptica (cats, dogs, guinea pigs, and humans); Toxoplasma gondi (cats, sugar gliders, and humans); Salmonella spp. (rodents, sugar gliders, dogs, cats, and humans);

and Encephalomyocarditis virus (rats and mice to sugar gliders). In these cases, it is particularly important to identify agents in question that could be causing disease in shelter populations through careful observation of the animals and preventative measures such as separation of housing facilities, room sanitation equipment, cage housing environment, personnel training, and traffic patterns.

Maintaining quarantine procedures with physical and functional separation of species and individuals by known or suspected disease status would also be useful procedures to institute if group housing is used. One possibility includes isolating incoming individuals, pairs, or groups in a separate room in polycarbonate shoebox static microisolator housing. This would significantly decrease transmission of viral, parasitic, and bacterial disease in animal populations. Microisolator units are affordable and consist of a cage bottom, filtered cage lid, and wire rack for food and water presentation to rodents housed within the unit; usually water bottles, sipper tube, and stoppers must be purchased separately (Allentown Equipment, PA; Lab Products, MI) but should fit within the confines of the cage bottom and filter top lid to protect cage occupants. Microisolator housing densities will vary with animal size (ILAR Guide, 1998).

Isolating incoming individuals, pairs, or groups in a separate room (in a polycarbonate shoebox static microisolator if possible), using chlorine dioxide or a 1:32 dilution of household bleach during cage and rack sanitation and using disposable clothing (for example, shoe covers, masks, gloves, laboratory coats, and bonnets) may decrease spread of infectious disease agents during initial quarantine holding periods and assist in isolating specific diseased individuals, colonies, or rooms in the shelter. Species that require larger housing quarters or that are best housed in open caging could be treated as a group, and their health status managed at the room population level with modified entry and exit procedures similar to those noted previously.

Many small mammal or marsupial pets are derived from wild caught colonies or are bred and produced by breeders. These pet origin colonies are not considered to be free of specific pathogens but may be endemically and subclinically infected with a variety of different organisms (Prattis and Morse, 1990; Pakes et al., 1994; Harkness and Wagner,

1995; Wagner and Farrar, 1994; Small, 1994) and contain considerable genetic variability, including genes governing disease susceptibility. Pet rats and some mice classically are afflicted with bacterial and viral respiratory and gastrointestinal disease, endoparasitism and ectoparasitism. Hamsters have routinely exhibited gastrointestinal disease, most often manifested as diarrhea (and potentially zoonotic if due to agents such as Hymenlepsis spp tapeworm or Campylobacteriosis) and in aged animals, amyloidosis; guinea pigs carry opportunistic Bordetella spp. organisms in the oropharynx that can be exacerbated into frank pneumonia and sepsis and includes variants of Bordetella bronchiseptica, the causative agent of canine kennel cough and arguably part of the upper respiratory infection complex in cats; gerbils have variable penetrance of epileptiform seizure expression. There may be vast differences in severity of disease expression even among animals that become clinically ill depending on age, genetic strain, or stock background, and the presence of other concurrent infections (Small, 1994; Pakes et al., 1994).

Similarly, sugar gliders are susceptible to a simi-lar spectrum of bacterial disease as are encountered in larger species, as well as a range of fungal skin infections, Herpesviruses, and Encephalomyocardi-tis viruses. They are also stress susceptible and should not be exposed to overly warm or cool hous-ing areas but should be housed in room tempera-tures ranging from 64–74°F/18–24°C (Pye and Carpenter, 2002).

For some of the reasons already mentioned, a for-mal system of disease monitoring may be desirable in some shelter settings. The sentinel assessment programs that are used to monitor disease in labo-ratories with large populations of long-term resi-dential small mammal colonies typically require an-imals to be euthanized and would, thus, not be suitable for shelters whose mission is one of pro-viding for relatively short duration housing for ani-mal welfare. However, one application of a labora-tory program that might prove useful is to develop a disease risk analysis management plan based on Monthly Disease Frequency (MDF) data determi-nations (Akhtar and Khan, 1995). MDF is defined using the monthly incidence density (ID) method, as the following:

$$ID = \frac{\text{Number of cases of disease } x \text{ during month } k}{\text{Number of animals at risk at the end of the previous month} - (\frac{1}{2} \text{ withdrawals}) + (\frac{1}{2} \text{ additions})}$$

This method is especially applicable for dynamic animal populations featuring a high degree of ani-mal turnover and multiple cases of specific disease entities (Akhtar and Khan, 1995) as might be pres-ent in a shelter.

Disease exposure and transmission among colony animals are also decreased when instituting a quar-antine program, separate isolated housing area and dedicated personnel, materials, and procedures for handling and housing newly received rodents and small mammals of indeterminant health status. Be-cause infectious disease is frequently subclinical in nature, diagnosis may be facilitated through the use of relatively inexpensive in-house solid phase ELISA testing (Immunocomb, Charles River Labo-ratories, MA), cellophane tape examination of fecal egg shedding, and classical fecal parasitic examina-tion. More extensive commercial testing may be im-plemented as shelter finances and priorities allow, consisting of complete blood count and chemistry, serodiagnostic and nucleic acid testing, and viral, bacterial, or fungal isolation (Thigpen, 1989; Rehg and Toth, 1998; Otto and Talwani, 2001). Testing programs can be advantageous in that they can re-quire minimal amounts of physical space and rela-tively inexpensive housing equipment. One poten-tial drawback of testing programs may be their expense and the length of duration of sentinel expo-sure required to accurately and sensitively assess the presence of infectious agents in a closed colony; open colonies with fluctuating animal numbers should be considered to be conventional colonies, and their assessment needs may be less intense. Testing time period duration, diagnostic assessment extent, and accompanying expense may be altered and tailored by individual shelters in accordance with their caseload and the desired level of health status of their particular animal population.

HUSBANDRY CARE AND MANAGEMENT

Good animal husbandry is the basis of disease prevention and in some cases, treatment; is subject to governmental regulation (ILAR, 1998); and is a hallmark of humane animal care in any setting. In a shelter setting, most rodent species can be comfortably housed in clear plastic caging (polypropylene or high temperature that may be autoclaved) and on direct bedding. Use of inclusive microisolator caging systems consisting of a fitted, filtered cage lid, a cage for direct bedding, and an integrated food hopper, specially designed water bottle, and water bottle holder or automatic watering system outlet (Allentown Caging, PA; Lab Products, MI) allows for the receipt of new arrivals from differing health backgrounds in the same, or contiguous, colony housing area in the shelter facility.

Water may be provided through water bottles equipped with well–fitting stoppers and sipper tubes or through automatic watering systems, which must be checked daily to detect sipper blockage and ensure that they are working. Detecting small volumes of water ingested by these mammals or providing water–based drug treatments may be accomplished using a modified autoclavable sipper tube apparatus (Pan et al., 1986). Many rodents enjoy stuffing bedding materials into water sipper sites, resulting in a blockade or alternatively, cage flooding. It is particularly important to be sure that young animals can reach the sipper tube to obtain water while being weaned and afterward. It is also possible to acidify (pH 2.5) or chlorinate (10–12 ppm) water supplies to decrease bacterial contamination (Harkness and Wagner, 1995). A chlorine solution should be prepared using 2 ml of a 5.25 percent sodium hypochlorite solution in 10 L of water, resulting in a 10 ppm Cl_2 solution. Similarly, 2.6 ml of concentrated hydrochloric acid should be added to 10 L of water to prepare a solution measuring approximately pH 2.5; the specific resulting pH should be measured as variation in water composition across different locales (Harkness and Wagner, 1995).

Cage bedding should be changed a minimum of once per week, and preferably 2–3 times per week depending on animal size, physiological status, and cage population to meet cage sanitation standards and to contribute to animal well-being (Blom et al., 1996; Duke, 2001; ILAR, 1998). Mice and rats in particular appear to exhibit clear preferences for bedding materials consisting of easily manipulated, larger fibrous particles that do not produce high ultrasound production when disturbed, such as shredded filter paper or wood chips (Blom et al. 1966). While selecting areas for fecal and urinary deposition, the remainder of the direct bedding cage is used primarily for nest resting, digging, and additional shredding (Blom et al., 1996). Pine, cedar, and any other softwood bedding materials that produce elevated dust levels and act to induce liver P450 enzymatic systems should be avoided in rodents; exposure to these agents may result in the modified drug duration of action and decreased efficacy (Harkness and Wagner, 1995; Wagner and Farrar, 1994). These products may also be toxic in sugar gliders. A number of other low dust-producing products are appropriate for this use including corncob or paper pellets, hardwood chips, or artificial media. Chronic prophylactic treatment for skin mite infestation can be instituted in colony rooms using permethrin–treated bedding (MiteArrest, EcoHealth, Inc., MA) in addition to standard therapeutic intervention (see the following section).

Cage cleaning procedures in rodents that are not frequently handled can result in significant elevation in cardiovascular indices (blood pressure levels and heart rate) and modified arousal behavioral patterns (investigative ambulation, grooming, and rearing) immediately after completion of these tasks and for 45–60 minutes afterward (Duke et al., 2001). In some instances, it may be preferable to house rodents in raised hanging wire caging with excretory deposition on treated surfaces below the housing area. This type of animal housing may result in pododermatitis and traumatic injury especially in larger guinea pig boars and sows; some authors have recommended the use of rectangular mesh measuring 75×12 mm (Quesenberry, 1994).

Similarly, the absence of husbandry cage cleaning in hamsters, first-time murine (rats or mice) breeders, and in some individuals in other species during the week prior to, and after, parturition may decrease the incidence of litter cannibalism observed (Harkness and Wagner, 1995; Wagner and Farrar, 1994). Nest building materials should be provided for pregnant mice, gerbils, and hamsters, allowing them to engage in species–specific nest building periparturient behavior (Harkness and

Wagner, 1995; Wagner and Farrar, 1994). An unusual and characteristic behavior frequently observed in hamsters is stuffing their cheek pouches with food; an alarmed dam may also sequester her neonates in this same fashion, with later deposition to the nest.

NUTRITION AND HOUSING

Some rodents are omnivorous, with wild species ingesting a variety of plant foodstuffs, seeds, fruits, and meats, and others (chinchilla, guinea pigs) are herbivorous cecal fermenters that require roughage and exhibit intestinal physiological similarities to species such as rabbits and horses. Pet rodents can be easily and well fed using commercial rodent chows. Guinea pigs are especially susceptible to vitamin C deficiency (Scurvy), which can be avoided by using freshly milled, refrigerated vitamin C-containing feed specifically for this species. Because vitamin C is degraded by heat, and with time, such food should be discarded after 60 days. Guinea pigs require 5–20 mg vitamin C per kg bodyweight, and pregnant or lactating sows require at least 20 mg/kg vitamin C daily (Quesenberry, 1994). This requirement can be met by feeding commercial guinea pig chow, which contains an average of 800 mg ascorbic acid per kg of feed (Quesenberry, 1994).

Younger mice and some specific mouse strains are unable to eat commercial pelleted food because it is too hard for their teeth to effectively crush or grind; in these instances, food may be moistened and placed in a container on the cage floor, being careful to remove that which is not eaten or becomes contaminated with excretory materials. Alternatively, young mice may be fed a diet that is packaged as kibble and not in hardened pellets (Ralston Purina, MO). Hamsters should be fed from receptacles that have especially wide and blunt slats to accommodate their broader nasal anatomy and to prevent the onset of nasal dermatitis.

Rodents and other small mammals benefit from the presence of enrichment devices that should be items that are impervious to chewing, easily sanitized, and consistent with the normal species behavioral patterns such as PVC piping (to provide runways and hiding spots), exercise wheels, nest boxes, and chew toys. Well-washed fruit, vegetables, and other treats presented in a puzzle feeder or by dispersion to facilitate foraging behavior can

also serve this purpose (Cheal, 1987). It is also possible to introduce chronic medical treatments to a small mammal colony using food as a vehicle; an example commonly in use is medicated feed, with the addition of 150 ppm fenbendazole (Harlan Teklad, WI) alternated on a biweekly basis with standard rodent chow to eliminate pinworm infection in rodent colonies (Otto and Talwani, 2001). Reproductive indices may be affected by nutritional support, and commercial rodent diets (Ralston Purina, MO) provide enhanced content for pregnant and/or lactating rodents.

Sugar gliders are best housed in modified aviary flight cages lined with shredded paper or a similar material to allow them to climb and in larger units, exhibit gliding behavior. They are social animals and seem to thrive in captivity more easily with members of their own species; young sugar gliders can become acclimated to human interaction if handled regularly from the time that they exit from their dam's pouch (Lightfoot, 1999; Pye and Carpenter, 2002). Those that are housed as single pets can develop unusual behavioral patterns (Lightfoot, 1999).

Because this is a nocturnal species, it is advantageous to provide nest boxes for hiding and sleeping during the day; adding a sock, or other cloth material that can be easily sanitized would be preferable (Pye and Carpenter, 2002). Inverted drinking water sipper tubes are appropriate for use in this species as are hanging enrichment device toys. Sugar gliders are insectivorous and have short digestive tracts similar to carnivores. They can ingest sweet liquids (nectars) but are usually maintained on commercially available sugar glider pellets and insectivore diets (Exotic Nutrition, VA); monkey chow (Mazuri primate diets—Purina Mills); or bird pellets, crickets, and mealworms (Pye and Carpenter, 2002; Johnson–Delaney, 2000). Useful supplements include manna, gums, and honeydew melon; small freshly dead vertebrates such as mice or cooked chicken; and arthropods (Pye and Carpenter, 2002; Johnson–Delaney, 2000). Pregnant or lactating animals should be supported with increased nutritional plane. Maintenance nutritional feeding levels are typically offered daily at 15–25 percent of the sugar glider's body weight with average weights being 140 gm (males) to 115 gm (females) (Pye and Carpenter, 2002). It is particularly important to change nectar sources regularly and frequently and to sanitize feeding containers for this species because the highly concentrated sugar–based foods that they ingest are a rich media for support of microorganism growth. Sugar gliders should not be fed dry dog food, or they will develop hypervitaminosis D.

Hedgehogs, while variably social as young animals, can become increasingly aloof and more difficult to handle as they mature to adulthood (Lightfoot, 1999); continued extensive and gentle handling is necessary to ensure that this does not occur. All hedgehogs currently obtained as pets originate from captive breeding colonies; special permits may be required to hold these species. Two states do not currently allow hedgehogs as pets (Arizona and California).

Hedgehogs are also an insectivorous species but can ingest other types of foods with a tendency toward significant weight gain with age; because they are a nocturnal species, they should have fresh food made available at night (Lightfoot, 1999). Many hedgehogs will also exhibit an unusual foaming hypersalivation reaction on tasting new items, including normal dietary components, medications, and toys; this is a normal phenomenon in this species. Hedgehogs can be housed on direct bedding in a similar manner to rodents as described previously. The addition of nesting boxes or similar hiding areas, running wheels, and other enrichment devices within the cage housing area is helpful; extremities trauma, observed as lameness or other gait abnormalities, has also been reported previously when held under these conditions.

SMALL MAMMAL AND MARSUPIAL THERAPEUTICS

All therapeutic drug usage in these small mammals should be considered to be extra label usage. Although marsupials such as sugar gliders are considered to exhibit lower metabolic rates than mammals, similar liver and enteric metabolic responses suggest that pharmacological doses of common agents used in these species are similar to those used in mammals. Allometric scaling can be used to calculate a questionable drug dosage based on the basal metabolic rate using drug dosages that have been pharmokinetically determined for a model species, although some authors have asserted that this approach can be insensitive to species-specific adaptations in gastrohepatic physiology and dietary preferences (Johnson–Delaney, 2000). Sugar glid-

ers can be treated using empirical drug dosages as those used for ferrets or cats (Johnson–Delaney, 2000; Adamcak and Otten, 2000).

The African/Asian hedgehog (*Atalerix albiventris)* and the European hedgehog (*Erinaceous europaeus)* do not necessarily require the same drug dosages due to differences in size, seasonal physiological variation, and diet (Lightfoot, 1999; Lightfoot, 2000). Parenteral drug administration is most commonly used; due to a significant subcutaneous fat layer, a tendency toward obesity in adult hedgehogs, and protective balling behavior, such injections are frequently deposited in subcutaneous sites underneath the quills (Lightfoot, 2000); increased drug and fluid absorption from these sites can be induced by incorporating hyaluronidase or Wydase (Wyeth Laboratories, PA) into the injected volume (Lightfoot, 2000). Topical and ocular drug access in the hedgehog is difficult due to grooming habits and avoidance, although they do respond well to shampoos and topical rinses. Intravenous drug access can be obtained by using the cephalic vein (26 gauge needle, insulin/TB syringe or butterfly) (Lightfoot, 2000).

Systemic antibiotic usage (Johnson-Delaney, 2000; Harkness, 1994; Wagner and Farrar, 1995; Adamcak and Otten, 2000; Antinoff, 1998) and management of postoperative pain (Antinoff, 1998; Wagner and Farrar, 1994) can be indicated with most small mammals and marsupials when afflicted with conditions that would respond to such intervention. Delaney–Johnson has published an excellent formulary for use in marsupial species (Delaney–Johnson, 2000).

Abundant citations document drug dosages, routes, and responses in rodent species, and several standard formularies are in general use (Adamcak and Otten, 2000). Parenteral drug administration in rodents most commonly utilizes subcutaneous (SC), intramuscular (IM), or intraperitoneal (IP) sites; careful restraint is required in all instances to ensure correct drug delivery and to avoid being bitten. Commercial plastic rodent restraint tubes are also available for this purpose (Plas-Lab, MI). Subcutaneous drug administration is frequently placed into the dorsal neck region, with intramuscular injections being given in the quadriceps or triceps muscle groups. Intraperitoneal injections should be administered in the left abdomen, with the animal's head tilted down to avoid puncturing viscera. Oral gavage using an insulin or TB syringe, or variably sized blunt-ended probes made specifically for that purpose according to the size of the rodent species being treated, is quite common as is venous superficial lateral tail vein injection in rats (Antinoff, 1998). The cephalic, lateral saphenous or femoral veins are also accessible in chinchilla, guinea pigs and rats (Antinoff, 1998). As noted previously, orbital venous sinus/plexus venipuncture to obtain a blood sample (*eye bleeding*) in rodents is no longer recommended in the absence of anesthesia. In emergency or critical care settings, an intraosseous catheter, consisting of a 18-, 20-, or 22-gauge needle, may be placed in larger rodents, mammals, and marsupials through the trochanteric fossa (femur) or tibial crest (tibia); this procedure may be used for large volume drug and fluid administration under sterile conditions for up to a 72-hour period (Antinoff, 1998; Hoefer, 1992).

Chinchilla and guinea pigs are both hindgut fermenters that require both roughage and bacterial microflora action for digestion; hamsters also are quite dependent on bacterial and protozoan species activation for normal digestive physiological activities (Harkness and Wagner, 1995; Wagner and Farrar, 1994). Typical microflora populations include *Bifidobacterium* spp., *Bacteriodes* spp., *Eubacgterium* spp (chinchilla), *Streptococcus* spp. (guinea pig), and *Lactobacillus* spp. (hamsters, guinea pigs, and chinchilla). Using contraindicated antibiotic agents in guinea pigs, chinchilla, and hamsters especially results in gram-negative and clostridial bacterial overgrowth, diarrhea, and death (Harkness, 1994; Johnson–Delaney, 2000; Adamcak and Otten, 2000). Milder cases can be alleviated partially by using a strong basic anion exchange resin such as cholestyramine to combat clostridial toxin release in the bowel (Adamcak and Otten, 2000).

Therapeutic doses used in chinchilla may be empirical and may include those commonly used in treating other fermenters such as guinea pigs and hamsters who are susceptible to antibiotic–induced enterotoxemia. Antibiotic toxicity in guinea pigs, chinchilla, and hamsters has been associated with administration of antibiotics targeting predominantly gram (+) bacteria (Hawk and Leary, 1995; Quesenberry, 1994; Adamcak and Otten, 2000). Classical examples of these medications include the penicillins (amoxicillin, penicillin, ampicillin), macrolides (erythromycin, lincomycin, strepto-

mycin); lincosamides (clindamycin, lincomycin), chlortetracycline and oxytetracycline, bacitracin and vancomycin; and occasionally with other antibiotics, including cephalosporins, chloramphenicol, trimethoprim sulfa combinations, and enrofloxacin, in which immediate withdrawal of therapeutic doses from individuals exhibiting diarrhea will stop the progression of the disease (Quesenberry, 1994). Mice, rats, and gerbils do not exhibit sensitivity to most commonly encountered therapeutic agents; however, species–specific fatal toxicities have been noted: streptomycin, dihydrostreptomycin, and procaine containing medications produce neuromuscular blockade-induced fatalities in mice, rats, and gerbils; and, ivermectin will cause neurological abnormalities at high doses in rats and mice through stimulation of gamma–aminobutyric acid pathways in these species (Adamcak and Otten, 2000). In most instances it is useful to provide additional support for commensal bowel populations by adding a lactobacillus probiotic product to the diet during periods of drug administration (Adamcak and Otten, 2000).

Drugs that may be considered safe to use in guinea pig and chinchilla include anti-ectoparasitic agents, such as DDVP (Vapona pest strip 1-inch segment attached to a cage lid and changed at weekly intervals), pyrethrin dusts applied in dose rates normally used for kittens or cats, and permethrin used on a cotton ball (5 percent active permethrin, and placed in the cage for 4–5 weeks), or, applied as a 0.25 percent dust; piperazine adipate, 4–7 mg/ml in drinking water, metronidazole 20 mg/kg sid subcutaneously (SC) or per os (PO), pyrantel pamoate 50 mg/kg PO, and ivermectin 200–500 μg/kg per os or 0.2–0.4 mg/kg SC (the author most commonly uses the smaller range of this dosage of ivermectin) once every 10 days for a minimum of three treatments (Harkness and Wagner, 1995; Hawk and Leary, 1995; Ellis and Mori, 2001).

Topical and/or systemic antibiotics are also appropriate, including Cefazolin 100 mg/kg SC bid, Cephalexin 50 mg/kg intramuscularly (IM) sid for 14 days, chloramphenicol succinate 20–50 mg/kg SC or IM, chloramphenicol palmitate 50 mg/kg PO bid–tid, tetracycline 20 mg/kg PO bid, and enrofloxacin 5–10 mg/kg PO (Hawk and Leary, 1985). Trimethoprim/sulfamethoxazole and ciprofloxacin can be administered at canine and feline doses (Quesenberry, 1994). Several excellent formularies and review papers may be consulted for additional information (Adamcak and Otten, 2000; Lightfoot, 2000; Hawk and Leary, 1995; Harkness and Wagner, 1995; Johnson-Delaney, 2000; Antinoff, 1998).

CRITICAL CARE, EMERGENCY PROCEDURES

Critical care and emergency procedures generally used in traditional small animal species are also applicable to small mammal and marsupial species (Antinoff, 1998). Debilitated animals or those with significant injuries or disease for whom manipulation could result in stress, respiratory, or cardiac arrest should be initially stabilized (hemostasis, SC, or IP fluid, oxygen cage, heat) prior to taking additional diagnostic or therapeutic measures. Hemostasis is particularly important in these species because loss of small blood amounts may constitute a significant proportion of their total blood volume; normal blood volume is 7.0–10.0 percent of the total body weight, with a maximum one time loss of 0.7–1.0 percent of the total body weight being tolerated by normal healthy animals (Antinoff, 1998). Transfusion guidelines are similar to those of larger animals (that is, indicated when packed cell volume [PCV] levels following acute blood loss fall below 20 percent, or a chronic nonregenerative anemia PCV of 12–15 percent) (Antinoff, 1998; Hoefer, 1992).

Common emergency conditions in small mammals (Antinof, 1998; Harkness and Wagner, 1995) include respiratory distress (traumatic or infectious pneumonia); cardiac distress (atrial thrombosis, cardiac myopathy in hamsters); bloat (guinea pigs, chinchilla and rodents); metabolic abnormalities such as hypoglycemia (manifest as seizures in sugar gliders and young rodents); hyperglycemia (diabetes mellitus); hypothermia; soft stool or diarrhea including those of zoonotic potential such as *Salmonella* spp, *Campylobacter* spp., *Giardia* spp, *Cryptosporidium* spp. among others (Harkness and Wagner, 1995; Davies and Way, 1995); intestinal intussusception and prolapse (hamsters especially); reproductive disease including fur ring paraphimosis (chinchilla), dystocia (guinea pigs and chinchilla), urinary obstruction secondary to urolithiasis (guinea pigs, hedgehogs) or fur ring obstruction (chinchilla); and neurological emergencies such as seizures (epileptiform in 29–40 percent of gerbils; hypocalcemia and pregnancy toxemia in guinea pig

sows; thiamine deficiency, *Listeria monocytogenes,* and cerebral nematodiasis in chinchilla; and various toxins). It is beyond the scope of this text to discuss the therapies for these various conditions; consult the reference list for more information.

SELECTED SIGNIFICANT ZOONOSES

One significant zoonotic cause of seizures in rodents is lymphochoriomeningitis virus (LCMV), which also causes a meningitis in susceptible rodents, guinea pigs, chinchilla, and humans; adult hamsters affected as neonates become chronically infected, asymptomatic shedders (Antinoff, 1998; Wagner and Farrar, 1994; Harkness and Wagner, 1995). More recently, Hantavirus has been isolated and identified as a human pathogen originating in wild *Peromysscus* spp. (deer mice) populations (Calisher et al., 2002; Hjelle and Glass, 2000; Nichol et al., 2000; Wichmann et al., 2002) and causing Hantavirus infection in humans (Hantavirus Pulmonary Syndrome, HPS). It is not yet completely apparent how Hantaviruses become established and persist within a rodent reservoir population, and there appear to be differences in disease infectivity and pathogenesis in deer mice infected transiently or persistently as adults (Nichol et al., 2000). Human exposure has been associated with increased deer mouse populations (Calisher et al., 2002), and activities bringing contact with airborne excretory material containing viable virus (Hjelle and Glass, 2000; Nichol et al., 2000). Experimental infection can cause fatal neurological disease in laboratory mice (Wichmann et al., 2002). Accordingly, it is prudent for shelters to be aware of this specific pathogen and to avoid wild mouse invasion of shelter spaces, including those housing domestic murine strains.

Small mammals and insectivores may also serve as biological vectors in transmission of *Mycobacteria* spp among livestock and swine and potentially human populations; *M. chelonae, M. vaccaem, M. avium,* and *M. fortuitum* isolates have been identified in small mammal and insectivore populations and are known to induce human disease (Fischer et al., 2000). Salmonella, Mycobacteria, and Hantavirus may all be present in normal stool and/or organs in mice and European hedgehogs carrying these organisms. As discussed earlier, several rodent parasitic organisms are capable of infecting humans and may also serve as biological vectors for significant zoonotic diseases, including Coxiella burnetti (Q Fever) and Yersinia pestis (Plague). These two diseases are also listed as biosecurity hazards because of concern over their possible use as biological weapons.

Appropriate sanitation (see chapter 6), disinfection, and husbandry procedures will lessen the possibility of cross species zoonotic infections (for example, hand washing, protective clothing, and the use of agents such as phenolics, quaternary ammonium, and halogen disinfectants). (The Center for Disease Control—www.cdc.gov—has information on its Web site about hand washing.) Similarly, an employee occupational health program should be in place to detect potential zoonotic disease agents.

RADIOLOGICAL AND SURGICAL CONSIDERATIONS

Although most shelters will not have the opportunity or resources to radiograph small mammals or marsupials unless involved in a cruelty investigation, they are amenable to radiographic assessment; as in larger species, there should be bilateral symmetry of axial skeletal structures and normal soft tissue densities (Williams, 2002; Silverman, 1993). Chemical restraint with appropriate anesthetic monitoring may be required for patient positioning, which may be improved through the use of acrylic plastic devises and tape and by elevating small patients on solid supports and separating them from the radiologic cassette to sharpen the resultant image (magnification radiography) (Williams, 2002). Radiographic cassettes should not contain grids for animals measuring less than 10 cm in thickness; larger animals may require a grid, in which case recommendations include the use of one with ratios of 8:1 and greater than 100 lines per inch (Silverman, 1993). A combined technique incorporating a minimum of two orthogonal views, high detail film and screen combinations (Cronex 10 film, E.I. Dupont, DE; Lanex Fine intensifying screens with TMG film, Eastman Kodak, NY); use of increased kVp (at least 50–60 kVp) and mA levels, and very short exposures (less than 1/60 second) should yield good routine radiographs (Williams, 2002; Silverman, 1993). Very small structures or patients may be best examined using small products similar to those noted previously (Min R system, Eastman Kodak, NY) or nonscreened film, for example, dental or other single emulsion film, which must then

be accompanied by significantly elevated mAs exposure factors (Williams, 2002). Radiologic interpretation is especially helpful in cases of pneumonia or pulmonary neoplasia; bloat or gastric tympani; generalized enteric or systemic disease resulting in abnormal abdominal gas patterns, especially in guinea pigs; cardiac disease; pododermatitis (guinea pigs, rats, occasionally other rodents); traumatic or pathological fracture secondary to cage housing accidents, osteomyelitis, or bony tumors; and nutritional disorders such as scurvy (guinea pigs) (Williams, 2002; Silverman, 1993; Harkness and Wagner, 1995). Ultrasonography is useful in detecting urinary calculi (Silverman, 1993) while availability of molecular imaging modalities such as Positron Emission Tomography (PET scans) of anesthetized patients in medical or veterinary regional facilities would enhance detection of neurological and cardiac disease, carcinogenesis, or other diseases using glucose metabolic or reporter molecules expressed during in vivo imaging due to their high spatial resolution and interaction data provided (Chatzilonannou, 2002). Attempts are in progress to combine physiological information gathered using PET or single PET techniques with anatomically based noninvasive methodology such as Computerized Tomography (CT), Magnetic Resonance Imaging (MRI), and conventional radiography.

Rodent aseptic surgery is commonly performed in developing experimental models and in exotic animal medicine practice and should be very accessible for application in shelter practice settings as well. Many procedures are performed in rodents that are similar to those encountered in larger species (for example, gonadectomy, and excisional tumor removal among others). In general, rodents demonstrate an earlier return to normal physiological states following surgical intervention with substitution of inhalant anesthesia for traditional pentobarbital parenteral anesthesia, careful attention to body temperature maintenance through the use of heated rodent surgical boards or supplemental heat packs and the incorporation of fluid and analgesic therapy during or immediately following surgical intervention with continuing attention for a minimum of a 4–6 hour postoperative period (Hampshire et al., 2001). Analgesics can be incorporated into gelatin cubes or other oral medication vehicles for direct ingestion or administered parenterally (Hampshire et al., 2001; Adamcak and Otten,

2000). As has been the trend in traditional small animal patients, administering postoperative analgesic relief prior to the end of the surgical procedure results in enhanced and prolonged pain relief.

CONCLUSION

In conclusion, small mammals and marsupials are interesting, lively pets that have begun to increase in popularity, and so will begin to become a larger proportion of shelter hospital case loads. Disease, facility, and personnel management are core areas in which shelter veterinarians and their colleagues may make a difference in animal well-being for these species in shelters and in educating the public about conditions in which they will grow and thrive.

REFERENCES

Adamcak, A., and Otten, B. 2000. Rodent therapeutics *Veterinary Clinics of North America: Exotic Animal Practice*; 3(1): 221–237

Akhtar, S., and Khan, M.Q. 1995. An on-farm health monitoring of small ruminants: design, data and disease frequencies. *Revue Scientifique et Technique (International Office of Epizootics)*; 14(3): 831–840

Antinoff, N. 1998. Small mammal critical care *Veterinary Clinics of North America: Exotic Animal Practice;* 1(1): 153–175

Blom, H.J.M., Van Tintelen, G. et al. 1996. Preferences of mice and rats for types of bedding material. *Laboratory Animals*; 30:234–244

Calisher, C.H., Root, J.J., et al. 2002. Assessment of ecologic and biologic features leading to hantavirus pulmonary syndrome, Colorado, USA. *Croatian Medical Journal*; 43(3): 330–337

Chatzilonannou, A.F. 2002. Molecular imaging of small animals with dedicated PET tomographs. *European Journal Nuclear Med.*; 29(1): 98–114

Cheal, M. 1987. Environmental enrichment facilitates foraging behavior. *Physiology and Behavior*; 39:281–283

Davies, R.H., and Wray, C. 1995. Mice as carriers of Salmonella enteriditis on persistently infected poultry units. *Veterinary Record*; 137:337–341

Dillehay, A.L., Lehner, N.D., and Heuerkamp, M.J. 1990. The effectiveness of a microisolator cage system and sentinel mice for controlling and detecting MHV and Sendai virus infections. *Laboratory Animal Science;* 40:367–370

Duke, J.L., Zammit, T.G., and Lawson, D.M. 2001. The effects of routine cage-changing on cardiovascular and behavioral parameters in male Sprague—Dawley rats. *Contemporary Topics;* 40(1): 17–20

Ellis, C., and Mori, M. 2001. Skin diseases of rodents and small exotic mammals *Veterinary Clinics of North America*; 4(2): 493–542

Fischer, O., Matlova, L., et al. 2000. Findings of Mycobacteria in insectivores and small rodents. *Folia Microbiology*; 45(2): 147–152

Hampshire, V.A. 2001. Handheld digital equipment for weight composite distress paradigms: New considerations for rapid documentation and intervention of rodent populations. *Contemporary Topics*; 40(4): 11–17

Hampshire, V.A., Davis, J.A., et al. 2001. Retrospective comparison of rat recovery weights using inhalation and injectable anesthesics, nutritional and fluid supplementation for right unilateral neurosurgical lesioning. *Laboratory Animals*; 35:223–229

Harkness, J.E. 1994. Small rodents. *Veterinary Clinics of North America: Exotic Pet Medicine II;* 24(1): 89–102

Harkness, J.E., and Wagner, J.E. 1995. Biology and husbandry in *The Biology and Medicine of Rabbits and Rodents*. Philadelphia, PA: Williams and Wilkins Press, 13–74.

Harkness, J.E., and Wagner, J.E. 1995. Clinical procedures in *The Biology and Medicine of Rabbits and Rodents*. Philadelphia, PA: Williams and Wilkins Press, 75–142

Harkness, J.E., and Wagner, J.E. 1995. Clinical signs and differential diagnosis in *The Biology and Medicine of Rabbits and Rodents*. Philadelphia, PA: Williams and Wilkins Press, 143–170.

Hjelle, B., and Glass, G.E. 2000. Outbreak of hantavirus infection in the Four Corners region of the United States in the wake of the 1997–1998 El Nino—Southern Oscillation *Journal of Infectious Diseases*; 181:1569–1573

Hoefer, H.L. 1992. Transfusions in exotic species *Problems in Veterinary Medicine* 1992; 4(4): 625–635.

Institute for Laboratory Animal Resources (ILAR), 1998. Guide for the Care and Use of Laboratory Animals; National Academy of Sciences.

Johnson-Delaney, C.A. 2000. Therapeutics of companion exotic marsupials *Veterinary Clinics of North America: Exotic Pet Practice*; 3(1): 173–181

Konsman, J.P., Parnet, P., and Dantzer, R. 2002. Cytokine—induced sickness behavior: Mechanisms and implications. *Trends in Neurosciences*; Vol. 29 (3): 154–159.

Lightfoot, T.L. 2000. Therapeutics of African pygmy hedgehogs and prairie dogs *Veterinary Clinics of North America: Exotic Pet Practice*; 3(1): 155–172.

Lightfoot, T.L. 1999. Clinical examination of chinchillas, hedgehogs, prairie dogs and sugar gliders *Veterinary Clinics of North America*; 2(2): 447–469.

Nichol, S.T., Arikawa, J., and Kasaoka, Y. 2000. Emerging viral diseases *Proceedings of the National Academy of Sciences* 97(23): 12411–12412

MacPherson, C. 1997. Sugar gliders: Everything about purchase, care, nutrition, behavior and breeding. *Barron's Educational Series* Hauppage, NY: Barron's, 5–77.

Otto, G., and Tolwani, R.J. 2001. Use of microisolator caging in a risk–based mouse import and quarantine program: A retrospective study. *Contemporary Topics*; 41(1): 20–27

Pakes, S.P., Lu, Y.S., and Meunier, P.C. 1994. Factors that complicate animal research in *Laboratory Animal Medicine*; New York, NY: Academic Press, 649–697.

Pan, H.P., Gaddis, S.E., and Crane, K.A. 1986. A glass drinking tube for small birds and mammals. *Laboratory Animal Science*; 36(1): 77–78.

Percy, D.H., and Barthold, S.W. 2001. *Pathology of Laboratory Rodents and Rabbits* 2002; Ames, IA: Iowa State University Press, 3–315.

Prattis, S.M., and Morse, S.S. 1990. Detection of mouse thymic virus (MTLV) antigens in the thymuses of infected mice using competition immunoassay *Laboratory Animal Science*; 40(1): 33–36.

Pye, G., and Carpenter, J.W. 2002. A guide to medicine and surgery in sugar gliders. http://www. Hilltopanimalhospital.com/sugarglider.htm; *Glider Science* — www.sugarglider.com/GliderPage/aramaic/diseases.html; Chicago IL: Lincoln Park Zoo, – www.lpzoo.com/mammals/hedgehog.

Quesenberry, K.E. 1994. Guinea pigs *Veterinary Clinics of North. America: Small Animal Practice*; 24(1): 67–87.

Rehg, J.E., and Toth, L.A. 1998. Rodent quarantine programs: purpose, principles and practice. *Laboratory Animal Science* 48:438–447.

Silverman, S. 1993. Diagnostic imaging of exotic pets. *Veterinary Clinics of North America: Small Animal Practice* 23(6): 1287–1299.

Small, J.D. 1994. Rodent and lagomorph health surveillance — Quality Assurance in *Laboratory Animal Medicine*, New York NY: Academic Press, 709–724.

Wagner, J.E., and Farrar, P.L. 1987. Husbandry and medicine of small rodents *Veterinary Clinics of North America: Small Animal Practice*; 17(5): 1061–1067.

Wichmann, D., Grone, J-H., et al. 2002. Hanta virus infection causes an acute neurological disease that is fatal in adult laboratory mice. *Journal of Virology*; 76(17): 8890–8899.

Williams, J., 2002. Orthopedic radiography in exotic animal practice. *Veterinary Clinics of North America: Exotic Animal Practice*; 5(1): 1–22.

10

Domestic Rabbit Care in the Animal Shelter

Susan M. Prattis

INTRODUCTION

Originally discovered by the Phoenicians in Spain by 1100 B.C., the rabbit was domesticated at some time in the sixteenth century (Fox, 1984). Rabbits have long been important participants in human concerns, serving families, businesses, research, and educational institutions through its diverse roles as a pet, involvement in food and pelt–related commerce, and as a human disease model research subject, the latter stemming from extensive similarities in physiological mechanisms existing between human and rabbit species (Fox, 1984). New organizations, such as the House Rabbit Society, have increasingly come to the foreground in the general community and provide accurate information regarding rabbit housing, pet ownership, and adoption. The domestic rabbit has become a more common pet species and one that has increasingly become a part of shelter animal populations. In fact, some shelters have such large rabbit populations that February has been designated Adopt a Rabbit month by the ASPCA. This brief review will provide an overview of biological health management concerns commonly found in this species for application in the shelter environment. It is not intended to replace clinicopathological or epidemiological reference materials.

BIOLOGICAL AND ANATOMICAL CHARACTERISTICS

General Characteristics

The domestic rabbit, *Oryctolagus cuniculus*, a lagomorph species, is the only member of the European rabbit genus (Cooke, 2002; Fox, 1984; Harkness, 1995; Von Holst, 1999). A member of the family Leproidae, it is a separate genus from hares (*Lepus spp.*) or cottontails (*Sylvilagus spp.*), with which it

cannot breed (Cooke, 2002; Fox, 1984; Harkness, 1995; Von Holst, 1999). Wild rabbits should not be confined and kept as pets. (See chapter 13 on wildlife management.) A small to moderately sized animal, rabbits are available in many different breeds with an estimated lifespan of 5–6 years, with pets living for appreciably longer (Cooke, 2002; Fox, 1984; Harkness, 1995; Von Holst, 1999). Certain breeds are more commonly found as pets; whereas others are raised commercially for laboratories, meat, or their pelts. Dentition consists of open-rooted, continuously growing teeth (10–12 cm per year) in the following formula: 2/1 incisors, 0/0 canines, 3/2 premolars, and 3/3 molars; *peg teeth* are evident and form the additional set of incisors in the upper jaw behind the front incisors, which are found only in rabbits (Harkness, 1995). Both cheek teeth and incisors may exhibit overgrowth and malocclusion if not worn or clipped (Harkness, 1995). Many of the characteristics of rabbits that differ from other species have clinical significance. The following are among some of the more prominent features (Table 10.1):

- The rabbit has an extremely small thorax that can be easily compressed manually or following intestinal dilation (Harkness, 1995), resulting in a predisposition toward developing respiratory compromise under certain conditions.
- They also have a characteristically small heart, with bicuspid rather than the usual tricuspid right atrioventricular valves observed in other animals (Harkness, 1995).
- Instead of a uterine body, the uterus in rabbits is bicornate, consisting of two separate horns that each opens into the vagina (Fox et al., 1984; Donnelly, 1997).

Table 10.1. Normal Rabbit Values

	Temperature	101.3–104.0°F	
	Heart rate	180–250 beats/minute	
	Respiratory rate	30–60 breaths/minute	
	Dental formula (hypsodonts)	2/1 incisors, 0/0 canines, 3/2 premolars, and 3/3 molars	
	Weaning age	4–6 weeks	
	Life span	5–6 years	
		Female (doe)	Male (buck)
	Age at sexual maturity[a]	4–9 months	6–10 months
	Weight	2–5 kg	2–6 kg
	Reproductive cycle	Induced ovulator	
	Gestation	32–35 days (avg. 33)	
	Litter size[b]	6–8 kits	

Source: Donnelly, 1997; Johnson-Delaney, 1996.
[a] Onset of breeding varies according to breed size.
[b] Average litter size for medium-size breeds.

- Another striking anatomical structure is the large paired outer pinna, which function in sound detection and heat regulation, are generously supplied with arterial and venous supply, and serve clinically as a prominent venipuncture access site (Harkness, 1995). They represent 12 percent of the total body surface of a rabbit (Donnelly, 1997). The ears of lop-eared rabbits may reach the ground when they are standing.
- One key rabbit characteristic is the very light skeleton, consisting of no more than 8 percent of the overall body weight, less than the comparable proportion in the domestic cat (Harkness, 1995; Percy and Barthold, 2001). Rabbit airway diameter is also quite small in comparison to their body size and approximates 5.81 mm by 5.41 mm at the level of the cricoid apparatus (Kok-Mun, 1999).

Gastrointestinal Characteristics

Rabbits are herbivores that typically nibble continuously. They require large amounts of fiber in their diet to stimulate intestinal motility, prevent obesity, reduce hairball formation (trichobezoar), and reduce hair-chewing vices (Fox, 1984; Gres et al., 2000; Harkness, 1995). Fiber does not serve as a primary source of nutrition (Brooks, 1997). Maintenance nutrient requirements of adult domestic rab-

bits are as follows: 45–55 percent carbohydrates, 15 percent protein, 15 percent roughage, 3–5 precent fat, 0.7 percent sodium chloride, and 7 mg vitamin E (Inglis, 1980). The following items are also required although daily nutrient requirements have not yet been identified: calcium, phosphorus, and vitamins A and B1 (Inglis, 1980). Rabbits do not require vitamins C and D to be present in their diet (Inglis, 1980).

As is the case with other herbivores, they are cecal fermenters (Harkness, 1995; Percy and Barthold, 2001; Small, 1994); their extensive intestine contains a large cecum and glandular stomach to facilitate this process. There is a prominent enteric lymphoid functionality through the presence of the cecal appendix and sacculus rotundus (Harkness, 1995; Percy and Barthold, 2001; Small, 1994). Two different fecal pellets are customarily produced. Cecotrophs are moist, irregularly round pellets produced in the early morning by most rabbits that contain abundant vitamins and minerals (26–29 percent protein, 14–18 percent fiber); these fecal pellets are typically reingested, sometimes directly from the anus, and their nutrients recycled (Harkness, 1995). Coprophagy is, thus, normal in the rabbit. The second fecal pellet, round, drier than the first and deposited into the cage, is less nutritive (9–15 percent protein and 28–30 percent fiber) and is one that is normally produced throughout the day as a consequence of digestion.

Urinary Systems

They absorb calcium through their bowel, maintaining high blood calcium levels (12–16 mg/l) and efficient primary renal excretion (compared with biliary excretion in most other species), renal reabsorption, and bony reabsorption (Benson, 1999; Harkness, 1995; Von Holst, 1999). Rabbit urine is filled with calcium phosphate crystals and, consequently, is both turbid and alkaline (pH = 8.0). The color of normal rabbit urine can vary from yellow to red depending upon the presence of porphyrin pigments that are related to the ingestion of certain plants. The red color generally lasts for a few days, is intermittent, and normal (Paul-Murphy, 1997). It must be distinguished from hematuria. Urolithiasis has been reported in rabbits and occurs as a consequence of nidus formation (such as infection), supersaturation, elevated calcium excretion into urine, and stasis (Benson, 1999; Harkness, 1995; Von Holst, 1999).

Sexual Characteristics and Reproductive Behavior

Sexual dimorphism occurs in many breeds and individual rabbits, with females and some males developing larger dewlap folds under the chin, males exhibiting larger heads and hairless scrotal sacs that are evident adjacent to the penis; glands in these sacs are used by males particularly in scent marking, along with urine marking to define territories and in agonistic display (Harkness, 1995; Von Holst, 1999). The penis overlies the anus in male rabbits, which also exhibits a penile sheath and rounded opening; the penis can be extruded from the sheath from eight weeks onward (Harkness, 1995). Male rabbits do not have an os penis, the testicles descend at about 12 weeks of age, and they have an open inguinal canal (Donnelly, 1997). Female rabbits exhibit a vulvar slit in the anogenital region. Inguinal pouches are found laterally on either side of the urogenital opening and have a strong smelling, dark, glandular secretion (Johnson-Delaney, 1996).

Rabbits are induced ovulators and, thus, do not have an estrous cycle. They have a short gestation period (32–35 day range, average = 33-day gestation), producing 6–8 young per litter for medium-size breeds, and provide lactational support through the 8–10 mammary glands present along their thorax and abdomen (Harkness, 1995). Male rabbits have smaller nipples; their inguinal canal remains open throughout life; and the testicles can be voluntarily withdrawn (Harkness, 1995).

Behavior

In the wild, rabbits form colonies composed of different individuals, most of whom are genetically related, and whom defend a territory composed of a large group of underground interlocking dens (Von Holst, 1999). Domestic rabbits held in captivity exhibit many of these same characteristics; multiple individuals can be housed in one area, and does (female rabbits) commonly exhibit less social stress and better relations than do mixed gender or male housing groups (Harkness, 1995; Von Holst, 1999). Group housed rabbits construct dominance hierarchies similar to those found in wild rabbit colonies (Von Holst, 1999) with bucks (male rabbits) supporting reproduction in a small number of does culminating in spring gestational seasons; conspecific fighting tends to diminish over time. To be safe, rabbits should always be observed for fighting when first housed together. Rabbits will breed on an ongoing basis throughout the year (Fox, 1984; Von Holst, 1999); thus, male rabbits should be separated by gender, and in some cases, into compatible and/or individual housing, at weaning, which occurs at 4–6 weeks of age. Females can be separated at 12 weeks of age. Group housed rabbits should undergo neutering if males are housed together to prevent fighting, or if both males and females are housed together to prevent breeding. Female rabbits may be housed together in most instances without difficulty, although mixed gender groups should be carefully observed at first to assess dominance hierarchy behavioral patterns. In general, group housing is preferred to single occupancy cage housing if facilities are available to support this husbandry function. Ovariohysterectomy and castration surgeries are commonly performed as routine procedures in the rabbit (Fox, 1984; Harkness, 1995). (See chapter 22 on spaying and neutering.) They can be performed beginning at 4–6 months of age. Many of the same reasons for neutering dogs and cats apply to rabbits—it reduces the incidence of mammary gland tumors, prevents ovarian and uterine cancer in females, and reduces objectionable behaviors such as spraying, mounting, and territorial aggression in males.

As a prey species, rabbits have developed aversive means of defending themselves (for example, acute senses, flight, and burrowing) (Von Holst, 1999). They are extremely susceptible to stress. They respond poorly to change and may lose their appetites or develop diarrhea as a result. Although most rabbits do not exhibit aggressive behavior, it may be observed during intraspecific agonistic display or in interactions involving territorial individuals, in which it consists of biting, rushing to the front or side of a housing enclosure, tail flagging, urination, squealing, thumping with both hind limbs, and in some instances, frank fighting (Fox, 1984; Harkness, 1995; Von Holst, 1999). Dutch rabbits are considered to be more aggressive than other breeds (Harkness, 1995). Sexually maturing individuals (three months and older) will also exhibit a tendency to fight and so may require separate individual housing during these periods.

In a shelter environment, rabbits should be provided with regular exercise and toys to alleviate boredom. Rabbits need to play, and staff and volunteers should be encouraged to gently stroke, pet, and carefully handle rabbits to help socialize them to human handling as they prepare to be adopted into a home environment.

HUSBANDRY AND HEALTH CARE MANAGEMENT

Handling

Rabbits are stressed easily and injured if handled roughly or without adequate preparation; best results are obtained by approaching the animal quietly prior to attempting to pick them up or handle them in any way. They should be lifted by the scruff or fur at the back of the neck while supporting their hind legs and back throughout; alternatively, an individual rabbit may be placed with their head buried in the crook of an arm, which has the advantage of calming the animal and shielding its vision. Never pick up a rabbit so that the abdomen and back are not supported or to allow them to struggle in any way—the combined bowel and ingesta are heavy enough to serve as a fulcrum whose swinging may result in a spinal fracture, as could contraction of the powerful skeletal muscles (Harkness, 1995). Rabbits should never be picked up by their ears (Fox, 1984; Mader, 1997).

Failure to maintain control of a rabbit can also lead to serious injury. The exam table should be covered with a nonslip surface because if the rabbit slips and kicks while trying to gain its footing when frightened, it can also break its back. They should be returned to their cages rear end first to prevent them from kicking away from the handler, which can also lead to spinal injury.

Environment

Rabbits should be maintained in 30 percent relative humidity conditions and on a regular light cycle (14:10 or 12:12 hours light:dark) at temperatures ranging from 4–29°C (40–85°F), with the best temperature holdings being between 16–21°C (61–70°F) (Harkness, 1995; Institute for Laboratory Animal Resources, 1998). Exposure to colder conditions will increase food and water intake while elevated temperatures will decrease feed intake and increase water intake; feed and water supplies should be adjusted accordingly (Harkness, 1995; ILAR, 1998). Rabbits adapt better to cold than heat and are highly subject to heat stress at temperatures greater than 72°F if they are not accustomed to seasonal changes in the ambient conditions (ILAR, 1998). Rabbits that are housed outdoors in hot weather must have free access to cool water, shade, and good ventilation (Harkness, 1995), or they should be moved indoors to a cooler environment. If the rabbit must be transported in hot weather, it should be in an air-conditioned vehicle.

Housing

Most rabbits adapt very well to standard cage housing, providing that the cage is sufficiently large, of strong quality construction, and does not contain rough or sharp edges. They may be housed in the same stainless steel cages as dogs or cats in the shelter, with a towel, straw, or textured paper on the bottom of the cage, or with a bottom rack so that urine and feces can fall through the mesh. Do not use newspaper (Mader, 1997) unless the ink is soy based or nontoxic. This is good for short-term housing. Suspended caging with removable trays underneath are the most convenient systems for rabbit cage housing; trays should be removed twice weekly, with regular cage and rack sanitation (two weeks and monthly, respectively, and as needed on an individual basis) (ILAR Guide, 1998). In general, for longer term housing, rabbits need more space to exercise or daily opportunities to exercise outside of the cage environment. Some shelters house rabbits outdoors in a hutch, and others convert a dog run or other enclosure such as a pen if they receive a sufficient numbers of animals. The space should be large enough that the animals can complete three hops, which would be a length of about two meters for the average rabbit, and the cage should be tall enough for them to stand on their hind legs (ILAR Guide, 1998; Love, 1994). If a hutch is built, wire construction may be used, with the proviso that there must be a resting board platform provided for the rabbit and that floor wiring should be of wider, heavier grating material and pattern to lessen the possibility of fractures or subluxations due to appendages slipping between the slats, or, in larger heavier individuals, of developing pododermatitis (see following discussion). The mesh opening should be no greater than 1 by 2.5 cm in size, and 14-gauge wire should be used. If an outdoor hutch is used, it must be secure from outside predators, especially in a rabies endemic area. In general, shelters should refrain from using wire floors because of the dangers to the rabbit's feet, and from housing rabbits exclusively outdoors because of danger from predators, human intervention, and temperature fluctuations.

In group housing, sufficient bedding should be made available to allow the colony to use one area as a latrine, and bedding should be changed several times per week and as needed on an individual basis. Rabbits tend to be very clean and can be trained to use a litter box. Litter box fillers include pelleted paper, pelleted grass products, or other organic materials. The material should be nontoxic and digestible; avoid clay; corncob; shavings such as cedar, pine, or any other aromatic wood or walnut shells (Johnson-Delaney, 1996).

Rabbit cage sanitation is best achieved with mechanical cleansing, aided by detergents, hot water (180°C for three minutes duration exposure), or chemical sanitization, and the use of commercially available urine descaling agents to remove deposits resulting from calcium and phosphate crystals in rabbit urine (Harkness, 1995; ILAR, 1998). Manure must be removed frequently to prevent the buildup of ammonia in the air. Sodium hypochlorite or bleach, which is commonly used as a disinfectant in other animal areas of the shelter, can also be used. It should be diluted 1:10 to 1:32 with water with a maximum of 10 minutes contact time (Fox et al., 1984). In all instances these agents should be rinsed

thoroughly from caging surfaces after use and prior to direct exposure to housed rabbits.

Rabbits should not be housed with cats or dogs if at all possible. In a shelter environment not only is it stressful to a prey species to be housed with a predator, it should be remembered that some diseases may cross species lines. Syndromes of special concern include dermatological disease such as ringworm and *Bordetella bronchiseptica*, which can cause respiratory disease in all dogs, cats, rabbits, and guinea pigs, especially. Care should be taken to minimize fomite transmission. See chapter 6 on sanitation.

Nutrition

Rabbits drink copious amounts of water compared to other animals. A 2-kg rabbit may drink as much water as a 10-kg dog (Inglis, 1980; Donnelly, 1997). Rabbits require 120 ml/kg bwt on average, and those on high-fiber or protein diets will ingest more water (Inglis, 1980; Harkness, 1995). Automatic watering systems can be used in rabbit housing as can water bottles; attention is required with both systems because many rabbits will play with their watering systems, resulting in overly wet dewlap conditions that can lead to superficial and fold dermatitis. If sipper water bottles are used, make certain the rabbit knows to use it. Rabbits may chew on the tip of the bottle's sipper, so water bottles should be inspected regularly when they are cleaned, which should be daily. If water bowls are used, the sides must also be high enough to prevent the dewlaps from getting wet and causing *wet dewlap* disease, infection with *Pseudomonas* (Fox, 1984; Mader, 1997). Bowls are easily contaminated and must be cleaned and disinfected daily.

Feed is commonly provided in J hoppers, but any container that will prevent fecal and urinary contamination while allowing access to fresh feed should be appropriate for this use. Rabbits are hindgut fermenters with additional microbial digestion; they require 2500 Kcal during growth and 2100 Kcal during the maintenance phases of their lifespan, and these requirements are best supported using a once daily feeding of 90–120 g (1/2–1 cup) of pellets (Harkness, 1995; ILAR, 1998) for a 3.5–4.5 kg rabbit. Free-choice feeding can be accomplished by weighing the pellets prior to putting them in the J feeder and using a high-fiber food to keep the rabbits from gaining weight; rabbits should be weighed quarterly to ensure appropriate housing dimensions and weight maintenance. Free-choice feeding of hay and vegetable supplements should be avoided because it may lead to nutritional problems and illness due to contamination of hay and vegetable food stuffs with various fungal or bacterial agents. Treat supplements, typically sweet foods or fresh legumes and leafy green vegetables, are encouraged as a form of environmental enrichment as long as the total caloric intake does not exceed that needed by the rabbit, resulting in increased body weight (Harkness, 1995). Avoid human treats, especially chocolate. Fiber supplements, such as good-quality alfalfa or grass hay or cubes, help to alleviate vices and pathophysiological conditions that are commonly noted in rabbits, including obesity, urolithiasis, enteropathies, and hair chewing (Harkness, 1995). A fiber content of 10–15 percent appears to be best for optimal growth, with diarrhea occurring at dietary fiber levels below 10 percent; high-fiber foods in excess of 17 percent may cause weight loss in obese rabbits and retarded weight gain in more sedentary adults (Harkness, 1995). Hair balls (trichobezoars) are not prevented by this method but are reduced in size and morbidity; trichobezoars are commonly found in most rabbit stomachs at necropsy regardless of the presence or absence of clinical signs of enteric disturbance (such as inappetance, lack of normal stool, or diarrhea). Rabbits appear to be less sensitive to mineral ratio variation and excrete calcium in their urine; use of grasses other than alfalfa will also serve to dilute ingested calcium. Optimal protein food levels in rabbits range from 15–19 percent; high protein foods are indicated in some situations (for example, during lactation [25 percent protein] or pregnancy) and usually are provided by including cereal grains and milling by products into food pellets (Harkness, 1995).

CLINICAL EXAMINATION AND SELECTED COMMON DISEASES

Clinical Examination

A clinical examination for the rabbit begins with an examination of the overall body condition, including musculoskeletal integrity; extremities and nails; integument and hair coat; brightness and turgor of the eyes, presence or absence of oculonasal discharge, and, external pinna/ear canal examination for evidence of ear mite infection; and dentition.

The rabbit should also be scanned for a microchip. Rabbits have a long, narrow mouth with restricted movement, and copious lingual membranes; thus, an extensive oral examination may require sedation, a mouth gag, and a good light source. Thoracic auscultation and abdominal palpation are also important and may reveal the presence of occult cardiovascular or pulmonary abnormalities or the (expected) presence of a trichobezoar in the stomach; an assessment of intestinal motility may be gained by auscultating the abdomen and listening for gut sounds. Hypomotility is associated with diarrhea in the rabbit, and normal active digestion is associated with auditory presence.

In the event that venous access is required, the most easily obtained sample originates from the outer pinna, followed by the cephalic vein, using small-gauge needles and syringes (for example, 25 gauge and 1.0 ml maximum), and lateral saphenous vein. Alternatively, a jugular venous sample may be obtained; this route is recommended for large volume samples (Harkness, 1995) but may require sedation. To do so, the rabbit should be placed in a position similar to that of a cat, with head tilted up and forelimbs extended, or placed on its side with neck extended; these maneuvers are best accomplished with the rabbit being well wrapped in a towel or commercially available rabbit restrainer (Plas Lab, MI). Rabbit blood volume varies between 57–78 ml/kg (Benson, 1999; Harkness, 1995) depending on breed, age, and size; aside from the New Zealand White Rabbit, a commonly encountered commercial and laboratory rabbit breed, fewer reports address normal hematological and clinical chemistry value variation across the varied rabbit breeds (Benson, 1999).

No vaccinations are recommended for pet rabbits; killed rabies vaccination may be administered in endemic areas. Because rabies vaccines are not approved for use in rabbits, this should be considered to be extra label usage, and legal authorities should be consulted as needed prior to instituting this policy. Unlike in dogs and cats, routine prophylactic deworming is generally unnecessary. If endoparasites are detected on fecal examinations, appropriate anthelmintics should be administered. See table 10.2 for common drugs and dosages. Healthy rabbits that are accepted for adoption should be microchipped in accordance with the manufacturer's guidelines and neutered before placement.

Table 10.2. Common Antiparasite Drugs for Use in Rabbits

Drug	Dosage	Duration
Amprolium 9.6 percent solution	1 ml/15 lbs per os	5 days
Carbaryl 5 percent powder	Apply as dust	
Fenbendazole	20mg/kg per os	5 days
Mebendazole	10 mg/kg per os	5 days
Piperazine citrate	100mg/ml in drinking water	1 day
Piperazine adipate	0.5 mg/kg per os	2 days
Praziquantel	5mg/kg SC or 10mg/kg per os	
Pyrethrin 0.5 percent	Apply as dust	

Source: Hawk and Leary, Formulary for Laboratory Animals, 1995.

Dermatologic Diseases

Several different causes of moist dermatitis in rabbits have been identified. These include malocclusion or dental disease, in which they drool constantly resulting in a disease known as *slobbers*; acute or chronic diarrhea; urinary incontinence; or following water apparatus play, resulting in wet dewlaps and *dewlap disease* (Harkness, 1995). The clinical presentation ranges from a superficial suppurative fold dermatitis to a severe ulcerative dermatitis and is treated with cleaning and debridement of the affected area, antibiotics, and analgesia. Common microorganisms infecting this area include *Staphylococcus aureus, Pseudomonas aeruginosa, Streptococcus spp, Fusobacterium spp, Corynebacterium spp,* and others (Harkness, 1995; Percy and Barthold, 2001; Small, 1994). (The dewlaps may appear green in color if infected with *Pseudomonas.*)

Urine scald results from constant exposure to urine and can result from poor husbandry, urinary incontinence, excessive urination, cystitis, obesity, urolithiasis, posterior paresis, and so on. The treatment is to keep the area dry and to correct the underlying cause. The hair can be clipped from the area and Domeboros solution or a similar drying agent applied twice daily; some animals also benefit from the application of topical disinfectants, such as betadine or nolvasan ointment, and in very severe cases, the use of systemic antibiotics. Urine scald can be confused with *Treponema cuniculus*, a venereal disease (vent disease) caused by a spirochete.

Ulcerative pododermatitis or *sore hocks* is a chronic, ulcerative dermatitis found on the plantar surface of the metatarsus and volar metacarpal area, not the hock. The ulcer often becomes infected with *Staph aureus* because of skin contact with soiled bedding and dirty cage floors. It occurs more commonly in animals housed on wire floors but has a multifactorial etiology, including inadequate space, obesity, heredity (large feet), and so on. Treatment can be difficult. It consists of applying topical antibiotics after cleaning the area with an antiseptic, maintaining a clean cage, and keeping the rabbit on a solid floor; analgesia may be indicated in severe cases (for example, longer duration acting buprenorphine). Bandaging, although not usually well tolerated by rabbits, may help (Gentz and Carpenter, 1997).

Among the most commonly observed ectoparasitic diseases observed in rabbits are ear mites (*Psoroptes cuniculi*), which initially are observed as pruritis, cores, and casts of material within the outer ear pinna, extending into the ear canal, and complications by secondary bacterial infections (Harkness, 1995; Percy and Barthold, 2001; Small, 1994). Psoroptes is considered to be potentially zoonotic (Johnson-Delaney, 1996). In severe cases, head tilt, torticollis, circling, and inner ear infections are also observed, although in the rabbit these are most commonly caused by *Pasteurella* multocida infection (Harkness, 1995; Percy and Barthold, 2001; Small, 1994). Ear mites are treated in a manner similar to that observed in other species (that is, extensive cleaning, crust debridement, and ivermectin 200 µg/kg sc repeated once at a 14–18 day interval or once every two weeks for three treatments). If ivermectin is not available, mineral oil or other topical acaricides that are safe in cats can be used. The environment must be cleaned (Hillyer,

1997). Other skin and fur mites that may be observed in rabbits include *Cheyletiella parasitivorax* and *Listrophorus gibbus*, both of which are fur mites and cause dandruff/scaling, alopecia or easy depilation, superficial dermatitis, and scaling; *Demodex cuniculi*, the follicular mite that is primarily asymptomatic in rabbits; *Notoedres cati* and *Sarcoptes scabiei*, both of which are rarely observed nonspecies—specific burrowing mites (Harkness, 1995). Treatment of these agents may be accomplished using ivermectin as noted previously; a less desirable application is the use of weekly lime sulfur dips (Harkness, 1995; Hillyer, 1997).

Dermatophytosis or ringworm in rabbits is primarily caused by *Trichophyton mentagrophytes* and is observed in rabbits as small alopecic areas with heavy crusts distributed around the nares, face, forelimbs, or ears; mycotic pododermatitis has also been reported in rabbits, and as in dogs, it appears to be most amenable to treatment early in the progress of the disease (Harkness, 1995). *Trichophyton mentagrophytes* is also contagious to humans, guinea pigs, rats, and mice (Fox, 1984). Ringworm may be treated in rabbits using topical or, in severe cases, systemic antifungal treatment (griseofulvin 25 mg/kg bwt per os in water, or, at 20 mg/kg bwt per day, in food); ketoconazole 10–40 mg/kg/day per os for 14 days; and long soaks in iodine solution, accompanied by environmental sanitization (Harkness, 1995; ILAR, 1998; Percy and Barthold, 2001) with regular household bleach, diluted 1:10 with water, for a maximum of 10 minutes surface contact time; the surface should be cleaned prior to disinfection because bleach may be inactivated by the presence of organic material. These eradication efforts should be accompanied by speciation to determine the zoonotic potential of the agent. Diagnosis of all dermatological disease is best accomplished using skin scrapings, skin swab, or hair culture, and in severe cases, skin biopsy and histopathology. Ringworm can be very difficult to eliminate from a rabbit colony, and humans and/or cats can serve as a primary source of infection for a previously uninfected rabbit colony.

Rabbits also get fleas, and, in general, the same products used to treat fleas on cats and kittens may be used on rabbits (Hillyer, 1997). The environment must be treated as well. When in doubt about the product's safety for use on rabbits, check with the manufacturer of the product or the ASPCA Poison Control Center (888-426-4435 or www.appc.aspca.org). (There is a fee.)

If rabbits are group housed, barbering, or in females, mounting behavior may be a problem. Dominant rabbits are responsible for pulling the hair and/or mounting of subordinate rabbits; if this behavioral pattern is observed, the dominant rabbit (that is, the one doing the barbering) should be identified and removed from the colony, and the remaining group observed to ensure that the resulting hierarchy rearrangement does not result in a similar occurrence of this problem.

Precautions should be taken to avoid spreading potentially cross-species infecting organisms such as Sarcoptes, Notoedres, Cheyletiella, or Trichophyton to dogs, cats, and other shelter residents. Most of these organisms are spread primarily through direct contact so transmission is unlikely if the species are kept separate. Fomite transmission is still a possibility. (See chapter 6 on sanitation for methods of minimizing fomite transmission.)

Respiratory Diseases

The primary infectious agent responsible for the majority of respiratory disease in rabbits is *Pasteurella multocida,* a gram-negative bacterial agent that results in chronic smoldering infections that are in many cases asymptomatic (Harkness, 1995; ILAR, 1998; Percy and Barthold, 2001; Small, 1994). Rabbit colonies tend to be infected with the same isolate, even though there is some colony heterogeneity during culture. *P. multocida* (the cause of the disease commonly known as snuffles) infection results in either peracute fatal septicemia, or persistent infection, most notably of respiratory tract structures resulting in chronic rhinitis, bronchopneumonia, and through systemic infection, severe fibrinopurulent lesions in a variety of different organs. Disease is worsened with the presence of *Bordetella bronchiseptica* isolates, which also infect guinea pigs, dogs, and cats, as well as with environmental predisposing factors including elevated ammonia levels, poor sanitation, poor ventilation, and environmental controls; increasing age; stress and reproduction (Harkness, 1995; ILAR, 1998; Percy and Barthold, 2001; Small, 1994). *P. multocida* is highly contagious, and rabbits may be asymptomatic carriers of the organism. Transmission occurs through respiratory droplet dispersion as well as direct contact, fomites, and, in pregnant rabbits, through transuterine and putative transovarian routes (Harkness, 1995; Percy, 2002). Infected rabbits may present with sneezing, snuffling, and discolored forelimbs; head tilt and circling secondary to middle ear infections; suppurative skin, conjunctivitis, and ocular and nasal discharges featuring thick white creamy pus. There may be excessive tearing and scalding of the face. There are no permanent cures for this disease, and rabbits develop little effective immunity after infection (Fox et al., 1984; Harkness, 1995). Symptomatic therapies typically used in adults may temporarily ameliorate this disease (nasolacrimal flush; topical ophthalmic ointments; enrofloxacin 5 mg/kg SC q 12 hours for 14 days.) Rabbits treated with penicillin for this disease may subsequently die from enterotoxemia, so penicillin use should be avoided in rabbits whenever possible; if no other antibiotic is available, this may be modulated in part by placing the individual rabbit on high-fiber feed prior to administration and treating them with gentamycin 4 mg/kg bid for three days after penicillin, ampicillin, or lincomycin administration (Harkness, 1995). Other effective antibiotics include chloramphenicol, erythromycin, trimethoprim-sulfa, and oxytetracycline (Hillyer, 1997). Young rabbit kits may be treated with 0.05 percent sulfaquinoxaline in water to decrease the incidence of enzootic pneumonia prior to weaning (Harkness, 1995). *Pasteurella* must be differentiated from other infectious diseases, including pneumocystis, *Staph aureus*, *Corynebacteria spp.*, *Francisella tularensis*, and others.

Gastrointestinal Disease

Trichobezoars

Trichobezoars (hairballs) can cause gastric stasis in rabbits resulting in a variety of symptoms including anorexia, depression, weight loss, and decreased water consumption. A firm mass may sometimes be palpated in the cranial abdomen, or gas may be palpable in the stomach or intestines; however, the presence of such a mass is not necessarily indicative that a hairball is responsible for clinical signs observed—most rabbit stomach contents will contain a trichobezoar, in many cases without any clinical disease or asymptomatic pathological problem (Fox, 1994; Harkness, 1995; Percy and Barthold, 2001). Trichobezoars are believed to be formed by the accumulation of excessive amounts of hair in

the stomach and occur most commonly in bored, stressed caged rabbits fed low-fiber diets. In general, experience is required to interpret clinical examination and radiographic results in rabbits when referring to abdominal disease in connection with trichobezoar incidence and prognosis. Various treatment options include intestinal lubricants such as cat lax; pineapple juice so that the active ingredient, papain, will partially degrade the trichobezoar; plain unflavored yogurt with active cultures (or any flavor the rabbit will ingest) to repopulate intestinal flora; vegetable and fruit purees, and pineapple juice, to stimulate appetite; and fluid replacement therapy. Antibiotic therapy with trimethoprim sulfa (30mg/kg PO q 12 hours) is sometimes helpful to reduce bacterial overgrowth. Surgery is generally not recommended for the treatment of hairballs.

Parasites

Coccidia

Rabbits are commonly infected with enteric parasites, including hepatic coccidiosis (*Eimeria steidae*) and intestinal coccidiosis (*Eimeria magna, E. performans, E. media, E. exigua and E. irresidua*) (Gres et al., 2000; Harkness, 1995; Percy and Barthold, 2001; Small, 1994). *E. exigua* is the only reported coccidian affecting lagomorphs that is reported to undergo intranuclear endogenous development during the protozoan lifecycle (Gres et al., 2000). These agents all cause clinical disease in rabbits, and in the intestine, may predispose toward bacterial enteritis due to *E. coli* and *Clostridia perfringens* enterotoxemia (Fox et al., 1984; Gres et al., 2000; Harkness, 1995). They are diagnosed through direct fecal examination. Transmission is associated with direct ingestion of oocysts, so good environmental sanitation is an important way to prevent infection among housed rabbits. This includes prompt removal of fecal material, keeping the cage dry, cleaning and disinfecting food and water bowls daily, and so on. Typical signs of disease include peracute death or diarrhea in weanling to young adult rabbits (1–3 months), coupled with bloody mucus-filled feces, depression, inappetance, weight loss, hypothermia, and polydipsia (Fox, 1984; Gres et al., 2000; Harkness, 1995; Small, 1994). Chronic intestinal infection is associated with pasty stools, intermittent inappetance, and intussusceptions in adults (Fox, 1984; Gres et al., 2000; Harkness,

1995; Percy and Barthold, 2001; Small, 1994). Hepatic coccidiosis may be asymptomatic, but with the ingestion of large oocyst numbers, is associated with anorexia, weight loss, enlarged liver in the upper abdomen, icterus, diarrhea, debilitation, and death (Fox, 1984; Gres et al., 2000; Harkness, 1995; Percy and Barthold, 2001; Small, 1994). This form of the disease is only curable if observed early in its progress and can be controlled with moderate success after that time. Necropsy examination reveals the presence of enlarged, rigid bile ducts and gallbladder walls, as well as the presence of yellow–green raised irregular focal nodular cysts in the liver; rupture of these nodules with concomitant release of coccidian lifecycle forms is associated with severe granulomatous hepatitis (Harkness, 1995; Percy and Barthold, 2001). A number of coccidiostats have been suggested for use in rabbits, including sulfaquinoxaline .25-1 g/L for 30 days (Johnson-Delaney, 1996) or 125–250 ppm in feed and sulfadimethoxine 75–100 mg/ kg per os (Harkness, 1995).

OTHER PARASITES

A few other parasites can cause clinical signs of GI disease in rabbits, but rarely do. They include *Giardia duodenalis*, which is not considered pathogenic; *Passalurus ambiguous*, a pinworm that is also considered to be nonpathogenic and nonzoonotic; and a few species of cestodes. *Baylisascaris procyonis*, the roundworm found in raccoons and dogs has also been found in rabbits. This parasite is also zoonotic, causing visceral larval migrans (Jenkins, 1997; Gentz and Carpenter, 1997).

Enteropathies

Enteropathies are a major cause of morbidity and mortality in this species and, when observed, are difficult to treat in most rabbits. Young rabbits (3–14 weeks) are most susceptible; predisposing influences are highly variable but have been reported to include genetic background, intestinal microfloral population, dietary shifts, environmental stress, antibiotic administration, and other factors (Fox et al., 1984; Harkness, 1995). Clinical signs include sudden death, anorexia, depression, dehydration, weight loss, tooth grinding (presumably due to discomfort), and diarrhea; clinicopathologic abnormalities include those referable to metabolic abnormalities and reduced hepatic and renal function

(Benson, 1999; Fox et al., 1984; Harkness, 1995; Henke, 1990). In their advanced stages, these diseases are difficult to treat successfully, but improvement may be noted by using symptomatic therapy (for example, fluids, analgesia, maintaining body temperature, manual stool removal, or enema to remove intussuscepted mucus stool plugs) increasing fiber content in the diet, and by decreasing the amount of energy/protein that affected animals ingest (Harkness, 1995).

Enterotoxemia is a more severe clinical entity than mere enteritis. The primary cause of this group of diseases are the *Clostridial* enterotoxemias (*Clostridium Spiroforme*), which cause anorexia, depression, brown and watery diarrhea, hypothermia, and death within 48 hours. This must be differentiated from Tyzzer's disease (*Clostridium piliforme*), which is characterized by diarrhea, depression, and death. Enterotoxemia may be treated with supportive care, a high-fiber diet (force fed if necessary), cholestyramine (to bind bacterial toxins) 2g per 20 ml of water by gavage and metronidazole 20mg/kg q12 hours (Jenkins, 1997). Tyzzer's can be treated effectively with oxytetracycline (0.1 gal/liter for 30 days); tetracycline, 10 mg/kg in repeated five day on and off schedules; or any of a range of other antibiotics (Benson, 1999; Fox, 1984; Gres et al., 2000; Harkness, 1995). Coccidiosis and Colibacillosis are also considered to be differential causes of this syndrome (Harkness, 1995). Salmonellosis (*S typhimurium*) is not common in rabbits; *Cryptosporidium parvum* can cause sporadic diarrhea in young rabbits.

Prevention is an important part of managing enteropathies, including 1) maintaining dietary fiber between 17–23 percent, which will dilute grain content and will optimize intestinal motility; 2) gradual changes in dietary grains and starches when taking rabbits into the shelter; 3) a high-fiber post-weaning diet, supplemented with intestinal microorganism preparations for young rabbits (Harkness, 1995); and 4) reducing stress.

Oral Diseases

Rabbits are prone to developing malocclusion, and a good oral examination is indicated in any animal developing inappetance or anorexia. In this species, malocclusion occurs as mandibular prognathism as a consequence to genetic factors (autosomal recessive related shortness in the skull) or a lack of oppositional wear from abnormal occlusion patterns (Harkness, 1995). Incisor overgrowth is customarily treated by clipping the teeth using a large nail clipper, and by giving additional food treats to stimulate interest in eating.

Significant Viral Diseases

MYXOMATOSIS

Several viral diseases naturally affect rabbits. The first, Myxomatosis, is caused by myxoma poxviruses with variable virulence disease phenotypic expression patterns (Harkness, 1995; Percy and Barthold, 2001; Small, 1994; Smith, 1985); transmission is by mechanical means from arthropods, mosquitoes, flies, plants, and fomites, with increased levels noted in North America between August and November (Harkness, 1995; Smith, 1985). Clinical signs include lethargy, reddened and swollen eyelids, pyrexia, and ocular discharge, followed by chronic changes including reddening and swelling of ears, eyes, face, lips, and anogenital areas (Harkness, 1995), and death. Necropsy lesions are characteristic and consist of extensive subcutaneous edema and visceral hemorrhage, and histologically, ballooning epithelial proliferation, hyperkeratinization, and large eosinophilic intracytoplasmic inclusion bodies in the stratum germinativum (Harkness, 1995; Percy and Barthold, 2001; Wasson, 2000). Surviving rabbits undergo lesion regression over a period of months; in subacute infections, this disease appears to be complicated by *Pasteurella spp* infections (Harkness, 1995; Percy and Barthold, 2001; Wasson, 2000). Because no treatment exists, controlling this disease relies on vector control of premise/perimeter properties in which rabbits may be affected if housed outdoors.

Oral Papillomatosis

Oral papillomatosis is caused by a viral disease in *Oryctolagus spp*, a rabbit papillomavirus that is a different virus than the Shope papillomavirus or cottontail rabbit papillomavirus, both of which predominantly affect skin (Percy and Barthold, 2001; Smith, 1985). As with other papillomaviruses, the oral disease is caused by infection of epithelial cells, resulting in hyperplasia, acanthosis, and tumor (Harkness, 1995; Percy and Barthold, 2001; Smith, 1985). The lesions are small, grayish white pedunculated warts found under the tongue or on the floor of the mouth. Domestic rabbits are susceptible to Shope papilloma infection but usually develop tumors that contain fewer virions (Smith, 1985). Shope papillomas are warts found on the neck, shoulders, ears, or abdomen. Treatment is not necessary, and the lesions usually resolve on their own.

Viral Hemorrhagic Disease

A third viral hemorrhagic disease in wild rabbit populations has been attributed to Calicivirus (Capucci, 1991; Cooke, 2002; Harkness, 1995; Kok-Mun, 1999; Nian-Xing, 1991; Percy, 2002). Rabbit Hemorrhagic Disease—also known as RHD, Rabbit Calicivirus Disease (RCD), Viral Hemorrhagic Disease (VHD)—is an acute, highly infectious disease in rabbits that results in acute death and mild bloody nasal discharge (Capucci, 1991; Cooke, 2002; Percy and Barthold, 2001). The disease progresses in 1–3 days after infection, and mortality rates approach 90 percent. It typically affects rabbits over two months of age. Affected young rabbits exhibit splenomegaly, hepatic discoloration, major hemorrhages of the lung, and more restricted abdominal visceral surface hemorrhages (Capucci, 1991; Cooke, 2002; Percy and Barthold, 2001). Other clinical signs include fever, lethargy, anorexia, dyspnea, orthopnea, diarrhea, opisthotonos, congestion of the eyelids and rapid flips, turns, convulsions, and shrill cries. Blood may be found on the floor of the cage. Survivors become carriers of the virus and shed virus for four weeks, spreading it to other rabbits. Transmission is thought to occur via *Phormia, Lucilia sericata,* and *Calliphora vicina* fly species, direct contact, and fomites, and it appears to require very few infective particles (Capucci, 1991; Cooke, 2002; Smith, 1985; DiGiacomo, 1994). RHD shares some homology with minute virus of mice (Kok-Mun, 1999), and may be diagnosed using immunological and molecular techniques (ELISA, HA; Western Blot; RT-PCR; electron microscopy). Disinfect the environment with bleach. Suspected cases of this disease should be reported to state or federal animal health authorities (www.aphis.usda.gov).

Neurological Problems

Encephalitozoon cuniculi species are the major microsporidial pathogens in rabbits (intracellular single cellular, spore-forming protozoan organisms containing a polar filament) (Fox, 1984; Gres et al.,

2000; Harkness, 1995; Percy and Barthold, 2001; Small, 1994; Wasson, 2000). These organisms have been found in many different species, including dogs, guinea pigs, rats, and mice. It has received increased attention following increased identification in immune–compromised persons, where it has been documented to cause chronic disease and wasting (Wasson, 2000). In rabbits, *E. cuniculi* causes head tilt, lethargy, tremors, and local or generalized paresis; ataxia, opisthotonos, torticollis, hyperaesthesia; and nonspecific signs, including failure to thrive and weight loss (Harkness, 1995; Small, 1994; Wasson, 2000); it is present in high numbers in kidney and brain and is shed in urine (Harkness, 1995; Percy and Barthold, 2001). Transmission occurs following ingestion of protozoal life forms in spore-contaminated urine, and in rabbits, is thought to occur following transplacental transmission (Gentz and Carpenter, 1997; Harkness, 1995). At necropsy, renal lesions grossly appear as multiple, white pinpoint areas scattered over the surface or as minute 2–4mm indented gray areas on the surface of the cortex (Pakes, 1994). Although the target tissues of this infection are brain and kidney, it is possible to also observe lesions and/or parasites in lung, lens, liver, and heart tissues from infected rabbits (Percy and Barthold, 2001; Wasson, 2000). As microsporidians must be differentiated from other parasitic/protozoal infections, demonstration in tissues using Gram's stain to identify gram positive rod-shaped organisms within an inflammatory focus or intracellular parasitophorous vacuole within endothelial cells, epithelial cells, or macrophages is definitive (Percy and Barthold, 2001; Wasson, 2000). Other infections that must be differentiated from *E. cuniculi* include Pasteurellosis, Listeria monocytogenes, Baylisascaris procyonis, and Toxoplasma gondii among others (Getz and Carpenter, 1997; Gres et al., 2000; Harkness, 1995; Percy and Barthold, 2001; Small, 1994; Wasson, 2000). No effective treatment exists for encephalitozoonosis.

Congenital Abnormalities

Two main genetic diseases afflict rabbits that shelter personnel should become most familiar with in their work with this species. The first, *splayleg*, results in a familial inheritance pattern of developmental abnormalities of the spine, pelvis, coxofemoral joints, or long bones that leave a bright,

alert but affected rabbit in ventral recumbency with the inability to adduct their limbs and stand (Fox et al., 1985; Harkness, 1995). It is usually observed shortly after birth or in early development and results in significant morbidity in surviving rabbits (Fox et al., 1985; Harkness, 1995). No treatment exists for this disease, and affected rabbits should be euthanized at their initial presentation.

Bupthalmia is analogous to congenital glaucoma in humans and results in hydrophthalmia, due to expression of an autosomal recessive gene spectrum; the disease phenotype is incompletely penetrant, so variable expression of the disease occurs among affected individuals (Fox et al., 1984; Harkness, 1995). New Zealand White rabbits are especially affected, and ocular abnormalities may be observed from 3 weeks of age to 3–7 months of age as the sclera matures and become less compliant (Harkness, 1995). These consist of an enlarged, protruding, firm ocular globe, corneal clouding and scarring, vascularization and secondary bacterial conjunctivitis (Harkness, 1995); enlargement occurs due to increasing intraocular pressure. Bupthalmia has a very poor prognosis, so individual animals are treated only symptomatically (for ocular infection, irritation, and to provide analgesia); in exceptional circumstances, reduction in intraocular pressure may be attempted using a 25-g needle and humor extraction or through enucleation (Fox et al., 1984; Gres et al., 2000; Harkness, 1995).

POTENTIAL ZOONOTIC DISEASES

A few diseases of zoonotic potential affect the rabbit, but generally they are quite rare. These include diseases that are encountered in wild rabbit populations, including salmonellosis, tularemia, ringworm, and toxoplasmosis; plague, is commonly reported in western states, where rabbit fleas serve as vectors of this disease. In *Lepus* and *Sylvilagus spp.* serologic evidence of exposure to ectoparasites carrying the causative agents for Rocky Mountain Spotted Fever and Lyme disease has been reported in individuals residing in urban areas in association with human populations (Henke, 1990; Peavey, 1997), suggesting that exposure of these agents to *Oryctolagus spp.* could result in similar effects. It is less common to observe rabies in rabbit populations, and pet rabbits are not customarily prophylactically vaccinated for this agent unless there has been evidence of a high probability of exposure in local areas (that is, rabies outbreaks in other animal vectors in the immediate area, and outdoor rabbit housing conditions) (Harkness, 1995). Rabbits are susceptible to tuberculosis (Harkness 1995) and could bring this disease into the shelter, or could serve as a susceptible population for humans asymptomatically infected with this agent whom have been previous owners or whom may be working with the colony as veterinary, technical, or husbandry team employees. Pasturellosis is a rare cause of zoonotic disease in humans where it can cause dermatidities, arthritis, meningitis, periodontitis, pneumonia, and septicemia in susceptible persons (Harkness, 1995; Small, 1994). Encephalitozoon cuniculi is also considered to be a rare zoonotic cause of disease, most especially of concern for immunocompromised individuals (Wasson, 2000). Cestodiasis is a problem in rabbits that have been housed outside with the concomitant increased risk of serving as intermediate hosts for organisms such as *Taenia (Multiceps) serialis* or *Coenurus serialis* (Harkness, 1995). *Psoroptes, Sarcoptes, Cheyletiella,* and *Dermatophytosis* represent the most commonly encountered, potentially zoonotic skin conditions (Delaney-Johnson, 1996).

The most common human ailment associated with rabbits is allergic disease, which has been reported in persons owning rabbits and employees working with these animals (Botham, 1995; Khedr, 1979). Childhood allergic disease typically takes the form of perennial allergic rhinitis; in one study, 6.5 percent of reported cases were attributed to exposure to rabbit dander allergens (Khedr, 1979). Allergic disease among those working with animals in laboratory settings has an estimated overall worker prevalence of 11–30 percent, with first-year incident rates in several prospective studies reported as 12–13 percent (Botham, 1995; Khedr, 1979). Decreasing rates in one setting have been associated with improved operating conditions (for example, mandated use of personal protective equipment and educational programs, and occupational health monitoring through the use of skin prick tests and radioallergosorbent testing [RAST] analysis) (Botham, 1995; Khedr, 1979).

Miscellaneous Therapeutic Considerations

It is beyond the scope of this textbook to provide definitive treatment options for the many diseases that have been given cursory coverage here. The reader is encouraged to consult the various resources listed here. Of particular value is the *Exotic Companion Medicine Handbook* by Johnson-Delaney because of its clinical orientation with diagnostic tables and flow charts. A few key points will be mentioned here.

As discussed previously, rabbits must be handled carefully to avoid loss of control resulting in a lumbar fracture, an injury that can also occur in frightened or startled caged rabbits (Gentz and Carpenter, 1997). The most common site of injury is at L7 (Kraus et al., 1984). Clinical signs include posterior paresis, paralysis, and/or fecal and urinary incontinence. Radiographs should be taken, and a thorough neurological evaluation conducted. In mild cases in which the cord has not been transected, there may be improvement after a few days following diminished spinal cord swelling. Conservative medical management is indicated to reduce the inflammation, and supportive therapy must include manual expression of the bladder. It should be determined early in the course of therapy whether the expertise and resources needed to provide proper care to manage these cases are available within shelter staff or whether such animals should be referred to a clinical facility for more intensive medical management. Euthanasia is often indicated (Gentz and Carpenter, 1997).

Rapid diet changes can lead to anorexia and gastric upset. Dietary changes should be made gradually (Donnelly, 1997). Anorexia of even a short duration in an obese rabbit, and of longer durations in normal weight animals, can lead to hepatic lipidosis and ketosis. Food intake and appetite should be carefully monitored, which may not be easy in group housed rabbits. Animals that are depressed or lethargic should be isolated and a second physical examination performed, with prompt diagnosis being essential to keep minor problems from becoming major ones. Commercially available urine test strips should be on hand to check for ketones and other substances that may be excreted in the urine. The presence of calcium crystals and a basic pH level is normal in rabbit urine. Sick rabbits can often be encouraged to eat by offering sweet substances like molasses.

The administration of oral medication to rabbits can be very difficult. Liquids can be given by inserting a syringe in the corner of the mouth and giving small boluses (up to .5 ml at a time) allowing the rabbit time to swallow. Unless a pill is palatable enough that the rabbit will chew it, pills should be crushed, mixed with a more palatable substance or formulated by a compounding pharmacist into a suspension.

Care must be taken when taking blood samples from the lateral ear vein, as the skin can slough if there is thrombosis; IV fluid administration can also be performed through the cephalic, saphenous, or jugular vein if large volumes are required, and may be best administered under anesthesia. If the veins are collapsed, damaged, or not available, and in cases of an emergency therapeutic intervention, fluid can be administered intraosseously through the greater trochanter of the femur. Use Elizabethan collars if necessary to prevent rabbits from disturbing indwelling catheters.

With respect to injection sites, SC injection should be given over the scruff or laterally just cranial to the hip; IM injections can be given in the large lumbar muscles on either side of the spine just cranial to the pelvis. It is best to avoid giving IM injections in the rear leg as this may damage the sciatic nerve.

Antibiotics should be chosen carefully to avoid dysbiosis or enteritis secondary to disruption of the normal gut microflora. Some antibiotics to avoid include clindamycin, lincomycin, penicillin, ampicillin, amoxicillin, Clavamox, cephalosporins, and erythromycins (Hawk and Leary, 1995; Harkness and Wagner, 1995; Kraus et al., 1984).

RADIOGRAPHIC TECHNIQUES IN THE RABBIT

Rabbits differ from other domestic pets in that their skeleton is very light and more closely approximates that found in avian species than in other mammals. Accordingly, adjustments should be made in radiographic technique used for this species. Most rabbits should be sedated prior to radiographic examination, using protocols such as 1) propofol, 2–3 mg/kg IV supplements with 0.5–1.0 mg/kg as needed to achieve anesthetic planes for a duration of 15 minutes; 2) ketamine 20–25 mg/kg and xylazine or acepromazine 2 mg / kg IM; or, 3) ketamine 20–25 mg/kg and diazepam 5–10 mg/kg IM, for longer duration anesthesia (Fox, 1984; Gres et al., 2000; Harkness, 1995). A formulary with drug protocols specific for rabbits should be consulted for other anesthetic and analgesic regimens (Hawk and Leary, 1995). The margin of safety for use of barbiturates and narcotics is small in rabbits (Fox, 1984; Mason, 1997).

Positioning should occur directly upon the radiographic cassette, and standard views should parallel those normally encountered in small animal medicine (right lateral recumbent and ventrodorsal views for skull, spine, pelvis; dorsopalmar and dorsoplantar view for front and rear legs, respectively; and medialateral views for the appendicular skeleton) (Harkness, 1995). Although the radiographic technique is best established with the specific equipment available for use in the shelter and a step series, a useful guideline for rabbit radiography includes the following technique: short exposure times of 1/30 for the thorax, and 1/120 for the abdomen; 2–6 MAS; 45–60 kVp; focal film distances of approximately 90 cm, and use of a beam limiting device (Harkness, 1995). Radiographic film should combine high detail and short exposure (that is, high resolution, fast speed film with high detail intensifying screens present) (Harkness, 1995). When using these techniques in abdominal radiographs, which require some experience prior to definitive interpretation because of the range of overlapping abnormal and normal anatomical radiographic appearances, it is normal to observe that the stomach contains a putative hairball (observed using barium contrast agents as a soft tissue mass), and that the cecum will be large and filled with fluid (Harkness, 1995).

CONCLUSION

It is estimated that at least 5.3 million companion rabbits exist in the United States (Cotter, 2001). As more and more rabbits turn up at shelters, there will be an increased demand for resource allocation for their appropriate care. Adoption counselors must be educated about the common diseases and behavioral problems of rabbits (that is, digging and chewing and compatibility with other pets) for successful adoption into another home. More information about behavioral enrichment programs, appropriate housing, control of disease transmission, careful restraint, handling, and husbandry can be found in any number of other books or from the House Rabbit Society (www.rabbit.org).

REFERENCES

Benson, K.G., and Paul-Murphy, J. 1999. Clinical pathology of the domestic rabbit: Acquisition and interpretation of samples. *Veterinary Clinics of North America*; 2(3): 539–551.

Botham, P.A., Lamb, C.T., Teasdale, et al. 1995. Allergy to laboratory animals: A follow up study of its incidence and of the influence of atopy and pre-existing sensitization on its development. *Occupational and Environmental Medicine*; 52:129–133.

Brooks, D. 1997. Nutrition and gastrointestinal physiology in *Ferrets, Rabbits and Rodents Clinical Medicine and Surgery* by Hillyer, E. and Quesenberry, K. Philadelphia, PA: WB Saunders, 169–175.

Capucci, L., Scicluna, M.T., and Lavazza, A. 1991. Diagnosis of viral haemorrhagic disease of rabbits and the European brown hare syndrome. *Revue Scientifique et Technique (International Office of Epizootics)*; 10(2): 347–370.

Cooke, B.D. 2002. Rabbit haemorrhagic disease: Field epidemiology and the management of wild rabbit populations. *Revue Scientifique et Technique (International Office of Epizootics)*; 21(2): 347–358.

Cotter, M.E. 2001. Rabbits Revisited ASPCA *Animal Watch* Volume 21, No. 1 Spring.

DiGiacomo, R.F., Mare, C.J. 1994. Viral diseases in *The Biology of the Laboratory Rabbit* 2nd ed. Manning, P.J., Ringler, D.H., Newcomber, C.E. eds. Academic Press: San Diego, 171–204.

Donnelly, T. 1997. Basic anatomy physiology and husbandry of rabbits in *Ferrets, Rabbits and Rodents Clinical Medicine and Surgery* by Hillyer, E. and Quesenberry, K. Philadelphia, PA: WB Saunders, 147–159.

Gentz, E., and Carpenter, J. W. 1997. Neurologic and musculoskeletal disease in *Ferrets, Rabbits and Rodents Clinical Medicine and Surgery* by Hillyer, E. and Quesenberry, K. Philadelphia, PA: WB Saunders, 220–225.

Gres, V., Marchandeau, S., and Landau, I. 2000. The biology and epidemiology of *Eimeria exigua*, a parasite of wild rabbits invading the host nucleus *Parasitologia* 42:219–225.

Harkness, J.E., and Wagner, J.E. 1995. Biology and husbandry in *The Biology and Medicine of Rabbits and Rodents*. Philadelphia PA: Williams and Wilkins Press, 1–372.

Hawk, Terrance, C., et al. 1995. *Formulary for Laboratory Animals*. Ames, IA: Iowa State University Press, 3–99.

Henke, S.E., Pence, D.B., Demarais, S. et al. 1990. Serologic survey of selected zoonotic disease agents in Black-tailed Jack Rabbits from Western Texas. *Journal of Wildlife Diseases* 26(1): 107–111.

Hillyer, E. 1997. Dermatologic diseases in *Ferrets, Rabbits and Rodents Clinical Medicine and Surgery* by Hillyer, E., and Quesenberry, K. Philadelphia, PA: WB Saunders, 212–219.

Inglis, J.K. 1980. *Introduction to Laboratory Animal Science and Technology*. Oxford, UK: Pergamon Press, 128–153.

Institute for Laboratory Animal Resources (ILAR). 1998. Guide for the Care and Use of Laboratory Animals; National Academy of Sciences, http://dels.nas.edu/ilar/.

Jenkins, J. 1997. Gastrointestinal disease in *Ferrets, Rabbits and Rodents Clinical Medicine and Surgery* by Hillyer, E., and Quesenberry, K. Philadelphia, PA: WB Saunders, 176–188.

Johnson-Delaney, C. 1996. Rabbits in *Exotic Companion Medicine Handbook for Veterinarians*. Lake Worth, FL: Wingers Publishing, Inc., 2–14.

Khedr, M.S., Shehata, M., and Talaat, M. 1979. Domestic pets and perennial nasal allergy in children *The Journal of Laryngology and Otology*; 93:991–994.

Kok-Mun, T., Barnes, S.M., and Hunter, S.N. 1999. Polymerase chain reaction amplification and gene sequence analysis of a calicivirus from a feral rabbit. *Virus Genes* 18(3): 235–242.

Kraus, A.L., Weisbroth, S.H., Flatt, R.E., Brewer, N. 1984. Biology and diseases of rabbits in *Laboratory Animal Medicine* Fox, J.G., Cohen, B.J., Loew, F.M. eds. New York: Academic Press, 207–240

Loewen, M.S., and Walner, D.L. 2001. Dimensions of rabbit subglottis and trachea *Laboratory Animals* 35: 253–256

Love, J.A. 1994. Group housing: meeting the physical and social needs of the laboratory rabbit. *Laboratory Animal Science, 44.*

Mader, D. 1997. Basic approach to veterinary care in *Ferrets, Rabbits and Rodents Clinical Medicine and Surgery* by Hillyer, E., and Quesenberry, K. Philadelphia, PA: WB Saunders, 160–168.

Mason, D.E. 1997. Anesthesia, analgesia and sedation for small mammals in *Ferrets, Rabbits and Rodents Clinical Medicine and Surgery* by Hillyer, E., and Quesenberry, K. Philadelphia, PA: WB Saunders, 378–391.

Nian-Xing, D. 1991. Molecular biology of the viral haemorrhagic disease virus of rabbits *Revue Scientifique et Technique (International Office of Epizootics)*; 10(2): 325–336.

Pakes, S.P., and Gerrity, L.W. 1994, Protozoal diseases in *The Biology of the Laboratory Rabbit* (2nd ed), Manning, P.J., Ringler, D.H., and Newcomer, C.E., eds. San Diego, CA: Academic Press, Inc., 205–229.

Paul-Murphy, J. 1997. Reproductive and urogenital disorders in *Ferrets, Rabbits and Rodents Clinical Medicine and Surgery* by Hillyer, E., and Quesenberry, K. Philadelphia, PA: WB Saunders, 202–211.

Peavey, C.A., Lane, R.S., and Kleinjan, J.E. 1997. Role of small mammals in the ecology of *Borrelia burgdorferi* in a peri-urban park in north coastal California *Experimental and Applied Acarology*; 21:569–584.

Percy, D.H., and Barthold S.W. 2001. *Pathology of Laboratory Rodents and Rabbits 2002*; Ames IA: Iowa State University Press, 248–306.

Small, J.D. 1994. Rodent and lagomorph health surveillance—Quality assurance in *Laboratory Animal Medicine*, New York: Academic Press, 709–724.

Smith, K.T., and Campo, M.S. 1985. The biology of Papillomaviruses and their role in oncogenesis *Anticancer Research*; 5:31–48.

Von Holst, D., Huntzelmeyer, H., Kaetzke, P., et al. 1999. Social rank, stress, fitness and life expectancy in wild rabbits. *Naturwissenschaften;* 86:388–393.

Wasson, K., and Peper, R.L. 2000. Mammalian Microsporidiosis *Veterinary Pathology*; 37:113–128.

11
Avian Care in the Shelter Environment

Fern Van Sant

INTRODUCTION

The World Parrot Trust (WPT) estimates that there are currently between three and five million large parrots in captivity in the United States.[A] The Pet Industry Joint Advisory Council (PIJAC) estimates that each large parrot in the United States will have a minimum of seven homes in its lifetime (Murad, 1999). These parrots, as well as the smaller more common species, are now at the center of a growing crisis in which large numbers of parrots are being surrendered to veterinary hospitals, humane societies, and animal shelters.

Parrots are ending up in animal shelters for many reasons. Parrots are long-lived and can easily outlive their caretaker's lifespan, ability, or desire to care for a pet. New bird owners may underestimate the cost of owning a bird and the amount of time required to care for it. Some parrots can be loud, destructive, or aggressive, causing problems with neighbors as well as the owners themselves. It is not uncommon for uninformed bird owners to relinquish care of their bird when it matures from a compliant baby bird to an unruly adolescent one.

Prior to 1990, most parrots in the pet trade were legally harvested from the wild and imported into the United States. Since 1990, most pet parrots have been raised by aviculturists and sold to new owners directly or through pet stores. Some professional aviculturists produce healthy, well-socialized birds, which they carefully sell to motivated, informed owners. More commonly a not-so-healthy, poorly socialized, immature bird is sold to consumers who buy on impulse. Unfortunately, the quality of information available to most new bird owners is poor. Trusting that a salesperson is knowledgeable and informed, many new owners purchase inappropriate diets, caging, and health care products for their birds.

In addition to the problem of unwanted pet parrots, an increasing number of parrot aviculturists, having fallen on hard economic times, liquidate their collections to anyone with cash. In some instances, these collections contain species that are endangered or threatened in the wild. Although the buyers of these collections may at first entertain notions of easy profits from a unique and glamorous venture, the reality is often not so rosy. These collections often contain aging birds that have been poorly managed and not in the best of health. Some carry latent viruses that may be triggered by the stress of relocation. These birds may also end up being cared for by shelters and rescue organizations.

It may seem that the answer is to return these unwanted pets to their native ranges, especially in the case of endangered species. The tragedy is that, in most cases, the unique habitat that once supported healthy populations of parrots has been damaged beyond recognition by agriculture, timber harvesting, and development. Even if the habitat did exist, captive parrots are unable to fly and forage, making them unfit to survive in the wild. In addition, some of these birds carry diseases that could decimate fragile wild populations.

Many professional organizations that take in unwanted parrots have programs to place birds with appropriate caretakers. This often involves first educating the prospective owner on how to care for a parrot. Current efforts by numerous professional veterinary, avicultural, and humane associations focus on defining reasonable and humane standards of

Table 11.1. Common Neo-Tropical Psittacines

Neo-Tropical Psittacine	Weight	Species	Description	Common Problems
Macaws	200–1600 gms	Blue and gold, Scarlet, Military, Green-winged Hyacinth, Mini macaws	Large area facial skin, long tail, monomorphic, talk, may blush when excited or stressed	PDD, sinusitis, asthma in Blue/Gold Noise, very territorial when bonded, papillomatosis in older Green Wings
Amazons	150–750gms	Yellow nape, Blue front, Double Yellow head	Stocky build, shorter tail, no facial skin, monomorphic except white fronted, good talkers	Seasonal aggression, obesity, abnormal foot wear, papillomatosis in older Blue Fronts
Conures	60–390gms	Mitered, Sun, Jenday, Nanday, Blue Crowned, Patagonian	Long tail, peri-ophthalmic skin, monomorphic	Trauma, noise
Pionus	250–260gms	Bronze wing, Blue Head, White capped	Striking feather color contrasts, monomorphic	Make snuffly sound when alarmed
Parrotlets	30–35gms	Pacific	Body green, dimorphic wing and tail colors	Trauma, chronic breeding behavior
Caiques	145–170gms	Black Headed White bellied	Stocky, very animated, can be aggressive	Trauma, seasonal aggression

158

care for parrots. All efforts are made more challenging by the facts that most local, state, and federal statutes regarding companion pet issues specifically address domestic cats and dogs. Standards of humane and compassionate care for birds have been slow to evolve. As companion birds can, in the short term, adapt to almost any circumstance, commonly accepted standards of care often fall short of reasonable or humane.

Professional humane organizations play a vital role in caring for unwanted pet birds. At the local level, shelters will need to have effective protocols to accept, evaluate, house, rehabilitate, and place companion birds. As many long-standing traditions of bird care are now acknowledged to be inadequate and inhumane, the following recommendations will cover basic health assessment and care for birds. Any veterinarian can achieve these recommendations in almost any setting.

SHORT-TERM APPROACH

Species Review
Although many avian species are kept as companion and caged birds, most birds that end up surren-

dered to shelters or in rescue are psittacines (Table 11.1). This is possibly the result of the increased demands of these birds and their long lives. Historically the term "parrot" referred to birds with stocky bodies and shorter tails such as the amazon or African Grey Parrot (AGP) (Table 11.2). These days the term encompasses most psittacine species. Psittacines are characterized by their hooked beak and zygodactylus toes (two forward and two back). Psittacine species range in size from 25 grams (parrotlet) to 1,600 grams (large macaw).

Although more than 300 species of parrots exist in the world, parrots common to the pet trade can be divided into several recognizable groups. The ability to recognize common species will be helpful when considering housing needs, behavior, and disease risks (Table 11.3). Illustrated books are available to assist with the identification of the many species seen as pets (Forshaw, 1977) (Fig. 11.1).

Exam Room Set Up
As stress management is the single most important consideration in all aspects of dealing with avian patients, advance preparation is imperative. An exam room should be modified, or bird proofed,

Table 11.2. Common African/Asian Psittacines

African/Asian Psittacine	Weight	Species	Description	Common Problems
African Grey Parrot	300–550gms	Congo, Timneh	Vivid red tail (Congo) dull red tail (Timneh) very dusty, talk	Viral disease, feather disorders, respiratory disease
Senegals	110–130gms		Stocky, monomorphic, green/yellow, gray head	Aggressive to other birds
Meyers	120gms		Teal/yellow/black	Hearty
Lovebirds	50–65gms	Peach faced, Fischers, Masked	Often kept in pairs, monomorphic, may be territorial and aggressive to each other, females more aggressive	Chronic breeding/ overproduction, Viral disease carriers, megabacteria
Ringneck Parakeets	115–250gms	Indian ringneck, African ringneck	Neck ring in mature males, long tail, wildtype green, yellow and blue mutations	Hearty and excellent flyers

Table 11.3 Common Australian and Indonesian Psittacines

Australian/ Indonesian Psittacine	Weight	Species	Description	Common Problems
Cockatoos	200–900gms	Umbrella, Moluccan, Sulfur crested, Goffins	Crest, light build, dusty, loud, mature dimorphic Bi-eye color (reddish/ brown female)	Viral disease, dermatitis, chronic breeding behavior, nonfood ingestion
Cockatiels	75–110gms	Wildtype is grey and white w/ yellow head and cheeks, also lutino, pied, whitefaced	Crest (may have bald spot), long tail, dusty, mature dimorphic by feather pattern and vocalization	Chlamydia, giardia, chronic breeding, nonfood ingestion, hepatic lipdosis, renal disease
Budgerigars (Parakeets)	30–50gms	Wildtype is green, also yellow, blue, grey, white, English budgie larger head/body	Dimorphic by cere (m, smooth, usually blue/ f, rough, usually brown)	Chlamydia, megabacteria, Polyoma virus, obesity, neoplasia
Eclectus	400–600gms	Grand, Vos Mari, Soloman Island	Dimorphic by color male/green Female/red	Feather disorders, viral disease (PDD, polyoma, PBFD), obesity in Females

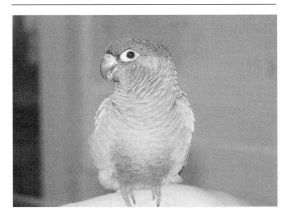

Figure 11.1. Green-cheeked conure (pyrrhura molinae). Conures are small neotropical parrots common in the pet trade.

and set up ahead of time for specific procedures. The room can be small and should be easy to darken, and windows and mirrors should be covered. It should be free of fans, heaters, light fixtures, open shelves, or open windows. Any containers, whether for trash, storage or instruments, should have fitted lids. The gap under the closed door must be small enough to not allow for a loose finch or other small bird to escape. The room should be equipped with a gram scale, light source, and magnification loupe. Cleaning agents used in this room should be unscented with minimal volatile and surface residues.[B]

Instruments and lab supplies should be sized appropriately for the patient. Blood collection is typically done by venipuncture with insulin syringes. Hematocrit tubes or microtainers and coverslips are necessary for correct sample handling. Sample collection into vials designed for larger volumes of blood will render the sample useless. Stethoscopes and otoscopes should have appropriate-sized pediatric bells and cones. Sterile swabs and clean slides should be readily available. Single or double strands of gauze should be precut for opening the mouth during oral exams. Small trays are helpful to safely transport samples to the laboratory area.

The gram scale should be equipped with a removable perch. Some birds will sit willingly on the flat surface of a small digital gram scale, but others will need a perch (Fig. 11.2). Small birds (less than 100 grams) can be weighed in a brown lunch bag. Uncooperative larger birds can be weighed in a container.

Birds are best handled with towels. Towels should be free of loose threads and holes that can trap appendages and feet. Small washcloths or hand towels are suited for birds lighter than 250 grams. Bath towels and beach towels work well for amazons, cockatoos, and macaws. A clean, disinfected towel should be used for each bird to avoid the

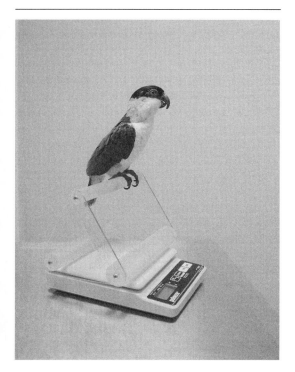

Figure 11.2. Black-headed caique (pionites melanocephala) perched on a digital scale.

spread of disease. Paper towels or shop towels can be used for small birds as an alternative to cloth towels.

Anamnesis

A thorough history of the bird as it comes into the shelter will likely provide more information about the bird's infectious disease risk than a battery of expensive tests will yield. Birds known to be kept as single pet birds for their life are much less likely to be an infectious disease risk in the shelter. In contrast, birds from larger collections (more than 10 birds), from dynamic populations that have seen the turnover of many birds, or from collections that have experienced unexplained or uninvestigated losses, must be treated very differently.

Intake forms should be designed to collect information about the species, age, sex (including how it was determined), length of time in this home, previous homes, history of veterinary care, major illnesses, diet, and environment. The history of where the bird has been and under what conditions serves to identify two principal things. The first is the relative disease risk to other birds. The second is the likelihood of age and management-related degenerative problems in an individual bird.

Physical Examination

There is no substitute for a good physical exam in determining the health of the avian patient. A thorough exam requires at least two people and careful handling of the patient. Although observing the bird in its cage will give the viewer information regarding feather quality, posture, character of respiration, and some behavioral traits, a comprehensive examination must also include picking up the bird and examining it from tip to tail. Birds are very unlikely to show signs of subclinical illnesses. Visibly sick birds attract predators, causing other flock members to drive them away from the group. Anyone attempting to ascertain the health status of a parrot must, therefore, understand the bird's adaptation to appear healthy and alert (Harrison and Ritchie, 1994).

CAPTURE AND RESTRAINT

Parrots should be carefully caught in a clean towel. Temporarily darkening the room can be a useful tool when approaching a recalcitrant parrot, as parrots' eyes do not adapt as quickly to low-light conditions as do ours. A psittacine of any size can be safely restrained by encircling the neck with the thumb and first finger. The secret is to gently extend the head and to lengthen the neck. The towel is used to control the wings and feet. It seems to be less stressful to insulate the bird from direct contact with hands by using a towel. It also causes less damage to the feathers. It usually helps to allow the bird to chew on the towel during the exam. As any process of restraint is stressful for birds, the patient should be monitored at all times for signs of decompensation.

THE PHYSICAL EXAM

Starting at the top of the head, examine the quality of the skin and feathers. The skin should be smooth, without scaling or crusting. Feathers should be glossy, without defects or retained feather sheaths. Feather loss on the head is usually the result of overpreening by another bird. Psittacine beak and feather virus will damage developing feathers so that they appear pinched. Head feathers showing these changes in solitary birds are significant. Many cockatiels have a large bald patch behind their crest feathers. Both the shaft (rachis) and the vane (plume) should be examined for defects of structure or color. Stress bars, horizontal bands of pigment loss, typically indicate underlying problems. Frequent handling by owners can result in black pigment changes on the feathers in areas of contact.

The eyes, nares, and oral cavity deserve close examination. The eyes should be bright and clear. Periophthalmic swelling or conjunctival inflammation can indicate underlying systemic disease. The nares should be open and free of debris or exudate. Although there is a great deal of species variation, both nares of a bird should be symmetrical. The operculum, a keratinized plate within the nares, should not be confused with debris. There should be no staining of the skin or feathers by exudate. The beak below the nares should be smooth and free of fissures. Some flaking of the beak is normal. The maxilla and mandible should meet and be bilaterally symmetrical. Healthy parrots in healthy environments will keep the steadily growing beak trimmed to a normal length. Any malocclusion is abnormal and may indicate a developmental abnormality, traumatic event, or chronic infection.

Otoscopic exam of the ears is often overlooked but can reveal a wealth of information. The ear canals house some of the few discrete exocrine glands in the bird. With active inflammation or infection, these glands can show impressive cystic inflammatory changes.

The oral cavity is best examined using two strands of gauze (Fig. 11.3). With one strand looped around the maxilla and another around the mandible, the mouth can be gently opened. Spike-like papilla are well developed in most species and line the margins of the choanal slit, the back of the oropharynx and the laryngeal mound. The mucosal surface should be free of plaques and exudate. Squamous metaplastic changes of the oropharyngeal mucosa are most often due to hypovitaminosis A.

Cockatoos, cockatiels, and African Grey Parrots (AGPs) produce an inordinate amount of feather dust, a white talc-like powder that aids in waterproofing. Without regular environmental cleaning and bathing of the bird, this powder can accumulate and become a significant respiratory irritant for the birds as well as for their owners. Very dusty birds may have secondary inflammatory changes of their nares, ears, choana, glottis, and lower airways.

After the head has been examined, proceed systematically down the rest of the body. The neck should be palpated for masses or abnormalities. The crop, on the right side of the thoracic inlet, is an esophageal pouch that stores food prior to diges-

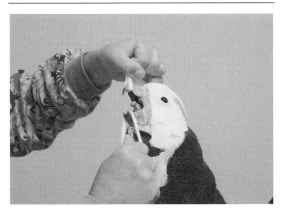

Figure 11.3. Exam of the oral pharynx is safely done with strips of gauze.

tion. Food and ingested materials are easily pal-pated through the crop. The crop should not contain accumulations of fluid or gas. Peristaltic activity may be seen, especially in juvenile birds.

The pectoral muscle mass should be symmetrical and species appropriate. Cockatoos tend to have less muscle mass. Flighted birds will have more developed muscles. Sedentary, poorly nourished birds may have flabby or poorly developed muscles. Parrots prone to obesity, like the amazon, may develop cleavage or the *Dolly Parton* look. Subcutaneous fat deposits are abnormal and may indicate hepatic disease and degenerative metabolic diseases. The feathers over the keel should be parted and the skin and keel examined. Birds that have severely clipped wings or excessively short nail trims can sustain injury from falls. Bruising, hematomas, and abrasions of the skin and tissues over the sternum are typical wounds sustained from falls.

The abdominal space should reveal no swelling, distention, or fluid accumulations. Liver disease, obesity, reproductive disorders, fecal retention, and neoplasia are the most common causes of abdominal enlargement.

Auscultation of the ventral and dorsal thorax will give information about the health of cardiac and pulmonary systems. Murmurs and arrhythmias are not common and, when present, may or may not reflect functional problems. Normal heart rates for parrots are fast, at 150–350 beats per minute (Harrison and Ritchie, 1994). Normal body temperature is 103–107°F as measured by tympanic thermometers, reflecting internal temperatures of 107–112°F. Febrile changes are uncommon, and measuring body temperature is rarely warranted (Harrison and Ritchie, 1994).

Careful examination of the feet will provide information about the age and nutritional status of the bird. The scales on the featherless part of the feet should be smooth and soft. Plantar surfaces should not show signs of wear or erosion, which manifests as loss of scale pattern. Parrots are designed to have sharp nails. Most normal birds will maintain healthy sharp nails. Long overgrown nails or nails that corkscrew are abnormal and may be attributed to poor nutrition, lack of activity, and inadequate perches. With articular gout, deposits of white uric acid form at the joints of the feet. Gout is seen primarily in budgerigars with end-stage renal disease.

Each wing should be carefully extended and examined. Feather loss, evidence of self-barbering, and clipping of flight feathers should be noted. Feather loss from the wing webs may indicate endocrine dysfunction. Each wing tip should be examined for evidence of repetitive trauma. Birds prone to "night frights," an intense startle reaction, will often traumatize their wings as they attempt to take flight in their cage. Large birds, particularly macaws that have been confined to small cages, may develop range-limiting degenerative joint problems that prevent normal extension of the wing. These lesions will predispose the bird to falls and to secondary trauma. Wing clipping is usually recommended unless a flight cage is available. The number of flight feathers clipped should be tailored to the birds weight, condition, and wing span. Most birds should have only five to eight primary flight feathers cut on each side. These should be cut about 3/4 inch below the dorsal coverts (Figs. 11.4 and 11.5). Severe wing clips that involve both primary and secondary flight feathers will predispose the bird to serious injury.

Examination of a parrot's droppings will provide you with important information on its health and nutritional status. Normal droppings are composed of fecal material, urates, and free water. The volume and frequency of droppings are good indicators of appetite. Small birds like cockatiels and budgerigars will have at least 15 droppings a day. The appearance of normal droppings varies by species and

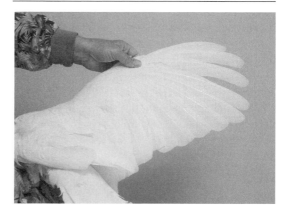

Figure 11.4. Unclipped wing of a moluccan cockatoo (cacatua moluccensis).

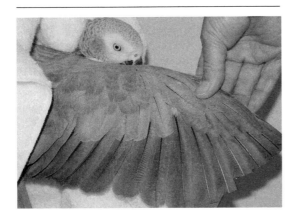

Figure 11.5. Clipped wing of an African grey parrot (psittacus erithacus). When wings are clipped to prevent flight, the number of feathers cut should take into account the weight and strength of the bird. In stocky, heavy bodied birds, it is usually only necessary to clip 4—6 primary flight feathers on each side.

diet. Evidence of profound thirst and an increased free water component in the dropping is usually a sign of severe metabolic dysfunction.

LABORATORY TESTING

Several quick laboratory tests can be very useful in assessing the general health of a bird and can be easily performed in the shelter. These include packed cell volumes (PCV), total solids, Gram stains, and fecal wet mounts. PCV and total solids provide excellent general information about an individual bird. A PCV of 45–55 percent in a hydrated bird is normal. Total solids usually range from 3.0–5.0 mg/dl (Lane, 1996). Gram stains of a choanal swab and of fresh feces are helpful screens for abnormal bacteria. A healthy bird will have small numbers of gram-positive bacteria in its choana and predominantly gram-positive flora in its droppings. A wet mount of recently voided feces is an easy way to screen for yeast, motile trophozoites, protozoal cysts, and megabacteria.

When signs of illness are present, a complete battery of tests for metabolic function and infectious disease is always worthwhile but is often cost prohibitive. When a minimum database is appropriate, samples are best obtained by venipuncture using a tuberculin syringe with an attached 25-g needle.

The medial tarsal vein is an accessible peripheral vein and is often preferable to the jugular for venipuncture. In a healthy individual, total blood volume can be estimated at 10 percent of body weight (6–12mls/100grams body weight). Most laboratories offering avian services can run a CBC and chemistry profile on slides, a spun hematocrit tube (to read PCV), an unspun tube (for red blood cell parameters), and .15–.20cc serum or plasma.[C, D, E, F] Serum can be harvested from microhematocrit tubes or commercial microtainers. Traditional glass vacutainer tubes should not be used as they are designed for larger volumes of blood. Many labs offer screening for infectious diseases including psittacosis, psittacine beak and feather virus (PBFD), and polyoma virus.[C, D, E, F, G, H, I] Polymerase Chain Reaction (PCR) probes for specific viral diseases are useful as long as samples are collected carefully. Fecal swabs and blood samples collected from toenails for viral and chlamydial disease can reflect environmental contamination rather than infection.

Despite the fact that psittacosis remains a serious issue as a contagious agent as well as a zoonotic risk, no definitive antemortem diagnostic test exists. Fecal swabs are useful for detecting shedding of *C. psittaci* into the environment and, therefore, the potential for human exposure. Some species of companion psittacines, such as cockatoos and AGPs, are inordinately resistant to the agent and can confound diagnostic efforts. Even when infected with *C. psittaci*, PCR and serologic assays may be negative in these species. Others, like amazons and macaws, will demonstrate classic signs and have measurable serologic titers. Cockatiels, lovebirds, and budgerigars are considered by some to be reservoir hosts. In these birds, an active psittacosis infection usually will be easily proven by testing swabs from conjunctival, pharyngeal and fecal sources (Fudge, 1996; Gerlach, 1994c; Grimes, 1996).

Routine cultures of the choana and feces of a bird are costly and may not accurately assess the general health of a bird. Cultures are indicated before antimicrobial medical management of any significant bacterial infection. This would include enteritis, sinusitis, dermatitis, or infected wounds. Cultures should be obtained prior to treatment even when empirical therapy is indicated.

Each individual bird should be permanently identified. Many birds will already wear a band or have a microchip, so they should be scanned when they enter the shelter. Birds that have been surgically sexed will have a tattoo of black ink in the wing web. Female birds are tattooed on the left wing and males on the right. Individuals without permanent identification should be banded or microchipped. The AVID microchips system is the one most commonly used in birds.[J] The microchip is usually placed in the left pectoral muscle mass with the syringe supplied by Avid. Although problems are rare, smaller birds (under 125 gms) may be banded instead of microchipped as the supplied needle is relatively large (18g). Identification of the individual is important for comprehensive record keeping.

Zoonotic Disease Risks

Several infectious diseases of companion psittacines pose a potential threat to humans. These include Chlamydophila psittaci (also called psittacosis, ornithosis, avian chlamydiosis, or Parrot fever), Mycobacterium avium, Salmonella spp., and Giardia spp. An awareness of these diseases is essential to minimize the risk of exposure to shelter staff and to ensure that birds placed in new homes will not endanger their new owners. Serious liability issues could result from exposures that cause disease in a human, especially when currently accepted screening protocols are not followed.

Psittacosis is caused by Chlamydophila psittaci (formerly Chlamydia psittaci), a nonmotile obligate intracellular bacterium. The elementary body is the infectious form. Infection is usually the result of inhalation of volatilized fecal debris or exudates. The infective agent can remain stable in dried feces for months. Conditions that produce immune dysfunction in humans, such as AIDS or chemotherapy, can increase susceptibility. The best protection is careful removal of all waste on a daily basis. When used in concert with an effective disinfectant, the risk of exposure is minimized (Carpenter and Gentz, 1997).

Symptoms of chlamydophila infections in parrots vary widely. Asymptomatic carriers are not uncommon in hardy small birds like cockatiels, budgerigars, and lovebirds. Clinical signs in affected birds can include upper respiratory signs, conjunctivitis, gastrointestinal dysfunction, and hepatitis (Gerlach, 1994c).

Several laboratory tests for Chlamydophila exist, including serology, PCR probes, ELISA, histopathology, and immunofluorescent staining (Grimes, 1996). Hematology and biochemistry panels may be suggestive but are not diagnostic. Chlamydophila is not usually cultured, although many state health agencies still recognize this test as diagnostic. Psittacosis remains a reportable disease, but laws vary from region to region. Learn current local protocols and follow them. Psittacosis in people may not be as common as once thought. Atypical pneumonias in humans, once thought to be caused exclusively by C. psittaci, have been found to be caused by other chlamydial agents as well. Psittacosis in humans is characterized by fever, headache, cough, myalgia, and pneumonia (Carpenter and Gentz, 1997). Current information can be accessed at www.avma.org.pubhlth/psittacosis.asp.

Treatment for birds infected with Chlamydophila psittaci is doxycycline for 45 days. Many formulations exist including oral suspensions, oral syrups, long-acting parenteral injections, and medicated feeds (Carpenter, Mashima, and Rupiper, 2001).

Avian mycobacteriosis (tuberculosis) usually is caused by Mycobacterium avium. This agent can cause serious drug resistant infections in immunocompromised people. Some species of older birds, such as amazon parrots, seem to be at increased risk. Unfortunately, antemortem diagnosis of M. avium infection is difficult. Acid-fast stains can be performed on fecal samples but are often nondiagnostic. Definitive diagnosis is via biopsy. Although published protocols for treatment of M. avium infections do exist, the liabilities associated with treatment are significant and must be considered. Mycobacterium avium is a ubiquitous organism and can survive in the soil of contaminated environments for years (Carpenter and Gentz, 1997; McCluggage, 1996).

Salmonella, although not a common infectious agent in companion birds, is the most widespread zoonosis in the world. Salmonella is a gram-negative, nonspore forming rod, classified as an *Enterobacteriaceae*. Domestic psittacines are most likely to become infected via contact with wild birds. Symptoms of Salmonella infection in birds may include diarrhea, depression, anorexia, weight loss, abscesses, and sudden death. Asymptomatic carriers can act as reservoir hosts. Fecal cultures may be used for screening and diagnosis. Antimicrobial therapy should be based on sensitivity testing. Salmonella infections in humans can cause vomiting, diarrhea, and fever (Carpenter and Gentz, 1997; Dorrestein, 1997; Gerlach, 1994b; McCluggage, 1996).

Giardia is a motile protozoan intestinal parasite. Giardia forms stable cysts that are shed in feces. The life cycle is direct, and infection results from the ingestion of cysts by a susceptible host. Birds infected with Giardia may be asymptomatic, or they may show signs of diarrhea, malabsorption, maldigestion, weight loss, eosinophilia, hypopro-teinemia, and, in cockatiels, feather picking. Giardia infections can be serious in young birds. Diagnosis is easiest with direct fecals but trichrome stains and IFA can also be used. Some cases are very refractile to treatment. It is important to differentiate chronic resistant infection from reinfection. All fecal matter must be removed on a daily basis, and an effective disinfectant regimen should be instituted. Although no specific evidence proves that transmission to humans from psittacine birds is possible, care should be exercised to prevent exposure to humans (Carpenter and Gentz, 1997; Greiner, 1997; Greiner and Ritchie, 1994; McCluggage, 1996).

Unlike the zoonotic diseases that can be passed directly from birds to people, West Nile virus (WNV) is a zoonotic disease spread by a mosquito vector. Many species of mammals, birds, and reptiles have been affected by this virus since it was first reported in the United States. Birds are the principal hosts of WNV. Humans, horses, and several other species are thought to be incidental end hosts. West Nile Virus has become endemic in the United States in the last several years. A commercially available vaccine has been successfully used in horses. This same vaccine has been used with variable success in a variety of avian species.

Psittacine Infectious Diseases

BACTERIAL DISEASES

Bacterial infections are the most commonly diagnosed and treated medical conditions of pet birds. It is important to recognize that the most common bacterial infections in pet birds are secondary rather than primary (Dahlhuasen, Aldred, and Colaizzi, 2002). Underlying causes, such as malnutrition or poor management practices, should be addressed. Unclean drinking water is a common management problem that can expose companion birds to high levels of bacteria. Contaminated seed mixes are not uncommon as most commercial seed mixtures contain animal grade seed. The designation of animal grade feed is given to food deemed unfit for human consumption, which is usually based on elevated levels of rodent fecal contamination and rancidity. Practices that involve the feeding of cooked food, previously frozen food, or finely chopped fresh food that is not removed from the cage promptly will also result in exposure to a wide variety of bacteria. In psittacine species, most gram-negative organisms are considered potential pathogens, and most gram-positive organisms are regarded as normal flora. Contagious bacterial disease is rare in parrots and is usually caused by Salmonella, Mycobacterium, or Chlamydophila (Gerlach, 1994b; Reavill, 1996).

Because many bacterial diseases in companion psittacines are a secondary problem, positive choanal or fecal cultures must be interpreted within the context of physical exam findings, laboratory findings, and management history. Bacteria cultured from wounds, abscesses, surgical sites, or from the choana or feces when enteritis or sinusitis exist, should be considered significant. Appropriate antimicrobial therapy should be started.

VIRAL DISEASES

Several viral diseases, including Pacheco's Disease, Polyoma Virus, and Psittacine Beak and Feather Disease (PBFD) have had a devastating impact on pet psittacines in the last decade. Two other significant psittacine diseases, papillomatosis and proventricular dilatation disease, may have a viral etiology. Generally, these diseases can be carried latently by some individuals and may have long and variable incubation phases between exposure and signs of disease. Symptoms can range from acute death to an asymptomatic carrier state. Acute episodes are more likely to occur in young parrots with a history of exposure to infected or suspect birds.

An avian herpes virus causes Pacheco's Disease. Multiple strains exist, and virulent strains are capable of causing significant losses. Parrots who survive infection are thought to become latent carriers capable of shedding virus intermittently. Many species of psittacines are susceptible. Today, as many large collections of older birds are sold and relocated, this disease must be regarded as a real risk. Older neotropical birds, especially those from large collections, should be regarded as potential carriers. Nanday conures, Patagonian conures, macaws, and Amazon parrots have been implicated in some outbreaks. As the stress of relocation may trigger latent carriers to shed the virus, suspect individuals should be isolated and tested. Screening tests for herpes virus can be difficult to interpret because of the large numbers of serotypes. PCR probes can be used to identify birds shedding the organism. The spread of this virus depends on many factors including hygiene, crowding, and air circulation. As the virus is an enveloped virus, it is unstable in the environment and sensitive to most disinfectants (Reavill, 1996).

Avian Polyoma Virus (APV) has been responsible for significant losses in parrot nurseries. This virus causes a disease in young budgerigars and is called budgerigar fledgling disease. The course of the disease is affected by the patient's age at the time of exposure. Birds exposed before 15 days of age usually die. Birds exposed after 15 days of age may survive but lack flight or tail feathers. These birds must be considered a reservoir for the virus capable of long-term shedding. Some birds with chronic APV infections are coinfected with PBFD (Gerlach, 1994a; Vriends, 1984).

Parrots other than budgerigars can also be infected by APV. Birds at greatest risk are juveniles or immunocompromised adults. Susceptible juvenile psittacines may develop peracute, acute, or chronic forms of this disease. Most survivors shed virus for 60 to 90 days before clearing the infection. PCR probes are available and are useful for diagnosis. A vaccine is available and is recommended in dynamic situations in which birds are housed together from different sources.[K] The virus is nonenveloped and stable in the environment. It is advisable to periodically submit swabs from hospital wards and exam rooms to help maintain a clean facility (Gerlach, 1994a; Vriends, 1984).

PBFD, caused by a circovirus, can be devastating for susceptible species such as cockatoos, eclectus parrots, AGPs, lories, and lovebirds. Most neotropical birds are fairly resistant to the virus, but the severity of the disease can vary based on age of exposure, amount of initial inoculum, and general health. In cockatoos, birds exposed as juveniles do not develop signs of disease until their first molt. Lesions result from abnormal feather development, resulting in feathers with a pinched appearance. The

disease often progresses to painful, disfiguring lesions of the beak as well. Some infected birds, like AGPs and eclectus parrots, can die suddenly before the development of beak and feather abnormalities. Lovebirds may refeather normally after showing transient signs and may become asymptomatic carriers (Vriends, 1984).

Birds infected with PBFD shed the virus from feathers and skin and should, therefore, be strictly isolated. The virus is extremely stable in the environment and resistant to most disinfectants. DNA probes have been developed to identify the virus in blood samples, tissue samples, and environmental swabs (Vriends, 1984).

The most important paramyxovirus (PMV) of birds is PMV-1, also known as Newcastle Disease virus (NDV). The lentogenic and mesogenic strains of NDV are common in domestic poultry and pose little risk. However, the velogenic strains, called Exotic Newcastle Disease (END), are foreign pathogens that pose a significant risk to commercial poultry enterprises. Wild-caught smuggled birds, especially young Amazon parrots, have been identified as infected with this virus in small but consistent numbers since the 1970s. Parrots infected with END can be asymptomatic or can have mild to severe disease involving the respiratory, gastrointestinal, and nervous systems. Outbreaks of the virus in states with extensive poultry operations are treated as emergency situations by state and federal authorities. Currently (2003), several counties in California, Nevada, and Arizona are quarantined, and at least a million birds have been destroyed. Awareness of this disease and of current regulations regarding shipping and testing of birds are important. Serologic testing is available, and definitive diagnosis is by histopathology and virus isolation (Gerlach, 1994a; Vriends, 1984).

Papillomatosis is a disease of unknown etiology that causes papilloma-like growths on the mucosa of the avian alimentary tract. Papillomatosis is most common in neotropical birds, producing wart-like, friable growths in the cloaca and oral cavity. In most cases, papillomatosis is best treated by improving the overall condition of the bird rather than surgical excision. Many birds can live for years with the condition, although there is a higher incidence of biliary and pancreatic carcinoma in these individuals. While the lesions are histologically similar to papillomavirus infection in dogs, humans, and cattle, the causative agent has yet to be identified (Gerlach, 1994a; Vriends, 1984).

Proventricular dilatation disease causes the progressive dysfunction of the gastrointestinal tract in many species of psittacines. Histologic changes involve plasmacytic and lymphocytic infiltration of central and peripheral nerve tissue (Vriends, 1984). This damage translates into a loss of gastrointestinal tone and function, leading to weight loss and wasting. Neurologic signs may occur with or without signs of wasting. Outbreaks have been more common and more devastating in indoor aviaries. A virus is suspected but has not been identified. Therapy with COX-2 inhibitors targets secondary inflammatory changes and can be beneficial in reducing clinical signs (Dahlhuasen, Aldred, and Colaizzi, 2002).

MYCOTIC INFECTIONS

Aspergillosis is by far the most commonly reported fungal disease of psittacines. A ubiquitous soil fungus, Aspergillus fumigatus, can cause severe respiratory disease. Infection occurs via the inhalation of spores. Aspergillus is considered to be opportunistic with clinical disease the result of overwhelming exposure or poor immune function. The high incidence of aspergillosis in companion birds is likely due to suboptimal management including poor nutrition, inadequate ventilation, poor hygiene, and stress (Oglesbee, 1997; Reavill, 1996). Aspergillus will grow easily in cages not cleaned daily. Corncob and walnut shell litter are particularly problematic as they often contain fungal spores, and the cost and mess discourage daily removal of feces. Aspergillosis is a noncontagious disease, but several birds housed together may develop the disease because of common predisposing factors. Diagnosis is best achieved with a combination of tests including anamnesis, hematology, physical exam, radiology, and serology. Treatment must include rectification of poor management practices. Oral antifungal therapy with itraconazole and nebulization, with an antifungal agent like clotrimazole, is useful (Carpenter, Mashima, and Rupiper, 2001; Oglesbee, 1997; Reavill, 1996).

Yeast infections, especially of the gastrointestinal tract, are not uncommon in parrots. Usually caused by Candida species, yeast infections should be considered opportunistic. Factors contributing to these conditions are suboptimal nutrition, stress, and an-

tibiotic usage. Infections of the pharynx, crop, ventriculus, and intestines are commonly reported. Juvenile birds are at greatest risk. Treatment may include fluconazole, nystatin, or ketaconazole. Underlying problems must be corrected. Yeast infections can be diagnosed with cytology, wet mounts, and gram stains. Ingested brewers yeast and yeast in leavened bread or crackers can appear in the feces, mimicking an infection. Exams are best run after these foods have been removed from the diet. Candida albicans may be identified by the classic pseudo-hyphae produced (Oglesbee, 1997; Reavill, 1996).

Megabacteria, or avian gastric yeast, is a recently recognized condition found primarily in smaller birds. When first observed, this organism was misnamed megabacteria due to its large size and rodlike shape. This organism is also considered an opportunistic invader. Avian gastric yeast causes increased pH and ulcerations in the proventriculus and ventriculus, leading to maldigestion and progressive weight loss. Budgerigars and cockatiels are most susceptible. Diagnosis is easiest with a direct fecal wet mount. Immune dysfunction is a common underlying theme. Treatment is with oral amphotericin B, which, as it is not absorbed orally, acts as a topical agent.

PARASITIC INFECTIONS

With the exception of protozoal infection, parasitic infections of companion psittacine birds are very uncommon. Although not uncommon in free-living populations, the incidence in carefully managed companion birds is rare. Infections in psittacines from many kinds of parasites, including helminths, protozoans, and arthropods, are observed in the wild. In captivity these infections usually are seen in birds whose cage has a dirt floor. Serious problems can also arise in mixed bird aviaries, especially those in which psittacines are mixed with poultry, pigeons, or doves (Greiner, 1997; Greiner and Ritchie, 1994).

One common parasitic infection, seen in young budgerigars, is scaly face mites. This infection, caused by *Knemidokoptes sp.*, may be seen on nonfeathered areas of the body, especially the face and cere. The beak deformities seen in young birds with this parasite usually resolve with treatment. Treatment with ivermectin is usually curative. All birds in an affected group should be treated. Underlying immune dysfunction due to malnutrition, crowding, or viral disease must be addressed (Greiner, 1997).

Biting lice are usually very host-specific. Occasionally, psittacines housed with pigeons or poultry will become infected. Lice are occasionally seen on young cockatiels from infected flocks. Treatment with safe topical insecticides, usually pyrethrins, will remedy the problem.

Infections caused by the flagellated protozoa giardia have been covered in the section on zoonotic disease. Infections caused by other motile protozoa, hexamitiasis, and occasionally trichomoniasis have been reported in cockatiels, budgerigars, and grass parakeets (Greiner, 1997; Greiner and Ritchie, 1994).

STABILIZATION AND REHABILITATION

Housing in the Shelter

Accommodating companion birds in the shelter environment is easy after the specific needs of avian species are recognized. A specific area of the shelter should be set aside for birds. This area should be insulated from the sights and sounds of dogs and cats and should be in a quiet area without walk-through traffic. A small room is ideal. The area used to house birds should be bird-proofed in the same way as the avian exam room. This will protect against the inevitable escapee, facilitating safe and easy retrieval.

Small birds can be temporarily housed in acrylic or Plexiglas aquariums (Fig. 11.6). Aquariums offer an inexpensive way to provide a suitable microclimate while preventing disease transmission by containing food, feather, and fecal debris. Most healthy birds do well at room temperature. Stressed or ill birds will require supplemental heat. Heat can be provided with a heating pad placed underneath the aquarium. Larger healthy birds are best accommodated in individual birdcages. Facilities anticipating avian patients should invest in a set of safe, high-quality cages (Fig. 11.7). Standard stainless steel small animal cages can be adapted to house birds, but daily care is cumbersome because the cage cannot be changed without removing the bird. With pet birdcages, kennel staff can offer food and clean the cage without disturbing its occupant. Cages should have a grate at the bottom well above the newspaper tray so that the bird cannot access droppings and food debris.

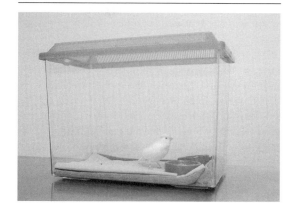

Figure 11.6. Plexiglass aquariums can be used to provide a temporary hospital cage.

Cages should be furnished with nonporous materials that can be effectively disinfected between occupants. Textured acrylic perches offer secure, non-slip surfaces and can be effectively cleaned. Acrylic toys, stainless steel toys, and hardware can be easily disinfected and are reusable. Single use, inexpensive wood toys are an alternative and are recommended to enrich the cage environment. If classic wood dowels are used, they should be single-use

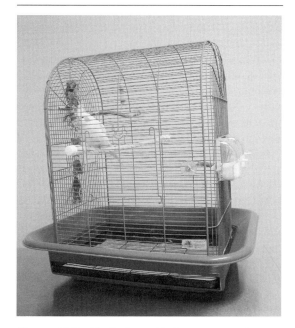

Figure 11.7. Typical pet birdcage setup for a cockatiel (nymphicus hollandicus).

items. Cages can easily be modified for rope or wood perches that can be replaced between occupants.

Most pet birds are comfortable in the presence of other birds, but each situation should be carefully monitored. Some psittacines, such as macaws and cockatoos, can be very loud. This noise can be stressful to other birds as well as to kennel attendants. Providing visual barriers and diversions, like toys, may help. Yelling at the birds will not work and will likely delight them, only encouraging the unwanted behavior. Soft music and background white noise may be helpful. Removal of a persistently loud bird to a quiet dark place for a short time out is the best remedy.

An efficient ventilation system is necessary to protect the health of birds in the shelter and to reduce the possibility of disease transmission. The feather dust produced by birds like AGPs, cockatoos, and cockatiels is considerable. The most effective way to reduce the amount of aerosolized dust is to give parrots a daily misting with water. If a bird is misted immediately before its cage is cleaned, the feather debris will be removed when the paper is changed. Changing the cage paper daily will also reduce exposure to airborne pathogens as well as the growth of saprophytic bacteria and fungi in cage debris. Tolerating days to weeks of fecal accumulation in birdcages is dangerous both to birds and their keepers.

Attention must also be paid to protecting birds in the shelter from common indoor air pollutants. Birds should not be housed in or near a kitchen as volatile oils and heated nonstick pans can kill birds quickly. Aerosols or pump spray cleaners can be noxious or irritating. Birds have an extraordinarily effective gas exchange mechanism and have been reported to die suddenly from air fresheners, carpet cleaners, and cleaning compounds.

Cleaning done in the presence of birds should be done with safe, nonaerosol application of an unscented disinfectant. Routine cleaning with soap and water and dilute bleach (1:32) will protect against most pathogens, but birds should be protected from direct contact and fumes. Dentagene® is a tamed organic chlorine solution commonly used to disinfect floors, surfaces, and cages.[B]

Cleaning floors with a sponge mop is the preferred method for bird rooms. Vacuums are best avoided because of the noise and because of the fact that they are ineffective at removing small particulate debris. Air cleaners with HEPA filters are useful to reduce airborne dust but must be regularly and fastidiously maintained.

Medical Support

Medical treatment of avian patients in the shelter should only be undertaken after careful assessment of the individual. Most psittacines surrendered to shelters will appear to be in reasonable health. Each case will require evaluation of known history and a physical exam. Birds with serious medical conditions will require stabilization prior to appropriate medical or surgical management. Stabilization efforts commonly utilized include supplemental heat, fluid support, and supplemental oxygen as needed (Jenkins, 1997).

True emergency situations include airway obstructions, egg binding, hemorrhage, lead ingestion, noxious inhalation, severe trauma, and gastrointestinal obstruction (Quesenberry and Hillyer, 1994). Tracheal obstructions are most commonly seen in cockatiels and result from seed inhalation or fungal disease. Tracheal obstruction can be remedied surgically by establishing an alternate airway with an air sac tube. Some cases of dyspnea are caused by accumulations of free fluid in the abdominal space. Centesis with a small needle (25g) will relieve signs of dyspnea and allow for diagnostics. Gastrointestinal obstruction is rare in psittacines, but can occur. Accumulations of feces that obstruct the vent are one cause of gastrointestinal stasis. Obstructions can also occur with fiber impaction or foreign body ingestion. Gastrointestinal bleeding may be due to enteritis, starvation, water deprivation, lead ingestion, foreign bodies, or neoplasia. Emergency medical support for melena or hematochezia should include thermal support, parenteral vitamin K_1, fluids, and oral barium. Standing radiographs are stress free and facilitate diagnosis of metallic foreign bodies.

Many cases of egg binding are due to calcium depletion. If a bird has a history of successfully passing eggs, then thermal support, parenteral calcium, and fluid therapy are indicated. First eggs, especially in older birds, may require manipulation in addition to medical support. Prolapse of the oviduct or cloaca may occur with dystocia and require surgical intervention.

Most avian patients with degenerative medical

conditions benefit more from improvements in management and nutrition than from medications. Companion birds suffering from a poor diet may be obese or have hepatic lipidosis. Medical support should address immediate concerns, and a diet change should be instituted as soon as possible.

It should be noted that very few pharmaceuticals are specifically approved for use in birds. Most drugs commonly used fall under the Food and Drug Administration's interpretation of the Extra-label Drug Use Act of 1994.[R]

Diet Change and Rehabilitation

Despite a wealth of scientific literature that clearly defines the risks and predictable disease syndromes associated with a seed diet, most birds remain on a seed ration. Many formulated diets on the market have proven to be successful at meeting long-term nutritional needs of many species. Ideally, birds should be fed an organic formulated diet that is well accepted by most species.[L] Some species of smaller birds are easier to convert and maintain on a pellet and seed cake diet.[M]

The process of diet conversion for a companion bird is often viewed as stressful and difficult. The reality is that, in most cases, these changes can be accomplished fairly easily. Mixing a new diet with the bird's usual ration rarely works. Most birds are naturally neophobic about foods and will try to live on a reduced amount of the old ration rather than accept new food. Instead, it is more effective to remove the seed altogether and to offer the new ration in addition to fresh fruits and vegetables (for larger birds) or spray millet (for smaller birds). Although it can be difficult to determine which foods have been chewed and dropped and which foods have been actually consumed, it is usually very easy to observe and roughly quantitate the fecal material produced. Obtaining daily weights and observing for regular droppings will take the mystery out of diet conversion. A bird that is eating will have regular droppings containing green fecal material. Smaller birds will usually produce about 20 droppings a day, and larger birds about 15. Birds should not be fasted into diet conversion as serious illness can result. If you have an avian patient who is resisting diet conversion, consult an avian veterinarian.[N]

Many pet birds are accustomed to irregular and unpredictable photoperiods. In the wild, parrots are diurnal. They get up with the sun and retire at dusk. Most companion psittacines are from tropical and subtropical parts of the world where a regular pattern of 12 hours of daylight followed by 12 hours of darkness exists. Even subtle changes in this photoperiod can trigger yearly molts and breeding behavior. Restoring the birds in your care to a regular recurring photoperiod is advisable.

Some exposure to sunlight or to full-spectrum lighting that provides both UVA and UVB is also necessary. Conditions such as hypocalcemia and osteoporosis are seen in birds deprived of natural or full-spectrum light. As most windows effectively block out UV light, birds housed for extended periods of time should be provided with full-spectrum lights. It is recommended that bulbs be changed yearly, as their effectiveness wanes over time.

In addition to diet conversion and photoperiod correction, a daily shower with a fine mist sprayer encourages normal preening, aids in removing powder and dust, and restores health to feathers and skin. Although some birds may be unfamiliar with routine baths, when lightly misted with warm water, most will quickly learn to enjoy the process. Many dusty birds will have accumulated plugs of particulate debris in their nares. A fine mist spray will often remedy this and will help resolve many secondary sinus infections and inflammatory conditions.

Euthanasia

Euthanasia should be considered as a last resort, reserved for birds with incurable conditions whose symptoms adversely affect their quality of life. As described in the 2000 AVMA report on euthanasia, the methods accepted for humane euthanasia in birds include inhalant anesthesia overdose, carbon monoxide, and barbiturate overdose. However, thoracic compression should be avoided. Care should be taken to avoid undue stress to the patient. Intracoelomic, intramuscular, or intravenous sodium pentobarbital is acceptable. If necessary, this can be preceded by inhalant or parenteral anesthetic. In general, a small injection of euthanasia solution into the pectoral muscle mass of a small bird will be effective within minutes. Intravenous injections that offer quick and simultaneous cessation of cardiac, respiratory, and brain function in mammals may not produce the same results in birds. Administration of euthanasia solution intravenously, particularly in large psittacines, is generally reserved for anesthetized patients. It is important to choose a route of administration that minimizes stress. The size of the bird, proficiency of handlers, and the skill of the veterinarian should factor into the decision.

LONG-TERM APPROACH

Outreach/Education

Humane organizations, shelters, and veterinarians will have to focus on specific aspects of the problem in order to achieve, or at least work toward, long-term solutions to the many issues of parrot rescue. It would be wise to have a plan in effect at a shelter or humane organization before a need arises. In practice, many shelters are already effectively dealing with small numbers of unwanted parrots. Throughout the United States and Europe, several organizations have distinguished themselves with their plans and methods. Time and money can be saved by relying on organizations like The Gabriel Foundation[o] or Parrot Education and Adoption Center (PEAC).[p] Decisions should be made as to whether each shelter should operate independently, placing birds back in suitable pet homes (as is typically the case now) or focusing on regional centers that can rehabilitate and educate prospective owners and ensure follow-up.

Adoption to a new pet bird home is the most common strategy in parrot rescue. Time and energy are required to establish a system that educates new owners, rehabilitates effectively, and supports the bird and the new owner successfully. Revolving door scenarios can be prevented with careful attention to education protocols and screening of prospective owners. Many organizations begin with a foster care agreement that, with time and success, develops into a permanent adoption. Both PEAC and The Gabriel Foundation use this approach.

Many people who have been involved in parrot rescue for years regard sanctuary as an alternative to individual pet homes. It is not uncommon for birds carefully placed in new pet homes to be surrendered again within months for the same reasons that placed them into parrot rescue in the first place. Education will always be the key to success and should be the foundation of any parrot rescue project. In a sanctuary, it is assumed that lifelong quality care will be provided to each bird. This approach is only possible when funding is available. Sanctuaries are becoming more common as the problem of unwanted birds escalates. Sanctuaries have been founded to meet the needs of hard to place or chronically ill birds. As the commitment to a group of birds can easily span several human lifetimes, careful planning to ensure uninterrupted funding is necessary. Clearly the overhead of a sanctuary far exceeds that of an organization that focuses on rehabilitation and placement.

Enforcement

Current federal law regarding the treatment of warm-blooded animals is covered under the Animal Welfare Act of 1966 (Public Law 89–544). This law defines acceptable care, neglect, and abuse but does not apply to pets. Unfortunately, birds (along with rats and mice) were arbitrarily excluded from the original version. In 2000, the U.S. Department of Agriculture modified its definition of animals to include birds, but that legal protection was reversed upon passage of an amendment to the Animal Welfare Act in the Agricultural Appropriations Act (Farm Bill) of 2002. Several federal laws, including the Endangered Species Act, the Wild Bird Conservation Act, the Convention on International Trade in Endangered Species of Wild Fauna and Flora (CITES), and the Lacey Act regulate the importation of wild psittacines. With rare exceptions, these laws do not pertain to privately owned birds in the United States. There are currently (2003) no federal laws pertaining to the care and well being of companion psittacines.

State governments have the authority to regulate captive bred birds, but most states neither have statutes that provide for basic care nor define negligence or abuse. Most states have commercial regulations regarding the sale of birds in pet stores, and a few states regulate and even license breeders, but the basic protections afforded most mammals do not extend to captive birds. Even when regulations exist, they focus primarily on issues of human health and safety. Although many states have animal protection statutes, the legal definition of animals, and whether or not it includes birds, varies significantly. The ability to prosecute neglect or abuse of parrots will depend on circumstance and location.

Historically, neglect and abuse were difficult to enforce because many accepted traditions of psittacine management tolerated conditions of crowding, filth, and improper nutrition. These attitudes were unfortunately reinforced by the apparent tolerance of these conditions by hearty psittacines. Current traditions of care are now based on scientific research and veterinary medicine.

In situations where neglect or abuse is a concern, standards of humane care applicable to other animals can serve as guidelines. Signs of neglect and abuse may include open wounds, fractures, environmental contamination from rodent or insect infestations, lack of appropriate food or potable water, or accumulations of excreta. Signs of abuse and neglect specific to birds can include severely overgrown beak or nails, degenerative changes, or plantar erosions due to inadequate perches and soiled or damaged feathers caused by contact with oil, filth, or other contaminants. Bird cages should be of appropriate size and construction for the species housed and should allow the occupant to move around, exercise, and spread its wings. Abusive or negligent conditions may include inadequate ventilation, exposure to noxious fumes, or exposure to extreme temperatures, either hot or cold. Birds should have access to natural light or full-spectrum UV lights and a regular recurring photoperiod of roughly 12 hours of daylight followed by about 12 hours of darkness. Fresh, nutritious food and water should be offered daily. Debris and excreta should be removed regularly, if not daily. Unfortunately, many birds endure and survive conditions that most thinking people would define as negligent. The most common defense offered is that of tradition. As more intelligent standards of care become usual and customary, it will be extremely important to recognize negligent and abusive situations for what they are.

The Model Aviculture Program (MAP)[Q] is a set of guidelines developed by aviculturists for aviculturists. This voluntary program has a set of minimum facility standards required for certification. The guidelines are general and applicable to commercial and hobby aviaries, sanctuaries, and rescue facilities. A working familiarity with the program is advisable because MAP guidelines have been accepted as a basic minimal standard of care in aviculture. In situations where either abuse or negligence was apparent but prosecution and enforcement were hampered by a lack of applicable laws, the program and its guidelines could conceivably be used as a standard.

The Association of Avian Veterinarians, a national professional organization dedicated to ad-

vancing the fields of avian medicine and surgery, has become an important resource for ethical issues regarding psittacines. Published position statements are available that clarify current veterinary opinion on issues of psittacine care.[N]

Several organizations currently are focusing on the development of protective legislation for companion birds. One of these organizations, the Animal Protection Institute (API)[R], is addressing these problems in several states. API has been instrumental in a current effort in California to prohibit the sale of unweaned baby parrots in pet stores and bird marts. The job of enacting effective legal protection for companion birds is an uphill battle, at least in part, because of a tough "no restrictions" attitude in commercial aviculture. Many organizations, including TGF, PEAC, WPT, and API are actively involved in educating the public, lobbying for better protections under law, and seeking innovative solutions to the current crisis of unwanted parrots.

CONCLUSION

Although there are regional differences in the population of animals that shelters typically receive, more and more shelters should be prepared to receive and care for birds that have been seized based on a cruelty complaint or other legal problem. This chapter provides an overview of some of the husbandry and medical issues that should be first addressed in order to provide appropriate care for them, but staff should identify support groups and avian veterinarians, and have other suitable resource materials available beforehand to provide assistance whenever faced with circumstances that require expert opinions.

REFERENCES

Bauck, L. 1994. Mycoses. In *Avian Medicine: Principles and Application*, Branson W. Ritchie, Greg J. Harrison, Linda R. Harrison, eds. Lake Worth: Wingers Publishing, Inc., 997–1006.

Carpenter, J., and Gentz, E. J. 1997. Zoonotic diseases of avian origin. In *Avian Medicine and Surgery*, Robert Altman, Susan Clubb, Gerry Dorrestein, Kathy Quesenberry, eds. Philadelphia, PA: W.B. Saunders Company, 350–363.

Carpenter, J. W., Mashima, T. Y., et al. 2001. *Exotic Animal Formulary*, 2d ed. Philadelphia, PA: W.B. Saunders Company, 109–249.

Dahlhuasen, B., Aldred, S., et al. 2002. Resolution of clinical PDD by Cyclooxygenase 2 inhibition. In *Proc. Annual Conference Association of Avian Veterinarians*, 9–12.

Dorrestein, G. M. 1997. Bacteriology. In *Avian Medicine and Surgery*, Robert Altman, Susan Clubb, Gerry Dorrestein, Kathy Quesenberry, eds. Philadelphia, PA: W.B. Saunders Company, 255–280.

Forshaw, J. M. 1977. *Parrots of the World,* Neptune: T.F.H. Publications, Inc.

Fudge, A. 1996. Chlamydiosis. In *Diseases of Cage and Aviary Birds*, 3rd ed. Walter Rosskopf and Richard Woerpel, eds. Baltimore, MD: Williams and Wilkins, 572–585.

Gerlach, H. 1994a. Viruses. In *Avian Medicine: Principles and Application*, Branson W. Ritchie, Greg J. Harrison, Linda R. Harrison, eds. Lake Worth: Wingers Publishing, Inc., 862–948.

Gerlach, H. 1994b. Bacteria. In *Avian Medicine: Principles and Application*, Branson W. Ritchie, Greg J. Harrison, Linda R. Harrison, eds. Lake Worth: Wingers Publishing, Inc., 949–983.

Gerlach, H. 1994c. Chlamydia. In *Avian Medicine: Principles and Application*, Branson W. Ritchie, Greg J. Harrison, Linda R. Harrison, eds. Lake Worth: Wingers Publishing, Inc., 984–996.

Greiner, E. C. 1997. Parasitology. In *Avian Medicine and Surgery*, Robert Altman, Susan Clubb, Gerry Dorrestein, Kathy Quesenberry, eds. Philadelphia, PA: W.B. Saunders Company, 332–349.

Greiner, E. C., and Ritchie, B. W. 1994. Parasites. In *Avian Medicine: Principles and Application*, Branson W. Ritchie, Greg J. Harrison, Linda R. Harrison, eds. Lake Worth: Wingers Publishing, Inc., 1013–1029.

Grimes, J. E. 1996. Detection of Chlamydial infections. In *Diseases of Cage and Aviary Birds*, 3rd ed.Walter Rosskopf and Richard Woerpel, eds. Baltimore, MD: Williams and Wilkins, 827–835.

Harrison, G. J., and Ritchie, B. W. 1994. Making Distinctions in the physical exam. In *Avian Medicine: Principles and Application*, Branson W. Ritchie, Greg J. Harrison, Linda R. Harrison, eds. Lake Worth: Wingers Publishing, Inc., 144–175.

Jenkins, J. 1997. Hospital techniques and supportive care. In *Avian Medicine and Surgery*, Robert Altman, Susan Clubb, Gerry Dorrestein, Kathy Quesenberry, eds. Philadelphia, PA: W.B. Saunders Company, 232–252.

Lane, R. 1996. Avian hematology. In *Diseases of Cage and Aviary Birds*, 3rd ed.Walter Rosskopf and Richard Woerpel, eds. Baltimore, MD: Williams and Wilkins, 739–772.

McCluggage, D. M. 1996. Zoonotic diseases. In *Diseases of Cage and Aviary Birds*, 3rd ed. Walter Rosskopf and Richard Woerpel, eds. Baltimore, MD: Williams and Wilkins, 535–547.

Murad, J. 1999. Unwanted birds: An alarming increase. In Proceedings Annual Conference Association of Avian Veterinarians, 255–259.

Oglesbee, B. L. 1997. Mycotic diseases. In *Avian Medicine and Surgery*, Robert Altman, Susan Clubb, Gerry Dorrestein, Kathy Quesenberry, eds. Philadelphia, PA: W.B. Saunders Company, 323–331.

Quesenberry, K. E., Hillyer, E. V. 1994. Supportive care and emergency therapy. In *Avian Medicine: Principles and Application*, Branson W. Ritchie, Greg J. Harrison, Linda R. Harrison, eds. Lake Worth: Wingers Publishing, Inc., 382–416.

Reavill, D. 1996. Fungal diseases. In *Diseases of Cage and Aviary Birds*, 3rd ed. Walter Rosskopf and Richard Woerpel, eds. Baltimore, MD: Williams and Wilkins, 586-595.

Reavill, D. 1996. Bacterial diseases. In *Diseases of Cage and Aviary Birds*, 3rd ed. Walter Rosskopf and Richard Woerpel, eds. Baltimore, MD: Williams and Wilkins, 596–612.

Vriends, M. M. 1984. *Simon and Schuster's Guide to Pet Birds*, New York, NY: Simon and Schuster.

NOTES
Products and Associations

[A] World Parrot Trust
P.O. Box 50733
St. Paul, MN 55150
651-275-1877
www.worldparrottrust.org

[B] Dent-a-gene
Oxyfresh
P.O. Box 3723
Spokane, WA 99220
509-924-4999

[C] Avian and Exotic Lab
2712 N. US Hwy 68
Wilmington, OH 45177
937-383-3347
www.avianexoticlab.com

[D] IDEXX Laboratory Service
2825 KOVR Drive
West Sacramento, CA 95605
www.idexx.com

^E Antech Diagnostics
17672-A Cowan Ave. Suite 22
Irvine, CA 92614
800-745-4725
www.antechdiagnostics.com

^F California Avian Lab
P.O. Box 5647
El Dorado Hills, CA 95762
877-521-6004
www.californiaavianlab.com

^G Infectious Disease Laboratory
College of Veterinary Medicine
University of Georgia
Athens, GA 30602-7386

^H University of Miami
Comparative Pathology
Avian and Wildlife Laboratory
P.O. Box 016960 (R-46)
Miami, FL 33101

^I Research Associates Laboratory
14556 Midway Road
Dallas TX 75244
972-960-1997
www.vetdna.com

^J AVID
3179 Hammer Ave.
Norco, CA 92860
800-336-2843
www.avidid.com

^K Biomune Vaccines
913-894-0230
www.BiomuneCompany.com

^L Harrison's Bird Food®
7108 Crossroads Blvd. Suite 325
Brentwood TN 37027
800-346-0269
www.harrisonbirdfood.com

^M Lafeber Company
Cornell IL 61319
800-842-6445
www.lafeber.com

^N Association of Avian Veterinarians
P.O. Box 811720
Boca Raton, FL 33481
www.aav.org

^O Gabriel Foundation
P.O. Box 11477
Aspen, CO 81612
970-963-2620
www.gabrielfoundation.org

^P Parrot Education and Adoption
Center
(PEAC)
P.O. Box 6000423
San Diego, CA 92160

^Q Model Aviculture Program
PO Box 6287
Auburn, CA 95604
www.Modelaviculture.org

^R Animal Protection Institute
P.O. Box 22505
Sacramento, CA 95822
www.animalprotectioninstitute.org

12
Reptile Care in the Animal Shelter

Jörg Mayer and Janet C. Martin

INTRODUCTION

With the ever-growing popularity of reptiles as pets, hospitals and shelters are receiving an increasing number of reptiles as patients. Not only must the shelter provide the basic care required, but many times these animals are presented with severe health problems due to previous mistakes in basic husbandry. It will be seen that often the most important key to success in dealing with sick reptiles is a knowledge of the natural history of the species. Luckily only 20–30 of the approximately 6500 existing reptilian species are commonly presented to the clinician or the shelter. It is recommended to have some of the books mentioned in the suggested reading list (at the end of this chapter) on hand for an in-depth coverage of the topics presented here.

We will discuss reptile care in the shelter setting, highlighting the most important aspects of commonly seen reptile health problems. This chapter merely provides an introduction to the basics of reptile medicine to the clinician who may not feel particularly familiar with managing the reptilian patient.

INITIAL ASSESSMENT

In a few cases when reptiles are surrendered, the original owner may be available for questions regarding the medical history of the animal; however, when dealing with reptiles that present with an unknown medical background, an initial assessment of the overall health status of the animal is of utmost importance.

Sexing

The sex of the reptile should be determined immediately if possible, as knowledge of the gender will help determine appropriate husbandry, rule out certain medical problems, and can be of additional help when the animal is placed in a new home.

Secondary sexual characteristics are prominent in some species and less so in others. It can be difficult to use them to be sure of the gender if one is not familiar with the species, if the maturity of the animal is unknown, or if only a single animal is being examined.

SNAKES

Special snake sexing probes should be used by the examiner in order to prevent damaging the cloaca and reproductive organs. These are inexpensive and readily available from several sources. The probe should be lubricated with a water-based lubricant, such as K&Y jelly, as petroleum-based products are toxic to sperm and can cause temporary infertility in males. The probe then is carefully inserted into the cloaca pointing cranially and then reoriented to point caudally and moved gently toward the tail. In a male animal, the probe usually can be inserted into the hemipenal pocket as deep as 6–8 rows of scales. In a female snake, the probe will only enter to a depth of 2–4 rows.

LIZARDS

In juvenile lizards, sex determination can be difficult; however, most adult lizards have some external features that aid in sex determination. Most male lizards have pronounced femoral pores consisting of the openings of a row of glands lined up along the ventral side of the hind leg in a linear pattern. Females may also have a row of pores; however, they will be much smaller and harder to see than those of the adult male. In addition, bulges formed by the two hemi-penes may be seen just caudo-lateral to the cloaca in the adult male. The hemi-penes can sometimes be everted from the cloaca with the application of gentle pressure just caudal to the bulge.

Secondary sexual characteristics might also be used for sexing. Some include the length of the dorsal spines in the iguana, the large jowls (cheeks), and body size. Males usually exhibit larger growth of these structures.

TORTOISES

Tortoises can be difficult to sex. As a general rule, males have a longer tail than females of the same species, with the opening of the cloaca located caudal to the caudal edge of the carapace. The female has a shorter tail, and the opening of the cloaca is located between the margins of the plastron and carapace. In most species of terrestrial tortoises, the shape of the plastron can also be used to determine the gender. A concave plastron is usually seen in male animals, and a flat plastron is more indicative of a female. In some aquatic turtles, the males have very long nails on the front feet that are used in courtship displays to the female. Eye color may vary between the sexes in some species as well, but it is difficult to use unless there is an animal of known sex for comparison.

Nutritional Status

An assessment of the nutritional health of the animal is critical to include in the initial examination of the reptile patient. A physical examination can reveal much about current nutritional status, but radiographs often will be needed to demonstrate problems caused by long-term nutritional inadequacies in an individual reptile.

SNAKES

Body scoring in the snake can be assessed by observing the status of the longissimus dorsi muscles that run parallel to the spinal cord. In the healthy, well-nourished snake, an imaginary cross-section of the animal should produce an oval shape. However, if these muscles are wasted due to malnutrition, the cross section will take on an abnormal triangular shape with the spine being the dorsal apex.

LIZARDS

Body scoring in lizards should be based on the state of the muscles of trunk and limbs of the animal. A healthy animal should be strong enough to lift the trunk of its body off the floor when moving. Also, most lizards assume a threat posture by pushing up with the front limbs and lifting the cranial part of the body. This should be easily accomplished by a healthy lizard. In animals with chronic malnutrition, locomotion can be seriously impaired due to generalized weakness or skeletal deformities. Some animals may not be able to ambulate at all due to partial or generalized paresis, and others may show gross postural deformities when ambulating. If limb or vertebral fractures are suspected, radiological evaluation is necessary.

TORTOISES

Tortoises are a true challenge to judge for body score. For a few species, the Jackson-ratio has been established. The Jackson-ratio is obtained by comparing the weight of the animal in relation to the length of the carapace and is more useful for accurate body scoring than the single factor of body weight alone. Therefore, it is a good idea to record these two measurements whenever a turtle is handled. It is useful information and can be especially helpful as a standard to quantify health status when one seeks advice from a third party. Work has been done involving 11 species in order to generate an equation to assess the adequate weight in a better way:

$$\text{Bodyweight} = 0.0191 \, (\text{SCL}^3)$$

The SCL is the length of the carapace (midline) in centimeters. This can give you a rough estimate of the turtle's weight.

A healthy turtle should resist the examiner's attempts to extend the head or the limbs from the flexed position. Seriously weakened animals will try to avoid the handler but won't really be able to resist manipulation. Care must be taken to avoid excessive force when trying to extend the head or a limb, as joints can be dislocated easily if pulled too hard. Very obese animals can have problems retracting all their extremities into the shell. Radiographs are again useful in assessing any gross shell deformities noted during the exam.

Hydration

Reptile physiology has evolved with unique and efficient water conservation mechanisms. Clinical signs can be helpful in judging the state of dehydration in reptiles but may be misleading. Skin tenting is somewhat unreliable in reptiles but can be used to some degree. A dehydrated reptile may also have sunken eyes and/or dry mucus membranes. However, the best choice for accurate evaluation of the hydration status of the reptile patient is to determine the hematocrit and total solids values from a blood sample.

FURTHER ASSESSMENT

In order to fully assess the reptile patient, a full clinical examination should not only include the physical exam, but hematology and a blood chemistry evaluation, as well as at least one form of diagnostic imaging (that is, radiography, ultrasound). If abnormalities are detected, supportive care should be initiated immediately.

Phlebotomy

As a general rule, blood samples that constitute approximately 0.5–1 percent of the animal's bodyweight can be collected for diagnostic purposes. The lower value should be used in tortoises, in consideration of the large amount of bony material contributing to their body weight. Usually lithium heparin is the anticoagulant of choice for reptile blood. As with all species having nucleated red blood cells, it is good practice to immediately prepare 2–3 blood smears in order to avoid any artifacts in blood cell morphology caused by storage or transport of the samples. The hematological assessment should be made by someone familiar with reptilian blood cell morphology in order to avoid common lab errors and misinterpretations.

Other basic principles of phlebotomy (for example, aseptic technique and good hemostasis at the site) apply to reptiles to the same degree as other animals. Care must to be taken in reptiles to avoid contamination of the blood sample with lymph during phlebotomy, as lymphatic vessels will frequently be closely associated with blood vessels and may be inadvertently sampled. If this occurs, and another sample cannot be obtained, the dilution effect of the lymph must be taken into account when interpreting the hematocrit value.

SNAKES

The most common site for obtaining blood from a snake is the coccygeal vein in the tail, using the same basic principle as obtaining blood from the tail of a cow. The snake should be restrained by the handler with the ventral side facing the phlebotomist. As most ground-dwelling snakes have poorly developed venous return mechanisms, holding the snake in an upright, vertical position will aid the phlebotomist by allowing blood to pool to some extent in the caudal vessels. This is not as helpful in arboreal snakes however. The central tail vein is located on the ventral surface of the vertebral bodies. A small-gauge needle and a small-sized syringe (22–25 gauge needle, 1–5 cc syringes) are usually necessary to obtain the sample. The needle should be inserted about 8–10 rows of scales caudal to the cloaca in order to avoid potential damage to the reproductive organs or the scent glands. The needle should be inserted at a 30–45 degree angle to the body surface until contact is made with the bone of the vertebra. Applying slight negative pressure, the needle should be retracted slowly until blood fills the syringe. Blood flow may be very slow, and negative pressure on the syringe should be intermittent to avoid vessel collapse.

A second method for obtaining blood is to obtain it directly from the heart by cardiac puncture. The heart is generally located within the first cranial third of the snake's body, and its position can be located easily with a Doppler probe or by observation of the heartbeat beneath the ventral scales. A small-gauge needle can be inserted between the ventral scales and into the heart. Even repeated sampling appears to be well tolerated by the tissue.

Another commonly mentioned superficial vessel is the palatine vessel, which can be used for blood collection in large snakes. Although this vessel can easily be seen during inspection of the oral cavity, this method requires sedation of the patient and practice to be successful.

LIZARDS

In lizards, the vein in the tail is also the vessel of choice for phlebotomy; however, more approaches are available. One approach is the ventral stick, exactly the same as mentioned earlier in the snake (see "Snakes"). However, some clinicians have more luck with a lateral approach. This is very similar to the ventral approach except that the vessel is accessed from the side. An advantage to this approach is that the animal can be maintained in ventral recumbency with the tail gently restrained by the handler. The lateral midline of the tail usually is visualized easily by the presence of a slight groove. The needle is inserted along this groove, perpendicular to the tail, until contact with the bone is made, and then under slight negative pressure, the needle is slowly retracted until blood flows into the syringe.

The jugular vein is also available in lizards and is located roughly between the maxillo mandibular joint and the scapula. A few necropsy observations are a good way to get familiar with the location. Again, sedation of the patient is preferable and decreases the chance of laceration of this vessel.

TORTOISES

The tortoise is perhaps the most difficult reptile from which to obtain blood. In larger tortoises, the dorsal coccygeal sinus can be used for phlebotomy. To access this area, extend and straighten the tail caudally and insert the needle exactly on the dorsal midline, directed cranially at a 30-degree angle. However, in smaller animals the tail is simply not large enough to use this location for successful phlebotomy. Other venous sinuses exist at the back of the elbow and behind the knee joints. The limb must be at least partially extended, and the vessel penetrated blindly. Excessive lymph contamination is often encountered with this method.

The jugular vein can be used in all tortoises when the head can be fully extended for this procedure. A small risk of lymph dilution exists with this method. The jugular vein can sometimes be visualized, but often a skin fold will mimic the vessel. The best landmark for jugular access is the midline of the tympanic membrane. The needle should be inserted caudal to the tympanic membrane and directed straight backward. This site can also be used to place an indwelling venous catheter. In larger species, a cut-down to this vessel might be required to accurately visualize its location.

In an uncooperative, conscious turtle, another option for obtaining blood is the use of the subcarapacial venous sinus (Fig. 12.1). This sinus is located roughly where the first vertebra is fused with the carapace. For access, the needle should be inserted on the centerline under the edge of the carapace at the border of the attachment of the skin to the cara-

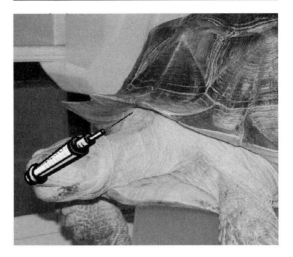

Figure 12.1. The subcarapacial sinus is located roughly where the first vertebra fuses with the carapace. Photo courtesy of Jörg Mayer.

pace and directed dorsally. The advantage of this technique is that it is completely independent of the animal's head position. Whether the head is retracted or fully extended, the location of the sinus always remains the same. Caution must be taken, however, as many animals will try to bite during this procedure. There is also the possibility of lymph contamination with this method.

RADIOGRAPHS

Radiographic images should be routinely obtained of every reptile entering the shelter. Two views, both dorsoventral and lateral, should always be taken in order to obtain a true three-dimensional assessment, which is lost when just a single view is taken. Radiographs often reveal much about current and past medical problems even in cases in which no medical history is available.

Snakes

In most cases, snakes do not have to be anesthetized for radiographs. An initial whole body view can be obtained with the snake restrained in a pillowcase or a plastic container. For a more concentrated view of a certain segment, the snake can be restrained in a plastic tube to hold the desired segment straight. This also facilitates rotation of the animal to obtain a lateral view of the body. Multiple images obviously will be needed if the snake's body is longer than a single cassette, so care must be taken to label the images correctly for future interpretation.

Lizards

Lizards can be placed directly on the cassette to obtain a dorsoventral image. Most animals will hold still for the brief time required. Smaller specimens can be secured on the cassette with a few strips of tape across the neck and the dorsum. If the animal is large or especially active, the front and hind limbs can be taped caudally along the lateral body wall and tail for restraint. With the hind limbs in this position and the fore limbs taped together in front of the body, animals can be placed easily in lateral recumbency for the lateral image. A third method of restraint is the use of the vago-vasal reflex. Digital pressure applied to both eyes for a few seconds will elicit this response, and the animal will remain in an immobile state for 3–5 seconds. This window of time is often just enough to position the animal and obtain the radiographic image needed. A cotton swab placed over each eye and secured with self-adhesive tape will maintain a constant pressure and might prolong the frozen state if more time is needed. This method will not work with every species or with every individual.

Tortoises

Smaller tortoises can be taped to the cassette in the same way as small lizards, but most of the time even small specimens' powerful legs will interfere with this method of restraint. Alternate restraint of a conscious tortoise can be obtained by placing them on top of a radiolucent object, such as a plastic jar or roll of tape that is tall enough to prevent their legs from contacting the cassette, thus, keeping the animal stationary.

Three separate images are necessary for the complete radiographic assessment of a tortoise. In addition to the usual dorsoventral and lateral views, a craniocaudal view is also needed. This image is primarily used to evaluate the individual lung fields. Pneumonia tends to be localized in tortoises due to the anatomy of their respiratory system. This view can help to determine the location and extent of any lesions.

A horizontal beam is necessary for both the lateral and the craniocaudal radiographic images in order to avoid artifact production. The radiograph machine rather than the animal should be manipulated to obtain these images. Because reptiles do not have a diaphragm, if the animal is tipped on end or placed in lateral recumbency, the coelomic contents will be displaced toward the lungs distorting them. Also, if there is free fluid in the lungs, it will move in response to the positioning, making the image useless for diagnostic evaluation.

HOUSING

In order to provide a reptile with the best care, identification of the species and knowledge of the natural history is the key element, especially for setting up optimal housing. Species-specific behavioral traits are important factors; for example, some species may react differently to con-specifics in terms of aggression. Some species are very aggressive toward any intruder; others will challenge only males of the same species; whereas others will hardly ever show aggression toward other individuals. In a shelter situation, where animals come from different backgrounds and often with unknown histories, isolation of individuals, even of the same species, is the best solution in terms of quarantine and prevention of aggression.

An area dedicated to reptiles only will also be useful in preventing the spread of pathogens to and from these animals. The topic of salmonella in reptiles has received plenty of media attention, and even when dealing with the simple facts of this disease, it is good practice to consider all reptiles as salmonella risks. Therefore, when caring for animals in the shelter, it is best to minimize contamination by caring for the reptiles in the facility last and protecting yourself by always using disposable gloves when handling reptiles or their equipment.

Principles of quarantine should apply to housing any new acquisitions. Unfortunately, valid time periods for quarantine of reptiles have not been established. The incubation periods of many pathogens in reptilians have not been studied or are simply longer than practicality would allow (for example, up to 6 months for some diseases such as the Inclusion Body Disease in pythons and boids).

Substrate and Cage Furniture

Of all the different substrates available today, newspaper is probably the best. Newspaper is readily available and cheap. It is also nontoxic, easily replaced when soiled, and not easily ingested by the reptile.

Other necessities include an appropriate water source, a hide box, and some branches for climbing for arboreal species. The hide box can be made of a plastic container, cardboard box, flowerpot, and so on. Choose a container that the entire animal can fit into fairly snugly. Many reptiles like to hide in crevices and feel most secure when their body touches more than one side of the hide box. This box can also function to provide a small area with its own microclimate. During shedding for example, animals benefit from an increase in humidity, and this can easily be maintained inside the hide box. Natural branches (make sure no pesticides have be applied), driftwood, or PVC pipes can be used to provide arboreal species the necessary vertical comfort zones. Artificial flowers and plants should be avoided, however, as they could be toxic or cause obstructions if ingested.

For housing aquatic reptiles, it is important to keep in mind that basic concepts of an aquarium will still apply (that is, water quality, aeration, filtration, and so on), but a site for drying on land also has to be made available. Nearly all aquatic reptiles love to bask in the sun out of the water. This gives them a chance to heat up their system and to dry off. Make sure the animal can easily climb out of the water onto the dry dock without much effort. Keep gravel size large enough so no accidental ingestion of the pebbles can occur.

All cage furniture should be cleaned regularly, preventing the buildup of bacteria or noxious gases from waste. Reptiles rely to a great degree on their olfactory sense, and an unclean environment will most likely cause stress to the animals. Chlorhexidine, iodophores, and quaternary ammonium compounds are generally regarded as safe to use on the enclosure and the furniture.

TEMPERATURE AND HUMIDITY

These environmental factors are of utmost importance to the captive reptile; however, they are often neglected in spite of the ease of monitoring. Every reptile housing setup should include two thermometers, one set at either end of the thermal gradient, and one hygrometer as part of the basic equipment. The aim is to keep the reptile healthy by imitating the natural environment as closely as possible in the captive setting.

Temperature must be carefully controlled, and achieving an appropriate temperature gradient within the captive setting is of utmost importance. The gradient usually should consist of a variation of about 10–15°F. The appropriate temperature range for each species can be estimated by dividing environmental niches into roughly three types: desert, tropical, and temperate conditions. The optimal temperature for most desert and tropical species will be around 90–95°F at the hot spot and 75–80°F at the cool end during the day. For temperate zone species, the high end should be approximately 75–85°F. At night, the temperature should fall to 75°F for desert and tropical species and 65°F to 70°F for the temperate species. Water temperature for aquatic turtles and crocodiles should be around 75–80°F, and the air temperature can be 10°F higher.

Humidity should also mimic the natural environment of the animal, with the desert species being kept at the low end of about 50 percent humidity and the tropical species at the high end with 80–90 percent humidity. The temperate zone animals should be housed at about 60–75 percent humidity. In humid regions of the country, use of a dry heat source will help regulate any excess humidity; however, in dryer regions of the country, providing adequate humidity can be more challenging. An ultrasonic humidifier, a simple misting from a plant spray bottle several times during the day, or the presence of a large surface area water source can be used to increase the humidity. Inadequate humidity can lead to medical problems such as incomplete shedding (dysecdysis), dehydration, and respiratory problems. However, it is important to note that with increased humidity, proper air circulation becomes vital, as many deleterious pathogens thrive in humid conditions.

HEAT AND LIGHT

The natural cycles of heat and light should be considered in designing the captive reptile environment. The sun provides heat, light, and UV-B radiation from above and follows a regular cycle of light and dark periods. In tropical countries, the sunset and dawn are approximately 12 hours apart, so a 12/12 hour on/off cycle should be maintained in captivity.

Some debate exists as to whether all reptiles need UV-B irradiation on a daily basis for vitamin D_3

synthesis, but it seems best to provide a light source capable of irradiation at the 290–320 nm wavelength to all captive reptiles. Note that fluorescent UV-B light sources (for example, Reptisun 5.0 by ZooMed) must be changed after every 12 months of use as their UV-B output decreases over time. Newer products provide both incandescent light and heat and will provide heat and UV-B irradiation up to six feet away (for example, UVHeat by T-Rex). These lamps also claim to provide three years of UV-B irradiation without the need of replacement. Care has to be taken when purchasing a light source, as some reptile lamps on the market claim to be full spectrum but completely lack the UV-B wavelength. Heating elements such as hot rocks are unnatural, providing active heat from below, and are a dangerous potential source of burns and should not be used.

SEDATION AND ANESTHESIA

In most cases, reptiles will not need to be sedated for the physical exam or the initial assessment. However, in rare cases, sedation is needed in order to prevent injuries to the animal and/or handler. All procedures involving sedation or anesthetic protocols must be conducted at the preferred optimal temperature zone (POTZ) of the animal. Induction and recovery will be significantly prolonged if the animal is not at the ideal temperature. Chilling the animal down is not an acceptable way to quiet any reptile.

If venous access is available, induction should be performed with Propofol intravenously at 5–10 mg/kg. This short-acting hypnotic produces a rapid, smooth, and excitement-free anesthesia induction. The onset of effect will be about 2–3 minutes after the injection. This will allow the animal to be intubated and ventilated. Isofluorane at 2–3 percent usually will provide anesthesia at a surgical plane. Recovery from inhalation anesthesia will be more rapid if room air is used rather than pure oxygen, preventing respiratory depression due to oxygen-saturation.

If neither venous access nor gas anesthesia are available, an intramuscular injection of ketamine at 50 mg/kg can produce effective sedation. Ketamine alone should not be used for painful procedures due to its questionable analgesic effects. Ketamine can be combined with other drugs to achieve surgical anesthesia with analgesia. Please see Carpenter 2001 in the suggested reading section for an extensive list of anesthetic drug combinations.

Injectable anesthetics usually result in a much more prolonged recovery than the assisted gas inhalation protocol. It has also been mentioned in the literature that snakes have become permanently aggressive after a ketamine injection (Bennet, 1991).

FLUID THERAPY

Due to their slower metabolic rate, reptiles need fewer fluids per kg bodyweight per day than birds or mammals. As a general rule 25–35 ml/kg/day is a normal maintenance rate. Fluids can be given SQ, IV, IO, ICe, PO, or by soaking.

Soaking the animal in lukewarm water is a very stress-free way to provide hydration to noncritically dehydrated animals. Chelonians (turtles and tortoises) especially benefit greatly from soaking, as they both drink the water and absorb fluids through the cloacal membranes. Soaking for up to 8 hours will also stimulate the GI tract, and defecation is commonly observed. The depth of the water should be shallow enough to prevent drowning of a weakened animal. Chin height in chelonians is a good measure. Lizards and snakes also seem to benefit from a warm soak bath.

Enteral hydration follows the same principles as force-feeding as discussed in the following section. The parenteral routes provide more aggressive forms of hydration. The SQ route is practical only for small amounts of fluids, because reptiles do not have the same skin elasticity as mammals. Larger fluid boluses can be given intracoelomically (ICe), but this route has potential risks. Due to the fact that reptiles lack a diaphragm, care must be taken when administering the fluids ICe not to enter an air sac or lung and drown the animal. In chelonians, the needle should be introduced into the ventral inguinal fossa and angled downward, in order to avoid the dorsal lungs or the bladder. In snakes, the caudal third of the body should be selected to avoid the lungs. The coelom is entered at the point where the ventral scutes meet the dorsal scales. Usually one-third of the daily maintenance dose can be given as a bolus. For long-term hydration, an intraosseous (IO) catheter should be placed. In tortoises, the IO catheter can be placed in the bridge, the shell structure that connects the carapace with the plastron. In lizards, the IO catheter can be placed easily in the tibia or the femur. Because IV catheter placement often requires a cut-down procedure, the IO route is usually preferred. The rate of fluid administration IO can be the same as IV, and usually drugs suitable for IV injection can be used readily via the IO route.

The types of fluids used for reptiles can be very different from those used in mammals or birds. The authors' fluid of choice is Plasmalyte A (Normosol), but a mixture of 1 part Lactated Ringers Solution (LRS) + 2 parts 0.45 percent NaCl with 2.5 percent Dextrose, or LRS + 2.5 Dextrose are suitable. All fluids should be warmed to the patient's preferred temperature before administration.

NUTRITION AND FORCE-FEEDING

Basic nutrition in the class reptilia is challenging as many species have unique requirements, and many of the factors involved are not yet completely understood. This section will focus on a few key points of nutrition necessary to maintain a small population in the shelter.

Snakes

All snakes are carnivorous and need prey animals as their main diet. A common presentation in snakes is anorexia and severe emaciation. The use of live prey should be avoided for both welfare and medical reasons. A snake should always be trained to accept dead prey. However, in a shelter environment, it is highly likely that some animals will refuse to eat. Large snakes can go for a month without having to eat. Determining the limits of a normal, physiological episode versus an abnormal, pathological episode of anorexia can be difficult. As a rule of thumb, a decrease of 10 percent bodyweight can be normal during a state of physiological anorexia. If the animal loses more than 10 percent of its bodyweight, supportive care should be initiated. If the animal refuses to eat previously frozen prey, warming the prey animal in chicken broth might help to stimulate a feeding response. The prey animal can also be cut open to expose viscera, as this has also some positive effect on the feeding response. If there is still no success, the next step is to offer a freshly killed (still warm) animal. In some cases, snakes respond when the animal is gently slapped at the snake's face. If everything else fails, the snake can be placed in an empty container with a *pinkie* mouse (newborn naked mouse before it grows fur) and left overnight. The use of live animals should be the last resort and car-

ries a potential danger of injury to the weakened animal. If a live rodent is placed in the snake's environment, the situation must be supervised, and the prey animal should not be left unattended with the snake. Rodents can inflict serious harm to their potential predators by biting them or even eating them.

If the animal has to be force fed, a dead prey animal can be forced down the throat with the help of long, padded feeding tongs. This procedure can be very stressful for the animal and regurgitation may occur after the attempted force-feeding. Sedation of the snake for this procedure is sometimes helpful.

Lizards

Nutrition of lizards in captivity is not straightforward and presents several potentials for disaster. Lizards can be divided into three main nutritional groups. Herbivorous, omnivorous, and carnivorous/insectivorous lizards each have different nutritional requirements, and malnutrition is probably the most common health problem encountered in captivity in all three groups.

The herbivorous lizard can be maintained exclusively on vegetable matter. Common herbivorous species in captivity include the green iguana and the prehensile tail skink. A salad of mixed dark greens (for example, kale, collards) and flowers (for example, dandelion) is usually offered with a vitamin/mineral supplement added. A few good commercial products that claim to be complete diets are currently available. The advantages of using these products are obvious. They have a longer shelf life than fresh produce diets, and the risk of an accidental imbalance inducing malnutrition is minimized. Two products recommended by the authors are the Mazuri Iguana Diet (Mazuri) and the Complete Iguana Diet (Walkabout Farms).

Carnivorous lizards, most commonly *monitor spp.*, are similar to snakes in their nutritional needs; however, a few differences apply. For example, a carnivorous lizard needs to be fed more often than a similarly sized snake. Overfeeding is a common problem because most lizards readily accept food on a daily basis, leading frequently to obesity problems. Appropriate prey should be offered according to the size of the animal. Usually, the length of the prey's body should be approximately equal to the width of the lizard's mouth. If whole prey is fed, supplementation of minerals and vitamins is usually not necessary. However, if only pinkies or other juvenile animals with incompletely calcified skeleton are fed, calcium supplementation may be needed. Raw meat or commercial dog/cat food can be used on a short-term basis but should be avoided for longer maintenance, as these feeds will lead to metabolic problems. Again, as with snakes, the animal safety issues and ethical concepts of feeding prekilled prey also apply.

For insectivorous lizards (geckos, anoles, and so on), farm-raised insects such as mealworms, wax worms, crickets, or fruitflies are usually sufficient. Wild invertebrates can also be collected but care has to be taken to make sure that these animals have not been exposed to pesticides. Before any invertebrates are fed, they should always be supplemented in some way with calcium. Invertebrates have much more phosphorus than calcium in their system due to the chemical composition of the exoskeleton. Dusting the insects with a calcium supplement (for example, ReptiCal by Terra Fauna) or gut-loading the insects with calcium enriched food and/or water (for example, Cricket Diet—High Calcium and Cricket Quencher by Fluker Farms) is necessary.

For omnivorous lizards (for example, uromastyx and bearded dragon), a mixture of the herbivorous diet and the insectivorous diet is best. Most of these species have a higher invertebrate content in their diet during the juvenile stages of their life and as adults tend to consume more plant materials. It is advisable to mimic this in captivity.

Tortoises

Tortoises can also be divided into three groups according to their nutrition: herbivorous, omnivorous, and carnivorous. Commonly encountered species within the herbivorous group include: desert tortoises, gopher tortoises, spur-thighed tortoises, and Hermann's or Greek tortoises. The omnivorous species commonly encountered are the box turtles. The carnivorous species are mostly aquatic and include the snapping turtle, pond turtles, map turtles, red-eared sliders, and so on.

Herbivorous tortoises can be maintained on selected greens and hay. Commercial foods are available and can be used either as supplementation or as the sole diet (for example, Mazuri, Walkabout Farms). Omnivorous turtles need to be fed a mixture of greens and some invertebrates. A healthy box turtle usually will respond positively to a moving invertebrate. All invertebrates fed to omnivorous reptiles should be enriched with a calcium supplement (see previous discussion of insectivorous lizards) prior to feeding out. A few commercial diets for box turtles are available (for example, Walkabout Farms). The carnivorous species can be maintained on commercial products alone or with supplementations of invertebrates.

Force-feeding is indicated if the animal refuses to eat despite supportive care (that is, rehydration, vitamin therapy—Vitamin B complex, Vitamin E, and Selenium—and treatment of underlying disease) or if signs of severe weight loss are evident. For force-feeding chelonians, the authors recommend the products from Walkabout Farm, as this specially designed formula will pass easily through a 3.5 French rubber catheter, making the force-feeding an easy and nutritionally complete treatment. Prior to the initial feeding, the animal's head should be extended and the distance from the mouth to the stomach measured by holding the feeding tube end at the middle section of the plastron and marking the tip of the mouth on the tube. The tube then can be inserted into the mouth through a speculum, making sure that the animal can't bite off the tube. Usually 10–15 ml/kg/day of food should be fed. This dose is best divided into two equal portions for twice a day (BID) feeding.

SIGNS OF ABUSE AND NEGLECT

More often than not, reptiles are the victims of neglect, due to their exotic needs and the ignorance of their owners who are uneducated about their proper care, rather than abuse. The most common problems encountered with neglected reptiles include nutritional secondary hyperparathyroidism and renal secondary hyperparathyroidism commonly referred to as metabolic bone disease, UV-B dependant disease, and over/under supplementation of vitamins and/or minerals.

If the animal has been kept in suboptimal conditions for a prolonged period of time, it is very likely that irreversible damage has been done. With immediate correction of the husbandry problems, the animal's life may be saved, but the underlying damage may be permanent. Kidney failure and bone malformations are the two most commonly detected permanent sequelae of poor husbandry. Radiographs can give immediate information regarding skeletal problems, and blood work to obtain the Ca:P ratio will reveal kidney damage. The optimal

Ca:P ratio=2:1 and Ca*P<70. Both of these diagnostic tests should be performed as soon as the animal is presented to the shelter.

Other signs of neglect include skin wounds, usually due to heat burns or rodent aggression. Fresh injuries or old scars are easily picked up by the initial physical exam. A detailed examination of the skin can be very informative in determining the level of care the animal received. Neglected skin wounds often become infected and don't heal completely. These wounds should be thoroughly examined, as chronically infected skin wounds can serve as a constant source of bacteremia in the animal. Even completely healed skin wounds can become a problem during sheds. These scarred areas do not shed skin as easily as the rest of the skin, and an incomplete shed or dyecdysis can be the result. In these cases the unshed skin should be soaked to soften and then be removed manually.

Injuries are common in snakes that are fed live rodents. In the authors' opinion, feeding live prey is not an acceptable practice and constitutes animal cruelty. Shelters may also find this alternative unacceptable, and a decision must be made as to what lengths to go to in order to save the life of the animal. Damage from prey species is often extensive and severe, and the basic principles of open wound management should be applied. Thermal burns are also frequent presentations of neglect. Hot rocks or unprotected heat lamps are usually the culprits. While warming themselves, reptiles can inflict serious burns on themselves if they are allowed close contact with the heat source. They do not seem to connect the source of heat to the source of pain and stay close to the heat source until serious tissue injury results. Again, principles of thermal wound care apply to the same degree to reptiles as with other animals.

EUTHANASIA

Euthanasia is sometimes necessary due to the severity of the disease present. Euthanasia of reptiles can be challenging on occasion, as some reptiles appear to recover hours or days after they received a fatal injection of euthanasia solution. When performing euthanasia, the animal should be initially anesthetized, and then if IV access can be established, a dose of euthanasia solution should be administered. If IV access does not seem to be feasible, the euthanasia solution can be given ICe. The authors recommend the use of 2–3 times the usual recommended mammalian dose, in order to avoid failure and later recovery of the patient.

Verification of death is essential in these species as with any other species, and they should never be placed in the refrigerator or freezer until this has been done. Freezing is not a humane method of euthanizing reptiles. Respirations and the heartbeat should be monitored for cessation of activity. Turtles should be checked for limpness of the limbs and neck in addition to the cessation of the vital signs that may be difficult to assess (Rhoades, 2002). See chapter 24 for more information on euthanasia.

CONCLUSION

In general, reptiles are admitted to most shelters sporadically and only kept for short periods of time. However, some shelters may find they are receiving more exotic animals than they did in the past, and expectations are that they will provide quality care for them. The guidelines provided in this chapter are intended primarily for short-term and immediate care. Longer stays may result when reptiles are seized for animal cruelty or relinquished by owners unable to provide appropriate care. Treatment must be rendered while court cases are resolved, and the animals are rehabilitated for rehoming. Many shelters do not have the space or staff experience necessary to provide for long-term medical care for sick or injured animals. For example, many shelters lack the radiology equipment that is key to diagnosing certain conditions and must send the animals to local veterinary facilities to have the procedures performed. Unless the shelter veterinarian has experience dealing with reptiles, any shelter that receives reptiles frequently or holds them for long periods of time should contact a herpetological society, zoo, or veterinarian with a special interest in and experience dealing with exotics for additional advice on providing immediate and ongoing care when problems arise.

SUGGESTED READING

Bennet, R.A. 1991. A review of anesthesia and chemical restraint in reptiles *Journal of Zoological and Wildlife Medicine* 22: 282–303.

Beynon, P.H., Lawton, M.P.C., et al. 1992. *Manual of Reptiles* Cheltenham, UK: British Small Animal Veterinary Association.

Boyer, T. 1998. *Essentials of Reptiles A Guide for Practitioners*. Lakewood, CO: AAHA Press.

Frye F.L. 1991. *The Biomedical and Surgical Aspects of Captive Reptile Husbandry*. Malabar, FL: Krieger Publishing Company.

Frye, F.L. 1994. *Reptile Clinician's Handbook, A Compact Clinical and Surgical Reference*. Malabar, FL: Krieger Publishing Company.

Carpenter, J. W., Mashima, T. Y., et al. 2001. *Exotic Animal Formulary* 2nd ed. Philadelphia, PA: WB Saunders Co.

Johnson-Delaney, C.A. 1995. *Exotic Animal Medicine in Practice*. Lake Worth, FL: Wingers.

Mader, D. R. 1996. *Reptile Medicine and Surgery*. Philadelphia, PA: WB Saunders.

Messonier, S.P. 1996. *Common Reptile Diseases and Treatment*. Cambridge, MA: Blackwell.

Rhoades, R. H. 2002. *Euthanasia Training Manual*, Washington, DC: Humane Society of the United States.

Appendix 12.1:
Reptile Care Products

Mazuri
1401 S. Hanley Rd.
P.O. Box 19856
St. Louis, Missouri 63144
Phone: 314-768-4861 or 800-227-8941
Fax: 314-768-4859
Email: buymazuri@buymazuri.net or mazuri@purina-mills.com

T-Rex
T-Rex Products, Inc.
1124 Bay Blvd., Suite A
Chula Vista, CA 91911
Phone: 619-424-1050 or 800-991-8739
Fax: 619-424-1051
http://www.t-rexproducts.com/

ZooMed
Zoo Med Laboratories, Inc.
3100 McMillan Rd.
San Luis Obispo, CA 93401
Phone: 805-542-9988
Fax: 805-542-9295
zoomed@zoomed.com

Walkabout Farm
P.O. Box 625
Pembroke, VA 24136
Owner: Susan Donoghue, VMD, DACVN
Phone: 540-626-3081
Fax: 540-626-3564

Fluker Farms
1333 Plantation Rd.
Port Allen, LA 70767
800-735-8537
info@flukerfarms.com

13

Temporary Care of Wildlife in the Animal Shelter

Scott Diehl and Cheryl Diehl

INTRODUCTION

Animal shelters may be limited in their ability to assist wildlife in their communities by either mission or lack of resources. Nevertheless, they are often called upon by their communities to assist wildlife in distress. A survey of nearly 100 animal shelters in the United States found that over half of them deal with injured, orphaned, or nuisance wildlife over 500 times each year (Kirkwood, 1998). However, many of the critical needs of wild animals in rehabilitation are much different than the needs of sheltered companion animals. Therefore, being a well-equipped companion animal shelter with a highly capable staff does not automatically make a shelter a humane and effective wild animal care facility.

This chapter is intended primarily for shelters that do not have a full-service in-house wildlife rehabilitation center. It is intended to help shelters that accept wildlife on a limited or temporary basis or are considering doing so. Establishing an effective, well-planned wildlife program for your shelter can decrease animal suffering and enhance community confidence in your organization.

PREVENTIVE MEDICINE

The authors consider public education that reduces the occurrence or likelihood of injury, illness, needless disruption, or death for wildlife in one's community to be preventive medicine. As important as it is to provide humane care for injured, sick, and orphaned wildlife, how much better it would be if we could *prevent* these sufferings.

Tracking the causes of injury, sickness, and death for wildlife in your community may reveal one or more key issues upon which you can have a positive

impact through public education. In this way, even shelters without an in-house wildlife rehabilitation capability can reduce injury and suffering for wild animals in their communities.

The public can be educated about these key issues in a number of ways, including media stories, brochures, facility displays, automated telephone tip-lines, and stories in shelter newsletters or on the shelter's Web site. The authors discuss these methods in greater depth elsewhere (Diehl and Diehl, 2001).

MAKE CONNECTIONS

What resources exist for wildlife in your service area? Are the services you plan to provide for wildlife already available from another organization or individual in your area? Are the services that are already available humane and effective?

The idea that you will be providing temporary care for wildlife means that you have somewhere else to transfer wildlife in need of help. This "somewhere else" really means a capable, licensed wildlife rehabilitator or wildlife rehabilitation center.

To begin, compile a list of the wildlife rehabilitators, humane societies, wildlife veterinarians, state and federal agencies, and others who provide wildlife services in your community. A good place to start is to contact your state Department of Conservation, Fish and Game, or Natural Resources (DNR). This agency should have a list of the licensed wildlife rehabilitators in your area. Also ask the agent about your state's wildlife rehabilitation permitting process. Ask them what requirements they have for your shelter to be a temporary holding facility for wildlife. Ask what this agency has to offer the wildlife you are called upon to help; for instance, will they help transport wildlife to a local wildlife rehabilitator?

Also ask what species are considered rabies-vector species in your state and about any restrictions the DNR has on the handling of these species.

Your DNR should be able to provide you with a list of endangered species in your state. Ask them what they would like you to do if a client finds and brings an endangered animal in to your shelter.

Ask what limitations they have on your shelter staff performing euthanasias on wildlife that cannot be rehabilitated.

Find out how these various agencies and individuals view and work with one another. What types of services for wildlife does each provide? Ask them how they think your shelter fits in and how you can work together. The ideal situation would be to have all of these parties meet together to establish or redefine the network of services for wildlife in your community.

Create an Operating Framework

With this list of available resources, you will be able to establish an operating framework for your shelter's wildlife program (Parker, 2000). An operating framework will help take the guesswork out of what your shelter will and will not do. It will help provide answers for the questions about "who," "what," "when," "where," and "why." For example, if a call about an injured hawk comes in to the shelter, who will handle the call? What happens to calls for help after you are closed? Will shelter staff answer the caller's questions, or will these calls be directed to a local licensed wildlife rehabilitator? What hours is the rehabilitator available? Who will capture the bird, transport it, and ultimately provide care? What if it needs euthanasia? What if it is an endangered species?

Also, check with your shelter's insurance carrier to find out whether they will cover your wildlife program, or whether changes to your insurance policy are needed.

Admission Protocols

One important aspect of your operating framework will be admissions protocols. Work with your consulting wildlife rehabilitators to create a list of indicators that will help your staff determine which animals need help and which animals are actually exhibiting natural behaviors that are unfamiliar to the caller. For example, many fledgling birds do not fly well when they leave the nest, and they spend the first several days on the ground being fed by their parents. The parent birds are busy foraging for food and are often not in the immediate vicinity of the fledglings. People will find a fledgling, see that no parent is immediately nearby, and assume that the bird is orphaned. A well-designed admissions protocol for these situations will prevent the intake of healthy, unorphaned birds.

Legalities

Most states require permits, even for veterinarians and animal shelters, to care for wildlife. State rehabilitation permits generally cover mammals, reptiles, amphibians, and nonmigratory birds.

The requirements necessary to get a permit vary widely from state to state. Some states simply require the applicant to write a letter describing their experience and facilities, while other states have formal applications and examinations. Forty-three states require an inspection of the proposed wildlife facilities (Casey and Casey, 2000a). It may be possible for you or your facility to be subpermitted under the license of a local wildlife rehabilitator.

A federal permit issued by the U. S. Fish and Wildlife Service (USFWS) is required to care for migratory birds, and a rehabilitation permit issued by your state will be needed in order to get a federal permit. A federal permit is not required to care for Rock Pigeons (feral pigeons—*Columba livia*, formerly Rock Dove), House Sparrows (*Passer domesticus*) or European Starlings (*Sturna vulgaris*).

Both state and federal permits may have limits as to the species for which the permittee is allowed to provide care. Special permits will be needed to care for or euthanize federally endangered species and are likely to be needed to care for or euthanize species on your state's endangered and threatened species list. However, state or federal conservation officers may grant permission for the euthanasia of an endangered or threatened animal on a case-by-case basis.

Obtain a list of your state's endangered and threatened species from your DNR and get a list of federally endangered species encountered in your state from the USFWS. Some states limit the rehabilitation of rabies-vector species. Also, some states will not allow the release of some rehabilitated non-native (invasive) species (Casey and Casey, 2000b).

Authorities will sometimes allow an unlicensed individual a brief time period (for example, 24 hours) in which to transport an injured wild animal that they have found to a licensed wildlife rehabilitator.

It is also prudent to check into local ordinances (for example, zoning) regarding the keeping of wildlife in your community.

Moore and Joosten (1997) provide a list of regional USFWS offices and addresses for the various state's DNRs.

Parker (1997) provides information about obtaining permits in Canada.

Training

The authors highly recommend the training offered by The National Wildlife Rehabilitators Association (NWRA) and International Wildlife Rehabilitation Council (IWRC). (See Appendix 13.1.) For example, the latter offers classes such as "Wildlife Rehabilitation Basic 1AB" that includes basic anatomy and physiology, calculating drug dosages, handling and physical restraint, gavage (tube-feeding), giving injections and much more. However, as valuable as these classes are, hands-on training with a licensed wildlife rehabilitator is still essential for gaining experience with animal identification, handling, housing, wild animal behavior, and natural history.

Classes in bird identification and the natural history of your area's wildlife, such as those offered by nature centers and community colleges can be helpful. Correct identification of species handled by the shelter is necessary for properly selecting handling techniques and housing, for identifying endangered species and for accurate record keeping. Natural history information is needed for determining whether animal behaviors observed or reported to shelter personnel on the telephone are normal or indicate that an animal is injured, sick, or orphaned.

Reference Materials

Reference materials that the authors believe are essential for shelters handling wildlife on a temporary basis are listed in Appendix 13.2.

STRESS

Controlling stress for wildlife in your facility is essential. Unlike most companion animals, wild ani-

mals view humans as a threat, even predators, and exposure to us through handling, petting, hearing, seeing, and even smelling humans can be very stressful to them.

Stress is cumulative (Fowler, 1986b), and all wild animals presented to an animal shelter for care are already stressed. In addition to somatic stressors such as injury, infection, parasites, heat or cold, ination, and dehydration, they have also experienced psychological and behavioral stress from fear, anxiety or even terror, and frustration.

The authors have seen injured or sick wildlife, already under great cumulative stress, die almost instantly from simply being picked up by a human.

Furthermore, wild animals also view companion animals as predators. Therefore, wildlife must be housed with companion animals out of their view and hearing.

To minimize stress for wildlife in your facility do the following:

1. Eliminate unnecessary handling. Do not "pet" wild animals.
2. Eliminate unnecessary talking and other noise (for example, radios, intercom loud speakers, and barking). Communicate necessary information to coworkers in a quiet voice.
3. Avoid prolonged direct eye contact with an animal.
4. Use visual barriers such as towels or sheets draped over cages (see "Temporary Housing") to prevent wild animals from viewing humans, companion animals, or other wild animals that may be natural predators.

ANIMAL HANDLING

First, a word about public safety. In the interest of human and animal health and safety, do not allow clients that are bringing a wild animal into your facility to handle the animal once they are in your shelter. This will eliminate the chance of a member of the public being bitten, reduce the chances of animal's escape, and will ensure safe and humane handling for the animal.

The use of proper animal handling techniques and equipment will help protect the animal handler from injury and bite-transmitted zoonotic disease (for example, rabies) and will help protect the animal from further injury and excessive stress. In the case of possible rabies-vector mammals, preventing bites will also protect the animal from euthanasia required to test for rabies (see "Zoonoses" that follows).

Because animal handling is almost invariably stressful for the wild animal patient, handling must be kept to a minimum. The animal should be handled only when absolutely necessary to render essential care. Patients must also not be physically restrained unless actually being handled for an essential procedure. Such unnecessary restraint is very stressful and can cause profound physiological changes, which may result in death (Spraker, 1982; Schulz, 1997).

When handling wild animals, remember that they fear humans and perceive the handler as a threat. Consequently, they will use their bill, teeth, talons, or claws to protect themselves. It is not true that a wild animal will sense that the handler is trying to help and, therefore, not injure the handler.

Shelter personnel who will be handling wildlife should receive hands-on animal handling training from an experienced wildlife rehabilitator. A veterinarian with experience handling exotic animals may be able to provide additional training in animal handling and restraint.

General Guidelines for Birds

Use a towel or bed sheet (for large birds) to wrap the bird loosely but securely around the body with its wings folded against its body in a natural position. This wrap must be secure enough to limit the bird's movements but must not be too tight; birds lack a diaphragm and excessive restraint will impair respiration. When handling a bird's bill, be certain not to cover the nares (nostrils). Drape the bird's head with a cloth during handling to minimize visual stimuli for the patient (see Figs. 13.1 and 13.2). This often helps calm the bird and reduces struggling.

A bird loose in the facility should be captured by noting the location of the bird in the room and then turning off the lights and approaching and capturing the bird in the dark. Most birds other than owls (Strigiformes) and nightjars (Caprimulgidae: nighthawks, Whip-poor-will) are reluctant to fly in the dark and usually can be captured in this manner with a minimum of stress to the patient or handler.

This technique should also be used when capturing a smaller bird in housing for examination or treatment. Attempting to capture a bird in a cage or box with the lights on will often result in the bird fluttering frantically, trying to avoid capture. Turn the lights out and feel around in the container to capture the bird.

HERONS AND CRANES

The handler and anyone assisting should wear a plastic face shield. These birds defend themselves by jabbing at the handler, usually at the face and eyes, with their sharply pointed bills.

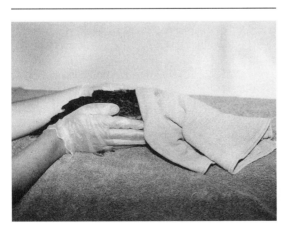

Figure 13.1. Covering a bird's head with a cloth during restraint reduces visual stimuli and often reduces struggling. Photo credit to Scott and Cheryl Diehl.

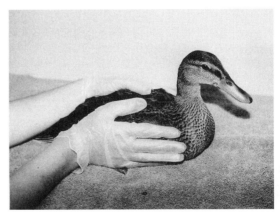

Figure 13.2. Proper restraint for a bird. Photo credit to Scott and Cheryl Diehl.

When approaching the bird for handling, hold open a large sheet or towel in front of you at arm's length and drape it over the bird. The handler should control the bird's head and neck by using a hand protected by a lightweight leather glove to grasp the tip of the bird's bill. Be careful not to block the bird's nares (nostrils), usually located on the proximal one-third of the maxilla (upper bill) (see Fig. 13.3).

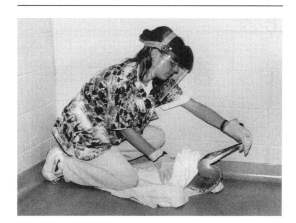

Figure 13.3. Proper restraint for a Great Blue Heron (*Ardea herodias*). Note the handler's protective face shield and leather gloves. Photo credit to Jessica Orlofske.

HAWKS AND OWLS

Heavy leather, gauntleted gloves are required for handling large birds of prey (raptors) such as Red-tailed Hawks (*Buteo jamaicensis*) and Great Horned Owls (*Bubo virginianus*). Even wearing these gloves, the handler and others assisting with procedures must use caution when handling these birds. Raptors protect themselves by grasping with their very powerful, sharply pointed talons, although they also sometimes bite. Their talons are sometimes capable of piercing heavy handler's gloves, so skilled handling and control of the bird's feet is essential to prevent injury to the handler and to keep the bird from grasping and injuring one of its own feet. Smaller birds of prey such as Screech Owls (*Otus* sp.) and American Kestrels (*Falco sparverius*) should be handled with lightweight leather gloves.

Good control of birds of prey is afforded by grasping one of the bird's legs in each gloved hand, as high up on each upper leg as possible. Drape the bird's head and body with a towel. If necessary, the bird then can be "cast" (laid) on its back on a table, while still maintaining good control of its legs and talons, for examination or treatment. Schulz (1997) discusses raptor restraint and transport in greater detail.

MISCELLANEOUS BIRDS

Most small nonraptorial birds require no special protective equipment other than perhaps latex or vinyl exam gloves. However, some grosbeaks (family *Cardinalidae*), shrikes (family *Laniidae*), crows and ravens (family *Corvidae*), and gulls (family *Laridae*) bite very hard; wear lightweight leather gloves when handling these birds. Small nonraptorial birds are best handled by grasping them around the body and holding the wings against the body in their naturally folded position (see Fig. 13.4).

Keep some small- and medium-sized, fine-mesh (butterfly) nets on hand for capturing small- to medium-sized birds that may escape inside the shelter. Fine mesh (1/4-inch or smaller) is required to prevent birds from becoming entangled in the mesh, causing injury or feather damage.

Small and Medium-Sized Mammals

Avoid directly handling untranquilized biting mammals such as adult raccoons (*Procyon lotor*), foxes and coyotes (family Canidae), woodchucks

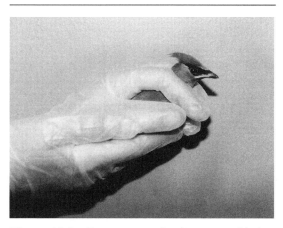

Figure 13.4. Proper restraint for a songbird. Photo credit to Scott and Cheryl Diehl.

(*Marmota* sp.), and squirrels (*Sciurus* sp.). A good-quality pole snare (approx 1.3m in length) is essential for handling some of these animals. For wild mammals other than canids, the snare is placed so that the animal's neck and one front leg are through the loop of the snare. This will minimize the chance for the animal to back out of the snare, and it affords greater animal control and comfort and prevents restricting or damaging the animal's airway. With the snare properly positioned as described, the handler can lift the animal off of the ground if necessary.

If recaging of these animals is needed, one can often get the animal to move from cage to cage on its own by placing the cages door to door with both doors open. Cover the cage you want the animal to move into with a towel and uncover the other cage. The animal will often voluntarily move from the uncovered cage to the covered cage.

The authors have found that chemical restraint using a 5:1 mix of 100mg/ml Ketamine HCl and 100mg/ml xylazine HCl or Telazol® (tiletamine HCl and zolazepam, Fort Dodge) is often required for thorough examination and first aid for these creatures.

The handler should increase their level of protection against bites and scratches by wearing heavy leather gauntleted handler's gloves when working with these animals. However, even heavy leather gloves designed for animal handling are usually inadequate to provide complete bite protection: careful handling and prudent use of a pole snare and/or chemical restraint are essential for the safe handling of these animals.

RECORD KEEPING

Thorough and accurate information taken at the time of admission can provide very important clues to an animal's problems. Moreover, accurate records regarding the species of animal admitted, its injuries or illness, the date of admission, and date of transfer to a wildlife rehabilitator or other final disposition will be needed for year-end reports required of wildlife rehabilitation permit holders.

The information gathered at the time of admission should include the location the animal was found; the cause of its illness or injury (if known); the name, address, and phone number of the finder; when the animal's distress was first noticed; when the animal was captured; any food, water, or prior care the animal has received; and in the case of mammals, whether or not anyone was bitten or scratched (see the discussion of "Rabies" that follows).

Pass a copy of this information, along with your findings from your examination of the animal and a record of any care given while at the shelter, to the cooperating wildlife rehabilitator when the animal is transferred to their care.

THE INITIAL EXAMINATION

Upon admission examine the animal quickly to identify any serious problems that need to be addressed right away. These problems include shock, hypothermia, serious bleeding, or severe injuries that would warrant immediate euthanasia. Work with your cooperating wildlife rehabilitators to establish a list of injuries and illnesses for various species that would require immediate euthanasia.

Beyond the initial exam, because the wildlife presented to you for care will already be stressed by the time you receive it, forgo any more handling (unless emergency intervention is needed) until the animal has had a chance to rest. Let the animal rest in a dark, warm (provided the animal is not hyperthermic), quiet place for 30–60 minutes. While the animal is resting, review the patient's history for clues to its problems.

After the animal has rested, it is time for a more thorough examination. If possible, observe the animal in its cage to look for abnormal behaviors, attitude, posture, and perhaps gait. It will be important for the examiner to have a good knowledge of the natural history and behavior of the animal in question in order to accurately evaluate the animal.

Proceed to restrain the animal (physically or chemically) to continue the examination. Of course, do not stop with the first significant problem found, but continue on to give the animal a complete physical examination. In the author's experience, multiple injuries/illnesses are commonplace. Be prepared to stop the exam temporarily if the animal shows signs of excessive stress.

A national survey of licensed wildlife rehabilitators showed the following categories as the nine most frequently seen problems in wildlife admitted for rehabilitation:

1. Shock and dehydration
2. Head trauma (concussion, bruising, swelling)
3. Wounds (punctures, lacerations, bites)

4. Neurological injuries (head or body tilt, paralysis, damaged nerves)
5. Diet and nutrition problems (emaciation)
6. Musculoskeletal problems (fractures, sprains, muscle tears)
7. Blood-related concerns (severe blood loss, bleeding from orifices, anemia)
8. Ectoparasites
9. Emotional states (fear of others, general fear, aggression) (Casey and Casey, 2000a)

SUPPORTIVE CARE AND TREATMENT

Shelter personnel treating wildlife, whether veterinarians or technicians, should be prepared and trained to render appropriate emergency medical care to manage stress, shock, dehydration, and mild hypothermia. Staff often are reluctant to do so because of their inexperience handling wildlife, even though the basic principles of emergency care remain the same.

Bleeding

If it is safe to do so, wear latex or vinyl gloves and use gauze and direct pressure to stop any serious bleeding.

Shock

Animals that are admitted to shelters are often seen by the nonveterinary staff initially.

In fact, many shelters do not have veterinarians on staff and must transport sick or injured animals to the nearest veterinary facility or utilize on-call veterinary services. Nonveterinarians should immediately notify their consulting or shelter veterinary staff about animals that are in shock. Veterinarians should establish a written treatment protocol and training for other shelter personnel for dealing with shock if animals are being admitted to the shelter when veterinary personnel are not on-site. Veterinarians should train staff to recognize the signs of shock (that is, prostration, apathy, rapid, thready pulse, rapid, shallow respiration, low body temperature, and poor peripheral circulation—cool extremities, pale mucous membranes, slow capillary refill rate), and how to initiate treatment until professional care is available. Staff should be taught to slowly warm the animal, ideally in an incubator or isolette; eliminate further stress (for example, excessive noise or visual stimuli); stop any bleeding; and make sure that the animal has a clear air passageway.

Medications

Few drugs are actually approved for use in wildlife, therefore, nearly all of the drugs used in wildlife medicine are used extra-label. The Willowbrook Wildlife Center Pharmaceutical Index (Brown, 2000) is an extensive formulary of drugs and dosages used in wildlife medicine. Many other veterinary references are available that also contain exotic animal formularies (Fowler, 1986; Merck Manual, 1998; Johnson-Delaney, 1996). Every shelter that receives wildlife, even if only occasionally, should have at least one of these texts in its library.

Hypothermia

Hypothermia is very common in wildlife presented for care. Warm the animal slowly in an incubator or isolette, or with one half of the animal's box or cage placed on a heating pad set on low. Placing only half the animal's cage on the heating pad allows them to move to the unheated side of the cage if they get too warm (see Fig. 13.5). Animals that are unable to move on their own should be checked and moved periodically to make sure they do not get too warm.

If the bird or terrestrial animal is also wet, if possible, gently blot or wipe the animal dry with a clean cloth or paper towel. Dry a bird's feathers by wiping them in the direction of feather growth only. Doing otherwise will break or damage feathers.

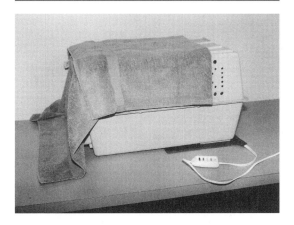

Figure 13.5. Plastic pet carrier covered with a towel to reduce visual stimuli. Note the heating pad located under half of the pet carrier. Photo credit to Scott and Cheryl Diehl.

Dehydration

Like hypothermia, dehydration is another very common problem. Proper methods and fluids for fluid therapy vary depending on the species of animal and its degree of dehydration.

Generally speaking, for mildly to moderately dehydrated patients, a glucose and electrolyte solution such as Pedialyte® (Ross), or Electramine® (Vitae) should be used. The fluid should be warmed so that it feels warmer than your body temperature, but not hot.

If not hypothermic, unconscious, or highly stressed, songbirds can be offered oral fluids by using an eyedropper to place a drop at a time on the seam of the bill (where upper and lower bill meet) and waiting for the drop to be swallowed before more is given. Tickling the bird's throat may help to stimulate swallowing. If the bird shakes its head to reject the fluid, too much is being placed into the mouth at one time.

Infant and juvenile mammals that are not hypothermic, unconscious, or highly stressed can also be offered this same warmed solution using a dropper or 1-ml syringe.

Do not give fluids in a bowl to an unconscious or semiconscious animal, or to an infant or young juvenile as they may drown or get wet and become hypothermic. Larger birds will benefit from being gavaged with fluids (see Fig. 13.6). This is often the only way to get the volume of replacement and

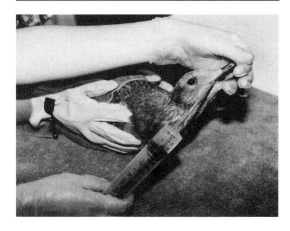

Figure 13.6. Gavaging a juvenile Herring Gull (*Larus argentatus*). Photo credit to Scott and Cheryl Diehl.

maintenance fluids they need into them. Consult with your cooperating wildlife rehabilitator for instruction in gavaging various species of birds.

For weak, debilitated patients, start with a volume of 0.01ml of fluids per gram of patient body weight. A volume of 0.025ml/gm patient bodyweight is an average stomach or crop capacity for patients that handle the initial volume well or are not badly debilitated. For most animals, 0.05ml/gm bodyweight is considered a maximum stomach or crop capacity.

The volume of fluids administered per day must provide for the patient's maintenance requirements while beginning to compensate for any fluid deficit. Clinical signs corresponding to varying degrees of fluid deficit are shown in Table 13.1. Daily maintenance fluid requirements are computed and given at a rate of 50ml/kg/day for birds and 55ml/kg/day for mammals. Fluid deficit is computed by estimating the percent of dehydration as shown in Table 13.1. This deficit is stated as a decimal: for example, 8 percent dehydration is written as 0.08. This figure is multiplied by the patient's body weight, in grams. If the patient is underweight, the patient's normal body weight is estimated, and the latter figure is used in computing the fluid deficit. The figure that results from multiplying the estimated fluid deficit stated as a decimal (for example, "0.08") by the patient's estimated normal bodyweight (in grams, for example, "1000g.") is the volume of fluid deficit. In the case of a 1000g (1kg) bird that is estimated to be 8 percent dehydrated, the volume of fluid deficit would be 80ml ($0.08 \times 1000 = 80$ml). The goal should be to replace this volume of fluids over the next 48 hours, while providing maintenance fluids. Additional fluids will need to be given to replace ongoing losses (Wolf, 1993; Redig, 1993).

Although often preferred or even essential for some patients (for example, in the case of shock), intravenous fluids can be difficult to administer in some wild animal patients. Animal restraint during the procedure and the small size of the patient's veins can make IV fluid administration difficult or even impossible. However, bolus IV fluids for birds can be administered, often with very good effects (Redig, 1993).

FEEDING

Because the wild animals you take in at your shelter may only be with you for a few hours, with the

Table 13.1. Clinical Signs of Dehydration

% Dehydration	Clinical Signs
<5%	History of fluid loss; no detectable clinical signs; normal mucous membranes; normal skin pliability; skin turgor (return time of tented skin to normal position): ≤1 sec.
5%	Clinical signs first appear; slight dryness of mucous membranes; skin turgor: 1–2 sec.
6%	Moderate and obvious fluid deficits; dry, red, "tacky" mucous membranes; skin turgor: 2–5 seconds; eye orbits slightly sunken; slight concentration of urine; oliguria (reduced urine output)
8%	Severe fluid loss; dry, red, tacky mucous membranes; skin turgor: 2–5 seconds; eyes sunken in orbits; oliguria; pulse may be weak, slight prolongation of capillary refill time; overall depressed condition
10–12%	Extremely serious, may be life-threatening; dry mucous membranes; skin turgor: >5 seconds or no return, eyes sunken in orbit, signs of shock possible, (tachycardia, cool extremities, rapid and weak pulses)
12–15%	Life-threatening; definite signs of shock, death imminent

Source: Linda Wolf, D.V.M. 1993. *NWRA Quick Reference*, p.72.

exception of nestling and fledgling birds (see the following discussion), feeding is generally not needed. Feeding an emaciated animal too soon can actually be quite detrimental. Many species of wild animals have very specialized dietary needs and feeding techniques, which are far too many to be addressed here. Ask your cooperating wildlife rehabilitators for specific guidelines about feeding wildlife at your shelter.

Most species of young songbirds such as jays, robins, crows, and cardinals need to be fed every 30 minutes (nestlings) to 60 minutes (fledglings) throughout daylight hours. Generally, these birds will do well on *very* moist, tiny bits of canned, or soaked dry cat food *gently* placed well back into their gaping mouths using the blunt end of a flat toothpick (for very small birds) or a plastic coffee stirring stick. Consult with your cooperating wildlife rehabilitator for their preferred feeding techniques.

TEMPORARY HOUSING

House wildlife in an area separate from those used to house companion animals. This separation can help minimize the risk of animal-to-animal disease transmission and reduce stress for all of the animals involved. The wildlife holding room should also be isolated from the sounds and activities associated with other shelter operations.

The ideal wildlife holding room will be well ventilated, though warm. It will have a counter or other workspace, a sink with running water, a gram scale for weighing animals, and a small refrigerator for storing fluids and nutritional items such as food for baby birds.

The holding room's floor should be sealed concrete, epoxy, tile or other hard, washable surface. The room should become dark when the lights are switched off to facilitate capturing an escaped bird in the room. Eliminate gaps between items such as cabinets and walls to prevent escaped animals from entering these gaps where they may become difficult or impossible to recover. Make sure that the room is secure so that escaped wild animals cannot get into the ceiling, ventilation system, or other parts of the shelter where they may become irretrievably lost, injured, or do considerable facility damage.

Caging

A cardboard box makes a good temporary holding container for most types of birds. The box should be large enough to hold the bird without cramping it into an unnatural position, but not so large that the bird can make large movements that may cause further injury.

The box should have enough pencil-sized air holes to provide adequate ventilation. Avoid large holes as they may permit escapes or allow the bird's head to get caught. A three-sided door cut into the side of the box and secured by tape will make it easier to capture the bird in the box for necessary procedures.

A cardboard box can also be used for many types of infant and juvenile mammals. Boxes can also work well for bats and nonvenomous snakes, but you must make sure that these containers are very secure, as these animals are escape artists! Double caging (that is, the box placed inside a ventilated, securely covered glass aquarium) is highly recommended for these creatures.

Plastic pet carriers make good containers for holding medium-sized songbirds, larger birds, and nongnawing mammals. Be advised that a determined woodchuck or tree squirrel can gnaw their way out of a plastic pet carrier in a matter of minutes.

A sturdy wire cage will be needed for alert, active gnawing mammals such as woodchucks. *Do not* use wire cages for wild birds as feather damage and serious injury can occur! Cover the cage with newspaper or a cloth to afford the animal a sense of security and to minimize visual stimuli. Make sure to allow for adequate ventilation.

Nestling birds should be placed on multiple layers of clean facial tissue or toilet paper in a clean plastic nest such as an empty margarine tub. This should be placed inside a warm box or incubator. Do not use plant material or material from the original nest, as they may be damp or harbor parasites.

Caging Substrate

Provide newspaper or soft ravel-free (without loose strings or loops) cloth on the cage floor. Loose strings or loops can wrap around the animal's neck or a limb and cause strangulation. Mammals appreciate shredded newspaper on top of sheet newspaper for bedding. Do not use strips torn from the edges of computer paper. These strips can cause entanglement.

For a bird that cannot stay sternally recumbent, roll up a towel or other suitable cloth and form a ring of this cloth around the bird. The bird's head should rest on the edge of the ring of cloth. Birds should not be deliberately laid on their back other than for necessary examination or treatment procedures.

DISEASE TRANSMISSION

The following are general guidelines for the prevention of wildlife disease transmission in the shelter. Disease transmission is also discussed in several other chapters in this textbook.

1. Become aware of wildlife diseases prevalent in your area by talking with area wildlife rehabilitators, your state DNR, and your local and state health departments.
2. House wildlife in a room separate from companion animals.
3. Disinfect wild animal housing and equipment such as pole snares after each use.
4. Don't house animals that appear overtly ill (ocular or nasal discharge, sneezing, coughing, seizuring, and so on) near other animals, wild or domestic.
5. Protect your staff against animal bites by getting them trained in wild animal handling techniques and providing them with proper equipment.
6. Develop written shelter safety equipment protocols and handling instructions.
7. Consider pre-exposure rabies vaccinations for your staff.
8. Wear latex or vinyl gloves for wild animal cleanup and for handling animals that don't require other handling equipment (for example, leather gloves).
9. Wash your hands thoroughly with disinfectant soap and water after each animal is handled. Wash up before eating and when entering or leaving the wildlife area from another part of the shelter.
10. Keep a pair of "sick gloves": leather handler's gloves used only on animals suspected of having a transmissible disease.
11. Keep a set of animal handling equipment for use exclusively with wildlife.
12. When handling wild animals, avoid holding them close to your body. This will reduce the potential for transmission of fleas, ticks, and mites.
13. Outside of the shelter, don't wear shoes and clothing worn while working with wildlife.
14. Consider establishing a disinfecting footbath between your companion animal and wildlife holding areas.

15. Inspect incoming wildlife for fleas, ticks, and mites. Spray adult animals with fleas or ticks with pyrethrin flea spray. Debilitated adult mammals and juvenile mammals should be sprinkled lightly with a pyrethrin flea powder. Nestling and fledgling birds with nest mites should have their feathered areas (avoid bare skin) *lightly* sprinkled with pyrethrin flea powder, with excess powder gently brushed (with a clean, dry cloth) out of their feathers. Alternately, spray pyrethrin flea spray on bathroom tissue or paper toweling and wrap this treated paper around the bird's body for a few minutes at a time. Remove the wrap and wait about 30 minutes before applying more treated wrap. Repeat until the bird is free of mites.

ZOONOSES

Like domestic animals, wild animals can carry a wide variety of diseases that are transmissible to humans. A partial list of possible zoonotic diseases includes rabies Leptospirosis, Lyme disease, salmonellosis, aspergillosis, dermatophytosis (ringworm), chlamydiosis, hantavirus, hydatidosis (echinococcosis), plague, and sarcoptic mange (Wolf, 1997; Fowler, 1989). An in-depth discussion of zoonosis is beyond the scope of this text. However, a number of points about zoonosis and wildlife deserve emphasis here.

Rabies

According to Porter (1997), "The incubation period [for rabies in wildlife] varies from nine days to greater than one year depending on the virus strain, host species, dosage, and site of inoculation." Therefore, unlike domestic dogs and cats, no rabies quarantine and observation periods have been established for wild animals. A mammal of a species considered a rabies vector in your area that has bitten someone will need to be euthanized for rabies testing. Contact your state and local public health departments for specific information about rabies-vector species in your area and how and where to submit specimens for rabies testing.

Visceral Larva Migrans

A number of carnivore ascarids, like *Toxacara canis* in dogs and wild canids and *Toxacara cati* in cats and wild felids, can cause visceral larva migrans.

The one receiving the most attention in wildlife rehabilitation circles is the raccoon roundworm *Baylisascaris procyonis*. However, skunks, badgers (*Taxidea taxus*), fishers and martens (*Martes* sp.), and bears (Ursidae) can also carry their own *Baylisascaris* species (Fowler, 1986a; Kazacos and Boyce, 1989).

As transmission is via the fecal-oral route, shelter personnel are advised to promptly pick up and properly dispose of carnivore feces—*Baylisascaris* eggs are reportedly not infective for 3–4 weeks after they are shed (Kazacos and Boyce, 1989); wash up thoroughly after working in animal care areas, especially before eating or drinking; wear disposable gloves when cleaning up after carnivores; and restrict humans from eating and drinking in animal care areas. The authors deworm raccoons staying in their facility for rehabilitation and maintain them on a deworming schedule throughout their stay in captivity.

CONCLUSION

The continued encroachment of cities into wild animal habitats and the adaptation of some wild species (for example, raccoons, coyotes, and deer) to living in close proximity to humans will continue to result in many thousands of injured, sick, and orphaned wild animals being brought to shelters and wildlife rehabilitators in the coming decades.

Through public education, sheltering practices adapted to the special needs of wild animals, and working with nearby licensed wildlife rehabilitators and other wildlife professionals, a shelter can play an important role in preventing and alleviating suffering for wild animals in its community. An added bonus can be increased community confidence in your organization. Like all shelter programs, effective planning and management, trained staff, a properly equipped facility, and adequate financial resources are essential to success.

REFERENCES

Brown, C. M. 2000. *Willowbrook Wildlife Center Pharmaceutical Index,* 3d ed. Willowbrook Wildlife Foundation.

Casey III, A. M., and Casey, S. J. 2000a. A survey of conditions seen in wildlife admitted for wildlife rehabilitation. In *Wildlife Rehabilitation,* Vol. 18, Daniel R. Ludwig, ed. St. Cloud, MN: National Wildlife Rehabilitators Association, 143–160 .

Casey III, A. M., and Casey, S. J. 2000b. A study of state regulations governing wildlife rehabilitation during 1999. In *Wildlife Rehabilitation,* Vol. 18, Daniel R. Ludwig, ed. St. Cloud, MN: National Wildlife Rehabilitators Association, 173–192.

Diehl, S., and Diehl, C. 2001. Education: No time? No talent? No problem! In *Wildlife Rehabilitation,* Vol. 19, Daniel R. Ludwig, ed. St. Cloud, MN: National Wildlife Rehabilitators Association, 161–168 .

Fowler, M. E. 1986a. Ursidae (bears). In *Zoo and Wild Animal Medicine,* 2nd ed., Murray E. Fowler, ed. Philadelphia, PA: WB Saunders Co., 811–816.

Fowler, M. E. 1986b. Stress. In *Zoo and Wild Animal Medicine,* 2nd ed., Murray E. Fowler, ed. Philadelphia, PA: WB Saunders Co., 34–35.

Fowler, M. E. 1989. Zoonoses of concern to volunteers and staff of wild animal rehabilitation centers. In *Current Veterinary Therapy,* Vol. X, *Small Animal Practice,* Robert W. Kirk, ed. Philadelphia, PA: WB Saunders Co., 697–703.

Johnson-Delaney, C. 1996. *Exotic Companion Medicine Handbook for Veterinarians,* Lake Worth, FL: Wingers Publishing.

Kazacos, K. R., and Boyce, W. M. 1989. Zoonosis update: *Baylisascaris* larva migrans. *Journal of the American Veterinary Medical Association* 195(7): 894–902.

Kirkwood, S. 1998. Answering the call of the wild. *Animal Sheltering* 21(2): 4–5.

Merck Veterinary Manual, 8th edition, 1998. Whitehouse, NJ: Merck and Co. Inc.

Moore, A. T., and Joosten, S. 1997. State and federal permits. In *Principles of Wildlife Rehabilitation,* Adele T. Moore and Sally Joosten, eds. St. Cloud, MN: National Wildlife Rehabilitators Association, 31–35.

Parker, K. 1997. Getting started in Canada. In *Principles of Wildlife Rehabilitation,* Adele T. Moore and Sally Joosten, eds. St. Cloud, MN: National Wildlife Rehabilitators Association, 39–46.

Parker, K. 2000. Creating an operating framework for wildlife rehabilitation. In *Wildlife Rehabilitation,* Vol. 18, Daniel R. Ludwig, ed. St. Cloud, MN: National Wildlife Rehabilitators Association, 163–171.

Redig, P. T. 1993. *Medical Management of Birds of Prey,* 3rd ed. revised. St. Paul, MN: The Raptor Center at the University of Minnesota, 49–53.

Schulz, T. A. 1997. Raptor restraint, handling and transport methods. In *Principles of Wildlife Rehabilitation,* Adele T. Moore and Sally Joosten, eds. St. Cloud, MN: National Wildlife Rehabilitators Association, 105–119.

Spraker, T. R. 1982. An overview of the pathophysiology of capture myopathy and related conditions that occur at the time of capture of wild animals. In *Chemical Immobilization of North American Wildlife,* L. Nielsen, J.C. Haigh, M.E. Fowler, eds. Milwaukee, WI: Wisconsin Humane Society, 83–118.

Wolf, L. 1993. *National Wildlife Rehabilitators Association Quick Reference.* St. Cloud, MN: National Wildlife Rehabilitators Association, 83–85.

Wolf, L. 1997. Zoonoses: What you don't know can hurt you. In *Principles of Wildlife Rehabilitation,* Adele T. Moore and Sally Joosten.. St. Cloud, MN: National Wildlife Rehabilitators Association, 143–152.

Appendix 13.1

1. Wildlife Rehabilitation Organizations

National Wildlife Rehabilitators Association (NWRA)
14 North 7th Avenue
St. Cloud, MN 56303-4766
Phone: 320-259-4086
www.nwrawildlife.org
E-mail: nwra@nwrawildlife.org

2. International Wildlife Rehabilitation Council (IWRC)

4437 Central Place, Suite B-4
Suisun, CA 94585
Phone: 707-864-1761
www.iwrc-online.org
E-mail: iwrcinreach.com

Appendix 13.2

Essential Wildlife Rehabilitation Reference Materials

Principles of Wildlife Rehabilitation. Edited by Adele T. Moore and Sally Joosten. National Wildlife Rehabilitators Association, St. Cloud, MN. 1997.

Minimum Standards for Wildlife Rehabilitation, Third edition. Edited by Erica A. Miller, D.V.M. National Wildlife Rehabilitators Association, St. Cloud, MN. 2000. [Note: This document may be viewed at www.iwrc-online.org/standards.html.]

National Wildlife Rehabilitators Association Quick Reference. Compiled by Linda Wolf, D.V.M. Edited by Ginny Pierce, V.M.D., and Linda Wolf, D.V.M. National Wildlife Rehabilitators Association, St. Cloud, MN. 1993.

Willowbrook Wildlife Center Pharmaceutical Index, Third edition. Compiled by Catherine M. Brown, D.V.M., MSc. Willowbrook Wildlife Foundation. 2000.

Field Guides to the identification of birds, mammals, and reptiles and amphibians, such as the Peterson's series (Boston: Houghton Mifflin Company).

14
Equine Care in the Animal Shelter

Holly Cheever

INTRODUCTION

One outcome of the successful prosecution of a cruelty complaint is the removal of the horses in question from their current environment of neglect, misuse, or abandonment in order to place them in a humane sheltering or foster care system, wherein their rehabilitation and long-term needs must be addressed. This chapter will discuss the optimal protocol for promoting and maintaining herd health in the newly seized animals, which includes vaccination and deworming programs and recommendations for feeding the starved and debilitated individuals. It will also cover proper euthanasia techniques for those animals who are deemed too ill or debilitated to salvage, or for whom old age and severe arthritis finally cause an irreversible decline in the quality of life.

All animals seized during cruelty case investigations or surrendered voluntarily to a shelter or sanctuary must be evaluated for their physical health, their current vaccination status, and their previous anthelmintic history, if any and if known. In many cases, this information is not available. An effective shelter herd health program must include: (1) an initial evaluation of the animals' condition and history; (2) administration of an initial series of vaccines, required blood tests, and deworming agents (once the horse is deemed healthy enough to be treated); and (3) a regular herd health maintenance program to keep endoparasitism and disease transmission under control for long-term occupants. Preferably, the newly seized animals should be isolated from the pre-existing shelter residents to minimize the possibility of disease transmission. If space permits, isolation for two to four weeks is ideal, permitting the newcomers to be monitored for diseases that they may be incubating, and allowing them to be vaccinated and to develop protective titers from two initial vaccinations given two to four weeks apart. This period of isolation also permits at least one deworming treatment (two is better for severely parasitized animals), so that new arrivals do not contaminate the shelter's pastures and herds.

OUTLINE FOR AN OPTIMAL SHELTER HEALTH PROGRAM

Vaccinations

Vaccination protocols will be highly variable, depending on the region of the country in which the shelter is located and the year, because diseases such as Potomac Horse Fever and West Nile Virus encephalitis are spreading rapidly. Vaccinations should not be administered until an animal is assessed and found to be healthy enough to be immunocompetent and able to withstand any additional minor stresses. In a weakened animal, one should consider giving a battery of vaccinations separately as much as possible to minimize the chance for adverse reactions. Dr. Belinda Thompson (personal communication) recommends a core program including seven vaccines for horses in the northeast region of the country. Tetanus (*Clostridium tetani*), eastern and western encephalomyelitis, and equine influenza (A1 and A2 variants) are usually available in an affordable five-way combination vaccine and form the backbone of any vaccination program. Alternately, the influenza vaccine may be given separately in the intranasal form. In addition, vaccination against rhinopneumonitis (*Equine*

Herpes Virus type 1) is highly recommended, and rabies *(Rhabdovirus)* protection is essential in endemic areas (Thompson 2002).

For shelters situated on the West coast, Dr. W. David Wilson (personal communication) recommends a three-way vaccine containing tetanus and eastern and western encephalomyelitis protection. In addition, he recommends the use of an intranasal influenza type A2 vaccination and rabies vaccine if the horses might be exposed to skunks (the primary Californian vector) (Wilson 2002). Dr. Brett Scott (personal communication) recommends a basic core vaccination program for shelters in Texas, including tetanus, eastern and western encephalomyelitis, equine influenza, rhinopneumonitis, and rabies (Scott 2002). In Texas, as in California, skunks are the primary rabies vector, whereas in New York the current rabies epidemic is in raccoon populations. The practitioner must assess the potential for contact with these carrier species and abide by the recommendations of local health departments for rabies control.

Other diseases prevalent in specific regions may require additional vaccines to combat regional disease trends, such as Potomac Horse Fever *(Ehrlichia risticii)* in the northeastern United States, in northern California, and southern Oregon, and the West Nile virus (an arbovirus in the genus Flavivirus) along the northeastern coastline. Dr. Wilson notes that California veterinarians are advised to start vaccinating against the West Nile virus in 2003 in preparation for a projected influx of the virus in 2004. Similarly, Dr. Scott states that some Texas shelters might need to add vaccinations against Potomac Horse Fever, which arrived in the state in 2000 and the West Nile virus, which has been added to the recommended list of vaccines for transient horse populations starting in 2002. Venezuelan equine encephalomyelitis vaccine is not necessary for horses residing in the United States at this time because it has not been seen in this country for over 20 years. It remains a problem in South and Central America, but even the states bordering Mexico are not currently recommending this vaccine (Association of Equine Practitioners [AAEP] 2001a). Strangles *(Streptococcus equi)* vaccine is generally recommended in a shelter where the disease is already a problem or where separate quarantine housing is not available.

Consultation with leading equine practices in each region should help shelter veterinarians decide which vaccines are essential for their specific locations. Equine vaccines are licensed for annual boosters, although influenza vaccines may be given more often in stables where the disease is prevalent and where there is a high degree of flux (for instance, in show barns where horses travel extensively and contact other equine populations regularly). This is not likely to be the case in a shelter situation. Cost will be a limiting factor for most shelters whose financial constraints may prohibit an all-inclusive vaccination policy. In such cases, vaccinating with the previously suggested core vaccines, minimizing exposure to transient horse populations, and practicing vector control (mosquitoes for the West Nile and encephalomyelitis viruses, and trematode parasites of freshwater snails for Potomac Horse Fever) should provide reasonable control of disease transmission in shelter populations (AAEP 2001b).

Hematology

The requirements for blood testing horses coming into a shelter are mercifully simple. At this time, every state requires a negative Coggins test for Equine Infectious Anemia as its sole blood-testing requirement. States vary, however, as to the interval within which the test must be performed (six or 12 months for the continental United States, three months for Hawaii and Guam). Contact your state's Department of Agriculture and Markets or Bureau of Animal Industry for the specific regulations in your area.

Anthelmintic Treatment

Deworming protocols will vary enormously, depending on the number of animals housed per unit space, the ability to rotate pastures and paddocks, and the feeding system (i.e., whether horses prehend a significant amount of their feed communally from the ground as opposed to eating exclusively out of individual mangers and feed buckets). The age of the horses is also a critical factor because young stock and geriatric individuals are much more susceptible to the deleterious effects of endoparasitism. Seasonal and reproductive factors also play a role in the severity of parasite loads; egg counts and infestation rates are much higher during springtime and foaling season, so anthelmintic administration should focus on these periods for optimal control. Although it is recommended to perform microscopic fecal analysis on the new arrivals, particularly for legal evidence in a cruelty case seizure, do not rely on the results of the fecal examination to determine if parasites are present or not. Occult endoparasitism is common, for example, in horses loaded with prepatent—not yet egg-laying—adult worms. Therefore, every new arrival should be dewormed at least twice regardless of the results of fecal analysis, with two to four weeks between treatments, to minimize infestation of the premises.

Particular care must be exercised when deworming horses that have been chronically starved or carry a high parasite load; inappropriate choices of anthelmintics or an excessively aggressive protocol can be fatal at worst, and at best, may cause colic symptoms if the numbers of dead adults and larvae are very high. A general rule is to use a narrow spectrum dewormer or a partial dose of your chosen anthelmintic agent so that there will not be such a massive kill rate as to cause intestinal blockage. Dr. Thompson recommends that compromised animals be given one of the milder deworming agents once they are eating and beginning to improve their health parameters. Anthelmintics such as pyrantel tartrate and fenbendazole have a wide margin of safety and are good choices for the debilitated individual, but are not effective against all larval stages. Therefore, products that are effective against larvae such as ivermectin should be used as a follow-up after the previous initial treatment of debilitated animals. Pyrantel tartrate has also been developed as a daily feed additive, effectively reducing the *Strongylus vulgaris* (i.e., large strongyle) larval loads responsible for the mesenteric artery damage implicated in many colic cases.

If the animals are strong enough to be treated with a broader range of anthelmintic products, ivermectin is a good choice for the first treatment, followed by any of the previously cited products plus pyrantel pamoate, oxibendazole, and moxidectin. Moxidectin is an effective product currently available for the elimination of both the adult and larval strongyle stages as well as all stages of a broad spectrum of other endoparasites. It should be used with caution because its margin of safety is narrower and the potential for a massive die-off of the worm populations is high in an untreated animal with a large parasite load. Do not use it initially in a debilitated horse requiring supportive nutritional care.

For specific parasite loads, use fenbendazole at a dosage five times higher than recommended to eliminate encysted strongyle larvae and administer a double dose of pyrantel tartrate for tapeworms. Stomach bots can be eliminated with ivermectin, fenbendazole, and moxidectin, while the parasites causing "summer sores" (Habronema and Draschia) require the use of ivermectin. The best deworming programs use a rotation of chemical agents to minimize the development of parasite resistance, and include treatments given every six weeks (in a crowded paddock with youngsters and/or seniors) or every 3 to 4 months in a management system with a lower population density consisting of healthy mature animals.

Feeding Protocols

Good nutrition is fundamental to good health. As a general guideline, a horse needs 1½ to 1¾ pounds of good quality hay per 100 pounds of body weight to maintain good condition. Mares that are lactating or are in advanced stages of pregnancy should receive 1½ to 1¾ pounds of grain per 100 pounds of body weight. These guidelines should be adjusted for the individual animal, and grain added in proportion to the amount of work the horse may be performing (Haynes 1994). A trace mineralized salt block and fresh potable water should be available at all times.

Unfortunately, a depressing majority of horses seized in cruelty cases are chronically starved or malnourished due to abandonment, owner ignorance, insufficient income, or seasonal variation in available forage and water (Witham and Stull 1998). These animals require a very precise "refeeding" program to bring them back to normal body condition and good health without causing a potentially fatal metabolic collapse. Carolyn Stull, Ph.D.,[7] has done extensive research in this challenging area. To summarize it briefly, an emaciated horse suffers from the loss of body fat stores and muscle tissue, resulting eventually in the depletion of fat, protein, and electrolytes, as well as anemia. If the horse is offered an excessive amount or the wrong types of feed sources, it can experience a resultant excessive insulin secretion, hypophos-phatemia, hypomagnesemia, and hypocalcemia. These profound metabolic imbalances can result in death due to cardiac, respiratory, or liver failure, as well as in convulsions and coma, within three to five days (Withum and Stull 1998). The aim of a refeeding and reconditioning program is to provide a feed source that won't provoke the insulin surge and the depletion of electrolytes and ions in the blood observed with diets based on a high carbohy-drate content. In addition, the diet must be relatively high in nutrients so that it can provide sufficient en-ergy, protein, and minerals while being fed in the small volumes with a low fiber content necessary for the chronically malnourished animal's dimin-ished gastrointestinal capacity. Dr. Stull's research, comparing refeeding programs utilizing alfalfa hay (low fiber content), oat hay (high fiber content), or a commercial concentrate fed with oat hay, shows that an optimal refeeding program consists of using leafy alfalfa hay fed at the rate of one pound of hay (approximately 1/6 of a flake) every four hours for the first three days, increasing to four pounds of hay in each of three feedings by Day 6. From Day 10 on, horses can be fed as much alfalfa as they can consume in two daily feedings, withholding grains and other concentrated feeds until they are well on their way back to good health. Access to a trace-mineral salt block and clean fresh water should al-ways be available (UC Davis 1998).

An alternative protocol, summarized by Harold F. Hintz, Ph.D., recommends the initial correction of dehydration and electrolyte disturbances by of-fering water and electrolyte solutions via nasogas-tric tube if necessary, followed by a slurry made of concentrates (a complete pelleted feed) mixed with corn oil and water (Hintz 1999). Optimally, it would be beneficial to monitor the horses' blood chemistry parameters on a regular basis with any of the sug-gested refeeding protocols, but this will be imprac-tical in a shelter situation with budget constraints. Therefore, it will be safest to introduce feed conser-vatively in terms of energy density, and to aim for a slow reconditioning program. Typically, it takes three to 10 months for chronically malnourished horses to regain their normal body condition (Withum and Stull 1998).

One other specialized diet that may prove useful for the veterinarian dealing with cruelty cases is the low-carbohydrate, high protein and fat diet pro-posed by various investigators for the treatment and prevention of Polysaccharide Storage Myopathy (PSSM), which causes exertional rhabdomyolysis ("tying up"), primarily in the draft and quarter horse breeds. A practitioner investigating a carriage horse's stiff gait or collapse should include PSSM in the differential diagnosis list, and should advise the owner or caregiver to change the diet to one with high protein levels, a low carbohydrate con-tent, and 20–25% of its calories derived from fat. One suggested diet includes alfalfa pellets with added corn oil or rice bran (Valentine et al. 1997). A review of the cited articles will provide the prac-titioner with specific diets to counteract this meta-bolic imbalance and prevent its recurrence (Valberg et al. 1997, Valberg and Mickelson 1997, Valentine et al. 1997).

Dental Examinations

Bringing a chronically starved horse back to health represents one of the greatest challenges a shelter veterinarian will face. Clearly, the correct diet is only one facet of the recovery program, which must also provide for regular dental exams and the cor-rection of malocclusion and oral pain from irregular dentition; these are significant risk factors for the development of colic and become increasingly problematic in the geriatric horse. Because neg-lected horses often have a long history of malnutri-tion, their incidence of dental problems and tooth loss may be higher than would be seen in a well-cared for animal, and may necessitate a more fre-quent oral examination program. The shelter staff should be advised to look for signs of dental prob-lems, including weight loss, excessive salivation, refusing feed, the presence of whole grains in the stool, and mouthfuls of partly chewed hay dropped onto the ground instead of being swallowed.

Hoof Care

Regular hoof care is an essential part of any long-term horse health program. All horses should have their hooves examined and cleaned regularly, daily if possible. The frequency with which farrier care should be provided will vary, depending on the age and health of the horse, as well as the footing to which he/she is exposed. Unless a chronic laminitis exists requiring frequent trims, most horses do well with trims performed every 6 to 12 weeks. Shoes are not recommended unless corrective shoeing is required to minimize the pain of a chronic lameness from, for example, navicular disease or laminitis.

One of an equine shelter's best resources is a farrier willing to assist in improving the condition of these animals on a regular and affordable basis.

Behavioral Needs

In addition to eliminating parasites as discussed previously, any stressors in the horses' environment must also be eliminated as much as possible because they may interfere with achieving the desired weight gain. Therefore, a horse's behavioral needs for companionship, comfort, and sufficient foraging time should be addressed and met in addition to the physical or medical needs. The best situation provides a run-in shelter with complete protection from cold, windy, or inclement weather. Manger space should be ample to allow subordinate members of a band to eat with ease without being chased away by the dominant members. If pasture rotation is available, the horses will be less plagued by internal parasites and will have increased opportunity to forage as they evolved to do so, (i.e. with the constant grazing pattern described in the chapter on investigating equine abuse). Clearly, any environment that permits the greatest degree of natural equine physical and behavioral activities will provide the healthiest setting in which to keep the shelter's equine population in optimal condition.

EUTHANASIA

Realistically, not every case will have the ideal ending in which the rescued horses regain their health and condition and live to a respectable and happy old age. Inherent in every cruelty case seizure is the sad reality that some horses may be too elderly, ill, or lame to be rescued and salvaged. For this reason, it is advisable for the initial search warrant, whereby animals will be seized and removed from the owner's property, to include a statement providing for humane euthanasia *on the premises* for those horses that have little hope for a humane recovery, or for whom rehabilitation will be a painful and unrealistically expensive process. It is essential that the search warrant include permission to perform the euthanasia *in situ* to spare these animals any more stress and suffering due to the need to transport them elsewhere before giving them a humane death.

Whether the euthanasia will be performed on the premises or in the more private and controlled environment of the shelter, there are several critical factors that must be addressed first. Equine euthanasia is very different from the euthanasia of a house pet whose body mass is much smaller and whose temperament is very different; many abused or neglected horses are very skittish in the presence of strange people and situations and will therefore require restraint by knowledgeable, experienced personnel. In addition, their large body mass makes their death much more dramatic to the observer due to the body's collapse as unconsciousness occurs, with the accompanying sound and vibration caused by the fall of a heavy body to the ground. For these reasons, the optimal situation provides for complete privacy without public viewing of the act. The horse should be adequately restrained by a sufficient number of handlers to keep themselves and the horse from being harmed during the procedure. Ideally, the horse should be pretreated with a tranquilizing agent such as xylaxine or detomadine to minimize excitement, and then should be given a lethal dose of a barbiturate solution administered quickly and smoothly. The prior use of the tranquilizer permits a gentler fall with a minimal amount of thrashing.

If the horse cannot be adequately restrained, or if the use of a barbiturate overdose is either prohibitively expensive or unavailable, euthanasia can be accomplished humanely by gunshot (using the appropriate kind and gauge of firearm, such as a .22-caliber long rifle, or a 9mm, or .38 caliber handgun) or by the use of a penetrating captive bolt gun (which must be correctly maintained to ensure proper function) (Hullinger and Stull 1997). Obviously, only a person properly trained in the use of firearms and acting in compliance with local firearm laws should perform this kind of euthanasia. The proper site and distance from the target for each method is clearly detailed in *The Emergency Euthanasia of Horses* cited in the references section. This method is emphatically not recommended for public viewing. In addition to this source, a video and booklet providing instruction on humane and safe euthanasia techniques for horses are available from the Instructional Media Center at Michigan State University (Martenivk and Walshaw 1997).

One final practical consideration is to plan ahead for the removal of the body. It will facilitate disposal of the remains greatly if the euthanasia is performed in an area easily accessible to heavy machinery; therefore, the site should be selected with this consideration in mind, as well as the need for privacy.

CONCLUSION

The preceding discussions are intended as an elementary guide to assist the practitioner in dealing with horses in abuse cases and shelter situations. The veterinarian may well be the only one in these cases with the knowledge of how to proceed, and may find it necessary to instruct local animal control officers, law enforcement officers, and shelter personnel in the intricacies of the proper evaluation, management, and finally euthanasia of this species. The cited references should provide the veterinarian with the necessary tools to gain sufficient experience to become proficient in this field.

REFERENCES

American Association of Equine Practitioners. 2001a. Guidelines for Vaccination of Horses, Lexington, KY, p. 4

American Association of Equine Practitioners. 2001b. Guidelines for Vaccination of Horses, Lexington, KY, p. 10

Haynes, B. 1994. *Keeping Livestock Healthy: A Veterinary Guide to Horses, Cattle, Pigs, Goats and Sheep*. Storey Books, Pownal, VT.

Hintz, H. F. 1999. Chronic weight loss and refeeding. *Equine Practice* 21 (2):6.

Hullinger, P. and Stull, C. 1999. *The Emergency Euthanasia of Horses* Available from Veterinary Medicine Extension, School of Veterinary Medicine, UC Davis, at www.vetmed.ucdavis.edu/vetext/home. html

Marteniuk, J. and Walshaw, S. 1997. Equine Euthanasia. Available from Michigan State University at www.msuvmall.msu.edu/imc

Scott, B. 2002. Extension horse veterinary specialist for the state of Texas, telephone conversation with the author in June

Thompson, B. 2002. Senior Extension Associate for the New York State Animal Health Diagnostic Laboratory at the College of Veterinary Medicine at Cornell, Ithaca, NY, telephone conversation with the author in June.

UC Davis Center for Equine Health. 1998. Rehabilitating the Starved Horse *The Horse Report* 17 (3):6.

Valberg, S. J, J. M. MacLeay, et al. 1997. Exertional rhabdomyolysis and polysaccharide storage myopathy in horses *The Compendium* 19 (9): 1083.

Valberg, S. J. and J. R. Mickelson, 1997. Polysaccharide storage myopathy: One important cause of exertional rhabdomyolysis. *World Equine Veterinary Review* 2 (3):36.

Valentine, B.A., A.J. Reynolds, J. Wakshlag and N.G. DuCharme. 1997. Muscle glycogen, myopathy, and diet. *World Equine Veterinary Review* 2 (3): 28.

Valentine, B. A., J. W. Wakshlag, et al. 1997. Polysaccharide storage myopathy: Lessons from the draft breeds. Paper presented at the International Equine Neurology Conference, College of Veterinary Medicine, Cornell University, Ithaca, NY. July 11–13, pp. 74–78.

Wilson, D. 2002. Professor of Equine Medicine at the UC Davis School of Veterinary Medicine. Personal conversation with the author in June.

Witham, C. L., and Stull, C. 1998. Metabolic responses of chronically starved horses to refeeding with three isoenergetic diets. *Journal of the American Veterinary Medical Association* 212 (5): 694–695.

Section 3:
Disease Management

INTRODUCTION

Animal sheltering has come a long way since the days when any sign of clinical illness in a shelter animal resulted in immediate euthanasia. Shelters today are employing multiple strategies for maintaining healthy conditions in their facilities, building hospitals and clinics, and searching for resources to perform the diagnostic tests and treatment protocols mentioned in this section that, until recently, would have been virtually unthinkable for all but the wealthiest private shelters. Veterinarians are being strongly encouraged to provide cost effective yet sophisticated medical care and to apply current medical knowledge to herd health situations that differ from the circumstances encountered in most other veterinary facilities. These can be daunting tasks without the comfort of research data or financial resources to support their decisions.

Each chapter in this section is designed to provide veterinarians with pertinent information to help meet the challenge of preventing and treating disease in the shelter environment. Many of the problems that veterinarians face could be better managed if there were data available to help direct them to workable solutions. In chapter 15, Hurley discusses the importance of collecting data and its use in managing disease outbreaks. In chapter 16, Foley provides much needed information and insight into some of the unique problems of managing some of the common (and not so common) infectious diseases of dogs and cats in shelters. This information should be used in conjunction with conventional medical texts and drug formularies—not every disease is covered here, nor are drug dosages provided. For example, heartworm disease is not covered. Despite the fact that heartworm disease is encountered in shelter dogs, it is neither zoonotic nor directly infectious between dogs, and, thus, is not a true herd health or shelter problem. Diagnostic and treatment protocols are covered extensively in other texts. Althought not discounting its importance, zoonosis as a separate topic is covered only briefly because of the widespread availability of other clinical material. The AVMA is an excellent resource for information on zoonotic diseases, especially those diseases of concern for biosecurity reasons (www.avma.org). Ford discusses basic principles of vaccination while addressing the special issues concerning vaccinating shelter animals. Shelters that have problems with upper respiratory infections will find some of this information especially helpful. Finally, to complete this section on disease management, Hurley provides information in chapter 18 to help veterinarians assess the practicality of diagnostic testing, as well as implications for the use of such testing in the shelter environment.

15

Implementing a Population Health Plan in an Animal Shelter: Goal Setting, Data Collection and Monitoring, and Policy Development

Kate F. Hurley

INTRODUCTION

This chapter provides an overview of population health concepts as they apply to animal shelters and suggests a strategy for implementing and evaluating a shelter herd health program. The foundation of this chapter is a belief that, although our emotional investment is what drives many of us in this field, the animals we care so much about can best be served when we translate our compassion into a logical and systematic approach to medical care in a shelter.

WHY POPULATION HEALTH?

It is common to hear shelter medicine described as small animal herd health or population medicine. Key elements of population medicine include a focus on production goals; the identification of risk factors for negative outcomes such as disease or poor performance; the development of strategies to prevent disease and maximize health and production; and the systematic reassessment of the effectiveness of those strategies. This can be a very useful paradigm for an animal shelter, although our product may be healthy animals adopted to permanent homes, rather than gallons of milk or pounds of wool.

Developing a population health plan requires stepping back from the everyday demands of sheltering to assess the goals and health of the shelter population. This can be difficult to accomplish amidst the clamor of urgent requests to treat indi-

vidual animals or respond to crisis situations. The challenge of herd health monitoring in many shelters is still greater because of the large numbers of animals entering and leaving the group on a daily basis and the lack of sophisticated computer systems in some shelters. In spite of these obstacles, at least some data collection is vital. Attempting to manage a shelter population without accurate information regarding the magnitude of problems and response to intervention is like treating a very sick individual without performing any diagnostic or follow-up tests.

The need for record keeping is well recognized in other branches of population medicine (Lechtenberg, Smith, et al., 1998; Teare, 1991; Munson and Cook, 1993; Reneau and Kinsel, 2001). A case could be made for even greater importance in a shelter setting, where not just profits but the very lives of the animals we care for are at stake. Formalized research is scarce in this emerging field, so a method by which various management or treatment strategies can be reliably evaluated within the shelter is crucial. In addition, shelters vary greatly one from another. A strategy that works well for one shelter may prove disastrous for another, so each shelter ultimately must assess the effects of various strategies in its own population.

Ideally, data will be collected in the context of a systematic population health plan, and establishment of such a plan will be the focus of the first part of this chapter.

Benefits of Data Collection and Analysis in Animal Shelters

IDENTIFICATION OF BASELINE DISEASE/PROBLEM LEVELS AND TRACKING PATTERNS
For instance, we all know that upper respiratory infection is a significant problem in many shelters. However, without a record of the magnitude and pattern of cases, it is impossible to assess progress objectively. "Disease" may be interpreted broadly to include excessive numbers of incoming animals or other evidence of irresponsible pet ownership.

IDENTIFICATION OF RISK FACTORS FOR DISEASE, ADOPTION, EUTHANASIA, OR OTHER OUTCOMES
This allows targeting intervention at highest risk animals or groups. For instance, extra socialization could be provided for dogs at high risk for developing kennel stress, or cats at high risk of not being adopted could be placed in particularly prominent locations or otherwise promoted.

DEVELOPMENT OF INTERVENTION STRATEGIES
After baseline disease levels are known and a list of possible risk factors developed, an intervention strategy can be planned specifically targeting the problems identified.

ASSESSMENT OF INTERVENTION
This is one of the most important reasons for data collection. A shelter veterinarian is asked many questions that can be answered only by following disease (or health) levels before and after a change. Did upper respiratory infection (URI) levels drop or increase after a change in vaccination strategy? Did a switch to a new, donated brand of dog food lead to more diarrhea problems? Do dogs that participate in a socialization program get adopted more quickly? Without baseline data for comparison, we must rely on impressions and guesswork to answer these questions.

It is also valuable to assess the effects of policy or even structural changes. A move to a new facility, a change in holding period length, or implementation of volunteer animal socialization programs, all might be expected to affect disease and adoption levels. Sometimes considerable controversy may exist over the extent and direction of such efforts. An objective answer in such a case may save hours of argument and speculation, making the time spent in collecting the data well worth the effort.

IDENTIFICATION AND EFFECTIVE RESPONSE TO OUTBREAKS AND EMERGING PROBLEMS
Reviewing data collected over time may reveal an insidious pattern that emerged too gradually to be seen in the day-to-day care of the animals. For sudden outbreaks, the availability and analysis of data can be key to implementing damage control and preventing recurrence.

COMPARISON BETWEEN SHELTERS/ESTABLISHMENT OF GOALS AND BENCHMARKS
It can be surprisingly difficult in a shelter to answer the simple question, "How well are we doing?" Herd health practitioners for many large animal species have access to databases regarding herd health parameters, against which they can compare the performance of their own herds. Such information would be invaluable to shelter professionals. For instance, although we acknowledge that feline URI is a problem in almost all shelters, what levels can we expect? What are the characteristics of shelters with the lowest levels?

BUDGETING AND JUSTIFICATION OF PROGRAMS AND FUNDING
Being able to demonstrate the magnitude of a problem, or better yet the amount of progress made in addressing that problem, to board members, government officials, or potential donors may help develop funding for vital programs.

EDUCATION OF THE PUBLIC, VOLUNTEERS, STAFF AND COLLEAGUES
The challenges we face in shelters do not begin or end there, but reflect the community from which the shelter population is drawn. Our colleagues in private practice and the public can better support us when we clearly articulate the source and magnitude of the challenges we face. When we can pinpoint sources of unvaccinated or unaltered animals in the community, for instance, we can enlist the help of private practitioners to promote vaccination in those areas. When we understand why animals are relinquished to shelters in the first place, we can enlist the help of animal professionals and con-

cerned individuals to decrease the circumstances that lead to relinquishment. Demonstrating the benefit of a new program in reducing disease may help in the sometimes difficult process of encouraging staff and volunteers to accept changes and take on additional tasks.

ESTABLISHING A GOAL-ORIENTED HERD HEALTH PROGRAM

Step 1: Performance Goals

The veterinarian responsible for care of a herd must constantly weigh the costs and benefits of various possible investments and balance the benefit for one patient with the impact on the rest of the population. This is a challenge with which shelter workers are painfully familiar. Not only must individual needs be weighed against group needs, but the potential benefit of the medical program needs to be balanced against other uses of resources that also help meet the shelter's goals; although we take the best possible care of animals in the shelter, we must never lose sight of the equally important goal of getting the animals adopted out, or better yet never coming in at all. Articulating performance goals and understanding the barriers to achieving those goals forms the basis for rational resource allocation on an individual and herd level. These goals are established by the stakeholders in the agency, such as staff, management, membership, and board of directors. Table 15.1 compares examples of performance goals for a dairy and an animal shelter.

Step 2: Obstacle Assessment

Failure to meet performance goals can be thought of as herd level disease. As for any disease, treatment is directed by an understanding of pathogenesis. A dog presenting with acute renal failure may have ingested a toxin or may be suffering from an infection; the treatment strategy will differ greatly depending on which of these is the cause. Similarly, in a shelter we need to understand the pathogenesis of performance issues in *that individual shelter* before designing an optimally effective intervention plan. The symptom, such as euthanasia of adoptable animals, may be the same from one location to another, but the cause may be different.

For example, decreasing euthanasia in a community can be accomplished by decreasing the number of animals entering shelters and/or increasing the number of owner reclaims and successful adoptions. The best strategy depends on what factors are most important in determining those numbers. For instance, we need to know the following:

- How many stray versus surrendered animals does the shelter take in?
  - For strays, what are the most common neighborhoods, breeds?
  - For surrenders, what is the distribution of reasons for surrender?
    - Unwanted litters versus behavior problems
  - What encourages/discourages people from adopting shelter animals?
  - Concern about health versus inconvenient hours

Table 15.1. Performance Goal Examples in a Dairy Herd and Animal Shelter

Dairy Herd	Animal Shelter
Producing milk such that economic return for the farmer is maximized	Ending euthanasia of adoptable animals/ placing adoptable animals in good homes
Providing housing and care resulting in reasonable animal comfort and in compliance with applicable laws	Ensuring health and comfort of animals in the shelter's care, whatever the outcome
Preventing transmission of zoonotic disease in dairy products	Protecting public and animal health and safety in community
Minimizing pollution and environmental impact by proper storage and disposal of animal wastes	Providing adopters with temperamentally sound, healthy pets and a positive adoption experience
Avoiding drug residues in milk	Educating the public and modeling good animal care practices

- What is the distribution of reasons for euthanasia or limiting intake?
- Space versus behavioral concerns

The results of this foundation work will build a picture of the shelter population and issues specific to that community, and clarify the best use of resources. Veterinary care represents one of many tools available to address the problems of disease and death in shelters; it should be chosen only when it is the best and most cost effective tool for that purpose. If most surrenders are for behavior problems rather than unwanted litters, a behavior hotline may be a more urgent investment than a low-cost spay/neuter program (Salman, New et al., 1998). If a significant number of adopters are discouraged by concerns about shelter animal health, a medical program is an important investment. If, on the other hand, inconvenient hours are more of a concern, opening a few more weekend or evening hours might be a better use of resources. If many healthy animals are being euthanized or turned away for lack of space, a major investment in treating sick animals might be lower priority than a program to increase adoption of healthy animals.

Some of the population information described previously, such as reasons for surrender and euthanasia, can be collected as part of routine shelter operations. Other information will require a more concerted effort to collect. For instance, people who are choosing not to adopt from shelters by definition are unlikely to be found in a shelter and may have to be reached through informal or formal surveys, focus groups, or other means (Fennell, 1999; Savesky, 1999).

The dynamics of unwanted animals and euthanasia are rooted in the community, not the shelter, and each organization serving a community may see a different part of the problem. Ideally all shelters and rescue groups serving a single community will cooperate to gather data in a consistent way and share it with one another to form a complete picture. General principles of data collection, monitoring, and analysis are discussed later in this chapter.

Step 3: Establishing Performance Measures and Baseline Values

When treating an individual patient, veterinarians look for abatement of symptoms or changes in diagnostic test parameters as an indication that treatment is working. When practicing population medicine, we identify *performance measures*— quantifiable values that can be tracked to see whether progress is being made. Some of the data collected in step two can serve as performance measures. For instance, following institution of a behavior hotline the anticipated outcome is a decreased number of animals surrendered for behavior problems. Other examples of performance measures are listed in Table 15.2.

Once performance measures are identified, baseline levels can be measured and specific goals established. The dairy herd veterinarian has the advantage that systems have long been in place to track performance measures. The payoff of having such systems in livestock production has been well established (Ekes, Oltenacu et al., 1994; Lechtenberg, Smith et al., 1998; Reneau and Kinsel, 2001). Shelter management software can currently track many of the performance measures discussed previ-

Table 15.2. Performance Measure Examples in a Dairy Herd and Animal Shelter

Dairy Herd	Animal Shelter
Average pounds of milk produced per cow	Percent and number of animals adopted, reclaimed or euthanized
Incidence and prevalence of diseases such as mastitis, lameness, ketosis, displaced abomasum	Incidence and prevalence of important diseases in shelter/frequency of disease immediately post-adoption
Reproductive performance—number of days open (days between pregnancies) and pregnancy rate	Average turnover time (number of days each animal is in the shelter)
Calf health and survival	Frequency and reason for returns after adoption
Percent culled/herd turnover	Adopter compliance with spay/neuter policy

ously. Given the amount of staff time already spent entering data into such systems, it makes sense to extract as much value as possible out of existing shelter databases. When no commercial software system is available, hand tracking or an in-house database is a worthwhile investment, particularly immediately before and after instituting a new program designed to affect a particular measure. A few measures, such as frequency of disease or behavior problems after adoption, require follow up outside the shelter. This can be accomplished with a post-card system and/or phone calls. Following up on post-adoption medical status with area veterinarians has the added benefit of improving communication between the shelter and local veterinary community. A sample veterinary follow-up postcard is included in Appendix 15.1. Phone follow up with adopters can provide support as well as assessing adopter satisfaction, frequency of behavior and medical problems in recently adopted animals, and ensuring spay/neuter compliance if applicable.

Step 4: Intervention—Establishing a Preventive Medical Program in a Shelter

After it has been established how the medical program fits in with the shelter's overall goals, it is time to focus on the specific tools available to maintain population health. Establishing and maintaining a preventive health program should be a substantial part of the job of a shelter veterinarian. This topic is covered in depth in chapter 8. As new strategies are tried, performance measures should be revisited to assess progress.

MONITORING AND DATA COLLECTION

No single recipe exists for population health that fits all shelters. Even seemingly straightforward choices, like the best vaccine or disinfectant, will depend to some extent on the characteristics of the shelter population and facility. Data collected from other shelters (on the rare occasions when it is available) can provide a valuable starting point, but ultimately the magnitude of problems and benefit of solutions need to be assessed for each individual shelter.

The Potential Benefits of Record Keeping in Shelters

The potential benefits of record keeping in shelters have been covered previously in this chapter. Despite its many benefits, consistent data collection

is unlikely to be performed if it is overly burden-some or if those responsible for collecting the data never see the results of their work. A good population monitoring program should be simple and goal directed, with data collected as part of shelter routine whenever possible, and should include prompt data analysis and reporting. Some important data to collect include the following:

1. Unique identifier for each animal (number that will allow later filing and tracking, as well as a name)
2. Intake record including animal description, source, reason for surrender
3. Medical record including all vaccines, treatments, tests, physical exam results, diagnoses, and medical and surgical procedures
4. Results of behavioral assessments, behavioral record similar to medical record including diagnoses of disorders, treatment plan, and progress (or lack thereof)
5. Daily record (especially in long-term shelter) monitoring attitude, feces, urine, appetite, and behavior
6. Weekly to biweekly medical and behavior reassessments

For a more complete list of data to collect, see this chapter's appendices.

Data Measurement Concepts

We know that relying on personal impressions to determine disease levels or other important measures can be deceptive. Even data can be misleading; it is very important to be clear on what, exactly, is being measured, and what factors can interfere with reliability of the results. This is not always intuitively obvious. Bad data (data that gives false information) is worse than no data at all, as it may lead to false confidence in the results obtained. In order to avoid this peril, formal methods of measuring disease levels have been developed. Important data measurement concepts in shelters include case definition, number reporting, measures of disease, and statistical analysis. Similar considerations apply to tracking measures other than disease, such as adoptions, returns, or euthanasia rate.

CASE DEFINITION

In order to track disease, everybody involved needs to be measuring the same thing. If one staff member calls every mildly sneezing cat a case of URI, and another counts only cats with green ocular and nasal discharge, they will come up with very different numbers characterizing the same reality. All people involved in tracking a disease or other outcome need to agree on a written case definition for the disease in question.

A case definition is needed for anything to be counted and compared over time or between shelters, not just disease. Other examples include adoptions, euthanasia for various reasons, and describing "unadoptable" versus "adoptable" animals. For instance, counting an adoption as an animal that is adopted and not returned within a specified time period will result in a different number than counting any animal that is adopted, even if it is returned soon after. If the definition of "adoptable" changes over time, it will be impossible to assess true progress in placing all "adoptable" animals, and, thus, to judge how much closer we are to realizing this major goal of the sheltering community.

CATEGORIZING DATA

The case definition is used to categorize similar cases of disease or other factors of interest. Except when dealing with numbers on a continuum (such as body weight or temperature), some level of categorization is necessary for data collection and analysis. The appropriate level of detail depends on the anticipated purpose of data collection. For instance, the shelter manager may be interested in tracking how many dogs are surrendered for various types of aggression. If a different reason for surrender is recorded for each individual dog, such as "bit the meter reader," "bites the postman," and "bites kids on bikes," the information is too detailed to be tracked meaningfully. There is no point in comparing how many dogs were surrendered for biting meter readers versus postal carriers, but all these surrender reasons could potentially be grouped as "behavior problem," "aggression," or "aggression toward humans," increasing levels of detail depending on the intended use of the information. As another example, one could categorize cats with either conjunctivitis, sneezing, or oral ulceration and fever separately or group them all under the category of URI. If a new treatment is being tried specifically directed at reducing signs of conjunctivitis, then it makes sense to track these separately. If, on the other hand, a new air filter has just been installed in the hopes of reducing all forms of upper respiratory disease, it would be easier to group all URI cases together. When developing case definitions, think about the level of detail that makes most sense for your data collection purpose, keeping in mind that it is always possible to combine categories if less detail is needed, but not the reverse.

NUMBER REPORTING: NUMBERS, PERCENTAGES, AND FRACTIONS

Simple numbers can be deceptive when you don't know the size of the population from which the number was taken, and percentages can be deceptive when you don't know the absolute numbers to which they refer. Unless you're trying to fool people, the best way to express a number is generally as a fraction showing both the numerator (the number of animals affected) and the denominator (the number of animals at risk). For instance when tracking such measures as number of animals adopted or euthanized in a shelter or a community, it is important to know how many animals were cared for by shelters in that same community. A community that adopts out 990/1000 animals is much closer to realizing its goal than a community that is able to place 990/10,000 animals.

POPULATION AT RISK

By definition, expressing a number as a fraction requires knowing the size of the population at risk (the denominator of the fraction). Sometimes, this is fairly obvious: all live cats that don't already have URI can be considered at risk for developing URI. Sometimes the population at risk is the source of some controversy and needs to be clearly defined. For instance, the definition of animals at risk for adoption may vary substantially depending on shelter policy. In the previous example, does the denominator in 990/1000 animals adopted mean that there was a total of 1000 animals in the shelter, or that 1000 animals in the shelter were considered adoptable, but there were others that did not meet criteria for adoptability? As with a case definition, internally consistent definitions for population at risk should be articulated, and if numbers are to be compared between shelters, external consistency is required as well.

Population *time* at risk is a special way of counting the at-risk population required for measures taken over time in a fluctuating population. This is discussed in greater detail later in this chapter.

Measures of Morbidity

Morbidity refers to the proportion of animals in a population affected by a disease. Two methods are commonly used to describe morbidity: incidence and prevalence. Each measure has certain strengths and weaknesses. These measures are not only useful for infectious conditions, but for other outcomes of concern, such as the development of kennel/stress-related behavioral problems.

PREVALENCE

Prevalence is defined as the number of cases of disease present in a population at risk at a given point in time and can be thought of as a snapshot of disease. For example, 20 cases of URI out of a total of 100 cats in the shelter that day = 20/100 = .2 = 20 percent prevalence.

Prevalence is simple to calculate: simply count the total sick and total population in the shelter that day. This can be done on a regular basis and the results plotted over time. Unlike incidence (see the following section), the population at risk used for prevalence calculation includes both healthy and sick animals.

Prevalence goes up with an increase in either the number of *new cases* of disease or *duration* of disease. This creates some potential problems with relying on prevalence to measure disease levels. For instance, if a shelter becomes able to treat cats with URI rather than euthanizing them immediately, prevalence will increase because the cats will be present in the population longer, even if the number of new cases of URI does not change or even decreases. On the other hand, if a more effective treatment for URI is found such that cats recover more rapidly, prevalence will decrease even if the number of new cases remains the same.

Because prevalence is influenced by duration, it *should not be used* to measure a disease for which animals are frequently sent to foster care, adopted, euthanized, or otherwise removed from the population before recovery. In such cases, duration is controlled by shelter policy, not the time it takes animals to recover, and resulting prevalence levels will be misleading.

INCIDENCE

Incidence is defined as the number of *new cases* of a disease occurring in a population at risk over a period of time.

For example, 20 cats developed URI out of 1500 cat days at risk that month = 20/1500 = .013 cases of URI per cat day at risk.

An advantage of incidence is that, unlike prevalence, it is independent of disease duration. This is important in shelters where animals are often removed one way or another prior to recovery. A minor disadvantage of incidence is that it *can't simply be calculated based on the total number of animals present in the shelter* during the time period under consideration. Because the shelter population is not fixed (individuals are constantly leaving and entering), some method must be used to determine or estimate population *time* at risk. This is defined as the total disease free time contributed by all individuals in the shelter during the period under consideration.

Population Time at Risk

Population time, or number of animal care days, is a useful measure for many purposes in a shelter. Simply trying to anticipate costs or compare shelters based on total annual population, for instance, is more appropriately done based on population time rather than the absolute number of animals that spent any amount of time in the shelter during the year. Clearly, a shelter that cares for 1000 animals a year for an average of 10 days each will require a different budget and shelter capacity compared to a shelter that cares for 1000 animals a year for an average of 100 days each. It would be no surprise if the second shelter's animal care expenditures were significantly higher, even though the same number of animals pass through each year. Shelter software that tracks date of entry and exit can generally be persuaded to report not only absolute numbers but number of animal care days, and shelters equipped with such systems should take advantage of this fact.

Calculating population time for disease incidence requires one additional consideration—that only time contributed by animals *at risk for that disease* can be counted. Obviously, that means dogs would not be counted for calculating feline URI incidence, but it also means that animals that already have the disease in question must be excluded. Population time at risk can be calculated in several ways:

1. **Daily count** (most accurate): Count the total healthy population each day (or generate by computer). The sum of daily counts at the end of the

time period of interest gives the total population days at risk.

2. **Average count:** Count total healthy population at beginning and end of time period, or at regular intervals during time period. Take the average of these counts and multiply by the number of days in the time period of interest. The resulting value estimates total population days at risk. This method is acceptable if there is little fluctuation in the daily population during the time period considered.

3. **Cage count:** Estimate time at risk by multiplying the number of cages for healthy animals by the number of days in the time period of interest. This method is acceptable *only* in shelters where cages for healthy animals are almost always full.

See Appendix 15.2 for more information on how to calculate incidence.

A sample form for tracking disease incidence is attached in Appendix 15.3.

DURATION OF DISEASE

Duration is defined as the time from development of clinical signs of disease to recovery. Neither incidence nor prevalence indicates duration or severity of disease. Duration should be considered when assessing the benefits of some interventions. For instance, some vaccines claim to decrease duration and severity of disease, although a greater number of mild cases of disease/vaccine reaction may be seen. If only the increased number of cases (incidence) were considered, one might conclude the vaccine was hurting more than helping. However, taking into consideration an overall reaction in average disease duration would give a more realistic picture of the vaccine's benefit. Some shelter software systems are currently being designed to automatically track duration provided date of onset and recovery are entered. Note that duration cannot be calculated for animals that are adopted, euthanized, or otherwise lost to follow-up prior to recovery. Measuring severity is also helpful, although more difficult because of the subjective nature of this assessment and the need for consistent, at least daily, observations. Often, duration is an acceptable substitute, as shorter duration usually reflects milder disease. If severity must be measured, a written definition of levels of severity should be used, as with the case definition of disease.

SPECIFIC MEASURES OF MORBIDITY

Stratum-Specific Morbidity

Cause-specific morbidity (incidence or prevalence) measures all cases of a particular disease occurring in the total population at risk. Sometimes, it is also helpful to calculate *stratum-specific* morbidity based on age, breed, intake status (stray versus owner surrender), location in shelter, or some other factor that logically might be relevant to the likelihood of disease or other outcome of interest. For instance, the shelter vet may wonder how the rate of upper respiratory infection (URI) in kittens compares to adult cats. The shelter manager may wonder how length of average shelter stay varies by location in the shelter (for instance, whether an animal is group versus individually housed), or what breeds of dog are most at risk for developing kennel stress. Documenting frequency of infectious disease in strays versus surrenders may affect housing and quarantine decisions, and so on. Some shelter software systems can be programmed to generate stratum-specific reports, taking advantage of the wealth of information contained in these systems.

Attack Risk

Attack risk (AR) measures the frequency of disease in a population exposed to a particular risk factor. Attack risk can be used to compare disease occurrence in an exposed versus unexposed group and is often used in outbreak investigations. A related measure is the *relative risk* (RR), which is defined as the attack risk for the exposed group divided by the attack risk for the unexposed group. Relative risk measures the strength of association between a particular exposure and the development of disease.

For example: An outbreak of diarrhea has occurred in the shelter cat population. A bad batch of cat food is suspected. 17/25 cats fed from the suspect bag of food developed diarrhea (exposed group), and 4/16 cats fed from the previous batch of cat food also had diarrhea (unexposed group). So:

Attack Risk (exposed) = 17/25 = .68
Attack Risk (unexposed) = 4/16 = .25
Relative Risk = AR exposed/AR unexposed = .68/.25 = 2.72

So cats fed the suspect diet were 2.72 times more likely to have diarrhea than cats fed the other diet. Although these data would certainly be reason enough to try feeding a different food and see whether that helps, it's important to realize that *association* does not equal *causality*, as discussed further later in this chapter. In determining the cause of an outbreak, it is often necessary to calculate AR and RR for a number of possible associations and further investigate the strongest associations.

Measuring Mortality

Mortality is defined as the number of deaths over time in a population at risk. Overall mortality includes death from all causes combined; it is generally more useful to calculate *cause-specific* mortality rates. (Stratum-specific mortality, as for morbidity, may be useful as well.) In many communities euthanasia for various reasons remains the leading cause of mortality for sheltered animals. Mortality due to euthanasia can be further refined into subcategories reflecting various reasons for euthanasia. Even for shelters and rescue groups that do not perform euthanasia themselves, detailed information regarding mortality from this cause in all area shelters allows more effectively targeted intervention. At minimum, reasons for euthanasia should be divided to a level that allows determination of how many animals die for simple lack of adopters, and how many additional animals could be helped if prevention was more effective or more resources were available for treatment of disease or behavioral problems. One possible categorization scheme for euthanasia reasons is as follows:

- Lack of space (healthy, behaviorally sound animals)
- Medical noninfectious
  - Treatable—euthanized due to resource limitations (money, space, staffing)
  - Terminal—euthanized due to poor prognosis
- Medical infectious
  - Treatable—euthanized due to resource limitations (money, space, staffing, unable to house/care for without excess population risk)
  - Terminal—euthanized due to poor prognosis
- Behavior
  - Rehabilitatable—euthanized due to resource limitations (money, space, staffing)

- Terminal—euthanized due to poor prognosis or public safety
- Owner-requested euthanasia

In order to generate consistent data for analysis, a case definition for each euthanasia reason is important. For instance, if a dog is euthanized because there is no space in isolation to treat it for kennel cough, there must be general agreement on whether to describe this as euthanasia due to lack of space or due to disease (in the previous scheme, this would be categorized as medical-infectious-treatable). Recording reasons for euthanasia in further detail, such as the specific cause of infectious disease, allows even more precise targeting of prevention.

Case Fatality Rate

Another mortality measure that is sometimes useful is the *case fatality rate*, defined as the proportion of individuals with a specific condition that die of that condition.

For example: In shelter X in the month of May, 2/57 cats with URI died of the disease, while in June, 17/64 died:

Case fatality rate in May = 2/57 = .04.
Case fatality rate in June = 17/64 = .27

This represents almost a 700 percent increase in the case fatality rate. Such an increase would warrant a further investigation; perhaps the cats have become infected with an unusually virulent strain of viral URI, or perhaps there is an unidentified coinfection such as feline panleukopenia.

Establishing Associations between Factors

Measuring levels of disease, adoption, euthanasia, or other outcomes of interest is useful to establish the magnitude of problems and the direction and amount of progress being made, and to suggest areas for further investigation. However, simply measuring changes in disease levels does not give the reason for progress or lack thereof, nor predict the likelihood of an outcome in a given animal.

The likelihood of a particular outcome may be influenced by characteristics of the individual animal such as age or breed, as discussed previously under stratum-specific morbidity. These are factors over which we have little control, but knowing which animals are at highest risk can direct the most appropriate use of resources. Presumably, the likelihood of disease or health, adoption or euthanasia, is also influenced by management and husbandry factors. These are the things we manipulate in the hopes of improving the numbers we care about. Some of these factors, such as vaccination or choice of treatment for URI, may operate at the level of the individual animal (that is, not every member of the population is subject to the same vaccination or treatment protocol). Other factors operate at the population level, such as population density, cleaning protocol, or seasonal changes. Disease levels, likelihood of adoption, and other factors may also depend on such things as location in the shelter, participation in socialization or training, and other special programs. Teasing out the true effect of the many population and individual risk factors requires statistical analysis.

STATISTICAL ANALYSIS

A certain amount of variation between animals or within a population over time is expected due to chance alone. Additional variation is likely to be the result of more than one factor. A change in season, an increase in the average age of the population at risk, and a change in vaccination protocol could all contribute to a decrease in URI levels, for example. So although tracking disease levels is helpful in order to identify possible trends and factors that should be examined more closely, statistical analysis is required to establish whether the variation seen is greater than that expected due to chance alone and to establish the relative contribution of various factors.

When only one factor is being compared, fairly straightforward statistical analysis is possible. This is most often the case in a controlled experiment. For instance, if a group of cats with otherwise similar characteristics each received a different treatment for URI, it would be fairly easy to test whether the average duration of disease was significantly different for one group or another. Such "hood of the truck" techniques can be performed by anyone with a calculator and a few minutes of time, and the interested reader is referred to Slenning (2001).

Unfortunately, such straightforward analysis is not always possible in a shelter. When several possible factors are involved, multivariate statistical analysis often is required. This can quickly become

rather complicated, and consultation with experts is generally advisable. For shelters located near a university, graduate students in statistics or epidemiology may be lured into performing more complex analyses if the shelter can provide the necessary data. As shelter medicine increases in sophistication, and more shelters collect and analyze medical and performance data, more efficient computer based methods for data collection and analysis may become available, as has been the case in many other areas of population medicine.

ASSOCIATION VERSUS CAUSALITY

One final word of caution about data interpretation: Statistics cannot be used to demonstrate causality, only association. Two factors may be closely linked without being causally related. For instance, cats may be adopted more rapidly from a multiple cat room than from individual cages within a particular shelter. This could be due to a causal relationship: Maybe people see the cats interacting with one another in a more natural and spacious environment and are more likely to choose those cats. On the other hand, maybe only cats that seem healthy and get along well with others are chosen for placement in these rooms. Perhaps these same cats would be adopted more rapidly than the general population, even if they were in individual cages. Statistical analysis can be used to help determine whether cats with similar characteristics are adopted out more rapidly from one type of housing or another, but ultimately logical evaluation of underlying biological and management factors is required to decide whether an association is likely to be truly causal.

SPECIAL CASES FOR DATA COLLECTION: OUTBREAK INVESTIGATION AND POPULATION MANAGEMENT

Outbreak Investigation

Avoiding serious disease outbreaks is a major goal of a population health program, but should prevention fail, keeping careful records can help analyze the problem and suggest methods for control. Specific information should be collected whenever serious disease spreads within the shelter or a disease with the potential to cause an outbreak is diagnosed (for instance, information should be collected for every case of distemper, parvo, or panleukopenia seen in a shelter animal). An outbreak investigation establishes the cause of disease (if possible); the magnitude of the problem; risk factors for infection; whether animals entered the shelter already infected or contracted disease within the shelter; and whether control measures were adequate to prevent further spread of disease. Questions to be asked in an outbreak can be categorized as what, how many, who, when, and where.

1. **What** is causing the disease: confirmation of diagnosis and definition of suspect and confirmed cases. In a suspected outbreak of serious disease, diagnosis should be confirmed in at least one or two cases by the accepted gold standard test (see chapter 16 on infectious diseases and chapter 18 on diagnostic testing). If no single reliable method of diagnosis is available, multiple criteria (such as symptoms, test results, clinical pathology, and necropsy findings) should be used for disease confirmation. When diagnosis has been confirmed, a written *case definition* should be established describing what constitutes a suspect case or a confirmed case. For instance, a suspect case may have symptoms consistent with the disease, and a confirmed case may have one or more positive lab tests in addition to symptoms.
2. **How many** animals are affected. Document the number of suspect and confirmed cases and the method of diagnosis for each.
3. **Who** is affected: Characteristics of affected animals, including age, breed, sex, and vaccination status. This helps determine which animals are at high risk and may suggest which animals can be spared should rigorous quarantine or depopulation measures become necessary. For instance, if no cases have been documented in animals older than one year with a current history of vaccination, these animals may not need to be quarantined as long.
4. **When** did disease develop:
   a. **How many days since shelter entry?**
      i. If signs developed in fewer days than the typical incubation period for the disease, the animal probably contracted the disease in the community and entered the shelter already infected. Strict quarantine/cohort admission of incoming animals is indicated in the case of a community-wide outbreak.
      ii. If signs developed after the typical incubation period, the animal almost certainly contracted the disease within the shelter. Re-examination of sanitation, cleaning, and other disease control procedures is indicated in this case.
5. **How many days since the first case** was recognized and control measures established? This question is asked to determine whether initial control measure have been effective. (*For example: the incubation of parvoviral enteritis is typically 4–6 days. If parvo was diagnosed on May 1, the affected dog was removed, and the facility thoroughly disinfected, more cases might still be expected in exposed dogs within the next week. However, if a new case of parvo develops on May 15 in a dog that has been in the shelter since the first, initial control measures were likely insufficient.*)
6. **Where** did the animal come from in the community/where was it housed in the shelter? Graphically plotting the location of affected animals may be helpful in tracking spread of the disease within the shelter or, if the disease is suspected to originate outside the shelter, may help determine affected areas of the community.

SUMMARY: RECORD FOR EACH CASE IN AN OUTBREAK
- Date of diagnosis
- Method of diagnosis (for example, snap test, clinical signs, necropsy)
- Confirmed versus suspect case
- Date animal entered shelter
- Location from which animal originated (for example, street address, neighborhood, ZIP code)
- Location(s) in shelter where animal was held
- Vaccine history
- Age, sex, and breed of affected animal

A sample outbreak tracking form is attached in Appendix 15.4. Specific intervention strategies depend on the agent characteristics and shelter philosophy and resources, as described in the section on infectious disease policy and procedures in this chapter. Disease information is given in chapter 16.

Monitoring and Managing Population Density

Population density is one of the most important parameters to track in a shelter, hence a section of this chapter is devoted especially to the topic. *Controlling population density is the foundation of an effective shelter health care program.* If a single "magic bullet" exists to prevent disease, this is it. Unfortunately, overcrowding is a common problem in shelters. Although sometimes necessitated by a facility inadequate to hold animals even for the legally required holding period, overcrowding often occurs in an attempt to avoid having to euthanize or turn animals away. In fact, overcrowding reduces neither of these sad elements of animal shelter life. Euthanasia or turning animals away occurs when more unwanted animals exist than there are good homes available. This can be impacted only by decreasing the number of animals needing homes or increasing the number of successful adoptions. Neither of these problems will be mitigated simply by packing more animals into shelters.

OVERCROWDING AND ITS EFFECTS
The effects of overcrowding are numerous:

• Intensifies the effect of many other negative factors, such as inadequate ventilation, noise, and stress
• Increases the contact rate between animals and increases overall amount of disease in the population
• Increases the likelihood that asymptomatic carriers of disease will be present in the population and will be shedding disease at any given time
• Makes it hard or impossible to practice good husbandry and customer service
• Leads to ever more crowding if staff is so overwhelmed by the animals' daily care needs that crucial management tasks are delayed, leading to longer stays for animals

Crowding is not just a matter of cage space. Overcrowding occurs when the number of animals outstrips the shelter staff's ability to care for each animal appropriately, even if not every cage is full.

HOW MUCH IS ENOUGH? DETERMINING THE
APPROPRIATE NUMBER OF ADOPTABLE ANIMALS
Although it may seem a bit crude to think of animals in these terms, inventory management principles that apply to any retail business have applications to shelters. Potential customers want a range of choices, but simply offering more stock will not increase sales. The grocer who crams more and

more boxes of a few brands of cereal onto her shelves will not find more customers. Similarly, the number of animals available for adoption should reflect a reasonable variety of size, temperament, and breed and should be in proportion to the number of anticipated adopters. Beyond this number, more animals awaiting adoption will not lead to more adoptions and will not save lives. Lives may be lost if overcrowding and disease discourage adopters from choosing a shelter pet.

Unlike the hypothetical grocer, shelters do not have the luxury of deciding how much potential inventory comes knocking at the door. Where possible, plans should be made for fluctuations in supply and demand. For instance, foster homes can be used to care for special adult cats during the height of kitten season, for return to the shelter during the quieter winter months. Surrendering owners may be required or encouraged to schedule appointments, spacing out the flow of incoming animals. Overflow space or interagency cooperation can mitigate the effects of major legal cases resulting in a massive influx of animals.

MANAGING TURNOVER TIME
Turnover time is the time from when an animal enters a shelter until the time it leaves, whether by adoption, reclaim, rescue, or euthanasia. For open admission shelters, decreasing turnover time is key to managing population density while minimizing euthanasia. For limited admission shelters, decreasing turnover time maximizes the number of lives that can be saved in the available space. Following are some key principles of turnover time management:

• The goal in decreasing turnover time is not necessarily to change the outcome for any animal but to decrease the time it takes to reach any given outcome. For instance, adoptable animals should not be euthanized early simply to decrease turnover time, but animals that will end up being euthanized eventually (for instance for temperament or humane reasons) should be identified sooner rather than later.
• Increased turnover time (longer stays in the shelter) increases the likelihood that animals will develop medical or behavior problems. Treatment of medical and behavior problems leads to still longer shelter stays, perpetuating a vicious cycle.

- Turnover time includes all time spent in stray holding, awaiting temperament testing, awaiting surgery, and so on. Policies that build in slower turnover time are not necessarily wrong, but the implications for population health and crowding should be considered.
- Turnover time is decreased by speeding adoption, reclaim, or rescue, and by *alert, proactive animal management.*

Decreasing Turnover Time: Adoption, Reclaim, and Rescue

Turnover time is decreased by

- Any program that speeds adoptions—for example, adopter prescreening programs, wish lists, off-site adoptions, Internet, radio, TV, print publicity, posting photographs of animals in foster care or in isolation.
- Any program that speeds reclaims—for example, promotion of ID, scanning for microchips, and lost pet matching.
- Rescue partnerships if rescuers are contacted and can take the animal promptly. Rescue partnerships actually can contribute to overcrowding if animals must sit for extended periods awaiting rescue.

Decreasing Turnover Time: Management Considerations

Although programs to speed up reclaim and adoptions are important, alert management is the single most essential factor in minimizing turnover time. Ideally, adoptable animals for which it takes a little longer to find the right home will receive as much time as possible. To maximize the amount of time available for adoptable animals, *wasted* turnover time must be avoided. Wasted turnover time includes any time an animal spends in the shelter not *actively available* for adoption or reclaim, or actively being treated for a medical or behavioral problem in anticipation that the animal will be adoptable in the future. Possible points for delay include anything that must be accomplished for an animal to be reclaimed, adopted, rescued, or euthanized and include the following:

- Owner contact for reclaim or surrender
- Resolution of legal issues
- Behavioral or medical assessment to determine adoptability

- Spay/neuter surgery, vaccination, testing, or other medical procedures required before adoption
- Behavioral or medical treatment of conditions prohibiting adoption
- Rescue arrangements, including contact and pickup
- Transfer from stray or other holding areas to adoptable areas
- Making and carrying out euthanasia decisions

Avoiding wasted turnover time requires *daily* assessment of all animals to ensure that relevant decisions are made and action taken as soon as possible. Action lists should be generated regarding each of the applicable categories. Shelter software can be used in some cases to automatically generate such lists (for example, all animals with possible owners that need to be contacted, all animals that need spay/neuter surgery prior to being placed for adoption, all animals that just became available for temperament testing or medical screening that day). The time invested in daily walkthroughs will be amply repaid in more efficient operation.

In addition to daily checks to ensure timely decision making, animals awaiting adoption should be formally reassessed at regularly established intervals (that is, weekly, biweekly, and so on), even if no specific decisions are indicated. At this assessment, the following needs to be done:

- Recheck the animal's health and behavioral status
- Identify barriers to adoption and establish an action plan
- Determine who will take any needed steps, when those steps will be taken, and who will be responsible for follow up

To expedite the process, daily assessment needs to be a team effort. Specifics will vary from shelter to shelter, but the walkthrough should include at least one representative with knowledge and authority regarding reclaim, rescue, legal, medical, behavioral, and adoptability issues. If only one person walks through without full authority or responsibility for followup, valuable time will be lost.

Turnover Time: Considering Some Numbers and Calculating the Cost

The dairy manager knows each extra day a cow is *open* (not pregnant) costs about $3 in lost profits.

One day in a single cow does not make much difference, but a few days multiplied by several thousand cows quickly becomes very expensive. Knowing this, dairy managers carefully track average number of days open per cow and work to minimize this number. Similarly, even a small delay in turnover time in a shelter can be significant when multiplied by many animals. For example, consider a shelter that takes in 5,000 animals a year. If there is an average delay of two days per animal in making (and carrying out) adoption/reclaim/rescue/euthanasia decisions, that adds 10,000 animal care days per year. 10,000 days/365 days in a year = 27.4 kennel spaces effectively taken out of commission for the whole year with no benefit to the animals. At a rough estimate of $10 per day to care for an animal, that comes to $100,000 per year!

Turnover Time Calculations

The average turnover time that needs to be maintained to avoid overcrowding can be estimated by the following formula:

Average turnover time in days = (total cage or kennel spaces ÷ total animals per year) × 365 days

For example: Big shelter A is an open admission shelter that takes in 5000 dogs per year and has 200 dog kennels. 200/5000 × 365 = 14.6 days average turnover time per dog. If one dog stays longer, another must stay less. If one dog can get out in less than 14 days, that buys some time for another dog to stay a little longer.

Or, to put the formula another way:

Number of animals that can be served per year = (365 days per year × total spaces) ÷ average turnover time

For example: Little shelter B is a limited admission shelter with 50 cat spaces, with an average stay of about one month per cat: (365 days × 50 cat spaces)/30 days average turnover = 608 cats served per year). If turnover time could be cut down to two weeks, this shelter could serve 1,303 cats (365 days × 50 cat spaces)/14 days average turnover = 1,303 cats) with the same space and staffing. If turnover time increased to six months per cat, only 100 cats per year could be served. This illustrates the importance of being mindful of turnover time even in a shelter that does not perform euthanasia.

Keep in mind all of these examples provide rough estimates and do not take into account the occasional animal that will need to stay much longer due to legal issues, and so on. Also, not all cages/runs are created equal; if you are considering the length of time animals may be held for adoption, then it is inappropriate to count isolation, quarantine, and stray animal holding areas for the purposes of turnover time calculations. For shelters that house animals in groups or open rooms, cages are not necessary for these calculations. Total spaces simply represents the number of animals of that species that can be accommodated at any given time without overcrowding.

Decreasing Turnover Time: Summary

- Calculate the number of animals that can be accommodated and the average turnover time your shelter needs to maintain in order to prevent overcrowding.
- Assess current policies and eliminate unnecessary increases in turnover time.
- Determine all possible points for delay in processing, establish timelines, and assign responsibility for ensuring that timelines are followed.
- Perform daily walk-through: Check each animal to ensure that all needed action has been taken.

POLICY AND PROCEDURE DEVELOPMENT

As part of a population health plan, written policies and procedures should be developed for all diseases of importance in a particular shelter. Diseases may be considered important because they are relatively common, potentially severe/fatal, zoonotic, or a combination of the three. Developing such policies *before* a crisis or outbreak occurs provides an opportunity to gather all needed information, thoughtfully weigh risks, costs, and benefits of various choices and allows all interested parties to understand the decision making process. It is also easier to assess the success of a disease management plan if the same steps are followed each time. Necessary steps for each disease considered include the following:

1. Assess the level of threat posed by the disease agent to individual animals, to the population, and to human health.

2. Define what is needed to manage the disease, including recognition, treatment, and environmental control.

3. Decide whether the disease can be controlled reasonably and treated within *your* shelter, and determine general policy (see the following discussion).

4. Develop a written procedure addressing specific steps to take when the disease is recognized.

Questions to Ask When Developing a Policy and Procedure for a Specific Disease

1. How will disease be recognized?
   a. Is there a test available?
      i. How reliable is the test (sensitivity, specificity, predictive value in test population)?
      ii. What can interfere with accuracy of test results?
      iii. How rapidly are results available?
   b. What are typical signs of the disease, and what are possible atypical presentations?
   c. Is there a carrier state for the disease? (*Carrier state* is defined as persistent shedding of infectious agent by asymptomatic or seemingly recovered individuals.)

2. What is the risk to the population/how hard is it to manage the disease?
   a. Severity of disease in individual?
   b. Zoonotic potential?
   c. Mode and ease of transmission?
   d. Methods/ease of disinfection?
   e. Vaccination possible?
      i. How effective?
      ii. What are the side effects/risks of vaccination?
   f. What is the frequency of disease?
      i. Can the disease realistically be eliminated, or just controlled?

3. Course of disease/treatment of individual
   a. What is the incubation period?
      i. Incubation period determines the length of quarantine.
   b. What are the options for treatment?
      i. How effective is treatment?
      ii. How much does treatment cost?
      iii. Is treatment practical in *your* shelter?
   c. Is there prolonged shedding after recovery from clinical signs?

   i. Determines time at which animal can be reintroduced safely to the general population or adoptive home with other vulnerable pets

Note that population risk may be very different than severity in an individual animal. For instance, FIV is a very severe disease for the affected individual but poses a relatively low population risk because it is not very readily spread and is easily destroyed by disinfection. Ringworm, on the other hand, is not a very severe disease in an individual, but is zoonotic, readily spread, and very difficult to disinfect. Treatment is available but may not be practical in some shelters, continued shedding is possible after recovery from clinical signs, and an effective preventive vaccine is not available. All of this combines to make a usually mild disease a significant population risk.

Policy Development

Answers to the questions posed here determine the general policy and specific procedures for disease management. Policy should be based on the practicality of managing the disease in an individual animal while protecting population health in that particular shelter setting. No cookbook formula will fit every shelter; the right choice depends on the resources and mission of an individual agency and must take into consideration any legal or contractual obligations the shelter has. Policy options to consider include the following:

1. Test and remove (or exclude) from shelter (do not admit, foster, treat at outside vet clinic, euthanize).
   - Appropriate for diseases that pose a high population or zoonotic risk, and/or cannot be treated effectively with the resources available in that shelter.
2. Isolate and treat within shelter.
   - Appropriate for diseases that pose a moderate population risk, in a shelter with appropriate isolation facilities.
3. Treat in general population.
   - Appropriate for diseases that pose a low population risk but are detrimental to individual animal health.
4. Don't treat, don't worry (release for adoption or reclaim with documentation).

• Appropriate for diseases that do not pose an immediate threat to individual or population health but should be brought to the attention of potential owners.

No matter what the general policy is for a given disease, a specific procedure needs to be developed detailing how the disease will be managed in the shelter, including recognition, notification, treatment, housing, disinfection, adoption policies (if applicable), and documentation. A generic written procedure is included in Appendix 15.5.

CONCLUSION

This chapter has outlined some of the basic components of a population health monitoring program. Some shelters may already have put into practice much of what has been presented here, and others may feel that implementing all of this is an overwhelming task. The good news is that population health and infectious disease prevention does not have to be tackled all at once, and in fact is more appropriately approached as an ongoing process, a dialogue between where you are now and where you would like to be. Shelter medicine itself is an emerging discipline. As more and more shelters track and share information about what works and what doesn't in this unique and challenging setting, we can all benefit from a solid foundation of knowledge on which to base the choices that matter so much to us and our animals. When we consistently put the principles of population health into practice in a shelter, veterinary medicine can provide not only a powerful tool to keep animals healthy, but help get them out the door alive.

Summary: Shelter Population Health in a Nutshell

1. Define your shelter's goals and measure baseline numbers.
2. Consider medical, behavioral, outreach, adoption, facilities, and other aspects of your shelter:
   a. What are you doing now?
   b. What would you do in an ideal world?
   c. Decide which changes best use your resources to meet your goals.
3. Establish a timeline for improvement.
4. Develop policies and procedures for management of individual diseases.
5. Make changes, measure results.
6. Repeat as necessary

REFERENCES

Ekesbo, I., Oltenacu, P. A., et al. 1994. A disease monitoring system for dairy herds *Veterinary Record* (134): 270–273.

Fennell, L. A. 1999. Beyond overpopulation: A comment on Zawistowski et al. and Salman et al. *Journal of Applied Animal Welfare Science* 2(3): 217–228.

Lechtenberg, K. F., Smith, R. A., et al. 1998. Feedlot health and management. *Veterinary Clinics of North America Food Animal Practice* 14(2): 177–197.

Munson, L., and Cook, R. 1993. Monitoring, investigation and surveillance of diseases in captive wildlife. *Journal of Zoo and Wildlife Medicine* 24(3): 281–290.

Radostits, O. M. 2001. *Herd Health: Food Animal Production Medicine*, 3d ed. Philadelphia, PA: W.B. Saunders Company.

Reneau, J., and Kinsel, M. 2001. Record systems and herd monitoring in production-oriented health management programs in food producing animals. In *Herd Health: Food Animal Production Medicine*, O.M. Radostits, ed. Philadelphia, PA: W.B. Saunders, 107–146.

Salman, M. D., New, J. G., et al. 1998. Human and animal factors related to the relinquishment of dogs and cats in 12 selected animal shelters in the United States. *Journal of Applied Animal Welfare Science* 1(3): 207–226.

Savesky, K. 1999. Selling your organization's message: Social marketing. *Animal Sheltering*. Jan-Feb 99.

Slenning, B. 2001. Quantitative tools for production oriented veterinarians In *Herd Health: Food Animal Production Medicine*, O. M. Radostits, ed. Philadelphia, PA: W.B. Saunders, 47–107.

Teare, J. 1991. Medical record systems for the next century: the case for improved health care through integrated data bases. *Journal of Zoo and Wildlife Medicine* 22(4): 389–391.

Appendix 15.1
Post-Adoption Health Follow-up Postcard

This can be printed on a prepaid postcard with the shelter address on the reverse side and sent out with adopters to give their new veterinarian at the first visit. Adoption staff can fill in the animal identification and date of adoption at the time the animal is adopted out.

Dear veterinarian,

The health of our adopted animals is very important to us. Please fill out and return this card to help us keep track of how we're doing. Our veterinarian can be contacted at ＿＿＿＿＿＿＿ if you wish to report or discuss any special concerns. Thanks!

☐ Date Adopted:＿＿＿＿＿＿＿
☐ Animal identification: ＿＿＿＿＿＿＿
☐ No health problems noted
☐ Feline URI Mild, Moderate, Severe (if checked, please circle level of severity)
☐ Kennel cough Mild, Moderate, Severe (if checked, please circle level of severity)
Other findings:

＿＿
＿＿
＿＿

Appendix 15.2
Calculating Population Time
at Risk and Determining Incidence

Incidence rate can be calculated over any period of time: a day, week, month, or year. I use a month as an example here because it is a short enough time period to give a reasonable amount of detail, but not too short; a difference between July and January is likely to be of more interest than a difference between Monday and Tuesday. Population time at risk is defined as the sum of disease-free time for all individuals in the population during the period under study. Each day an animal is free of disease and in the shelter contributes one day to the total population time at risk.

Intuitively, we know that the amount of risk an animal experiences depends not only on whether it is in the shelter or not, but on how long it is in the shelter. Caring for 70 cats for one day each, one would not expect to see the same amount of disease as if one cared for 70 cats for 7 days each. In the first case, an average of 10 cats would be in the shelter on any given day in a week, but in the second case 70 cats would be in the shelter on each day of the week. It is inappropriate to simply count the number of animals cared for over the period in question.

Example

Consider a shelter with 50 cages for healthy cats that keeps all cages full most of the time. (This example presumes that sick cats are moved to an isolation area.) In the busy month of July, this shelter cared for 200 cats. In January, this shelter cared for only 50 cats. Suppose that 25 new cases of URI occurred in both January and July.

JULY

Average turnover time = number of cages/number of animals × number of days in a month

50 cages/200 cats × 30 days in a month = 7.5 days average per cat.

So each cat contributes, on average, 7.5 days to the total population time at risk. Total cat time at risk then is

200 cats × 7.5 days per cat = 1500 cat days at risk.

Incidence = # of new cases of URI/total cat time at risk = 25 cases of URI/1500 cat days at risk=.017 cases of URI per cat day at risk.

January

Average turnover time = 50 cages/50 cats × 30 days in a month = 30 days average per cat.

Total cat time at risk = 50 cats × 30 days per cat = 1500 cat days at risk.

Incidence = 25 cases of URI/1500 cat days at risk = .017 cases of URI per cat day at risk.

The incidence was the same in January and July. There were the same number of new cases and the same number of cat days at risk in each month.

Calculating incidence based on the absolute number of cats in the shelter during the month is the wrong way! Same scenario as preceding (50 cages, 200 cats in July, 50 cats in January).

July

25 new cases of URI/200 cats sheltered during July = .125

January

25 new cases of URI/50 cats sheltered during January = .5

Calculating incidence this way, based on number of cats sheltered rather than days at risk, gives a false impression that incidence was much higher in January than in July.

In a shelter that is virtually always full, as in the preceding example, it can be assumed that an animal is in almost every cage every day. Therefore, animal days at risk can be estimated by simply multiplying the number of cages for healthy animals by the number of days in the time period under consideration. *This is not accurate if sick animals remain in the general population.* In a shelter where spaces for healthy cats are not always full, either the actual daily count must be taken, or an average of daily counts taken at the beginning and end of the time period under consideration, as described in the chapter.

Appendix 15.3
Sample URI Incidence Tracking Form

Month/year_____

Animal ID	Date entered shelter	Date diagnosed with URI	Recovered yes/no, date if yes	Duration

Total cat days at risk this month:_____
Total cases of URI:_____
Incidence (# cases/total # of cat days at risk):_____
Average duration (total days duration/# of cats for which duration was recorded):_____

Appendix 15.4
Sample Outbreak Tracking Form

Animal ID	Date entered shelter	Date of vaccine	Date diagnosed	Cage/ run # at time of diagnosis	Animal description (sex, spay/ neuter, age, breed)	Symptoms[*]/ test results (SNAP test, necropsy, other)

[*]Symptom codes: D=diarrhea, V=vomit, B=blood in diarrhea/vomit, L=lethargy, N=no abnormal signs

Appendix 15.5
Generic Procedure for Disease Management

1. Disease description/case definition
2. How recognized?
   Who is authorized to perform test?
   Who is authorized to make diagnosis?
3. Who notified?
   When (immediately, within 24 hours. . .)
   How (paper, in person, and so on)
4. Where housed?
   Isolation, general population, not housed ever (euthanasia upon disease recognition)
5. How cleaned?
   Cage
   Environment
6. Treatment policy?
   Don't treat, leave in general population
   Treat in general population
   Treat in foster care
   Treat at outside veterinarian clinic
   Isolate and treat in shelter
   Euthanize
7. Treatment (if applicable)
8. Which animals will be treated?
   Only during legally required holding period?
   All animals?
   Decision making process if only some available animals are treated
   Who can initiate treatment?

If other than veterinarian can initiate treatment:
   Standard treatment
   Circumstances under which standard treatment initiated
   Side effects/precautions regarding standard treatment
   Who is responsible for daily treatment?
9. Recovery/treatment failure
   How defined?
   Who can determine?
   If other than veterinarian, standardize protocol for determining recovery/treatment failure
10. Adoption
   Will animal be adoptable prior to recovery? (Can actually go home while sick)
   Will animal be available prior to recovery?
   (People can see animal/photo, express interest, place holds)
   Adoption release required notifying adopter of medical condition
11. Documentation—where will the following be noted?
   Diagnosis
   Test results
   Treatment
   Rechecks
   Adoption release
   Home care instructions/prescriptions

Appendix 15.6
Shelter Data Collection Summary

* This is intended as a fairly comprehensive list of possibilities. Shelters can tailor this to their own needs and abilities. It may seem like a lot, but many shelters are tracking much of this information already for various purposes.

Data should be collected regarding:
- Disease levels
- Performance measures (animals in and out)
- Risk factors for disease
- Risk factors for good or bad performance (surrender, disease, adoption, euthanasia)
- Effect of intervention

INDIVIDUAL ANIMAL DATA

Unique identifying number—necessary for data filing, retrieval, and analysis

Possible risk factors
Species
Breed/mix
Age
Color
Location of origin (neighborhood where picked up or surrendered)
Location housed in shelter

Medical record
Vaccination history (prior to shelter)
Vaccines given in shelter
Prophylactic treatments given in shelter (deworming, flea control, and so on)
Test results (FeLV, FIV, fecal, and so on)
Surgery performed in shelter
Diagnoses and treatments given in shelter
Other conditions, for example, pregnant on intake

Daily individual animal monitoring
Urine
Feces
Appetite
Behavior/attitude
Abnormal symptoms (skin, GI, respiratory, other)
Weight/body condition score (weekly or biweekly)

POPULATION MANAGEMENT

* Much of this could be analyzed on a monthly or annual basis. For measures expected to vary with season, such as intake numbers, daily population, and disease incidence, monthly collection and analysis is preferable.

Intake data
By species:
    Stray
    Surrendered
    Shelter transfer
       Which shelter
    Adoption return
    Other

Reason for intake denial (for shelters that can accept some, but not all, over-the-counter intakes—as applicable, depending on individual shelter policy)

Lack of space in shelter
Medical noninfectious
    Treatable—not admitted due to resource limitations (money, space, staffing)
    Terminal
Medical infectious
    Treatable—not admitted due to resource limitations (money, space, staffing, unable to house/care for without excess population risk)
    Terminal
Behavior
    Rehabilitatable—not admitted due to resource limitations (money, space, staffing)
    Terminal/ excessive public safety risk
Adoptability issue—for example, breed restriction, size, age

Population burden
By species:
    Total animal care days
    Average animal care days to adoption in adoptable animals/no-kill shelters
    Average animal care days not adoptable or awaiting reclaim (awaiting temperament test, surgery, move to adoption, under medical treatment, and so on)

Surrender reason tracking (Modified from scheme used by National Council for Pet Population Study)
By species:
    Household animal population (can't find homes, too many animals)
    Behavior
        Aggression to humans
        Aggression to other animals
        Other behaviors (could certainly break down further—fear issues, separation anxiety, house soiling, excessive vocalization, disobedient, hyperactive, and so on)
    Housing issue (moving, landlord won't allow, no fence, and so on)
    Animal medical condition
    Animal characteristic other than medical or behavioral (too big/small, mellow, not protective enough, wrong color, and so on)
    Human lifestyle issue (allergies, divorce, new baby, owner death, and so on)
    Human preparation and expectation (litter box odor, cost of routine care, and so on)
    Owner requested euthanasia
    Adoption return
        Medical
        Behavioral
           Aggression
           Housebreaking
           Separation anxiety
           Destructive behavior
           Too energetic
           Other
        Other reason for adoption return (unanticipated allergies, change in owner circumstance)
    Other reason for surrender (doesn't fit any category already given, for example, a legal case)

Outcome data
By species:
    Reclaimed
    Adopted
    Rescued
    Euthanized
    Died
    Other

Euthanasia reason tracking (minimum level of detail—could break down further into specific disease diagnosis, behavioral problem)
By species:
   Lack of space (healthy, behaviorally sound animals)
   Medical noninfectious
      Treatable—euthanized due to resource limitations (money, space, staffing)
      Terminal—euthanized due to poor prognosis
   Medical infectious
      Treatable—euthanized due to resource limitations (money, space, staffing, unable to house/care for without excess population risk)
      Terminal—euthanized due to poor prognosis
   Behavioral
      Rehabilitatable—euthanized due to resource limitations (money, space, staffing)
      Terminal—euthanized due to poor prognosis or public safety
   Owner requested euthanasia

BEHAVIORAL HEALTH

Temperament testing results
Reasons for failure
   Depends on shelter policy
Numeric or subjective score if passes

Treatable behavioral issues noted in shelter (during t-test or other interactions)
Diagnosis (pulls on leash, fence aggression, repetitive behavior, and so on)
Time in shelter to diagnosis (particularly for kennel-stress related issues)
Treatment plan (drug treatment and behavior modification if applicable)
Outcome (no improvement, some, moderate, or marked improvement, completely resolved)

Post-adoption behavior issues
   Aggression
   Housebreaking
   Separation anxiety
   Destructive behavior
   Too energetic
   Other

DISEASE OCCURRENCE

Incidence (requires daily or estimated daily healthy population*)
URI
Kennel cough
GI disease/diarrhea
   Infectious
   Non-infectious
   Undiagnosed

Skin disease
   Infectious
   Noninfectious
   Undiagnosed
(Other frequent and significant diseases tracked separately depending on shelter, for example, parvo, ringworm, panleukopenia, distemper)

   * If daily population estimate is prohibitive, simply tracking number of cases and total shelter population over the same time period is still valuable.

Average duration (for animals which remained in the shelter system until recovery)
URI
Kennel cough

Disease cost
Average duration × estimated daily cost of treatment/housing × number of cases

Case fatality rate
Death versus euthanasia for
URI
Kennel cough
Other common conditions that lead to death or euthanasia in that particular shelter

Days in shelter to first sign of disease (Particularly important for shelters that quarantine, in order to determine appropriate quarantine duration)
Dogs
Cats

Test results (all that apply)
Number performed and number of positives for
   Parvo
   Panleukopenia
   FeLV
   FIV
   Heartworm
   Fecal exams (and what they were positive for)

Post-adoption health
Tally of complaints
If medical follow up offered, what type of complaints, how long after adoption
If follow up postcard, frequency of
   Healthy
   URI
   Kennel cough
   Parvo
   Ringworm
   Other zoonotic
   Other as needed for individual shelter

Descriptive impression of URI and kennel cough (what types of signs predominate, frequency of recurrence, description of refractory, or unusually severe cases). More detailed data could be collected regarding exact frequency of different signs but would be laborious without a good computer system set up. This level of detail would most likely be indicated only for a specified time to identify effect of a particular intervention, such as a new vaccine protocol. For instance, rather than just counting cases of URI, a graded system of severity from 1–4 could be used, and incidence of each level of severity could be tracked separately. Alternatively, a database could be set up to track frequency of specific symptoms of URI, as shown here.

Example

Of the feline URI cases, what is the frequency of the following symptoms?

Eyes
    Unilateral
    Bilateral
        Ulcers
        Discharge
            Serous
            Purulent
        Conjunctivitis
Nose
    Sneezing
    Discharge
        Serous
        Purulent
Other complications
    Lower respiratory
    Systemic involvement (fever, GI)
    Duration > 2 weeks

HUSBANDRY

For the time period under consideration:

Feeding protocol
Cleaning protocol
Vaccine protocol
Behavior enrichment program
Other husbandry/management factors expected to affect the outcome of interest (special advertising campaign, change in adoption policy, change in fees or hours, and so on)

Examples of Analysis

Outcome by individual risk factor examples:

Time to adoption by breed, color, location in shelter, temperament test results
Disease incidence by age, prior vaccination status, in-shelter vaccination type
Duration of disease by treatment received
Frequency of behavioral problem development by breed, temperament test results

Outcome by population risk factor examples:

Disease incidence by average daily shelter population (density)
Disease incidence before and after change in cleaning protocol
Disease incidence by location of origin/shelter of origin for shelter transfers
Adoption numbers before and after change in fees or hours

Outcome by time

Adoption numbers by season, day of the week (helps make decisions about staffing, open hours)
Disease incidence by season

16
Infectious Diseases of Dogs and Cats

Janet Foley and Michael Bannasch

INTRODUCTION

Infectious diseases are common in shelters and contribute to death by direct causes, euthanasia to manage infections, and reduced adoptions from the shelter due to public and local veterinarians' lack of confidence in the shelter animals' health. In addition to several almost universal infectious problems in shelters (kennel cough, feline respiratory infections, diarrhea), there are dozens of commonly and hundreds of rarely involved pathogenic bacteria, fungi, protozoa, arthropods, and other infectious agents targeting dogs and cats in the high turnover, densely housed environments characteristic of shelters. This chapter is intended as a companion medical guide for assessing and managing infections in shelters. It is meant to be used in a fully integrated management plan, utilizing concepts from the other chapters in this text extensively. This chapter is organized according to clinical syndromes, because that is how individual and population infectious problems present to the shelter medical staff. One goal is to briefly overview the possible contributing agents and give mention to noninfectious contributors where warranted, allowing the user to generate a "rule-out list" for possible etiological agents involved in a given clinical presentation. The next section under each syndrome is diagnosis; this information is presented with the full realization that extensive diagnostic testing may be beyond the practical or budgetary constraints of many shelters. Therefore clinical diagnoses are emphasized along with practical and possible diagnostic possibilities, as well as interpretations for when it becomes strongly advisable to incorporate diagnostic tests (for example, for ringworm surveillance). The last sections in each syndrome are herd and individual management of the syndrome, emphasizing preventive measures.

Again, rather than give treatment options for each different infection (information that is available in several other resources), We have tried to give a balanced, whole herd or whole animal treatment and management approach, recognizing that precise diagnoses often are not available. The final introductory word of caution: herd management comes before individual management *always* and prevention is cheaper, easier, and kinder to the animals than having to manage them after they become infected.

RESPIRATORY DISEASE

Overview

Respiratory tract disease represents the most prevalent, visible, and difficult to manage infectious problem in animal shelters. In dogs and cats, respectively, the major syndromes are kennel cough and upper respiratory tract infection. Less obviously (and less commonly), animals in shelters may develop lower respiratory tract infection. The upper respiratory diseases typically are due to infectious agents, while lower respiratory disease occurs due to some of the same pathogens, as infectious exacerbation of noninfectious medical problems, or due to extension of unique systemic or primary respiratory pathogens. Typically, epidemic spread and management difficulty are greater problems for the upper respiratory tract syndromes, with lower respiratory disease more typically incidental individual animal problems.

Feline Upper Respiratory Infections

BORDETELLA BRONCHISEPTICA

Bordetella bronchiseptica is a nonenteric Gram-negative rod-shaped bacterium which resides on the mucosa of infected animals and contributes to mild (cats) or more severe (dogs) respiratory tract infections, often in association with respiratory viruses (Wright et al., 1973; Bemis, Greisen, and Appel, 1977; Willoughby et al., 1991; Coutts et al., 1996; Welsh, 1996). *B. bronchiseptica* occurs commonly in pigs and rabbits, and sporadic bordetellosis has been reported in people, horses, and seals (Cross and Claflin, 1962; Goodnow, 1980; Magyar et al., 1988; Woolfrey and Moody, 1991). *B. bronchiseptica* is a zoonosis, causing disease primarily in immunosuppressed people. Cross-species transmission of *B. bronchiseptica* has been described, although genetic investigations document some host-species fidelity (Gueirard et al., 1995; Binns et al., 1998; Dawson et al., 2000; Foley et al., in press). If protected and kept moist, the bacterium can survive in the environment for weeks.

Bordetella bronchiseptica has virulence determinants that it shares with its more serious human pathogens, *B. pertussis* and *B. parapertussis,* including an adenyl cyclase that reduces the phagocytic competence of neutrophils and a cytotoxin which is damaging to ciliated epithelia. In cats, there are three forms of bordetellosis: very mild primary infection with conjunctivitis and mild oculonasal discharge, *Bordetella* pneumonia secondary to viral (caliciviral or herpesviral) upper respiratory tract infection and immunosuppression, and primary *Bordetella* pneumonia in young kittens (Jacobs et al., 1993; Coutts et al., 1996; Welsh, 1996). In dogs, the same strains of *B. bronchiseptica* can target the trachea, destroy the superficial epithelium, promote inflammatory infiltration and result clinically in a harsh honking cough that is refractory to treatment.

CALICIVIRUS

Feline calicivirus is an RNA virus that infects cats only. It is characterized by high rates of mutation and high antigenic and genetic diversity. The infection is acquired when a cat inhales or ingests calicivirus particles in the air, on fomites, or on other cats. The infection is transmitted by aerosol, and introduction of the virus into a cat is via the oral and nasal routes. Subsequently, the virus spreads systemically with viremia and high levels of virus secretion from many sites, including respiratory secretions, feces, and urine. At a minimum, shedding

occurs for 10 days to 2 weeks and commonly in shelters or in kittens, for months, during which time cats may have clinical URI or be asymptomatic. There are several disease conditions that can occur with calicivirus infection, including conjunctivitis and rhinitis with serous ocular discharge, vesicular stomatitis/faucitis (aphthous stomatitis), and pneumonia (Pedersen et al., 2000). Often on about the second day of infection there is a transient fever and limping with detectable polyarthritis, but starting about 10 days after infection there may be immune complex disease with polyarthritis and gingivitis. Immune-complex polyarthritis has been reported as a sequel to calicivirus vaccination. Recently, a very pathogenic series of calicivirus infections were reported, in which cats developed facial and limb edema, apparently due to vasculitis secondary to calicivirus, comparable to the hemorrhagic fever syndrome observed in rabbit hemorrhagic calicivirus infection.

Clearly, the effects of infection are both directly due to the virus and immune-mediated. Maternal immunity to protect the kittens can be short-lived, lasting from 3–9 weeks. Even cats that have recovered from earlier infections with calicivirus may not be protected if the challenge is with an antigenically dissimilar virus. However, as cats mature to about 3 years of age, their innate protective mechanisms appear to finally develop the capability to defend the cat against calicivirus, and many kittens that appeared chronically infected will finally stop showing clinical signs. Other cats, particularly those with immune-mediated gingivitis, may continue to have severe disease and may eventually be euthanized.

HERPESVIRUS

Feline herpesvirus is an enveloped DNA virus infecting felids only, but typical biologically of other herpesviruses in dogs, humans, and other species. The genome is double-stranded DNA coding for 6 proteins. Herpesvirus particles may be seen within host cell nuclei, cytoplasm, and extracellularly. The virus does not persist in the environment and usually is spread by close contact with an infected cat. Often, kittens acquire the infection very early in life, because the stress and hormones upregulated during parturition efficiently induce recrudescence of the virus. Later in life, transmission of the feline herpesvirus requires intimate contact among cats.

Following infection, the virus remains persistent in the trigeminal nerve with periodic or chronic activation manifest in the classical URI clinical signs, often described as rhinotracheitis. Activation occurs especially during stressful periods, parturition, or immunosuppressive events. Disease signs may include conjunctivitis, anterior uveitis, serous ocular discharge with secondary bacterial infection and mucopurulent discharge, or keratitis ± dendritic ulceration (Maggs et al., 1999). Ulcerative and necrotizing nasal dermatitis resembling shingles has been described in some cats with herpes (Hargis and Ginn, 1999). Herpesvirus infection is implicated as one cause of fading kittens and in older cats in chronic sinusitis, possibly with destruction of turbinates.

CHLAMYDOPHILA FELIS

Occasionally, URI signs in cats are due to infection with *C. felis,* an obligately intracellular bacterium, primarily of cats, but possibly (rarely) affecting humans as well (Dorin, Miller, and Goodwin, 1993). Previously, *C. felis* was classified in the same species as *Chlamydia (*now *Chlamydophila).* The reservoir for the feline pathogen is feline conjunctival and genital mucosa (and possibly GI). During infection, bacteria attach to target mucosal cells, elementary bodies are endocytosed into a phagosome, the bacterial bodies enlarge to form reticulate bodies, binary fission occurs, bacteria condense, and are released as elementary bodies. Chlamydial disease often is acquired shortly after weaning in cats. The typical signs include conjunctivitis, which is often unilateral. Chlamydial abortions have been reported, as has "pneumonitis," which probably reflect an unappreciated, underlying calicivirus or herpesvirus infection. Cats may be carriers of *C. felis.*

MYCOPLASMA SPP.

Mycoplasma spp. are degenerate, obligately parasitic bacteria with no cell wall, reduced genomes, and minimal ultrastructure. Mollicutes are technically Gram-negative (because there is no cell wall to uptake the Gram stain). The reservoir for mycoplasmas is respiratory and genital mucosa of several species, where the bacteria attach tightly to the epithelium via receptors. Transmission is direct via aerosol. Disease in cats attributed to mycoplasmas

includes URI, conjunctivitis, and arthritis (Haesebrouck et al., 1991). The two most commonly detected species are *M. felis* and *gatae*: arguably *M. gatae* is more commonly implicated in cases of arthritis (Moise et al., 1983). Mycoplasmas have a number of virulence determinants, but some of the secreted proteins can kill target cells and/or allow for chronic or latent infections. Nevertheless, many people remain unconvinced that mycoplasmas are primary URI pathogens in cats, given that they commonly are recovered from well cats.

DIAGNOSIS OF FELINE URI

Clinical Diagnosis

Individual cat and herd management protocols differ significantly depending on what agent(s) is present; thus it is important to obtain some level of confidence in a diagnosis. Often in a shelter, such a diagnosis is tentatively obtained by clinical evaluation. Clinically, the key features to observe in cats with URI include conjunctivitis, anterior uveitis, nature of the discharge from the eyes and nose, gingivitis, faucitis, stomatitis, glossitis, rectal temperature, and lymphadenomegaly. It is important to evaluate whether stomatitis and faucitis are vesicular. It is helpful to determine if the cat appears lame or painful in the joints, and to observe or listen for a cough. If there is a greenish or tenacious colored ocular or nasal discharge, there is bacterial contamination in the site, but this does not help determine the underlying pathogen. A cough suggests that the cat may have bronchitis (allergic or infectious) or pneumonia; far less commonly a cat with a cough may have "kennel cough" (that is, *Bordetella bronchiseptica* tracheitis). A cat with aphthous stomatitis probably has either calicivirus or herpesvirus infection, with faucitis indicative of calicivirus. Keratitis and corneal ulceration suggest herpesvirus infection. Chronic sinusitis often with turbinate destruction may have either herpesvirus or calicivirus underlying the problem, although it appears more typical with herpesvirus infection. Cats with serous or purulent ocular and/or nasal discharge without the other more specific diagnostic signs could be infected with any one or more of the URI pathogens. Fever occurs most commonly with the viruses; limping and polyarthritis are suggestive of mycoplasma or calicivirus infection.

Rapid laboratory confirmation of the etiologic agent is unlikely. However, cytology of conjunctival cells smeared onto a glass slide is helpful for identifying some cases of *Chlamydophila felis*. Direct antibody staining increases the sensitivity.

Culture-Based Diagnosis

All of the URI pathogens except *C. felis* can be cultured routinely, although samples need to be processed and routed differently for each and the expected agents need to be identified to the laboratory at the time of submission. More specific details of submission and testing should be obtained from the local laboratory directly. *B. bronchiseptica* is easily cultured from bacterial culturettes applied to the fauces, oropharynx, or trans-tracheal wash fluid, submitted for aerobic bacteriology. In our laboratory, we screen for *B. bronchiseptica* by growing on selective and differential MacConkey agar: most other nonenteric Gram-negative rods will not grow on MAC, and most enterics are lactose-positive (*B. bronchiseptica* is lactose-negative). *Mycoplasma* species may grow from bacterial swabs of the eyes and nose if plated appropriately (that is, it is important to request mycoplasma culture). Many laboratories routinely utilize thallium penicillin plates for mycoplasma isolation, and a positive colony has a typical "fried-egg" appearance. The low sensitivity of mycoplasma culture and unavailability of *Chlamydophila felis* culture motivate use of PCR for most routine diagnostics. Samples for bacterial culture should not be frozen.

In contrast, swabs for virus isolation may be frozen. Viral transport medium such as Hanks buffered salt solution often contains antibiotics, so the same swabs are not appropriate for bacterial isolation. Swabs may be taken from fauces and larynx area, eyes, and nose. For calicivirus, positive culture may be expected also from blood or feces. Samples need to be sent to a virology laboratory, where the same in vitro cell line (for example, Crandel feline kidney) may be used for both agents. If the infection is herpesvirus, cytoplasmic effect (CPE) occurs after 24-48 hours. Cells round up and detach diffusely from the monolayer with a moth-eaten appearance. Individual cells may appear connected by cytoplasmic streamers or may combine into giant or synctitial cells. In calicivirus infection, CPE occurs more quickly than herpesvirus (within 24 hours), with the whole monolayer becoming detached.

Cell clusters with an appearance similar to grapes appear in the tissue culture fluid.

PCR

Polymerase chain reaction (PCR) testing may facilitate diagnosis of URI pathogens, subject to availability, limitations due to sample handling, and expense. PCR detects nucleic acid, so a nonviable organism could yield a positive PCR test result. On the other hand, PCR typically is very sensitive, which can be a strong "plus" for diagnosing infections such as *Mycoplasma* sp. PCR for all of the pathogens except calicivirus is DNA PCR, so sample handling is less critical, but calicivirus is an RNA virus and samples must be sent immediately to the laboratory and/or deeply frozen to avoid RNA degradation. To collect discharge for PCR, a sterile swab can be applied to the ocular or nasal discharge or into the mouth and then transported in a small amount (just moistened) of sterile saline.

MANAGEMENT OF FELINE URI

Herd Management of Feline URI

The key concepts for managing URI are to expect and manage the frequent and chronic infections while protecting uninfected cats. URI is the most common infectious syndrome in shelter animals, and many cats harbor clinically silent or subtle calicivirus and herpesvirus infections. These cats will be entering shelters regularly, but many can be identified during quarantine, as the stress of being introduced to the environment often reactivates quiescent infections. At any point at which cats are identified as having URI, they should be evaluated for the severity of the infection. Obviously, severely infected cats should be isolated and treated. Mildly affected cats represent the biggest dilemma: some will stay mildly affected for months, and they probably should not remain in isolation that entire time (that is, they should go to a home, or foster care where the low cat density and low stress often will encourage recovery). On the other hand, there is a tendency in shelters not to remove the mild cases from adoption, thus ensuring that the well cats are exposed. Unfortunately, some of the modified live vaccines will induce mild to moderate URI that is clinically indistinguishable from disease caused by "field strain" pathogens. A balanced strategy for URI management is to separate cats into three populations: completely well, adoptable mildly affected, and isolation/treatment. If mildly affected cats are to be adopted, communication and client education must be excellent. It is *not* appropriate to treat all affected cats with antibiotics, as most are infected with viruses and antibiotic use adversely affects normal flora and promotes antibiotic resistance and susceptibility to further infection.

Environmental decontamination for URI should be focused on frequent cleaning and not so much eradicating difficult to kill pathogens, as most of the URI pathogens are susceptible to many commonly used shelter disinfectants. The main reservoirs for URI are the other cats in the shelters.

Herd immunity may be heightened with the appropriate use of vaccines. Commercial vaccines are available for feline bordetellosis, calicivirus, herpesvirus, and *C. felis*. The three main types of FVRCP (feline viral rhinotracheitis = herpesvirus, calicivirus, panleukopenia) are killed virus (KV), modified life virus (MLV)—traditional, and MLV-high antigen mass (HAM). In *KV*, the virus is inactivated and given with a chemical (adjuvant) to boost the immune response to the vaccine. The vaccine usually must be given at least two times (at least 2–4 weeks apart) before effective immunity is produced. Disadvantages include: 1) the adjuvant may be locally irritating and predispose the cat to later vaccine-associated sarcoma, and 2) the cat is *not protected* for 2 weeks or longer after the first vaccination. Advantages include 1) the cat does not experience "mild" (possibly mildly immunosuppressing) infection; and 2) there is far less chance of false positive virus culture or PCR tests.

Traditional MLV uses high passage virus to give animals a mild infection. Most manufacturers recommend a "booster" 2-4 weeks after the first vaccination. Advantages include: 1) possible earlier protection than KV vaccine, 2) less immunosuppression than HAM vaccine, and 3) less likelihood of false test-positives immediately after vaccination than HAM. Disadvantages include: 1) the cat needs to be given an injection, 2) the vaccine can lead to false positive tests approximately 1 week after vaccination, 3) the cat is not protected for the first week after vaccination.

HAM vaccines use lower passage numbers and less attenuated strains than traditional MLV vaccines. While these vaccines were originally described as HAM, some independent studies have re-

ported that there is not actually more antigen, but rather less avirulent virus. Another intent to these vaccines is their supposed ability to overcome maternal immunity, where antibodies from the queen prevent effective vaccination in young kittens. HAM vaccines are given mucosally, in the hope that a local mucosal antibody (IgA) may be produced that could block the attachment of the virus to receptors, thus aborting an infection if the cat were exposed. Advantages to HAM vaccines include 1) no needles required (although most cats hate having liquid squirted into their noses); 2) possibly earlier protection than traditional MLV vaccine; 3) possible protection in young kittens despite maternal antibodies; and 4) no predisposition to later vaccine-associated sarcomas. The disadvantages are 1) possibly insufficiently attenuated and can be immunosuppressive and facilitate opportunistic infections such as salmonella and 2) may be more expensive than traditional MLV and KV vaccines. Each shelter needs to develop vaccine protocols that work for it, preferably based on utilizing one strategy for a month or more while keeping accurate records of URI incidence, then trying other protocols and comparing.

Individual Cat Management, URI

Nursing care and maintenance of hydration are by far the most important components of care for individual cats with URI, especially since the majority of affected cats have viral infections for which antimicrobial drugs are unavailable. Cats with plugged noses, sore mouths, or any indication of inappetence may need to be encouraged to eat, especially if they are young kittens. This can best be accomplished by gently cleaning the nose and then offering warmed all-meat baby food (with no onion powder). Antibiotics should be reserved for cases where there is green purulent discharge, where there is a concern of sepsis, or where there is a strong suspicion of *Clamydophila, Mycoplasma* or *B. bronchiseptica*. The drugs of choice for each of these conditions differ. For purulent discharge, a good broad-spectrum drug with activity against pathogenic staphylococci is appropriate, such as cephalexin or amoxicillin/clavulanate. For possible sepsis, drugs with excellent broad and Gram-negative (enteric) spectrums should be included, such as amoxicillin or ticarcillin/clavulanate, enrofloxacin, or a penicillin with an aminoglycoside. The drug of choice for all three of the known bacterial components of URI is doxycycline. Other possibilities include enrofloxacin and azithromycin for mycoplasmas and *C. felis* and trimethoprim/sulfamethoxazole for *B. bronchiseptica*. Mycoplasmas are inherently resistant to penicillins (or any cell-wall active drug), and very high levels of resistance are seen in *B. bronchiseptica* isolates against many antibiotics. Cats with suspected *C. felis* or *Mycoplasma* spp. infection may be candidates for topical ophthalmic antibiotics, and would be expected to improve clinically within a few days.

Unlike calicivirus, there are several drugs available to mitigate infection with herpesvirus. None will actually cure the infection but may quickly terminate the active infection. These include idoxuridine (Herplex), trifluridine (Vira-A), vidarabine (viroptic), all given topically 5–7 times a day or practically as often as possible. These veterinary antiherpetics may be difficult to obtain, or may need to be purchased through a compounding pharmacy. Acyclovir is an excellent systemically active drug against human herpesvirus infection, but has much less efficacy against feline herpesvirus. Lysine sometimes is used to treat human and feline herpes, with the justification that it will antagonize utilization of arginine in herpesviral protein synthesis (provided dietary arginine is restricted). However, restriction of arginine is not safe for cats. Some clinicians report that lysine treatment improves the clinical status of some cats with herpes, while others consider this claim unjustified and cite the lack of controlled studies documenting efficacy in cats with herpes. Interferon and other immunotreatments are given in order to boost cats' natural immune defense against herpes and other pathogens. Alpha-interferon has direct antiviral properties and has been used with some success in feline herpes but is only available as a recombinant human protein, to which cats quickly become resistant.

Cats should be evaluated individually (Table 16.1). If they remain persistently severely ill despite treatment, their prognosis for being completely well long-term is poor. However, a cat with quick recovery or which has only minor clinical signs may be very adoptable given the high rates of herpesvirus carriage in completely well cats. See Table 16.1.

Canine Kennel Cough Complex

Kennel cough, caused by *Bordetella bronchiseptica* and/or co-infecting viruses or bacteria, is associated with significant morbidity and mortality in densely housed dogs, particularly dogs in animal shelters, breeding kennels, and research facilities. The disease is characterized by acute or chronic cough, ciliary impairment, local respiratory immunosuppression, and predisposition to secondary respiratory infections. Although antibiotic treatment may kill some of the pathogenic bacteria, the dog may appear clinically worse during antibiotic administration because of coinfection with viral agents, release of tracheal cytotoxin from dying *B. bronchiseptica* cells, and possibly intracellular bacterial localization. Even after clinical recovery, infected dogs may shed pathogens from their oropharynx for weeks. Among densely housed dogs, kennel cough represents a major management problem, because it is readily transmissible, reduces adoption and purchase rates for affected animals, and requires intensive medical management. It is not uncommon for shelter dogs with infectious tracheobronchitis to be euthanized. Many field cases of kennel cough may be due to more than one infectious agent, but prior techniques of testing and lack of interest in small animal herd health have resulted in poor ability to discriminate among the causes of infection and have seriously hindered breeders' and shelter managers' ability to manage this condition. Affected dogs may have a honking cough, may retch, and may develop life-threatening pneumonia. See Table 16.2.

B. BRONCHISEPTICA

See review in "Feline URI". Research has clearly documented that *B. bronchiseptica* has a role as a primary pathogen in kennel cough.

MYCOPLASMA SPP.

See review in "Feline URI". *Mycoplasma* spp. may exacerbate the kennel cough syndrome or be present with no clinical signs.

CANINE ADENOVIRUS-2 (CAV)

The canine adenovirus is genetically and clinically similar to the human adenoviruses associated with the common cold. It infects dogs only and can replicate in any part of the respiratory epithelium, from nasal and oropharynx to deep in the lungs. Adenovirus commonly is detected in dogs with kennel cough, either alone or in coinfection with *B. bronchiseptica* and can contribute to tracheobronchitis and pneumonia (Appel, 1987).

Table 16.1. Characteristics of Feline Upper Respiratory Pathogens

Organism	Mode of Transmission	Incubation Period/ Duration of Shedding	Asymptomatic Carriers?	Clinical Presentation, Typical	Diagnostic Optimal Tests	Optimal Therapy[a]	Zoonotic/ Herd Risk?
Feline calicivirus	Aerosol, fomites	1–2d/variable (mos)	Yes	Conjunctivitis, rhinitis, faucitis	VI	Nursing	H
Feline herpesvirus	Aerosol, direct[b]	2–6d/periodically indefinite[c]	Yes	Conjunctivitis, rhinitis	VI	Anti-herpetic[d]	H
Bordetella bronchiseptica	Aerosol, fomites	1–2d/20wks	Yes	Conjunctivitis	Culture	Tetracycline	Z
Chlamydophila felis	Direct	3–5d/2mos+	Rare	Conjunctivitis	PCR	Tetracycline	Z[e]
Mycoplasma spp.	Direct	2wks/3mos+	Yes	Conjunctivitis	PCR	Tetracycline	

[a] These therapies include off-label therapies and drugs that may present significant risk to some or all patients. Before use, shelter veterinarians are advised to read all of the relevant text in this book, consult a small animal medical text, and use proper medical judgment.

[b] Requires relatively close contact.

[c] Life-long infection with periodic recrudescence.

[d] Idoxuridine, vidarabine, and trifluridine equally recommended.

[e] Very rare.

[f] Agent is environmentally persistent, and contamination of the environment is a problem in herd management. None of the agents in this table have this characteristic.

VI: virus isolation

H: important threat to herd in shelters

Z: zoonotic

241

Table 16.2. Characteristics of Canine Upper Respiratory (Kennel Cough) Pathogens

Organism	Mode of Transmission	Incubation Period[b]/ Duration of Shedding	Asymptomatic Carriers?	Clinical Presentation, Typical	Optimal Diagnostic Tests	Optimal Therapy[a]	Zoonotic/ Herd Risk?
CHV	Direct, fomites	Up to 9d[b]/ 2–3wks	Yes	None[c]	PCR	Nursing + heat + acyclovir	
CDV	Aerosol, fecal-oral	9–14d/90d	No	Resp., GI, neuro	PCR + serology	None[d]	H
CPI	Aerosol	3–10d/8d	No	Conjunctivitis	PCR	Nursing	H, Z?
Bordetella bronchiseptica	Aerosol, fomites	1–2d/3mos+	Yes	Cough	Culture	Tetracycline	Z, H
CAV	Aerosol	3–6d/10d	No	Conjunctivitis	PCR	Nursing	H
Mycoplasma spp.	Direct	3–10d/3mos+	Yes	Conjunctivitis	PCR	Tetracycline	

[a] These therapies include off-label therapies and drugs that may present significant risk to some or all patients. Before use, shelter veterinarians are advised to read all of the relevant text in this book, consult a small animal medical text, and use proper medical judgment.
[b] Clinically affects pups as old as 9 days.
[c] Reported with poor support as part of canine respiratory disease complex.
[d] Euthanasia a strong consideration if diagnosis confirmed.
[f] Agent is environmentally persistent and contamination of the environment is a problem in herd management. None of the agents in this table has this characteristic.
H: important threat to herd in shelters.
Z: zoonotic.

CANINE PARAINFLUENZA VIRUS (CPI)

Canine parainfluenza virus, like other paramyx-oviruses, has an envelope, a peplomer with hemagglutinin-neuraminidase and fusion proteins involved in attaching to host cells, and a single negative-sense strand of RNA for the genome. Canine parainfluenza is in the genus Rubulavirus with mumps and human parainfluenzaviruses 2, 4a and 4b, and in the subfamily Paramyxovirinae with measles, distemper, and rinderpest viruses. It is closely related if not identical to SV5, which causes mild respiratory disease in monkeys (Randall et al., 1987). The virus persists in the epithelial cells of the proximal respiratory tract of dogs and causes direct damage to tracheal epithelium. Several cases have been reported of a systemic, more severe variant possibly infecting the central nervous system, prostate, or other tissues (Baumgärtner et al., 1982; Macartney et al., 1985; Vieler et al., 1994). Canine parainfluenza virus has been described in subclinically infected (carrier) cats. The ecology, genetic and serological relatedness, and host range of all members of the SV5-like virus group are not well understood, but one author describes the host range of canine parainfluenza to include dogs, people, and monkeys, and probably cats, cattle, sheep, swine, and chickens. Although reported in some cases of kennel cough, other pathogens such as *B. bronchiseptica* and adenovirus are far more common in kennel cough than parainfluenza.

CANINE HERPESVIRUS (CHV)

See review in "Genitourinary disease". Canine herpesvirus, primarily a systemic and genital pathogen of dogs only, has been described in association with canine kennel cough. In older pups or mature dogs, the virus replicates in the nasal and oropharynx (lymphoid tissue and epithelium) and possibly in the lungs. The significance of recovery of canine herpesvirus in dogs with kennel cough is unknown, but it is possible that coinfection with distemper or other kennel cough pathogens may result in more severe conjunctivitis or cough.

CANINE DISTEMPER VIRUS (CDV)

See review in "Lower respiratory tract disease". Undoubtedly, distemper virus co-occurs with primary kennel cough pathogens and dramatically worsens the prognosis for infected dogs.

DIAGNOSIS OF CANINE KENNEL COUGH

Almost always, a diagnosis of kennel cough is based on clinical observation and palpation of the trachea for sensitivity. At the most, testing for distemper and culture for *B. bronchiseptica* may be performed. It is important to note that kennel cough in shelters may be severe, and it is very difficult to distinguish between severe kennel cough and respiratory distemper. Most cases in shelters are not associated with infection with distemper virus. Kennel cough-associated viruses may be cultured or evaluated with PCR but rarely are. Also see "Feline URI" and "Lower respiratory tract" sections for information about diagnosis of *B. bronchiseptica* and distemper virus.

MANAGEMENT OF CANINE KENNEL COUGH

Herd Management of Canine Kennel Cough

Kennel cough is clinically distinctive, not environmentally resistant, causes high morbidity but not mortality, and has a duration of illness in most dogs of only a few weeks. Thus herd management of kennel cough should be straightforward, but the extremely high frequency of endemic and epidemic kennel cough in many shelters attests to the difficulty in managing the disease. There are several main reasons why failures of kennel cough management occur, including that the pathogens are moderately to highly infectious and difficult to contain in space. Also, dogs continue to shed kennel cough pathogens even after they appear recovered clinically: if such dogs are moved out of isolation, there is a good chance that they will expose other dogs.

Worthwhile practices for managing kennel cough include quarantine or separation of well from affected dogs, treatment of affected dogs, maintaining high air flow (or better yet exposure to outside), reducing stress, and minimizing dog density. Quarantine periods adequate to identify dogs that might be carrying kennel cough pathogens as they enter the shelter are at least 10 days long. If a shelter has higher turnaround times than 2 weeks for dogs, it will be unreasonable to quarantine incoming dogs, but dogs should be held if possible in small groups, so that exposure is restricted only to the other dogs in that group (this must be done in small rooms, not just separate kennels). After dogs develop signs of kennel cough, they should be housed in isolation with other affected dogs. If a shelter has a policy of only adopting well animals, then there needs be isolation space for affected dogs for 2–3 weeks *at least*. Alternatively, mildly affected dogs can be adopted out of the shelter, but they still need to be physically separated from well dogs, or kennel cough is guaranteed to be endemic. Recovered dogs are still shedding and should not go back to the main kennel with the well dogs for at least two more weeks, which is another reason why adoption out of isolation may be helpful. Improving air flow and reducing stress are two of the best means of prompting dogs to recover more quickly, which accounts for why, with respect to individual dogs, one of the best management plans is to get the dog out of the shelter and into a home. In the shelter, open windows, indoor/outdoor kennels, or minimally HEPA filters may help reduce pathogen density in the air. Vaccination may be helpful, but onset of protection is late enough that dogs may be infected early in their stay at the shelter, and vaccinated dogs may still develop disease, although hopefully with reduced severity.

Individual Dog Management of Kennel Cough

In homes, many previously well, immunocompetent dogs will recover from kennel cough in days to 2 weeks with little or no medical intervention. In shelters, treatment should focus on nursing care, reducing stress and concurrent disease, providing a suitable environment for recovery (that is, for appropriate air flow), and selective use of antibiotics. Antitussives are very helpful in kennel cough, unless the dog has pneumonia (in which case they are contraindicated). Despite regulatory difficulties of working with controlled substances in shelters, narcotic cough suppressants offer the best relief to coughing dogs. Antibiotics will impact normal flora, but justifications for their use are in controlling secondary pathogens such as streptococci, preventing or treating early pneumonia, and possibly in eliminating some of the *B. bronchiseptica*. Antibiotics with a good Gram-positive spectrum (such as cephalexin and clindamycin) are indicated if the animal has purulent ocular and/or nasal discharge, although it often is satisfactory to treat such dogs for only 2-3 days, after which the normal flora remains somewhat intact, the discharge may have reverted to mucoid or serous, and significant antibiotic resistance may not have been selected for. "Protecting"

dogs against pneumonia with antibiotics is a double-edged sword. If the dog currently is on antibiotics, most bacteria involved in the pneumonia will be resistant to that antibiotic, limiting further treatment options. Finally, antibiotics are not a panacea for treating *B. bronchiseptica*. *B. bronchiseptica* resides in mucus where low antibiotic levels occur, and it is routine to obtain positive culture results from dogs on appropriate dosages of antibiotics. Moreover, high levels of antibiotic resistance occur in *B. bronchiseptica* in shelters: currently the best choices for targeting *B. bronchiseptica* are doxycycline, enrofloxacin, and trimethoprim/sulfamethoxazole.

Lower Respiratory Tract Infection

Lower respiratory tract infection, commonly pneumonia, is a severe, sporadic condition in dogs and cats. Often, an underlying cause is present, such as preexisting calicivirus URI, which impairs local defense mechanisms and facilitates bacterial pneumonia. Other causes may occur secondary to septicemia in an immunosuppressed animal, during parvovirus infection or ascarid migration, and idiopathically. A few infectious agents may present with lymphadenopathy and pneumonia: while rare in North America, they are included here because of their serious zoonotic potential.

CANINE DISTEMPER (DV)

Canine distemper virus is an RNA virus in the morbillivirus group, biologically similar to the viruses that cause measles and rinderpest. Infection is acquired by dogs only orally and by contact with respiratory mucous membranes and initially localizes in lymphoid tissue, followed by systemic spread. Three basic clinical forms are seen in dogs: respiratory, gastrointestinal (GI) and neurological, with individual animals possibly expressing all three concurrently or serially (Greene and Appel 1998). Arguably, the most common scenario for shelter dogs is severe URI, generalizing to pneumonia ± vomiting and diarrhea. After several weeks, the dog may develop abnormal neurological signs such as seizures, changes in consciousness, deficits in proprioception, and so on. Additional clinical indicators for distemper include development of hardened pads on the feet and hypoplasia of the tooth enamel. The mortality rate in otherwise robust, well puppies is approximately 50 percent (and much higher in the stressed, previously neglected population of dogs often entering animal shelters). However those dogs that survive distemper may have permanent defects in local respiratory protective mechanisms and when aged, old dog encephalitis representing recrudescence of the possibly replication-defective virus (Rima et al., 1987; Axthelm and Krakowka, 1998).

Larva Migrans

Roundworms with a migration stage through the lungs of dogs and cats include *Toxocara canis* and *cati, Ancylostoma caninum,* and *Strongyloides stercoralis.* After these parasites enter the dog or cat via the oral route, they enter the GI epithelium, travel to the serosa, and then migrate through the body, typically to lungs, are coughed up into the oropharynx, and then swallowed, allowing larvae to exit in the feces. Reportedly, transmammary transmission is the main route of spread of *S. stercoralis,* while hookworms often are acquired across the skin and migrate to lungs. While in the lungs, nematode larvae can damage tissue, cause verminous allergic disease or pneumonia, and predispose the animal to secondary bacterial infection. Dogs and cats with nematodes migrating in the lungs may demonstrate ill-thrift, weakness, or no signs other than respiratory signs. Threadworm infestation (*S. stercoralis*) also may be associated with diarrhea and dermatitis, and hookworms are more likely to cause anemia (while in the GI tract). Very young puppies exposed to hookworm-infested milk may appear to "fade" and die, while slightly older puppies develop life-threatening anemia and chronic infestations manifest primarily as poor overall condition. Pups and kittens may become potbellied and have a poor quality coat.

Hookworm larvae may become arrested in dog muscles and often are reactivated during late pregnancy, efficiently ensuring that they will be present in milk to infest puppies.

Lungworms

The lungworms of cats and dogs are *Capillaria aerophila* (dogs and cats) and *Aelurostrongylus abstrusus* (cats). Both are associated with verminous bronchitis. Female lungworms deposit eggs in nests in the lung tissue; larvae migrate to the trachea, are swallowed, and then exit in the feces. *A. abstrusus* larvae pass through an intermediate mollusk host,

so infestation in cats is usually due to exposure to infected prey (secondary hosts). *Capillaria* may have direct dog-dog or cat-cat transmission or utilize earthworms as intermediate hosts. Both types of lungworms produce mild coughs and sufficient tissue damage and inflammation to increase risks for kennel cough, bronchopneumonia, and other lower respiratory tract syndromes.

Bacterial Bronchopneumonia

Bacterial bronchopneumonia occurs most commonly in dogs and cats with relative immuno-incompetence (for example, during concurrent infections) or with other underlying problems such as migrating grass awns, asthma, diabetes, and so on. A variety of aerobic and anaerobic bacteria are recovered from such cases, including (from University of California at Davis records): enteric species (*E. coli, Klebsiella*), *Pasteurella multocida,* anaerobes, streptococci, *Actinomyces viscosus* and *hordeovulnaris* (usually with migrating foxtails), and *Bordetella bronchiseptica.*

Francisella tularensis

Tularemia occurs in cats, less commonly dogs, and humans as a result of infection with the small Gram-negative *F. tularensis* biotype A (*tularensis*) and B (*palearctica*). The epidemiology of biotype A in the U.S. includes hare reservoirs and *Dermacentor* spp. and *Amblyomma americanum* tick vectors; biotype B is spread among a number of hosts by ticks, mosquitoes, spread in water, and direct contact. Cats and dogs may acquire the infection also by eating infected prey. Infected cats and dogs typically have fever, purulent ocular and nasal discharge, possibly lymphadenopathy of the nodes draining the site of inoculation, and bacteremia and abscessation of multiple internal organs.

Yersinia pestis

Y. pestis is a nonspore forming, facultatively anaerobic, Gram-negative bacterium in the family Enterobacteriaceae. It does not survive high temperatures or desiccation, but persists in the environment in carcasses. Infection occurs in nature primarily in rodent hosts such as prairie dogs and some ground squirrels among which it can spread via fleas or through aerosol discharge of heavily infected animals. Cats and less commonly dogs acquire the infection through direct exposure to these rodents or more commonly their fleas, and humans can be infected via fleas or respiratory secretions. In the U.S. plague occurs sporadically in the eastern Sierra Nevada, transverse mountain ranges of southern California, and Four Corners areas of Colorado, New Mexico, Arizona, and Utah, into Texas, Oklahoma, and Kansas (Chomel et al., 1994).

Infected cats develop bacteremia and high levels of infection in the oropharynx from 1-10 days after exposure. Mandibular and retropharyngeal lymph nodes become enlarged and eventually abscessed. Infection can spread to the lungs (pneumonic plague) or other organs where abscesses may develop, or the *Y. pestis* endotoxin can cause septic shock, DIC, or death. In endemic areas, cats with fever, lymphadenomegaly, pneumonia, or nonspecific systemic illness should be evaluated for plague.

Diagnosis of Lower Respiratory Tract Infection

In shelters, lower respiratory tract infection generally will only be diagnosed if there is an index of suspicion. Suspect signs range from cough (especially in cats) to elevated respiratory rate or dyspnea with or without open mouth breathing, to lowered energy levels and responsiveness to external stimuli. Most animals with lower respiratory tract disease just appear depressed, and the cause may not be identified until a physical examination with thoracic auscultation is performed. For cats, a major rule-out for dyspnea and cough is asthma. If abnormally quiet or harsh lung sounds are detected in dogs or cats, the animal has difficulty obtaining sufficient air, or even if mucous membranes appear pale or cyanotic, further diagnostic tests are important. Optimally, thoracic radiographs will be performed if at all possible. To evaluate for bacterial and fungal lower respiratory tract disease and parasitic larvae, trans-tracheal washing with parasitology, cytology, and bacterial and fungal culture is helpful. Given the high rates of verminous pneumonia in shelter animals, it is important to perform a Baermann fecal examination for larvae and fecal flotation for *Capillaria* eggs, although infested animals will only shed parasites intermittently.

If distemper is suspected (based on severity of respiratory disease, concomitant GI or neurological signs, hard pads or enamel hypoplasia, or known previous exposure), confirming or ruling out distemper can be difficult. Tests which can be run include serum IgG and IgM (and CSF titers if indicated), PCR on whole blood or ocular or nasal discharge, and cytology of conjunctival or bladder epithelial cells. However, since so many dogs receive a distemper vaccine early on admission to a shelter, it is expected that IgG titers may be positive and rising. Anecdotally, positive serum IgM is uncommonly detected in dogs even shortly after vaccination. Vaccine-positive PCR tests also occur, especially in the 1-2 weeks following vaccination. Cytology is a good technique for assessing for distemper but is insensitive; sensitivity is much better if more cells are obtained, either by vigorously swabbing the conjunctiva or traumatic catheterization of the bladder.

If the animal has signs of respiratory tract infection with lymphadenopathy, rule-outs may include plague, tularemia, or mycobacteriosis. Obviously, plague and tularemia are significant zoonoses and cannot be managed (diagnosed or treated) in most shelter environments. For diagnosis of plague and tularemia, fine needle aspirate and cytology and culture of lymph nodes, or culture of swabs of the throat, often will yield the diagnosis, but suspect animals should be transferred to a veterinary clinic for diagnostic workup.

Herd Management of Lower Respiratory Tract Infection

Given the sporadic incidence and significant role of host factors in lower respiratory tract infection in shelters, preventive management does not differ significantly from the plan for kennel cough and URI. It is important to have a standard protocol for assessing the obvious wellness of each animal routinely, since many cases of pneumonia are subtle and won't be picked up unless someone notices that the animal is depressed and reports it to the medical staff. Environmental decontamination is unique for ascarid contamination, given the extraordinary environmental resistance of ascarid eggs. It is recommended that contaminated dirt be sealed over with concrete, so new shelters might choose to guard play areas very well from dogs until they have been thoroughly dewormed. Thorough cleaning and strong bleach are used on concrete to loosen ascarid eggs, which can be depopulated with further cleaning. All new arrivals should be dewormed prophylactically. Prevention of transmission of distemper relies on identifying and removing infected dogs, vaccinating, keeping the environment clean, and keeping dog contacts to a minimum number.

INDIVIDUAL ANIMAL MANAGEMENT, LOWER RESPIRATORY TRACT INFECTION

Many animals with lower respiratory tract infection require hospitalization and serious medical treatment. Shelters without high-end medical facilities might consider transferring such cases to collaborating clinics or euthanizing affected animals. Dogs and cats probably will require intravenous hydration and possibly oxygen supplementation, intravenous antibiotics, and antiparasitic drugs. Antibiotics should be broad-spectrum or chosen specifically on the basis of culture and susceptibility of the affected animal. If plague or tularemia is suspected (and the animal is not euthanized), appropriate antibiotics include aminoglycosides, trimethoprim sulfonamide, or enrofloxacin, or doxycycline. For parasites, fenbendazole and ivermectin are appropriate for lungworms. Some clinicians add prednisone into a treatment regimen for lungworms but this may be risky in shelters. If *Strongyloides* is diagnosed, eliminating deep tissue stages may be difficult, although ivermectin at 0.2 mg/kg two times reportedly is effective. *Toxocara cati* and *canis* are effectively treated with most anthelminthic drugs, including piperazine for young puppies and kittens. See Table 16.3.

GASTROINTESTINAL DISEASE

Overview

In shelters, the most common manifestations of gastrointestinal disease are vomiting and diarrhea. Stress, diet change, and a few primary pathogens can instigate diarrhea, but there is also a long list of opportunistic organisms that can accompany primary pathogens or other bowel disruptions. The complicated etiology makes management difficult, including strategies for prevention, interpretation of diagnostic tests, and whether or how to treat affected animals.

Primary Pathogens

FELINE PANLEUKOPENIA VIRUS

Feline panleukopenia virus (feline parvovirus or FPV) is a small DNA virus that infects cats and can produce life-threatening diarrhea, vomiting, and immunosuppression. The disease in cats sometimes is called feline distemper. Characteristics of parvoviruses include prolonged environmental persistence, resistance to most chemical disinfectants, and tropism for rapidly dividing cells, such as epithelial cells of the gastrointestinal tract, white blood cell precursors in bone marrow, and cerebellar Purkinje cells in neonatal or very young kittens. The virus enters the animal through the nose or mouth and replicates initially in the lymphoid tissue of the throat. Then it is spread to systemic lymphoid tissue, including in the gut. The incubation period of parvovirus, from infection to clinical signs, is between 3 days to 2 weeks (usually 5–7 days).

Animals under 6 months of age are most likely to get severe disease. Adult animals may get mild disease that is indistinguishable from diarrhea of any other cause. Clinically, infection with parvovirus manifests as vomiting and diarrhea, leading to dehydration, usually accompanied by immunocompromise via loss of white blood cells as infection targets the bone marrow precursors. Lymph nodes may be enlarged, and the cat may have a fever. This can predispose the animal to septicemia, shock, and death. In the *neurological form* of feline panleukopenia, damage to the Purkinje cells results in poor gross motor control from the cerebellum although other peripheral nerves and the cerebrum remain intact. Kittens usually are born with this disease if the queen was infected (or received a modified live virus [MLV] vaccine while she was pregnant). The presence of the disease usually is evident only after kittens begin to ambulate around one week after birth. At that time, there are intention tremors, nystagmus (abnormal movement in the pupil in the eye), abnormal placement of legs and possibly rolling over rather than standing upright. If cats can feed themselves by nursing, they can survive this stage and eventually (over months), the cerebrum compensates, allowing the cats to function somewhat more normally. These cats can be placed for adoption and live relatively normal lives despite their balance problems. Adopters should be counseled to observe their activities to determine what their limitations are so they can provide adequate safeguards for them.

CANINE PARVOVIRUS

Canine parvovirus is a virus that infects dogs and is closely related (and actually evolved from a

Table 16.3. Characteristics of Canine and Feline Lower Respiratory Pathogens

Organism	Mode of Transmission	Incubation Period/ Duration of Shedding	Asymp- tomatic Carriers?	Clinical Presentation, Typical	Optimal Diagnostic Tests	Optimal Therapy [a]	Zoonotic/ Herd Risk?
Larva migrans	Fecal-oral[b]	4–6 wks/ indefinite	Yes	Cough	Fecal float	Pyrantel and others	H, Z
CDV	Aerosol, fecal-oral	9–14 d/ 60–90 d	Yes	Resp., GI, neuro	PCR + serology	None[c]	H
Lungworms	Fecal-oral	2 mos+/ indefinite	No	Cough	Baermann	Albendazole	Z
2° bacteria	Direct, fomites	Variable	Yes	Cough	Culture	[d]	
F. tularensis	Aerosol, water, arthropod	48 hrs/ 2 wks	No	Cough, lympha- denopathy	Culture, serology[b]	Fluoroquin- olone[c,e]	Z
Y. pestis	Fleas, resp.	1–10 d/ 2 wks	No	Cough, lympha- denopathy	Culture, serology[b]	Doxy- cycline[c,e]	Z

[a] These therapies include off-label therapies and drugs that may present significant risk to some or all patients. Before use, shelter veterinarians are advised to read all of the relevant text in this book, consult a small animal medical text, and use proper medical judgment. None of the agents in this table have this characteristic.

[b] Agent is environmentally persistent and the contamination of the environment is a problem in herd management.

[c] Euthanasia a strong consideration if diagnosis confirmed.

[d] Select antimicrobial therapy depending on culture and antibiotic susceptibility testing.

[e] If agent is strongly suspected, local public health authorities and diagnostic laboratories should be notified.

H: Important threat to herd in shelters

Z: Zoonotic

parental strain of FPV). The strain 2b of canine parvovirus has broad host tropism and, unlike most canine parvoviruses, can infect cats as well as dogs. Both canine parvovirus and FPV share characteristics of environmental persistence, resistance to most disinfectants, and tropism for rapidly growing cells. As for cats, infected dogs usually develop diarrhea and vomiting with profound leukopenia. Young puppies from 3-16 weeks of age may acquire parvovirus myocarditis and die. Rottweilers, Dobermans and mixes of these breeds are especially vulnerable. Viral incubation and age-related clinical disease are essentially as described for FPV.

CANINE CORONAVIRUS (CCV)

Canine coronavirus is closely related to feline corona virus (FECV) of cats, but only infects canids. The enteritis caused in dogs by coronavirus can be significantly more severe than that caused in cats by FECV. Villus tip epithelium cells are targeted by the virus, resulting in distortion and loss of microvilli and moderate self-limiting diarrhea. The infection is spread via exposure to infected feces. Although coronaviruses are susceptible to most disinfectants and survive only hours or a few days unless protected in moist environments, such high levels of virus are produced in infected dogs, and the infection is so contagious, that it is easily spread and maintained in shelters.

CANINE DISTEMPER VIRUS

See "Lower Respiratory Tract Infection" for review.

SALMONELLOSIS

Salmonella enterica serotype typhimurium is a zoonotic, Gram-negative, facultatively anaerobic bacterium in the family Enterobacteriaceae. *S. enterica* typhimurium has a broad host range and moderate invasive potential, and can be recovered from humans, birds, rodent, cows, pigs, horses, dogs, and cats. Many strains have a capsule (K or Vi antigen), lipopolysaccharide (consisting of 64 different O antigens), and flagella (H). Pathogenic salmonellae have R plasmids, containing a number of virulence determinants for transporting bacterial proteins, promoting macrophage apoptosis, replicating in macrophages, and reducing phagosome-lysosome fusion, tolerating GI acid, adhering to host cells, and scavenging iron.

Once *S. enterica* is ingested and adheres to host cells, it is intracellularized, inhibit phagosome-lysosome fusion, and may persist unless successfully treated, the host mounts an effective immune response, or the bacteria invade systemically. There are several mechanisms by which salmonella produces diarrhea. Protein kinase C is activated leading to sodium-channel blockage, spilling of chloride and water into the lumen, and diarrhea. There also are secreted cytotoxins that incite inflammation and salmonella enterotoxin that cross-reacts serologically with cholera toxin. Dogs and cats with salmonellosis may be asymptomatic, diarrheic, or systemically ill (particularly cats). They may have fever, characteristically a few days before the onset of the diarrhea. Hematological values in cats are sometimes reminiscent of panleukopenia with severe left shifted neutropenia and total neutrophils less than 2000/µl.

Septicemic salmonellosis occurs occasionally in severely affected cats. It may enter via infected umbilical cords of young kittens (omphalophlebitis). Salmonella endotoxin massively disrupts the host inflammatory mechanisms, resulting in release of acute phase proteins from the liver, fever, vasodilation, increased vascular permeability, thrombosis, reduced organ perfusion with blood, reduced blood pressure, disseminated intravascular coagulopathy, shock, and death.

There are several host immune responses that serve to protect animals or help eradicate the infection. Local IgA, IgG, and IgM help block bacterial-host cell interactions. IgA and IgG from colostrums are particularly important for protecting neonates. If macrophages become infected with salmonella, it is important for phagosomes and lysosomes to fuse, which can happen after macrophages become activated. Thus T-cells, NK cells, and cytokines play important roles in protecting animals from severe salmonellosis.

BRACHYSPIRA PILOSICOLI AND *CANIS*

Brachyspira spp. (formerly *Serpulina*) are Gram-negative, obligately anaerobic spirochetes and most cross host species (that is, can infect cats and dogs). The reservoir for these possibly zoonotic bacteria is the GI tract of pigs (*B. pilosicoli*) and possibly dogs (Duhamel et al., 1998). *B. canis* has not been associated with disease and may be a component of the normal flora of dogs, while *B. pilosicoli* is implicated in intestinal spirochetosis in weanling pigs, dogs, and immunocompromised humans. Occasionally, *Brachyspira* may invade GI epithelium or blood stream and produce local inflammation and spirochetemia. *Brachyspira*-induced disease at its most severe, extrapolating from porcine disease, may include microvillus loss following attachment to enterocytes, epithelial necrosis and ulcers, and grey to red diarrheic feces.

Campylobacter jejuni, C. coli, C. upsaliensis

Campylobacters are zoonotic Gram-negative, motile, curved rod-shaped bacteria. Many are common in juvenile or stressed animals. There often are asymptomatic carriers. Campylobacters are acquired by the fecal-oral route from the reservoirs, such as the feces and eggs of chickens and feces of healthy cattle. After ingestion, *C. jejuni* adheres via an adhesin to receptors in the lower small intestine and upper large intestine. The capsule is antiphagocytic and helps the bacteria evade host immunity. *C. jejuni* secretes toxins similar to those present in cholera. The cholera LT-like toxin is responsible for the watery diarrhea observed in campylobacteriosis, and a cytotoxin produces the cell debris, mucus, and blood observed in the feces of affected animals. Slightly less pathogenic than *C. jejuni* and *C. coli* are the CNW (catalase-negative or weak) *Campylobacter* spp. such as *C. upsaliensis*. *C. upsaliensis* has been detected in association with bloody diarrhea outbreaks in day care centers of children and groups of dogs and cats (Goossens et al., 1995; Hald and Madsen, 1997). Often, diarrhea associated with campylobacteriosis is self-limiting, but debilitated, dehydrated, or very young animals may die of the infection without extensive nursing care.

Yersinia enterocolitica

Y. enterocolitica is a Gram-negative rod in the family Enterobacteriaceae. The reservoirs for intestinal yersiniosis are the environment, food, and possibly water or water-associated vectors. The disease in primates (including humans), cats, hares, and dogs is a mesenteric lymphadenitis with ileitis occasionally leading to sepsis. Several of the virulence determinants include a Shiga-like toxin, which is not required to produce diarrhea, and V and W proteins, which are required to allow the bacterium to avoid being killed by the host macrophage. In people, infection with *Y. enterocolitica* mimics acute appendicitis with severe cramps, fever, diarrhea, and skin rash. Dogs and cats may be infected without clinical signs or may develop moderate bloody diarrhea but not septicemia (Fenwick, Madie, and Wilks, 1994).

Nematodes Associated with Primary GI Disease

Most nematodes in the GI tracts of dogs and cats are not associated with diarrhea or vomiting and either cause almost no signs or cause other forms of disease such as pneumonia or anemia. Several primary pathogens in the intestines include *Trichuris vulpis* (whipworms) and *Strongyloides stercoralis*. *S. stercoralis* can cause a severe watery diarrhea, particularly in young dogs. See also "lower respiratory tract infections" for discussion of this parasite's biology. Whipworms spend their entire time in the dog in the GI epithelium and have a prepatent period of about 3 months. Disease may range in severity from no signs to severe diarrhea with mucus and blood.

Primary Pathogenic GI Protozoa

Giardia lamblia is a zoonotic flagellate protozoan for which the taxonomy is not agreed upon and may include the species *G. canis* and *G. felis*. Commonly in dogs and cats, the trophozoites attach to the small intestinal epithelium via sucking discs, form infective cysts (from which eventually emerge 2 trophozoites) and are shed in feces. Frank trophozoite shedding only occurs with high gut motility (diarrhea). To a lesser extent, the apicomplexans *Cryptosporidium felis* and *parvum* are primary pathogens as well. *C. parvum* has a wide host range including wild mammals, cattle, and dogs and cats. Only a small number (10^3) of oocysts are necessary to produce patent infection. Oocysts are ingested and excyst in the GI tract, releasing sporozoites which invade the epithelium in vacuoles. Within the vacuoles, trophozoites reproduce asexually and spread to other cells or sexually, and zygotes are shed in feces. Diarrhea is most severe in young and immunosuppressed animals.

Tritrichomonas fetus also is a flagellate, better known as a parasite in cattle, superficially resembling *Giardia lamblia* in fresh feces. Recently, cases have been reported in cats with severe watery diarrhea (Gookin et al., 1999). The infection is spread cat to cat without an environmental reservoir.

GI Opportunists

HELICOBACTER SPP.

Most intestinal helicobacters produce either no signs or contribute to mild to moderate enteritis. A number of species have been diagnosed in dogs or cats, including *H. colifelis, canis, hepaticus, bilis, pullorum, fennelliae,* and *cinaedi. H. cinaedi* and *H. fennelliae* have been reported in colitis in immunocompromised humans. It is also possible that intestinal helicobacters also could be involved in some cases of hepatitis in dogs and cats. Possible mechanisms of disease are unclear, but intestinal helicobacters have been associated with inflammatory bowel disease and might exacerbate clinical disease during coinfection. Gastric helicobacters (*H. felis, H. bizzozeroni,* and others) are common in cats and to a lesser extent dogs, with associated lesions ranging from none to moderately severe, and with or without clinical signs. *Helicobacter pylori,* associated with gastric ulcers and neoplasia in people, has been reported in cats and is thought to be possibly a reverse zoonosis (an infection cats acquire from people).

CLOSTRIDIUM DIFFICILE

C. difficile is a zoonotic anaerobe associated with sometimes severe disease in dogs and cats. Human pseudomembranous colitis typically is considered a nosocomial infection in people given that infection usually is secondary to underlying disease and/or antibiotic usage. The bacterium is a large Gram-positive rod and produces bipolar spores that are very stable in the environment. Not all strains have toxin genes, but secreted products may include 2 cytotoxins (A and B) and an enterotoxin, which can activate small GTP-binding proteins leading to actin cytoskeletal rearrangement and large intestinal cell damage. The toxins are pro-inflammatory and lethal to macrophages.

COCCIDIA

The coccidian protozoa infesting the GI tracts of dogs and cats are *Isospora* species. Following sexual reproduction, the parasites produce oocysts that exit in feces and from which emerge 8 daughter sporozoites. They continue a complicated life cycle through a number of named developmental stages, during which they are intracellularized within GI epithelial cells and undergo asexual reproduction. GI cells become damaged when the *Isospora* progeny emerge. The number of asexual reproductive cycles appears to be programmed, such that only 2 or 3 occur in any one host individual and infection is self-limiting. Small numbers of coccidian oocysts in the feces of nondiarrheic dogs and cats are very common. Disease associated with large numbers of *Isospora* is a profuse watery diarrhea, often with concurrent bacterial pathogens such as *C. perfringens.*

Miscellaneous Pathogenic GI Flora

TOXOPLASMA GONDII

Cats are the only definitive hosts for *T. gondii,* a protozoan that is shed in cat feces without causing GI signs in the cat. Larvae in the feces are infective to alternate hosts (such as people), where they encyst in muscles. *T. gondii* can cross the placenta in pregnant women and cause devastating birth defects. This parasite is mentioned here because it can be detected in cat feces, but is described more thoroughly in "Vector-borne, bite-transmitted, and systematic infections".

ASCARIDS NOT ASSOCIATED WITH DIARRHEA

Most nematodes either cause no disease or are associated with miscellaneous problems not including diarrhea or vomiting. *Toxocara canis* is common in puppies and can cause severe abdominal pain and bowel rupture in heavily infested dogs. Additional characteristics of roundworms and hookworms are covered in "lower respiratory tract infections."

CLOSTRIDIUM PERFRINGENS

A second GI *Clostridium* sp., *C. perfringens,* can contribute to diarrhea but also is an important component of normal flora in dogs and cats (Marks et al., 1999). Diseases attributed to *C. perfringens* include food poisoning (in people), in which the enterotoxin is produced by clostridial spores after they reach the acid stomach environment. *C. perfringens* also is described in hemorrhagic diarrhea of many hosts, although it often is difficult to determine the relative contributions of stress, food change, and bacterial opportunists, given that *C. perfringens* toxin genes and toxins often are detected in unaffected animals as well.

FELINE ENTERIC CORONAVIRUS (FECV)

Unlike canine coronavirus, which is a primary pathogen in dogs, FECV infection does not result in clinical GI disease in cats (Pedersen et al., 1983). This virus localizes in GI villus tip epithelium and produces at most mild pathological lesions with no detectable clinical signs. The virus is spread directly among cats through exposure to infective feces. The significance of FECV in cats is that mutant forms of FECF arise frequently in cats and may acquire the ability to enter and replicate within feline macrophages (Vennema et al., 1998). When accompanied by a particular feline immune response, this can produce feline infectious peritonitis (FIP), which is covered in "Vector-borne, bite-transmitted, and systematic infections".

Diagnosis of Vomiting and Diarrhea in Dogs and Cats

Appropriate and efficient testing for gastrointestinal disease in shelters can be difficult, given that even animals infected with primary pathogens may not have clinical signs and "complete" testing for GI pathogens and opportunists is laborious and expensive. Further complicating the picture is the fact that the inappetance and diarrhea that can be caused by the changes in diet or stress that shelter animals experience may initially be indistinguishable from true clinical disease. (Shelters with high turnovers may be unable to wait several days for animals to make the adjustments that would result in an abatement of the symptoms.) A shelter-specific profile of diagnostic tests should be developed in each shelter for surveillance as well as to diagnose individual cases. Such a profile, applied to diarrheic animals almost always includes parvovirus testing, but can incorporate additional tests described in this text according to the shelter's resources, the magnitude of the problem, and the pathogens seen most commonly in that shelter.

VIRAL DIAGNOSTIC TESTS

Suspicion of viral GI infection often arises because of the severity of the clinical signs, with the most severe, life-threatening disease suggestive of parvovirus. Clinical evaluation might reveal dehydration (with reduced skin turgor and increased capillary refill time), changes in the bowel with fluid and gas distension, lack of response and reluctance to eat or drink, and if septic or in shock, pale mucous membranes, very delayed capillary refill time, increased heart and respiratory rates. The bowel movements are often profuse, very liquid, with increased frequency and foul odor. There may be little fecal mass if the animal has evacuated its bowels and is not eating, although many animals will continue to strain. There may be specks of blood or large amounts of frank blood in the feces. The character of the vomitus depends on the duration of vomiting, initially consisting of food then followed by bile and sometimes blood.

Animals with diarrhea and vomiting may have a zoonotic infection, so sampling and handling should be performed with care to minimize risk. (Wear gloves!) The most important of the laboratory tests is the complete blood count (CBC), in which most viruses cause mild to moderate reduction in white cell counts, while parvovirus infection causes severely depauperate or almost no white blood cells reflecting the viral infection in the bone marrow. Red blood cell and platelet numbers typically are within normal limits except late in the course of disease if the dog or cat develops sufficient GI blood loss (blood loss anemia) or disseminated intravascular coagulopathy (platelet consumption).

Necropsy findings reflect nonspecific viral enteritis except in parvovirus where classic lesions may be observed. A cat that dies with panleukopenia classically has segmental enteritis (that is, regions of small intestine that appear completely normal interspersed with severely affected regions even a few inches long). In affected regions, the bowel wall appears thin and yellowish-white and may be blood-streaked. These areas are filled with watery fluid. Mesenteric lymph nodes may be enlarged. If tissues are examined by microscopy, there may be normal regions of gut although most have some epithelial destruction, but within the grossly abnormal areas, there is almost complete obliteration of the architecture, with damage occurring because the crypt cells (where new epithelium is regenerated) are the primary targets. Parvovirus FA may be applied to these regions to document parvovirus or FPV antigen in tissue. In the spleen and liver, there may be microthrombi and there may be depletion of splenic lymphocytic foci. The bone marrow may have a normal or activated erythroid (red cell) series with almost complete loss of the myeloid (white cell) series.

Neurological panleukopenia and cardiac parvovirus often are suspected based on history and clinical signs and confirmed by pathology with FA.

If clinical signs and/or CBC suggest viral enteritis, further diagnostic tests may confirm the infection. For parvoviruses, some of the commercially available fecal ELISA tests designed for the detection of parvovirus antigen in canine feces can be used for dogs and cats. Because these are antigen ELISAs, the test will be positive only when there is virus in the sample. "False negative" test results may occur if the animal actually has an infection but is not currently shedding in feces (early in the course of infection or late when antigen is often tied up with specific antibody). There also are false positives, typically because of vaccination. The vaccine-positive results occur about one week after vaccination with a traditional modified live virus vaccine and within 3 days to a week with a high antigen mass vaccine. The occurrence of false positives is why animals generally should not be diagnosed with parvovirus enteritis unless they have appropriate clinical signs or a low CBC.

Serum antibody tests detect both natural (field) or vaccine strains of virus. IgG is not produced in detectably significant amounts until a minimum of 10 days after infection or vaccination, so the test is not appropriate to diagnose disease unless it is used to document convalescence (that is, used retrospectively to confirm an etiology). However the test is useful for evaluating herd immunity. There is no particular titer magnitude that directly indicates whether an animal is protected or not and whether the exposure was natural or vaccine. In order to evaluate exposure to FECV (for herd management of FIP, NOT diarrhea), the IFA should be run starting at a dilution of 1:25, where a titer < 25 indicates no previous exposure. Since some laboratories do not test at low dilutions, a result such as "negative at 1:400" does not rule out exposure.

PCR is a relatively new test that looks for DNA specific to a virus (commonly parvoviruses, FECV, canine coronavirus, and canine distemper virus). PCR can be run on any tissue where virus is suspected, including feces, gut, bone marrow, respiratory secretions, and brain/cerebellum. It is technically moderately demanding and the laboratory running PCR must make appropriate use of positive and especially negative controls to manage for cross-contamination. PCR also is used to test for cats carrying the clinically silent FECV, although five consecutive days of testing are required to accurately determine whether or not the cat is shedding.

The distemper, rotavirus, and coronavirus infections in dogs can be difficult to diagnose. Electron microscopy of feces reveals characteristic morphologies of viruses, but is rarely performed on dogs. Canine distemper tests such as IgM and IgG titers may yield false positive results in recently vaccinated animals. PCR also can be positive with vaccine strain depending on the particular protocol employed by the laboratory. Visualization of distemper virus inclusion bodies in epithelial cells has low sensitivity but is diagnostic. Many clinicians scrape the conjunctiva relatively aggressively and use traumatic catheterization of the bladder to obtain infected cells for cytology.

BACTERIAL CULTURE AND TOXIN IDENTIFICATION

To evaluate for bacteria involved in vomiting and diarrhea, feces or sputum should be Gram-stained and cultured aerobically, microaerophilically, and anaerobically. Aerobes may be identified using standard microbiological techniques including *Salmonella, E. coli, Yersinia,* and *Shigella* (dogs only, an anthroponosis). *Plesiomonas* does grow on MacConkey agar, but many strains are lactose-positive and such colonies often are not worked up in bacteriology laboratories. *Y. enterocolitica* grows slowly on MacConkey, and does better with cold enrichment. Enrichment is usually performed using a medium like selenite before plating for *Salmonella,* because there need to be at least 10^4 cells/gm in the sample in order to see colonies on a primary plate.

Campylobacter and *Helicobacter* generally must be cultured in reduced oxygen, because they have only a small amount of superoxide dismutase and can't tolerate more than about 10 percent O_2 (room air has about 20 percent). Routine microaerophilic culture on selective agar often is conducted at elevated temperature such as 42 degress Celsius and may miss less thermotolerant strains. However, the majority of pathogenic *Campylobacter* spp. will be detected, and additional infections can be identified if fecal Gram-stains are performed, especially if carbol fuchsin is used as a counter-stain. Identification of *Helicobacter* spp. may be much more difficult. Alternative diagnostic techniques for identification of fastidious helicobacters and some campylobacters include biopsy and molecular techniques.

To identify clostridial infection, anaerobic culture is coupled with clostridial toxin tests. On direct smear of feces, rods and spores often are seen and can represent normal flora. Positive cultures for these bacteria in the absence of clinical disease should not be considered diagnostic. Positive culture on selective media reveals whether the organism is lipase-positive (both species) or lecithinase-positive (*C. perfringens*). Immunologic assays also are available to determine whether protein toxins (*C. difficile* toxin A and *C. perfringens* enterotoxin) are present in feces. PCR may be performed to determine if a particular clostridial strain has toxin genes, but will not clarify whether the genes are expressed. Given the difficulty of determining whether *C. perfringens* isolates represent normal flora or pathogenic opportunists in a given situation, it is helpful to know whether genes are present and expressed in particular cases. *Brachyspira pilosicoli* is also an obligate anaerobe and can be cultured in reference laboratories. Key characteristics that differentiate pathogenic from apathogenic species are flagella number and hemolysis.

PARASITOLOGY

Thorough parasite evaluation includes microscopic examination of smeared fresh feces, flotation, and ELISA or FA testing. *Giardia, Tritrichomonas,* and sometimes coccidia can be seen in *fresh* feces smeared in saline. This method does not distort the morphology of the protozoa and has increased sensitivity because of their movement. Fecal flotation is a standard procedure for parasites, but caution should be employed when attributing many of the observed parasites as causes of diarrhea, since few actually contribute to diarrhea. The test specificity is determined by the skills of the reader. The test lacks sensitivity because many parasite eggs are shed intermittently; thus a single negative test does not rule out infestation. Early in the course of infection, few or no *Isospora* oocysts may be visible in feces, so failure to find them on float or direct smear does not rule them out as contributing to the diarrhea. Several different technologies are available for using antibodies against *Cryptosporidium* and *Giardia* to increase the sensitivity of examination of feces, but use of the FA kit requires a fluorescent microscope and the ELISA generally is available as a send-out test to a commercial laboratory. However, given the marked improvement of sensitivity these tests offer especially for *Cryptosporidium,* they are worth performing at least as part of surveillance.

PATHOLOGY FOR GI PATHOGENS

Biopsy for cats and dogs with refractory diarrhea often is performed to evaluate for inflammatory bowel disease. Such samples also should be stained with a silver-based stain such as Warthin-Starry and evaluated for bacteria including *Campylobacter* spp., *Helicobacter* spp., and *Brachyspira canis* and *pilisocoli*. An advantage to this technique, which may allow for identification of uncultivable pathogens, is that the degree of tissue damage and proximity to the bacteria can be evaluated as well. However, specific identification of the bacterial species will not be possible.

PCR

Quite a few PCR tests have been designed to identify pathogens and opportunists, although most are available only in research laboratories. Particularly useful targets, if and when available commercially, include *Brachyspira,* some campylobacters, helicobacters, and protozoa including *Tritrichomonas fetus* and *Cryptosporidium* spp.

Management of GI Disease

HERD MANAGEMENT OF GI DISEASE

Key ideas in managing GI disease include surveillance and outbreak investigations to understand the status of infection in the herd, and prevention of new cases by protecting innate defense and immune mechanisms of dogs and cats and by preventing transmission of infection. Surveillance should include regular quantification of how much GI disease is present in the shelter, as well as counts of how many cases are diagnosed (for example, number of parvovirus diagnoses, whipworms, and so on). Information also should be recorded on where cases are occurring in order to document environmental contamination in some areas, or areas where ongoing transmission appears to occur. For more information on data management, see chapter 15.

Animals can best resist GI infections when they are otherwise healthy and well-nourished, not stressed, have intact normal bacterial flora, and have been appropriately vaccinated. Each of these can be problems in shelters, as incoming animals often are coinfected, historically neglected, and have diminished normal flora due to stress and possibly antibiotic use at the shelter. Additional problems include high density and turnover of animals, highly susceptible breeds (such as Rottweilers for parvovirus), highly susceptible animals because of age, and changes in diet. If puppies or kittens are born in the shelter, it is important to ensure that they receive colostrum, particularly in preventing spread of infections such as *Salmonella.*

Even if vaccination is performed for all incoming animals, vaccines don't address most of the GI pathogens, puppies and kittens may not be protected due to maternal antibody interference and immunologic immaturity, and no dogs or cats will be protected for the first week or so after vaccination is performed. The available vaccines for gastrointestinal pathogens include parvovirus, coronavirus, and Giardia. Parvovirus vaccine is available as KV, MLV- traditional, and MLV-HAM, with the same advantages and disadvantages as described above.

Blocking transmission of GI pathogens obviously boils down to ensuring that susceptible animals are not exposed to infectious animals or to contaminated environments. The first step in population control is to realize that almost all animals are vulnerable to infection during the first week of residence in a shelter regardless of vaccination, and that some animals incubating the infections will enter the shelter from time to time. The cages and shelter structure should be cleaned in such a way that infectious agents do not persist: for GI pathogens except *T. gondii,* this requires bleach diluted 1 part in 32 parts of water. Members of the family Parvoviridae are very stable in the environment, can persist for months or years, and are resistant to most chemical disinfectants including chlorhexidine, quaternary ammonium, and betadine. Bleach will not kill parvoviruses in a porous surface, where the virus escapes contact, if there is fecal contamination, if the bleach is overly dilute, or if there is inadequate contact time. Coccidia are not susceptible to commercial disinfectants but will die if the environment is kept clean and dry or better yet, exposed to sunlight. Bleach will kill hookworm larvae on cement but not effectively in moist soil.

It is better to disinfect well, less often, than to disinfect cursorily every day. To prevent the casual spread of GI pathogens, bleach footbaths should be set up at entrances to kennels or better yet, built into the entranceways of shelters. There is no known way to truly disinfect contaminated dirt and grass, although sunlight and drying has some effect. Vulnerable dogs should not be allowed into contaminated yards for 3-6 months. Routine worming of

dogs as they enter the shelter can help prevent significant contamination of the soil, especially if drugs such as milbemycin or fenbendazole (effective against whipworms) are used. The Center for Disease Control (CDC) guidelines for the prophylactic deworming of puppies and kittens should be followed. The general recommendations are to deworm with an age appropriate anthelmintic on initial presentation, then every 2 weeks until they reach 8-12 weeks of age, then every month until they are 6 months, then institute routine monitoring and treatment as indicated. The full report can be found at www.cdc.gov.

Keeping animal numbers and density as low as possible are key to blocking transmission in some infections and may be most relevant to municipal shelters that work with foster care-givers. For example, one of the only ways to effectively stop transmission of FECV is to reduce the numbers of cats, especially kittens, in the environment. Cats can be isolated into smaller groups but not within a single building or under care of the same people, because with such a profoundly contagious virus, it is impossible to not spread the infection. Reducing the numbers of cats to 5 or less in a foster situation is the most important factor in controlling FECV and FIP. Similar principles of reducing density apply for less contagious GI infectious agents.

Similarly, movement control refers to keeping potentially infectious and susceptible animals from having any contact with each other. If possible, a 14-day quarantine could accomplish this, because the only animals allowed out of quarantine would be those that do not have infectious disease signs at the end of the quarantine. However, quarantine is a place for currently well animals (if they develop signs of disease, they should be moved to isolation), so animals in quarantine can and should be available for adoption. If there is simply inadequate space and holding time for a functioning quarantine, the next best option is cohort admission. This can be done by consecutively filling cages according to the date an animal enters a shelter and ensuring that there is no mixing among cats or with contaminated elements in the environment ("all in all out").

At any point if animals appear sick, they should be moved. Sick animals should *not* be with or near well animals. If there are too many sick animals, then "isolation" needs to be expanded, as opposed to the common procedure of tolerating sick animals in adoption. However, mildly ill animals may still be adoptable: if this is the shelter's policy, then it is important to find a way to allow potential owners to view mildly ill animals in an isolation area. If animals tend to stay for weeks or months in isolation, something is wrong. The managers and medical personnel should reevaluate whether such animals are receiving appropriate care or should be euthanized. Some infections, like kennel cough, can drag out for many weeks in a crowded shelter, while in a home the same dogs would recover within a few days.

INDIVIDUAL ANIMAL MANAGEMENT, GI DISEASE

Invariably, shelter resources are limited, and treating ill animals can seriously tax these resources. Also, every animal that acquires GI disease in a shelter represents a case that might have been prevented, and prevention is far less expensive and traumatic for the animal than treatment. Nevertheless, decisions to treat, adopt out sick, or euthanize depend on the transmissibility of each agent, the prognosis for each disease, and the potential adoptability of each animal. Additionally, individual animals may have abnormal GI signs but specific diagnostic tests are not run or are all negative. In such cases, empirical treatment may be advised. Many veterinarians have "favorite" empirical treatment regimens, often including antibiotics, motility modulators, bland diet, or anti-inflammatory and soothing agents. These may improve the clinical disease, but each also has some drawbacks. Antibiotics may adversely affect normal flora, particularly in an animal with viral enteritis where bacterial flora play an important role in competing against the virus. Drugs to reduce gut motility and diarrhea increase retention time of all luminal contents including pathogens, which can exacerbate the disease. On the other hand, anti-vomiting drugs such as chlorpromazine may provide relief from pain and allow for establishment of electrolyte balance. Bismuth subsalicylate should be used carefully in cats, which have a very low tolerance for salicylic acid. Even bland diet can be counter-productive if animals won't eat.

Before treatment or euthanasia is initiated for parvovirus, it is important to confirm the diagnosis. A good protocol is to have three separate areas: adoption areas for well animals, a transitional area for animals that have suspect parvovirus (diarrhea,

weak positive CITE test) but things don't add up (a CITE-positive dog that seems well, a dog with bloody diarrhea that has negative test results), and then a treatment area if desired. The status of animals in the transitional area should be clarified with a CBC; such animals may need to be monitored and retested until they are clearly not infected (and moved to adoption) or they clearly are infected.

If a positive diagnosis is made, many shelters euthanize the infected animals, while others consider treatment. The rationale for treatment is that mortality is only about 50 percent in kittens or puppies and less in mature animals, if the animal is otherwise previously well and if they receive excellent nursing care. The following should be considered with respect to treatment:

- Many animals entering a shelter are debilitated and thus mortality may exceed 75 percent.
- Infected animals can contaminate an environment, even after they appear to be recovered. If there is any doubt that the shelter can *completely* isolate the affected animals (preferably in a separate building or foster home), it is irresponsible to initiate treatment.
- Severely ill cats and dogs are candidates for euthanasia, and aggressive treatment is a misplaced kindness.
- Treatment requires a lot of resources (care by a veterinarian and veterinary technician, IV fluids, injectable [IV] antibiotics, extended nursing care, and biohazard precautions), which might better be employed in prevention.

Treatment for parvovirus includes nursing care, management of hydration and electrolyte status, prevention and management of secondary bacterial infection and septicemia due to loss of white blood cells, and facilitation of the recovery of the bone marrow. Cats and dogs may survive for days without nutrition but return to normal feeding may be delayed, necessitating "force-feeding" with warmed palatable food such as all-meat baby food (with no onion powder). Parvovirus-infected animals are very susceptible to secondary bacterial infection because the normal mucosal barrier between the blood and the bacteria in the gut is destroyed and because parvoviruses target the white blood cells, which are very important components of the immune system. Thus cats and dogs with parvovirus should receive injectable broad spectrum antibiotics and be monitored for septicemia. A good mainstay antibiotic combination would be a penicillin and aminoglycoside (only in a well-hydrated cat). In order to maximally stimulate the few WBC precursors that may survive parvovirus in the bone marrow, recombinant granulocyte colony stimulating factor (rGCSF) may be given as an injection at 20μg/kg body weight once a day until the WBCs are normal in the peripheral blood, but no longer than for two weeks. Not all cats or dogs survive parvovirus no matter how well treated. If, despite aggressive care, an animal appears unresponsive, does not improve within a few days, or in the opinion of the caretaker is suffering, there must be provisions for euthanasia and necropsy.

Other GI infections may have a better prognosis than parvovirus if identified and treated appropriately. Treatment of many parasitic infestations is straightforward and is covered in many medicine and infectious disease texts. Metronidazole and fenbendazole are the drugs of choice for *Giardia,* although treatment failure is common, particularly in Abyssinians, Bengals and some other purebred cats. Animals suffering from Giardia should be bathed with general shampoo, rinsed thoroughly, followed by a bath with a dilute quaternary ammonium product (rinse thoroughly to avoid skin irritation) as a matter of routine adjunctive treatment to help remove infective feces and cysts from their bodies and thus lessen environmental contamination (Barr, 1998). If treatment failure occurs, the feces should be reevaluated to determine if the protozoa are *Tritrichomonas* that have been misdiagnosed as *Giardia* and if other underlying diseases might be present. *Cryptosporidium* is considered self-limiting, but if treatment is necessary, possibilities include paromomycin and azithromycin (although both have low to moderate efficacy). Treatment of *Tritrichomonas* is quite difficult. Possibilities have reportedly included metronidazole and paromomycin, but the former has very little efficacy and the latter is toxic in cats (and not highly efficacious either). Coccidiastatic drugs such as sulfadimethoxine can reduce the number of asexual progeny produced until the "reproductive clock" for that species stops ticking and the host's epithelium can repair itself. Often animals with severe coccidiosis respond better to treatment when they also receive metronidazole, clindamycin, or ampicillin. The treatment

of parasites is discussed elsewhere in this chapter.

Treatment for bacterial diseases depends on whether the bacteria are primary pathogens (*Salmonella, Yersinia, Campylobacter,* and so on) in which case antibiotics appropriate to the bacterium identified should be utilized. For *Campylobacter* spp., erythromycin is often cited as the drug of choice. Other good choices include tetracycline, enrofloxacin, and tylosin. Triple therapy is helpful for severe or refractory cases, including bismuth subcitrate or subsalicylate (caution in cats), ampicillin, and metronidazole. We have found it helpful to substitute enrofloxacin for ampicillin in some cases.

Appropriate drugs for *B. pilosicoli* are tylosin, nitrofuran, and lincomycin. Antibiotic treatment for *Salmonella* has been controversial, because of older reports that patients receiving antibiotics developed a carrier state. With modern antibiotics, the greater concern is evolution of resistant strains, although there is a good probability of eradicating most infections, provided the antibiotic can penetrate cells (cephalosporins, chloramphenicol, enrofloxacin, tetracycline, and trimethoprim-sulfa drugs) and survive the acidic endosome (not aminoglycosides) and that the bacteria are susceptible. Antibiotic susceptibility testing often indicates susceptibility to amoxicillin-clavulanate, aminoglycosides, third generation cephalosporins, and enrofloxacin, of which all except the aminoglycosides are reasonable choices. Adjunctive therapy should include fluids as needed and possibly LPS hyperimmune serum.

If opportunistic bacteria are detected, further evaluation for underlying diseases should be performed and those diseases treated if possible (Table 16.4). If no underlying disease is found, antibiotics may or may not be appropriate. Many animals will experience self-limitation of opportunistic infection, and antibiotics only serve to scour the gut of normal flora and increase the likelihood of further problems. However, if the condition worsens or persists, antibiotics may be necessary. Good choices include tylosin, erythromycin, metronidazole, and ampicillin. If the animal is diagnosed with *C. difficile,* it is particularly important to address the underlying disease and decontaminate the environment. Animals may remain chronic shedders even after treatment. The two best drug choices are metronidazole and vancomycin, since many isolates are resistant to metronidazole. The public, public

Table 16.4. Characteristics of Pathogens Associated with Canine and Feline Diarrhea

Organism	Mode of Transmission	Incubation Period/ Duration of Shedding	Asymptomatic Carriers?	Clinical Presentation, Typical	Optimal Diagnostic Tests	Optimal Therapy [a]	Zoonotic/ Herd Risk?
Canine & feline parvovirus	Fecal-oral[b]	4–14d/10–12d	No	Diarrhea/vomiting	ELISA	Nursing	H
CDV	Aerosol, fecal-oral	9–14d/60–90d	No	Diarrhea/vomiting, severe resp.	PCR+ serology	None[c]	H
CCV	Fecal-oral	1–4d/14d+	Yes	Diarrhea	PCR	Nursing	
Salmonella	Fecal-oral	1–3d/3–6wks	Yes	None	Culture	Enrofloxacin	H
Brachyspira spp.	Fecal-oral	Unknown	Yes	Diarrhea	PCR	Tylosin	Z
Campylobacter spp.	Fecal-oral	Indefinite	Yes	Diarrhea	Culture	Triple rx	Z, H
Yersinia enterocolitica	Fecal-oral	None/50d	No	Diarrhea	Culture	TMS, doxycycline	Z
Trichuris vulpis	Fecal-oral	Wks	Yes	None—diarrhea	Float	Fenbendazole	Z
Strongyloides stercoralis	Fecal-oral, percutaneous	8d	Yes	None—diarrhea	Float	Ivermectin	Z
Giardia lamblia	Fecal-oral	5–12d	Yes	Diarrhea	Float + ELISA	Fenbendazole	Z
Cryptosporidium spp.	Fecal-oral	1 wk/indefinite	Yes	None—diarrhea	ELISA	None	Z
Tritrichomonas fetus	Fecal-oral	Days to wks/ unknown	No	Diarrhea	Direct smear	None[c]	H
Coccidia	Fecal-oral	Days/indefinite	Yes	None—diarrhea	Float	Albon	

[a]These therapies include off-label therapies and drugs that may present significant risk to some or all patients. Before use, shelter veterinarians are advised to read all of the relevant text in this book, consult a small animal medical text, and use proper medical judgment.
[b]Agent is environmentally persistent and contamination of the environment a problem in herd management.
[c]Euthanasia is a strong consideration if diagnosis is confirmed.
[d]Select antimicrobial therapy depending on culture and antibiotic susceptibility testing.
H: important threat to herd in shelters
Z: zoonotic

health veterinarians, and local veterinarians justifiably may be concerned about the use of vancomycin in shelter animals.

INTEGUMENTARY INFECTIONS

Overview

Unfortunately, many of the more severe dermatopathies of cats and dogs in shelters represent untreated or neglected conditions of animals before they came to the shelter. Some infections associated with integumentary disease are zoonotic and/or contagious to other animals, and management is important to reduce spread and to identify individual cases of noninfectious etiology.

Arthropod-Induced Dermatopathies

SCABIES

Scabies is a form of mange caused by the astigmatid mites *Sarcoptes scabiei* (dogs) and *Notoedres cati* (cats). They can cross infect rabbits and other species. These mites are acquired from contact with other infected animals or contaminated environments and tunnel through the skin depositing eggs and feces. They cause intense immune-mediated host reactions and pruritis even in small numbers. The animals may become so uncomfortable they traumatize themselves and stop eating. The skin is then susceptible to secondary bacterial and fungal infections. Animals with severe cases of scabies can be so debilitated that euthanasia for humane reasons can be justifiably considered. *Sarcoptes scabiei* is zoonotic.

DEMODEX CANIS

Demodectic mange is the generally milder mange caused by an overgrowth of the cigar-shaped, prostigmatid mite *D. canis* in a predisposed (relatively immunocompromised) dog. The disease often is arbitrarily characterized as either localized or generalized, depending on the extent of lesions. Dogs of any age with extensive lesions generally have significant specific immunocompromise, often will not respond to therapy, and have a poor prognosis. On the other hand, dogs under 12 months of age with only a few mild lesions usually just need to develop a mature immune system and likely will recover fully. The trick is to determine how extensive lesions need to be before they are considered

more than localized. *D. canis* lesions are nonpruritic unless secondarily infected with bacteria. *D. cati* is a rare mite causing similar problems in cats. *Demodex* is neither zoonotic nor contagious to other dogs, which already have small numbers of the mite in hair follicles as normal flora.

OTHER MITES AND LICE

Cheyletiella blakei and *yasguri*, the "walking dandruff" mites, are grossly visible among hair and skin debris of dogs (*C. blakei*) and cats (*C. yasguri*). They may also cross infect rabbits. Chiggers are trombiculid mites with free-living adult stages and parasitic larvae. The larvae invade the skin of dogs and people, protected in a hardened stylosome tube until they are ready to emerge. Chigger infestation is accompanied by intense pruritis.

Cats and dogs also may carry lice. *Felicola subrostratus* is the only louse species generally found on cats. Dogs can have *Linognathus setosus* (anopluran or sucking), *Trichodectes canis* (mallophagan or chewing), or *Heterodoxus spinger* (amblyceran) lice. Lice may cause irritation and hypersensitivity reactions and transmit tapeworms, although not as efficiently as fleas. Lice are host specific and not zoonotic.

FLEAS

Ctenocephalides felis and *canis* fleas are wingless insects that live on cats and dogs and feed on the blood of their mammalian hosts as adults. As larvae, fleas feed on defecated material from adult fleas, which is high in host blood content. Then the pupal fleas are protected in very environmentally resistant cocoons, from which they metamorphose into adults. Eggs are laid directly on the host. Although individuals in all three stages may remain on the host, numerous others will infest the environment and survive for several months without feeding (depending on the temperature and humidity). Dogs (and people) may be infested with *C. felis*.

Allergy to flea saliva is one of the most common causes of alopecia and dermal inflammation in dogs and cats. In severely allergic individuals, only a few flea bites suffice to trigger the immune response but many previously neglected animals present to shelters heavily infested. The clinical presentation includes erythema and alopecia, typically at the tailhead and caudal abdomen in dogs and ventral abdomen in cats. Fleas and flea dirt may or may not be apparent, and severely allergic and infested dogs may have obvious incisor wear from constantly chewing at themselves. Dog and cat fleas transmit tapeworms among animals and may transfer bartonellosis and typhus among people and animals.

TICKS

Ticks attach to the skin of dogs and to a lesser extent cats by biting mouth parts, cement themselves into the skin, and secrete inflammatory and vasoactive chemicals that ensure an influx of inflammatory cells and prevent clotting. Tick bites produce local irritation and may predispose the area to infection, but more significantly may introduce systemic infectious agents (ehrlichiosis, Rocky Mountain spotted fever, Lyme disease, babesia) or the toxin of tick paralysis. Tick paralysis, an ascending flaccid paralysis of dogs and children, is caused by a protein toxin elaborated most commonly by *Dermacentor variabilis* females after a few days of feeding. The common ticks that bite dogs and cats are *Ixodes scapularis* east of the Rocky Mountains, *Ixodes pacificus* on the west coast, *D. variabilis, andersoni,* and *occidentalis, Amblyomma americanum, A. maculatum,* and *Rhipicephalus sanguineous.* Only *R. sanguineous* is a "peridomestic" tick, meaning that it can develop through all three molts and lay eggs in and around human environments containing only dogs. The other ticks only appear on dogs in shelters that have been wandering in tick-infested environments. The ticks will feed for 2–5 days, and females can engorge to half or more of a centimeter in length. They are found most frequently in and around the ears and axillae. Invariably, tissue trauma accompanies removal of ticks, or fully engorged ticks will drop off the dog and seek a suitable microenvironment to lay eggs. Such environments are moist, dark, and protected by leaf litter and are rare in shelters. The larvae emerge months later and require rodents, birds, or some small reptiles to feed upon.

EAR MITES, EAR TICKS, AND INFECTIONS

Young cats are particularly susceptible to ear mites (*Otodectes cynotis*), an organism which is spread directly among cats or through exposure to infested fomites. Dogs occasionally also are infested in the external ear canal and adjacent skin. These mites cause pain and irritation, and most infested cats scratch at their face and ears, possibly to the point of bleeding. The mites may cause local inflammation and predispose the cat to an ear infection and can penetrate and lead to otitis media. Cats often develop some degree of immunity to ear mites. Older cats are more likely to suffer from ear infections, particularly if they have an allergy to components of their food, or underlying disease such as diabetes. This is not a condition contagious to other cats.

Dogs frequently have ear infections, especially if they have allergic skin disease and/or floppy pinnae. In both cats and dogs, flora in ear infections include yeasts (*Malassezia* and occasionally *Candida*), *Pseudomonas, Staphylococcus intermedius, Proteus mirabilis,* enteric species, and *Pasteurella multocida.* Dogs may also be infested with the spinose ear tick, *Otobius megnini,* which may remain in the external ear canal for months unless removed. Infected ears may be painful, the skin reddened and swollen, and frank purulent, malodorous discharge present.

Fungal Dermatopathies

DERMATOPHYTES

The dermatophytes are molds comprising the common species *Microsporum canis* (95 percent of cat and 65 percent of dog cases) and *M. vanbreuseghemi, M. gypseum,* and *nanum, Trichophyton equinum, mentagrophytes,* and *verrucosum, Epidermophyton* sp., and more rarely *T. rubrum, E. floccosum,* and a few others. The reservoir for the common species are cats for *M. canis,* soil for *M. gypseum,* soil or chickens for *M. nanum,* the horse for *T. equinum,* rodents for *T. mentagrophytes,* and cattle for *T. verrucosum.* All have septate, branching hyphae and develop into a mycelium. The conidia gain access to keratinized epithelium, often through a defect in the stratum corneum, then germinate with the mycelia entering cornified strata. Ectothrix growth involves mycelia following hair follicles along new hair growth. Arthroconidia develop in tissue, and clinical signs develop courtesy of virulence determinants including elastase, collagenase, and keratinase. Occasionally animals may develop dermatophytic onychomycosis (fungal infection of the toenails and nail beds).

In nature, the incubation period for ringworm is between 4 days and 4 weeks. About a week after the initial infection, there may be the development of secondary inflammation, termed a kerion. Classically there is a circular inflamed lesion with stratum corneum hypertrophy from which hair is lost and crusting develops. People and animals may have allergic responses to the fungi and develop a lesion termed a phytid. Infection finally may be terminated due to cell-mediated immunity in weeks to months, although chronically infected individuals may fail to eliminate the infection and function as carriers. Risk factors for more severe or chronic disease include age, with animals less than one year old or geriatric animals at higher risk; immunocompromise such as FIV and FeLV infection, pregnancy and lactation, malnutrition, use of anti-inflammatory drugs, cancer, and stress; and breed, with increased predisposition in Persian cats and Yorkshire Terriers. Ringworm, the disease produced by dermatophytes, is zoonotic.

MALASSEZIA AND CANDIDA

Yeast infections in the skin of dogs and cats usually are secondary to such primary conditions as allergies, arthropod infestations, immune-mediated disorders, keratinization defects, endocrinopathies, inherent conformational "defects" such as with Shar Peis, and antibiotic therapy for staphylococcal pyoderma. The two most common yeasts are *Candida* spp. and *Malassezia pachydermatis*. Both can be found in small amounts as part of the normal flora of skin, ear canals, and mucocutaneous junctions. With yeast overgrowth, the animal (most commonly dogs) becomes pruritic with seborrheic, erythematous, and alopecic skin. There often is an offensive odor and oily slime on the skin surface. The sites most commonly affected are any skin folds, neck, muzzle, ears, around the anus, and between the toes.

BACTERIAL FOLLICULITIS AND PYODERMA

Primary bacterial infection of the skin of dogs and cats is unusual. Pyoderma and folliculitis typically occur in animals with underlying disease such as fleas, mites, Cushings/other endocrine, atopy, seborrhea, or immune-mediated skin disease. The abnormal bacterial flora may include overgrowth of the skin's normal flora (*Micrococcus* spp. and non-pathogenic streptococci, *Acinetobacter* spp., and *Propionobacterium acnes*), as well as pathogenic flora including *S. intermedius, Pseudomonas,* and others. The infection may be superficial or invade

deep into the dermis, underlying fatty tissue, and into the blood stream. Most commonly affected areas are similar to those in yeast dermatitis, especially in the groin, axillae, and interdigital skin.

Diagnosis of Dermatopathy in Shelters

Accurate diagnosis of integumentary infection is very important in order to discriminate between animals with infectious conditions for which management could prevent extensive spread within the shelter, and/or treatable animals. The consequences of a false negative test for infections such as ringworm may be for an infected individual to spread disease within a facility or to a foster or adoptive home.

CLINICAL DIAGNOSIS

In severe dermatopathy, the clinical presentation gives a few clues but may not suffice to allow the shelter veterinarian confidence in the etiology. Ear infections and infestations may be primary conditions, in which case there may be obvious foxtails, ticks (in dogs), brown to black dry crumbly discharge (cats), or slimy greenish discharge (dogs and cats) in the ears, or secondary to other dermatologic disease, in which case the skin and general clinical condition of the animal need to be evaluated as parts of the whole disease.

If there is hair loss, chewing or scratching, bad odor or discharge on the coat, reddened exposed skin, or other such lesions in a dog or cat, all of the diseases listed above should be ruled out. In general, the most intensely pruritic of the infections is *Sarcoptes* or *Notoedres* infestation. Typically these mites produce crusting and hair loss on the tips of the ears, nose, and feet before generalizing, but extensive mange may cover most of the body. Briskly rubbing the pinna of a dog between the thumb and forefinger may elicit scratching with the ipsilateral hind limb (positive pinnal-pedal reflex) that is strongly suggestive of scabies. (Tilley and Smith, 1997).

Demodex canis lesions usually are well-circumscribed, reddened areas near the eyes and mouth, although they may extend to large areas of the body in generalized demodicosis.

The presence of ticks may be detected with a thorough examination although unfed nymphs or adults may be very small. Particular attention should be paid to ears, digits and axillae. Diagnosis of flea allergy is based on thorough examination of the coat, using a flea comb to search for fleas and flea dirt, evaluating the anatomic distribution of the lesions, ruling out other conditions, and evaluating response to a barrier-level flea protection program, including drugs to kill all of the fleas and topical products to discourage fleas in the environment from biting.

Severe ringworm may appear superficially as bad as mange, with discharge, crusting, skin wrinkling (lichenification), and so on. Mild cases of ringworm may be subtle, with small areas of hair loss or a few crusts. The most common locations include the face, ears, feet and tail. Because ringworm is such a mimic of other skin diseases, examination with a Woods lamp is warranted whenever feasible. The Woods lamp is an ultraviolet light at a wavelength of 253.7 nm. Exposure to this light causes a tryptophan metabolite of some (no more than 50 percent) strains of *M. canis* to fluoresce. Woods lamp examination should be performed correctly. The lamp should be turned on at least 15 minutes before use, and the animal should be examined in a dark room. Positive lesions are bright green. Low-level fluorescence should not be interpreted as a positive result. Some drugs, dandruff and other contaminants such as kitten milk replacer can also fluoresce more mildly.

Diagnosing pyoderma is straightforward clinically by observing lesions if there is purulent discharge. If pustules rapidly rupture, pyoderma may present clinically as crusts and papules. With vague clinical signs, it is important also to consider other underlying diseases such as mange or fleas and failure to respond to therapy.

SCRAPE AND MICROSCOPIC EXAMINATION

If the integumentary problem occurs primarily in the ears, swabs and microscopic examination of the direct smear may suffice to provide a diagnosis. In cats, the brownish dry discharge usually contains ear mites, while moister purulent discharge (heat fixed and Gram-stained) contains mostly bacteria and fungi and usually represents dermatitis involving more than just ears. A discharge from a dog's ear usually is due to ear infection that can be demonstrated by examining Gram-stained discharge for yeasts and bacteria. Ear mites may be identified by examining the discharge under the microscope at low power.

If mange or pyoderma is suspected, *deep* skin scraping at the periphery of lesions should be examined in mineral oil at low power for the mites and quick-stained and examined at high power for leukocytes and bacteria and yeasts. *Demodex* usually are present in large numbers if they are the cause of the clinical signs, and can be identified by their long "cigar-shaped" body shapes. *Notoedres* also usually is present in large numbers. In contrast, only a few *Sarcoptes* can cause severe disease, so these fat, round mites cannot be ruled out unless numerous scrapes and extensive examination are performed. "Scotch tape" preparations may be performed to identity *Cheyletiella* and lice. Clear scotch tape is applied repeatedly to the coat of the dog or cat and then laid down in mineral oil onto a microscope slide for examination at low power.

Microscopic examination for ringworm is performed on hairs plucked from the periphery of suspect lesions. Hair may be suspended in mineral oil and examined directly or cleared of keratin by suspending it in 10–20 percent KOH prior to examination. The slide is then gently heated for 15–20 seconds or allowed to stand for 30 minutes at room temperature. Infected hairs appear swollen, frayed, irregular or fuzzy in outline, and the normal structure of cuticle, cortex, and medulla is lost. Arthroconidia (beaded chains of small rounded cells) and hyphae can sometimes be seen. Hyphae are uniform in diameter, septate and variable in length and degree of branching. The morphology and presence of macroconidia and microconidia are essential characters for confirming and identifying dermatophytes; their characteristics are described in the package insert with the culture plates or in various microbiology texts.

CULTURE

Fungal and bacterial cultures often are helpful to determine if an animal has pyoderma or ringworm. For pyoderma diagnosis, the surface of the skin should be sterily prepped and the sample taken deeply (for example, by biopsy). In some severely affected animals, it is helpful to include bacterial culture of the blood. Finding pathogenic skin flora doesn't rule out other underlying diseases such as mange or fleas. However, positive culture of normal flora such as *Staphylococcus epidermidis* should be disregarded. Antibiotic susceptibility testing is very difficult to interpret, because of the difficulty determining what levels of drug likely are delivered to the affected area. To identify yeasts, skin scrape cytology, biopsy, and culture are helpful, with the cytology having the advantage of facilitating quantification of the yeasts.

Bacterial and fungal cultures sometimes are submitted to identify flora in ear infections. As for pyoderma, antibiotic susceptibility results for drugs given orally or via injection are not interpretable.

Fungal culture is the most reliable method of assessing the presence of ringworm. Samples are collected by plucking hair from the edge of the lesion or by running a new toothbrush through the coat. The hairs or toothbrush tines are placed onto an appropriate agar such as dermatophyte test medium (DTM), rapid sporulation medium (RSM), or "Derm Duets," which contain DTM and RSM. Dermatophyte media contain antibiotics and anti-fungal drugs to discourage growth of contaminants, although some nondermatophytes do grow. DTM contains phenol red, which turns red in the presence of alkaline metabolites produced primarily by dermatophytes (but not all) and not many saprophytes. Similarly, the bromothymol blue in RSM turns blue-green in the presence of dermatophytes. The plates should be incubated in air at room temperature for days to a few weeks, being observed for visible fungal mycelia and color change daily. When candidate dermatophytes are observed, a small amount of the hyphae should be removed and examined under the microscope for the characteristic conidia (most easily seen on RSM) to confirm the diagnosis. This step commonly is skipped in clinical practice and shelters but is essential. "False positive" test results can occur if there is dermatophyte contamination on the coat (that is, pathogenic fungi are present but not necessarily invaded in skin and hair). This problem can be minimized if free dermatophytes are eliminated through bleaching the environment and bathing of all in-contact animals with a good pet shampoo.

Management of Dermatopathy

Herd Management of Dermatopathy

Herd management for dermatopathy should focus on keeping the shelter as free as possible of arthropods, preventing spread of ringworm, and identifying animals with treatable and/or contagious disease. To manage and prevent arthropod infestations,

drugs such as ivermectin, Revolution (for scabies mites), Advantage, or other systemically active antiparasitics are highly effective if applied to all incoming animals. No specific herd management is required for *Demodex* spp., since these mites are common in normal dogs.

As for GI disease, herd management of ringworm should incorporate the assumption that infected animals periodically enter the shelter, and that minimizing movement and contact are important, together with control of infection in the environment. Ringworm-positive and suspect animals should be kept in a separate area of the shelter, ideally not in a common isolation with cats with URI. Staff should wear gloves and protective clothing (smocks/coveralls and boots or shoe covers) while working with or near affected cats and should not work with other cats until they have completely changed clothes and showered (that is, the next day). Animals can be treated as described in the next section, but should not be moved back into contact with uninfected cats for several weeks after apparent clinical recovery. Up to 10 percent of some breeds (for example, Persian cats) can remain asymptomatic carriers, so cats ideally should be culture negative for two weeks (two different culture tests) before moving to the main population.

Ringworm is extremely difficult to manage in herds and individuals: rapid, easy-to-use treatment protocols should be regarded with skepticism. The fungi are very durable in the environment. Shelter substrates, toys, grooming instruments, and so forth should be disposable or decontaminatable. Carpet should be avoided even in scratching posts. Dermatophytes are susceptible only to strong bleach (1:10 in water) or 1 percent formalin with prolonged contact time (preferably overnight). Quaternary ammonium compounds and chlorhexidine are not effective. A fog, spray, or rinse containing enilconazole has recently been reported as an option for reducing epidemic ringworm in densely housed cats and rabbits. In vitro, the drug inhibited fungal growth on infected hairs (White-Weithers and Medleau, 1995). However, in vivo studies have not been controlled and also failed to unambiguously document improvement in treated animals (Guillot et al., 2002; Hnilica and Medleau, 2002). Dishes and other washable items can be run through a dishwasher provided the water temperature reaches at least 43.3°C (110°F). Foster homes, once contaminated, may be virtually impossible to clean and may have to discontinue fostering. Asymptomatic carrier animals continually re-contaminate the environment with fungal spores. Because of the extreme difficulty managing ringworm, many shelters euthanize for this condition. Even though some animal care professionals may consider ringworm "no big deal", this is a zoonotic infection and a risk to the adopter's other pets, and represents a significant public relations and liability issue.

Secondary skin disease such as candidiasis, otitis externa, and flea allergic dermatitis don't require herd management per se other than to manage underlying disorders.

INDIVIDUAL ANIMAL MANAGEMENT, DERMATOPATHY

It is important to establish a strong clinical diagnosis for dermatopathy and perform testing as needed to guide treatment. For ear infestation or infection, treatment should address the primary problem, such as ivermectin or selamectin for parasites, allergy medication or restricted diet, removal of foxtails, etc, if possible. The ears should be thoroughly cleaned, using sedation if necessary. Topical drugs for ear infections commonly contain anti-inflammatory agents, analgesics, ceruminolytics, and drying agents. Topical neomycin, other aminoglycosides, chloramphenicol, and others are useful for bacteria, while nystatin, clotrimazole, miconazole, and thiabendazole are effective against yeast. The use of systemic antibiotics in animals with otitis externa is controversial, because very little drug gets into the ear canal where the infection resides; however dogs with deeper otitis require systemic therapy. There is significant concern about the role of drug-resistant *Pseudomonas* infection in the ears. Regardless of whether stronger and more targeted antimicrobials are used, the animal will continue to become reinfected with increasingly drug resistant *Pseudomonas* as long as underlying conditions with poor drainage and moisture persist. If and only if drainage and moisture are corrected, *Pseudomonas* infection may be cleared with Tris-EDTA or topical application of amikacin or enrofloxacin (diluted parenteral products). With chronic otitis, especially if associated with conformational problems as in Cocker Spaniels, it may be almost impossible for most shelters to provide the level of correction (such as surgical ear resection) that would be nec-

essary to eliminate the underlying problem.

As for ear infection treatment, pyoderma treatment is more successful if the underlying problem is addressed. Dogs and cats with pyoderma always do better with shampooing with a number of excellent medicated and soothing products available including some containing antibiotics. If the pyoderma is significant, the animal probably needs systemic antibiotics as well. Cephalexin is an excellent, inexpensive drug of choice. Other broad-spectrum options include amoxicillin-clavulanate, enrofloxacin, oxacillin, and trimethroprim sulfonamide. If there is secondary yeast overgrowth, treatment should address the primary problem, remove the oil, and reduce the fungal numbers. Shampoos are soothing and moderately effective; however some animals may require systemic antifungal treatment as well, with ketoconazole and itraconazole commonly recommended. Recent studies have documented that itraconazole levels remain elevated in skin for prolonged periods, so "pulse therapy" (5 mg/kg PO q25 hr for two days, then five days of no treatment, for three weeks) may be an effective option in shelters.

To treat mange and other arthropod infestations, ivermectin, although unapproved, is the least expensive commonly used systemically active drug and will kill most arthropods. There are a number of other choices for fleas, including topical permethrin (not on cats), nitenpyram, selamectin, fipronil, and milbemycin; of this group only selamectin kills mange mites. Lufenuron is an insect growth regulator and will not produce rapid kills of the fleas by itself. Topical insecticides with anthelminthics effect should be used cautiously in animals that might have heartworm, since death of the worms can cause inflammation, heart failure, and death. Check the label carefully before using any new or unfamiliar products. Where possible, it is helpful for arthropod-infested animals to be bathed. Topical acaricides or insecticides help eliminate arthropods immediately, and soothing agents and removal of serum and crusting help deal with secondary bacteria and provide comfort from pruritis. Some tick borne diseases such as Lyme disease are not efficiently transmitted until the tick is attached for at least 48 hours. Prompt tick removal will lessen the chances of disease spread. If an animal is heavily tick-infested, there is a temptation to remove all of the ticks, but this must be done carefully. Staff members should wear gloves and a technique should be employed to ensure that tick mouthparts are removed with the rest of the body. Sedation may be required. Vaseline, caustic agents, or recently burned matches applied to the ticks are not appropriate. Dogs that have been heavily infested may require hospitalization for observation and fluids and/or blood products if anemic. Sites of attachment may become infected with secondary bacteria and may benefit from treatment (see "pyoderma" section). In regions with endemic tick-borne disease, it is reasonable to check serology 2-3 weeks after tick infestation for borreliosis and ehrlichiosis.

Treatment of demodectic mange is a unique problem, in that the clinical problem represents an inadequate immunological response to a common commensal. Mild cases in dogs under a year are self-limiting. If the dog is older or lesions extensive, intervention is justified but the prognosis remains poor. Amitraz is a dip that can be applied to an affected dog after it has been clipped and bathed thoroughly. The drug can be given every 2-4 weeks if necessary but is toxic to personnel and should only be used by people with appropriate training. Both ivermectin and milbemycin have been used systemically with some benefit. Ivermectin is given orally at 0.4-0.6 mg/kg daily (higher than for other parasitic infestations) and can produce neurological and other adverse reactions, particularly in susceptible breeds. Successful outcome with high-dose ivermectin has been reported after *months* of daily administration. Milbemycin is used up to 2.2 mg/kg daily until no mites are seen in skin scrapings. Both systemic options become expensive over time; with the poor prognosis and severe discomfort associated with the disease, euthanasia often is a reasonable alternative. Dogs with mange may be adopted after they have been treated and the skin has demonstrated significant improvement (usually at least two weeks after treatment).

In order to implement individual animal treatment of ringworm, shelter veterinarians should understand that many animals spontaneously recover with or without treatment, that there is significant disagreement among infectious disease experts regarding efficacy of available treatments, and that no treatment has been found 100 percent effective. Many cats and dogs with ringworm will spontaneously recover in about 3 months with no treatment. Topical treatment is important in that it serves to reduce contamination of the environment; however, most such topical therapies arguably do not reduce the clinical severity or accelerate recovery of individuals. Clipping and discarding infected hairs removes them from the environment and should be performed *gently* with a #10 blade. Of the topical treatments available, 4 percent lime-sulfur dip (used twice weekly) is relatively effective, available and safe. Dip should be patted on using gauze sponges rather than rubbed into the coat. Treatment with creams and ointments is ineffective, and azole-containing shampoos produce disappointing results.

The drawbacks to systemic therapy are the relatively high cost of the drugs, the possibility of toxic side effects, the relatively long course of treatment required, and the reality that most do not reduce clinical severity or speed recovery. Griseofulvin and itraconazole are most often recommended. Griseofulvin is a fungistatic, less expensive than itraconazole but more likely to cause toxic side effects such as vomiting and diarrhea and bone marrow suppression. Itraconazole is the drug of choice in most human infections but does not efficiently resolve ringworm in dogs and cats. Adverse effects include hepatic disease and vasculitis. Getting either drug in a form in which an adequately small dose can be administered can be a problem, especially in kittens. Local pharmacies should be able to make up a suspension of itraconazole for this purpose. Daily oral lufenuron therapy is one example of a therapy that has garnered both enthusiasm and lack thereof, with some clinical trials reporting efficacy and others failing to do so. Similarly, there have been conflicting reports on the efficacy of the killed *M. canis* vaccine, which is marketed to speed recovery. See Table 16.5.

There is no clear time after which it is best to adopt out animals with a history of dermatophytosis. If the owner is made aware of the risks and responsibilities, is willing to continue therapy and diagnostic evaluation, and understands that some animals may become carriers, animals may be adopted at any time. If the owner (or shelter) requires a guarantee, the best approach is to ensure that the animal is culture-negative on 3 successive toothbrush cultures 3 weeks apart. An intermediate approach is to adopt out animals once clinical signs have resolved and the animal is culture-negative at least once, with proper owner information.

Table 16.5. Characteristics of Pathogens Associated with Canine and Feline Dermatopathies

Organism	Mode of Transmission	Incubation Period/ Duration Shedding	Asymptomatic Carriers?	Clinical Presentation, Typical	Optimal Diagnostic Tests	Optimal Therapy[a]	Zoonotic/ Herd Risk?
Sarcoptes scabiei	Direct, fomites	NA[b]/Indefinite	No	Mange	Skin scrape	Ivermectin	H, Z
Notoedres cati	Direct, fomites	NA[b]/ Indefinite	No	Mange	Skin scrape	Selamectin	H
Demodex canis	Commensal	NA[b]/ [c]	Yes	None to mange	Skin scrape	[d]	
Mites and lice, misc.	Direct, fomites	NA[b]/ Indefinite	Yes	Dermatitis	Scotch tape	Selamectin	H, Z[e]
Fleas	Direct, environment	NA[b]/ Indefinite	Yes	None to dermatitis	Comb	Fipronil, Imidacloprid, Selamectin	H, Z
Ticks	Environment	NA[b]/ 7 days	No	None to local lesions	Physical examination	Fipronil	Z[f]
Ear mites	Direct, fomites	NA[b]/ Indefinite	No	Otitis	Ear swab	Selamectin	
Dermatophytes	Direct, environment[g]	4+d/ Indefinite	Yes	Dermatitis	Fungal culture	Lyme sulfur	H, Z
Yeast	Commensal, direct	NA[b]/ [e]	Yes	Dermatitis	Skin scrape/ cytology	Itraconazole	

[a] These therapies include off-label therapies and drugs that may present significant risk to some or all patients. Before use, shelter veterinarians are advised to read all of the relevant text in this book, consult a small animal medical text, and use proper medical judgment.

[b] Concept of incubation period not applicable for this parasite.

[c] Small numbers of this agent present on all dogs.

[d] In dogs older than 1 year, euthanasia a strong consideration if diagnosis of generalized demodicosis is confirmed.

[e] *Cheyletiella parasitovorax* is zoonotic.

[f] Ticks will rarely if ever detach from a dog and then reattach to a human.

[g] Agent is environmentally persistent and contamination of the environment is a problem in herd management.

H: important threat to herd in shelters

Z: zoonotic

VECTOR-BORNE, BITE-TRANSMITTED, AND SYSTEMIC DISEASES IN SHELTERS

Bartonellosis

Bartonellas are Gram-negative intraerythrocytic bacterial parasites previously thought to be (and now known not to be) rickettsiae. Cats are commonly infected reservoirs for zoonotic *Bartonella henselae* and *B. clarridgeiae*, while dogs may be reservoirs for *B. vinsoni*. *B. henselae* and *B. clarridgeiae* are the agents of cat-scratch disease in people, as well as bacillary angiomatosis, relapsing fever, bacillary peliosis, and meningitis/neuroretinitis. Cats infected with *B. henselae* generally remain infected for months to years, yet are clinically well, although anemia, fever, and lymphadenomegaly have been reported following experimental infection. People acquire the infection directly from a cat bite or scratch or from being bitten by cat fleas. *B. vinsoni berkhoffii* is an important causative agent of endocarditis and granulomatous lymphadenitis in dogs; a single case of *B. clarridgeiae* endocarditis also has been reported in a dog (Chomel et al., 2001). In human endocarditis, *B. henselae* and *B. vinsoni berkhoffii* have been detected.

Diagnosis of active bartonella infection can be made by blood culture or PCR, although many laboratories do not offer the specialized techniques required for obtaining positive culture. Serological tests indicate whether a cat or dog has previously been infected; such animals may or may not still be infected. Additional tests may be necessary to evaluate dogs for endocarditis, including cardiac ultrasound and blood culture.

Several different antibiotics have been proposed to clear the bacteremia associated with *Bartonella* spp. infection, although none with 100 percent success, including tetracycline, amoxicillin-clavulanate, enrofloxacin, erythromycin, and rifampin. Given that a cat with *B. henselae* will probably remain well, the main justification for treatment is to prevent human infections, which can also be accomplished by careful matching of a possibly infected cat with an appropriate home that does not contain elderly people, young children, or known immunocompromised individuals. In dogs, treatment of *B. vinsoni berkhoffii* is aimed at managing a severe infection deep in the cardiac valves and is associated with a poor prognosis.

B. henselae and *B. clarridgeiae* are transmitted by fleas. The routes of spread of *B. vinsoni berkhoffii* are unknown but thought to be ticks. Many cases of cat scratch disease in people appear to be linked to cat bites or scratches, while others are related to flea bites. Management of these infections in shelters must include excellent flea control, minimization of bite and scratch wounds (primarily through staff training), and counseling of potential owners with regard to risks.

Tick-Borne Diseases: Ehrlichiae and Rickettsiae, *Borrelia burgdorferi*, *Babesia* spp., and Rocky Mountain Spotted Fever (RMSF)

Most of the tick-borne rickettsial and ehrlichial infections will be sporadic or rare in shelters. These include Rocky Mountain spotted fever in dogs (caused by *R. rickettsii*), *Ehrlichia canis* and *E. ewingii* (in dogs), *Anaplasma phagocytophila* (formerly *E. equi* or the canine granulocytic ehrlichiosis agent in dogs and rarely cats), babesiosis (due to several *Babesia* spp., and Lyme disease (*Borrelia burgdorferi*) in dogs. Additionally, ticks may produce local skin infection and tick paralysis.

EHRLICHIOSIS

E. canis is the most common ehrlichial agent found in clinically ill dogs. It is closely related but distinct from *E. chaffeensis*, the agent of human monocytic ehrlichiosis, although a case of human disease was reported in Venezuela in a patient infected with *E. canis* (Perez, Rikihisa, and Wen, 1996). This infection is transmitted by the peridomestic tick *Rhipicephalus sanguineous* and targets the canine macrophage, producing fever, lymphadenopathy, anemia and thrombocytopenia in its early stages. If the dog remains persistently infected, it eventually may enter a late stage of ehrlichiosis characterized by systemic disease, bone marrow suppression, and pancytopenia. Dogs may have vague generalized signs of systemic disease, including lethargy and weight loss, lymphadenomegaly and splenomegaly, uveitis and retinitis, and bleeding from eyes, nose, and in bowel movements. German Shepherd dogs are predisposed to more severe disease.

In some geographical areas of the U.S. such as New England, the upper midwest, and California, granulocytic ehrlichiosis in dogs is far more common than monocytic. In the U.S., *A. phagocytophila* is vectored by the Pacific black-legged tick, *Ixodes pacificus,* or the deer tick, *I. scapularis.* In contrast to canine monocytic ehrlichiosis, which is caused by an agent largely distinct from the human pathogen, canine granulocytic ehrlichiosis is caused by the same pathogen that infects people, horses, and a range of wildlife species. The clinical signs in dogs, horses, and people include fever, muscle and joint pain, and in people, headache. Hematological and biochemical abnormalities may include thrombocytopenia, anemia, leukopenia, and elevated liver enzymes. Horses particularly are susceptible to icterus, head pressing, and lower limb edema. However, in all species, most infections do not manifest any abnormal signs and go unnoticed.

Ehrlichiosis is diagnosed by direct visualization of the organism in target cells, serology, and PCR. *E. ewingii,* which is closely related to *E. canis,* may be seen in neutrophils as can *A. phagocytophila,* within small cytoplasmic, membrane-bound vacuoles called morulae. If monocytes contain morulae, these could be *A. phagocytophila* or *E. canis.* The sensitivity of this assay is increased if a buffy coat smear is examined. PCR is one of the most sensitive tests available for diagnosing active ehrlichiosis, because acute infections, especially with granulocytic ehrlichiae, often are resolved before the dog seroconverts. Serology is useful for documenting previous exposure to an ehrlichia, documenting four-fold rises in titer retrospectively, or documenting possible chronic infection with *E. canis.* There is sometimes weak cross-reactivity between granulocytic and monocytic ehrlichiae; it is best to run both titers, because typically one is much higher than the other (Dumler et al., 1995).

Acute monocytic and granulocytic ehrlichiosis respond well to treatment with tetracycline. Defervescence usually occurs within 24 hours. Even without treatment, most cases of granulocytic ehrlichiosis resolve on their own within about a week. In contrast, chronic monocytic ehrlichiosis is not easily treated and has a poor prognosis. Dogs require anti-ehrlichial drugs (doxycycline, or imidocarb), fluids and/or blood products, possibly erythropoietin or granulocyte colony stimulating factor, and steroids.

LYME DISEASE

Borrelia burgdorferi sensu lato is a spirochete that causes Lyme disease, a mild and nonspecific disease in most infected dogs and people, but which can be severe, with chronic arthritis, neurological and cardiac dysfunction and in dogs, nephritis. *B. burgdorferi* spp. Group 1 comprises a number of closely related genospecies, including *B. burgdorferi* sensu stricto, *B. bissettii,* and others. The bacterium is transmitted by the same ticks as granulocytic ehrlichiosis. Following inoculation into a susceptible host, the spirochete remains locally in skin and connective tissue, and eventually may disseminate particularly to joints and other areas with high concentrations of connective tissue. The infection in some dogs lasts months to years. Clinical signs are usually absent or may include fever, polyarthritis, or severe monoarticular arthritis. Severe nephritis with direct borrelial inflammatory and immune complex pathogenesis can lead to protein-losing glomerulopathy and fatal renal failure (Dambach et al., 1997).

Infection with *B. burgdorferi* should be considered in dogs with chronic arthritis or nephritis. Suspect sera should be screened by IFA, ELISA, or an equivalent test and the diagnosis confirmed with western blotting, because IFA alone has a high rate of false positivity. Another advantage of western blot confirmation is the ability to discriminate exposure to field strains from vaccination. In some cases, culture or PCR may yield positive results, especially in joint fluid, although most dogs are PCR-negative even while asymptomatic. If the diagnosis is accurate, acutely infected animals benefit from treatment with doxycycline, amoxicillin, or azithromycin. Chronic disease, particularly nephritis, has a poor prognosis. In human medicine, neuroborreliosis often is treated with IV ceftriaxone. There are 2 classes of Lyme vaccine available for dogs: whole cell preparations and recombinant OspA vaccine. In Lyme-endemic areas, shelters might consider Lyme vaccination of sheltered dogs, but more likely would leave the controversial decisions of using these vaccines to local practitioners.

ROCKY MOUNTAIN SPOTTED FEVER

The pathogen responsible for Rocky Mountain spotted fever is *Rickettsia rickettsii,* a bacterium transmitted by the ticks *Dermacentor andersoni, D. variabilis,* and *Rhipicephalus sanguineous.* Like other spotted fever rickettsiae, *R. rickettsii* is maintained in ticks transtadially and transovarially, which facilitates persistence of the pathogen in nature. Other reservoirs of infection include wild mammals and dogs. Despite the fact that RMSF was originally observed in the western U.S., cases in humans and animals are uncommon west of the Rocky Mountains but emergence of the disease is occurring currently in the American southeast.

R. rickettsii is inoculated into a mammalian host via the bite of an infected tick. It invades endothelial cells and leads to vasculitis, which causes especially severe lesions in skin, brain, heart, and kidneys. Classically, edema develops 2-10 days after the tick bite. Skin lesions may range from vesicular, hyperemic lesions to severe necrosis. There may be mucosal, genital, and retinal petechiae and hemorrhages. Ultimately, shock and CNS disease can be fatal.

If RMSF is suspected in a shelter dog, supporting diagnostic tests may reveal thrombocytopenia, leukopenia followed by leukocytosis, and possibly elevated protein in CSF. Antibody testing (especially with a four-fold rise in titer) may retrospectively confirm the diagnosis. However a low to moderate positive IgG does not confirm active infection as many animals may be seropositive animals and the antibodies cross-react with all spotted fever group rickettsiae (but not typhus group). Immunohistochemistry may be performed on biopsy samples (for example, skin), but not all laboratories offer the test. PCR testing is a good option where available.

Treatment should be initiated without waiting for confirmation of diagnosis. Appropriate antibiotics include tetracycline, baytril, and chloramphenicol. Concurrent steroid therapy is recommended to reduce the inflammation and vasculitis, and supportive care of gangrene and shock are necessary. Fluid treatment must be given slowly to avoid cerebellar/cerebral edema. The prognosis is fair, depending on how early disease is detected and how quickly it progresses. Prevention depends on tick control that generally would need to have occurred before the animal entered the shelter. It is unlikely that infection will spread to other dogs or shelter staff, but it is important to prevent environmental contamination of the peridomestic tick *R. sanguineous*.

BABESIA

Babesiosis is a tick-transmitted (*Rhipicephalus sanguineous*) disease attributable to one of several species of protozoa including *B. gibsoni* and *B. canis*. Occasional cases are due to transfusion with contaminated blood products. Most cases occur in the American southeast, Arizona, and Midwest (especially Oklahoma and Arkansas). The clinical presentation may be variable, generally manifest as a weak, depressed dog. The infection can cause splenomegaly, hemolytic anemia possibly with bilirubinuria, and thrombocytopenia. Dogs may eventually develop disseminated intravascular coagulopathy or immune-mediated glomerulonephritis. Subclinical carriers of *B. gibsoni* have been reported at a very high frequency in American Pit Bull Terriers (Macintire et al., 2002). The prevalence of *B. canis* in apparently well Greyhounds also is very high (Taboada et al., 1992). Coinfection with *B. burgdorferi, A. phagocytophilum,* or *E. canis* may exacerbate clinical disease. Diagnostic tests can include serology, evaluation of thick blood smears, or PCR. On evaluation of Giemsa-stained blood, *B. gibsoni* has a variable appearance but typically is a small (1–3 μm) piroplasm within erythrocytes, while the appearance of *B. canis* is larger (2–5 μm). There is some serological cross-reactivity among the *Babesia* spp. although PCR testing is species-specific. Treatment options include doxycycline, metronidazole, imidocarb dipropionate, clindamycin, and prednisone. Imidocarb appears particularly effective against *B. canis*. Supportive care, including blood transfusion, may be necessary. The prognosis for elimination of *B. gibsoni* is poor, with some dogs never recovering from the initial episode and others becoming long-term carriers or developing later episodes of hemolysis (Birkenheuer et al., 1999). Tick prevention is the most important preventive measure, although it is important to screen blood products before administering transfusions. Shelters that routinely rescue and place Greyhounds or American Pit Bull Terriers should always include this disease in their list of differentials when evaluating debilitated animals.

Rabies

Probably the greatest dog and cat bite-associated threat is rabies, which is emerging recently in a novel ecology, associated with strains endemic in populations of bats. Rabies virus circulates in a number of different enzootic cycles in different areas of the U.S.: most human and domestic animal cases in each given area are related genetically and serologically (detected by MABs against the N protein and by DNA sequencing) to the local circulating reservoir strains. Local reservoirs in the U.S. include several skunk species and raccoons along the eastern seaboard.

In 2000, five human cases were reported to the CDC: one in California, one in Georgia, one in Minnesota, one in New York (dog variant acquired in Ghana), and one in Wisconsin. With the exception of the dog variant, all were bat variants. In contrast, in dogs and cats in 1999, testing of 78 rabid dogs and 230 cats indicated that "nearly all animals were infected with the predicted terrestrial rabies virus variant associated with the geographic location of the submission". Bat variant rabies virus was found in a single cat from Maryland.

Rabies virus is usually inoculated into a host via a bite wound. The virus replicates locally in the myocardium and new particles bind with adjacent cell membranes, from which viral genetic material is infused into the target cell. Once virus is inoculated, it enters nerve cells and travels retroaxonally up to the CNS, unless eliminated by the host. Some host species and individuals are more resistant to rabies virus infections, with canids and felids having moderate to high susceptibility and opossums and birds being less susceptible. Also, if there is less virus inoculated or the individual is older, there is a greater chance of surviving. The speed with which virus enters the CNS depends on the distance it must travel from the inoculation site and the amount of innervation at the site. Reported incubation periods have ranged from weeks to, rarely, a few years. In the brain, lower motor neuron disease is associated with flaccid ascending paralysis and infection in the forebrain may produce behavior changes. Dogs tend to become fractious or docile if they previously were fractious. Cats tend to become very aggressive. Both dogs and cats may lick or mutilate the inoculation site. Later, dogs and cats become disoriented, may develop seizures and paralysis, and die. Especially in dogs, excessive salivation may occur, as well as masticatory muscle paralysis and the appearance of choking.

After infecting the brain, virus infects salivary glands and vibrissae, and virus particles are shed in the saliva of dogs and cats. If the animal is infectious at the time of a bite wound, the disease is already far-advanced and the rationale for bite quarantine of 10 days is that disease is expected to progress to the point of death within the 10 days. Ante-mortem diagnostic testing is not reliable; ac-

curate diagnosis requires brain tissue. If rabies infection is suspected in an animal, the animal should be euthanized only by trained personnel wearing heavy gloves and using catch poles or other protective gear. The head should be removed without generating aerosols, kept cool (but not frozen), and forwarded to the local appropriate laboratory as quickly as possible, accompanied by any history or other important information available. Commonly employed diagnostic tests include direct FA, virus culture, and PCR. If virus is detected, PCR or monoclonal antibody reactions may determine the strain (that is, probable host species). All shelters should develop a line of communication with local health officials *before* suspect cases of rabies develop. Additionally, state and federal laws regulate quarantine, vaccination protocols and so forth, so shelter medical staff should become familiar with all appropriate regulations.

Preventive management of rabies should include pre-exposure prophylaxis for staff, which will protect against bat rabies as well as the strains circulating in the traditional reservoirs. Staff in shelters must be well trained in universal precautions and safe handling of animals to avoid bite wounds. Following bites, wounds should be cleaned thoroughly (at least 10 minutes) with ethanol, hand disinfectant, or at least soap and water. Animals entering the shelter should be screened for rabies. This includes questioning clients whether the animal has bitten any one (or any animal) within the last 2 weeks or been bitten by wildlife or any other animal that could have had rabies within the last year. The animal should be examined on intake for bite wounds and neurological clinical signs. Requirements for quarantine are spelled out in the Compendium of Animal Rabies Prevention and Control (on the Internet at http://www.avma.org/pubhlth/rabcont.asp and updated annually in JAVMA). Especially in rabies-endemic areas, animals should be adopted with an information sheet informing clients to maintain a relationship with a veterinarian, monitor the animal for neurological signs and manage bite exposure appropriately.

Bacterial Bite Wound Flora

Animal bites may be sources by which zoonotic pathogens are introduced into people. Dog and cat bite wound flora usually are polymicrobial, including *Capnocytophaga canimorsus (DF-2),*

Pasteurella multocida, Staphylococcus spp., *Streptococcus* spp., *Bacteroides* spp., *Prevotella, Corynebacterium, Fusobacterium,* and *Peptostreptococcus.* Cat bites are far more likely to become infected with *Pasteurella* than dog bites. *Capnocytophaga canimorsus* is a slow-growing nonenteric Gram-negative rod that is found frequently in the normal flora of dog and cat mouths and has been linked to fatal septicemia in immunocompromised people following dog bites. Local cellulitis may develop initially, followed by fever, vomiting and diarrhea, endocarditis, dyspnea, thrombocytopenia, DIC, and death. Given the delay in obtaining a positive culture with this organism, it is helpful to inform the physicians that it is suspected based on the bite wound.

The initial approach to treatment of bite wounds is to manage bleeding and clean thoroughly with soap, running water, and antiseptics such as betadine. If the wound abscesses, maturation of the abscess should be facilitated with hot packs. When possible, the wound can be debrided, using universal precautions. Topical antibiotics are not as effective as systemically active drugs, but topical cleaning agents are useful when the wound is open. If the wound does not improve, systemic illness develops, or the lesion progresses, culture and antibiotic susceptibility testing may be indicated. Antibiotics should be chosen to be broad-spectrum, including activity against anaerobes. Good choices are amoxicillin, amoxicillin/clavulanate, and clindamycin.

Staff should always seek professional medical care for animal bites and avoid the temptation to self-treat.

Toxoplasmosis

Toxoplasma gondii is an obligate intracellular apicomplexans protozoan with a complex developmental cycle. *T. gondii* is usually acquired by cats via ingestion of prey and moves through the cat's GI tract. The protozoa penetrate epithelial cells, where both asexual and sexual development occur. Sexual reproduction occurs within 3-10 days and, within 18 days, fertilized macrogamonts develop into oocysts and are shed in feces. Members of the family Felidae are the only species in which sexual reproduction of *T. gondii* occurs. In other species, GI sporozoites reproduce asexually, and tachyzoites migrate to muscle and other tissue and encyst. Tachyzoites can be transmitted directly among animals by ingestion or congenital infection. Infected cats usually are asymptomatic and the primary significance is that the cat sheds oocysts that may lead to severe birth defects if ingested by a pregnant woman. Uncommonly, there may be clinical signs in cats if tachyzoites are encysted and the cat either fails to eliminate the infection, experiences tissue necrosis, or has inflammatory reactions to their presence. Main targets include the heart, lungs, CNS, liver, and eye. Disease is typically much more severe if the cat is immunosuppressed, such as with FIV or FeLV infection or FIP. Kittens are more likely to experience liver and CNS disease and pneumonia. Cats can acquire toxoplasmosis, and develop abnormal respiratory, GI, muscular, or neurological signs.

Diagnosis of toxoplasmosis in sick cats starts with abnormal physical exam findings or biochemical abnormalities reflecting the affected organ. Cytology of aspirates or biopsy of the affected organ may reveal the protozoa, often accompanied by lymphocytes. On serology, there are often false positives or false negatives in kittens with maternal immunity and IgG may be expected to be positive in many well adult cats. IgM is not always elevated during acute infection. If the cat has neurological or ocular disease, CSF/serum or ocular fluid/serum antibody ratio can be used to indicate infection locally. PCR shows promise in some cases. The indications for fecal evaluation are to diagnose cats that are currently shedding and may pose a public health risk, not to clinically evaluate sick cats.

Several drugs are used for cats with toxoplasmosis. Clindamycin is the drug of choice, and the ultimate prognosis of the cat may be determined shortly after drug treatment begins because those that will improve generally do so within 1-2 weeks. Other antibiotics with possible efficacy in toxoplasmosis include trimethoprim-sulfonamides and clarithromycin. Steroids may be used with caution to reduce inflammation. Monensin is used to treat cats that are shedding and has no effect on encysted tachyzoites.

The main role of shelter veterinarians in dealing with toxoplasmosis is to advise the public on the risk to pregnant women and their fetuses of exposure to infected cats. There are no absolute guidelines, and pregnant women always are advised to limit their exposure to undercooked meat that can contain tachyzoites and to soil or cat litter that may contain infectious oocysts. If a pregnant woman must clean litterboxes, she should be informed to clean the box daily, wear gloves, use a litter box liner, and wash utensils with boiling water. Oocysts must sporulate outside the cat's body for a minimum of 1-5 days before they become infective for humans, so daily cleaning greatly reduces the risk of transmission. A seronegative cat may become infected at any time and shed *Toxoplasma oocysts*. A seropositive cat with a low IgG titer has previously been infected. Most of the time such a cat will have eliminated the infection and would represent one of the safest cats in the home of pregnant women. To reduce the likelihood that cats will become infected, their exposure to raw meat, worms, and cockroaches should be reduced. It can be difficult to deal with environmental decontamination: the best bets are to hot-water treat or steam litterboxes and cover sandboxes to prevent roaming cats from defecating in them.

Retroviruses

Feline Leukemia Virus (FeLV)

Feline leukemia virus (FeLV) is a Gamma-retrovirus that infects members of the family Felidae only; it is not zoonotic. Cats transmit FeLV through direct contact: the virus is shed in many body fluids including urine, saliva, milk, and blood. Kittens can acquire FeLV in utero. The virus does not persist in the environment, so new cats can be adopted to a home that previously housed a FeLV positive animal without a lengthy waiting period. Many cats that are exposed to FeLV develop antibodies, eliminate the infection, and are healthy and immune. If the virus is not eliminated, infection may persist for months to a few years until the cat develops cancer, disregulated blood cell production, immunosuppression, or one of a number of rare bizarre FeLV-associated syndromes such as cutaneous horns. The most common neoplasia associated with FeLV is leukemia. Other affected cats may develop lymphoma or other sarcomas. FeLV infection often is immunosuppressive, and infected cats develop unusually severe concurrent infections. An infection of the ciliary body of the eye can cause the pupils to be unequal in some cats with FeLV. FeLV can induce deposition of antibody-antigen complexes in the kidney and joint tissue, resulting in kidney failure or arthritis.

Signs of FeLV infection can be vague, such as weight loss, vomiting, lack of energy, and so forth. The signs may be due to anemia, pressure from tumors, organ dysfunction, or others. Most FeLV infections are identified by antigen ELISA. Occasional cases are identified on complete blood count (CBC), with massive excesses of white blood cells and compensatorily reduced red blood cells and other cell lines. In the FeLV ELISA, antibodies in the test react with the p27 core protein from FeLV that is present in huge amounts in viremic cats. The FeLV ELISA test is direct evidence that the virus is present, as opposed to an antibody test that would only indicate previous exposure to an infectious disease. In-house FeLV kits can be run on cat blood in about 10 minutes; other samples (tears or urine) can be used but the test is not as sensitive using these samples. Of all diagnostic tests in veterinary medicine, the feline leukemia test is one of the best. If testing is performed, all individuals should be tested (that is, blood from kittens from a litter should not be pooled) because it is typical for some kittens to remain FeLV-free, even if the queen and/or littermates are infected.

After exposure to FeLV, a cat will become test-positive in blood within days to a week and will eradicate the virus within about 2 weeks if it is capable. If, after 3-4 weeks, the cat still tests positive, it is unlikely to ever become negative. It is statistically unlikely that one would happen to test a cat that would ultimately eliminate the infection during its few viremic days, although possible. To be sure, healthy FeLV positive cats should not be euthanized based solely on the results of one positive test—one should retest healthy cats in 4-6 weeks: if positive at that point, they are chronically infected.

Herd management of FeLV rests on preventing spread of the virus among cats. Cats transmit FeLV to other cats through direct contact, shared litter boxes, or water bowls. Feline leukemia positive cats should be isolated or kept only with other cats with FeLV. There is a commercial vaccine against feline leukemia, given yearly. Expert opinions differ as to how effective the vaccine is: certainly most vaccinated cats do not get feline leukemia, but neither do most otherwise well adult cats. The vaccine is safe.

At the individual cat level, FeLV is a fatal infection: at best, cats do well clinically for months to a few years. The only goals for treatment are to keep virus levels as low as possible, reduce the impact of

FeLV-associated disorders, and provide maximum quality of life. Cats with solid tumors like lymphoma often do well with chemotherapy to get the cancer into remission. On the other hand, cats with leukemia typically respond extremely poorly to cancer treatment. Anemic cats and cats with leukemia changes in their blood cells require supportive care including blood transfusions and antibiotics if there are secondary bacterial infections. Treatment usually fails within a few months.

Antiviral drugs have been assessed to target the virus itself. AZT inhibits the reverse transcriptase, an enzyme FeLV uses to insert itself into the cat's DNA. AZT can reduce the production of new virus but does not eliminate infection. The drug PMEA also reduces the viremia but has significant, unacceptable adverse effects. Some practitioners advocate immunomodulatory therapy in cats with FeLV, without a lot of controlled studies to document their efficacy. These range from herbal and homeopathic supplements to acemannan and cytokines to stimulate immunity. Human alpha and gamma interferon have immunostimulatory and antiviral activities but cats develop antibodies against the human recombinant products and derive no benefit after a few weeks. Each shelter should develop its own guidelines as to whether they will house FeLV-infected cats, and they should base decisions on euthanasia, housing, and adoption on the quality of life of the infected cats, the shelter's ability to minimize risk to other cats, resources, and mission-oriented philosophies. Healthy animals that are placed for adoption should be neutered.

FELINE IMMUNODEFICIENCY VIRUS (FIV)

Feline immunodeficiency virus is a lentiviral retrovirus of cats that is closely related to HIV, the virus responsible for AIDS. Domestic cats and some wild cat species are susceptible to FIV; the infection is most common in unneutered adult male cats. The main route of transmission of FIV is through biting and breeding. Cats may live together in one home without transmitting the disease. However, an important consideration when adopting out a cat with FIV is that bites occur most often during the initial introduction. After infection, FIV viral replication occurs within local lymphoid and thymic tissue, followed by viremia within a few weeks. Virus infects macrophages, B-cells, and T-cells, including CD4+ (T-helper) cells throughout the body.

Within weeks to months, host immunity leads to significant reductions in circulating virus load. Over time, progressive immunocompromise occurs, with an incompletely understood mechanism. Cats with FIV can live for several years without symptoms. However, most infected cats will develop "feline AIDS related complex" within 3-6 years of infection, with one or more secondary conditions such as severe oral disease, disproportionately severe URI, FIA, neoplastic disease, and others. Most FIV-positive cats develop full-blown AIDS within 6–8 years and die soon after. Cats that are showing clinical signs at the time of diagnosis will likely die much sooner.

The screening test for FIV is the ELISA (enzyme-linked immunosorbent assay), which can be quickly and easily performed in house. This test assays for antibodies to the FIV present in the blood of the cat. PCR for FIV is not sensitive enough for diagnostic use. If the FIV ELISA is positive, this result may be confirmed by Western Blot because in some cases ELISA may give false positive results. Each individual animal must be tested, as opposed to pooling blood from a litter. Maternal antibodies may interfere with FIV testing in kittens, although there is some disagreement as to when FIV screening becomes sensitive and specific in kittens. Maternal antibody interference rarely occurs at 4 months and is very unlikely by 6 months. A rational approach is to keep kittens in small groups until 6 months and then test and isolate cats according to results of the test.

After cats test positive for FIV, the decision as to how to manage these cats is difficult. If the cat is sick with an infectious disease, it is possible that the illness is exacerbated if the cat has FIV-associated immunosuppression. The level of immunosuppression can be investigated with a CD4+ T-lymphocyte count but this test is not available commercially. If the cat appears to have AIDS-related disease, many veterinarians counsel euthanasia. "Treatment" consists of good nourishment, protection from stress and infectious disease, and management of secondary conditions. Antiretroviral drugs have been researched extensively for HIV and FIV secondarily, but there remains no cure for FIV infection (or HIV infection). Drugs should be given in combination because retroviruses can become resistant quickly if exposed to only one drug. Drugs used in combination may include AZT, PMEA, ddI (didanosine) and others. Serious toxic adverse effects may be expected in cats.

The major dilemma for shelters regards whether to adopt or euthanize apparently healthy FIV-positive cats, because of the moderate rate of false-positive ELISA tests and the probability that cats may remain relatively healthy with a good quality of life in a home for years. However, because even moderately immunosuppressed cats are more susceptible to infection, FIV-positive cats may contribute disproportionately to the load of infectious organisms in a shelter environment, increasing risks for other cats. If euthanasia is not supported by the shelter's policies, cats with FIV should be housed only with other cats with FIV and not with FeLV-positive cats. If they are adopted, these cats should also be neutered, and prospective owners should be counseled extensively and should sign an acknowledgement that they have been informed of the cat's status.

There is a recently developed vaccine for FIV and new technology being actively researched which probably will result in additional vaccines within a few years. Unfortunately, widespread use of the current vaccine will make screening even more difficult because vaccinated cats likely will test positive on the ELISA test.

Hemobartonellas

The previously designated *Hemobartonella felis* and *canis* have been reevaluated phylogenetically and placed as a hemocytic clade within the family Mycoplasmataceae. The virulent large feline parasite has been renamed *Mycoplasma hemofelis* and a smaller low pathogenicity parasite *M. hemominutum* (Neimark et al., 2001). The organisms do not have cell walls and are technically Gram-negative. They live affiliated by filamentous bridges on the surface of red blood cells, and the mechanisms by which they spread among animals are not known.

In dogs, hemobartonellosis occurs only in splenectomized dogs and is characterized as an acute anemia with the organism easily visualized on the red cells. Infected cats often are completely asymptomatic especially if infected with the small form, or they may develop acute or cyclic anemia (feline infectious anemia or FIA). Signs of disease do not occur until after IgG is produced (at least 10 days after exposure), when splenic cleansing of parasitized cells leaves behind spherocytes with high osmotic fragility (Coombs-positive). Clinical signs

associated with hemobartonellosis include pallor, dyspnea with open mouth breathing, weakness, and fever. After primary infection, cats may enter a series of infection cycles of latency and recrudescence. Subsequent recrudescent attacks become increasingly less severe (in terms of percent parasitism, reductions in PCV, and clinical signs) with each attack. Alternatively, many cats become healthy carriers.

FIA is likely to be more severe in cats with other conditions including stress, pregnancy, intercurrent infection, neoplasia, and feline leukemia virus infection. Feline leukemia virus is a well-described potentiator of hemobartonellosis, although feline immunodeficiency virus (FIV) is not. Cats with concurrent hemobartonellosis and FeLV are usually much sicker, with more profound and refractory anemia, than cats with FIA alone. In cats coinfected with FeLV and *M. hemofelis* and *hemominutum*, hematological changes may reflect both the effects of FIA as well as the typical myeloproliferative disease, aplastic anemia, or various dyshematopoietic disorders of FeLV.

Hemobartonellosis is diagnosed on CBC or by PCR; testing is indicated in any cat that appears clinically anemic. Hematological changes in FIA may reflect frank blood loss (macrocytic anemia with reticulocytosis), although commonly the anemia is normocytic normochromic. The PCV may decline to 15 percent or lower. Clinical signs may become apparent once the PCV falls below about 20 percent. Leukocyte responses in FIA are variable, including leukopenia possibly with toxic neutrophils or leukocytosis. Hemobartonella organisms are readily stained by Wright-Giemsa or new methylene blue stains and appear as dark blue or Gram-positive variably shaped 0.3–0.8 μm bodies on the surface of feline erythrocytes. The fraction of erythrocytes that is parasitized is also highly variable, and hemobartonellosis may be overlooked in cats with low rates of parasitism. The fraction of parasitized erythrocytes in acutely ill cats can be as high as 95 percent, with 10 or more organisms observed in pairs or chains on the surface of erythrocytes. The parasites may be confused with Howell-Jolly bodies, but H–J bodies are at least twice as large as the *M. hemofelis* organisms and nonrefractile. Several different hemobartonella-specific PCR tests are available targeting the 16S rRNA subunit gene for both Hfsm and Hflg (Foley et al., 1998).

The treatment of choice for hemobartonellosis is one of the tetracycline class drugs (tetracycline, oxytetracycline, or doxycycline). Oxytetracycline is convenient because it can be given less frequently but is associated with pain on administration and local reactions at the site of injection. In anemic cats treated with tetracyclines, clinical signs may resolve within 24 hours and results of PCR tests become negative by 12 hours after initiation of antibiotic therapy. However, after discontinuation of antibiotics, PCR tests become positive again.

Some cases of FIA are refractory to tetracycline. As with mycoplasmas, *M. hemofelis* is resistant to antibiotics with activity against cell wall synthesis or integrity. Older recommended alternative treatments for FIA include thiacetarsamide, chlorpromazine, chloramphenicol, and a combination of spiramycin, metronidazole and chloramphenicol. More recent suggestions include enrofloxacin. Preliminary results demonstrate that enrofloxacin successfully improves cats' clinical conditions and PCVs but does not eliminate hemobartonella DNA.

In addition to antibiotic therapy, supportive therapy may be necessary to prevent severe hypoxia and death. Corticosteroids (for example, prednisolone at 1–2 mg/kg PO daily for the first 7–14 days) may be used to prevent the immune-mediated erythrophagocytosis of infected erythrocytes. Blood transfusion is frequently necessary, but transfused cells are very susceptible to parasitism and may need to be given repeatedly. An alternative might be transfusion with Oxyglobin (Biopure, Cambridge, MA), a polymerized bovine hemoglobin product licensed for use in anemic dogs, on the principle that the organism would not be able to parasitize the cells.

The epidemiology of hemobartonellosis is poorly understood. Risk factors for hemobartonellosis include age, sex, being indoor-outdoor, and presence of fleas. The incidence of FIA increases with age with a peak incidence from 4-8 years. Male cats may be at greater risk for FIA, and infection with *M. hemofelis* appears to be seasonal. The routes of infection may include *in utero* or lactogenic, iatrogenic, possibly oral, and hematophagous arthropod. *In utero* or lactogenic infection is suggested by detection of hemobartonellosis in very young kittens. Blood-sucking arthropods such as fleas might be natural vectors, although many cases have been identified in Salt Lake City, Utah, in the absence of fleas.

FELINE INFECTIOUS PERITONITIS (FIP)

Feline infectious peritonitis is a fatal disease of cats caused by infection with a mutant feline enteric coronavirus that has the capability to infect and replicate within feline macrophages. The disease is actually an immune-mediated response by the cat to the infection, in which immune complexes are formed and immunological reactions lead to the characteristic pathological and clinical abnormalities. In "dry" or noneffusive FIP, granulomatous masses form on kidneys, mesenteric lymph nodes, liver, spleen, and/or in the brain and eyes and may lead to organ failure. Cats with dry FIP may have ocular or neurologic signs. Cats with "wet" FIP develop a yellow fluid with high protein content in their chest or abdomen, causing dyspnea or abdominal distention.

The diagnosis of FIP should be based on a composite of history, signalment, clinical observations, physical exam, and laboratory findings. FIP is most common in 1-3 year old cats from multiple-cat households and shelters (Foley et al., 1997). The most common signs of FIP in young cats are cyclic, antibiotic nonresponsive fever, lethargy, and failure to grow. CBC abnormalities include elevated total protein (mainly globulin), increased numbers of total white blood cells and neutrophils, and decreased numbers of lymphocytes. Serum protein and globulin often are elevated.

Cats infected with FECV produce antibodies that cross-react with FIPV (Pedersen, 1995). Therefore, the diagnosis of FIP by antibody tests in a healthy cat is a serious error. Rising titers are not informative, because cats with FIP and FECV both cycle up and down in titer level. Very high titers (>1:16,000) are suggestive of FIP. New RNA-level tests, such as PCR, *cannot differentiate the FIPV from the FECV.* Their only usefulness for diagnosing FIP would be in odd anatomical locations, such as the brain (where FECV does not invade).

The fluid in wet FIP is characteristic, being yellowish, sticky or mucinous, high in protein, and containing numerous neutrophils and macrophages. Biopsies of masses in cats with dry FIP show granulomatous inflammation. There is only one way to confirm a diagnosis of FIP: that is to identify the FIPV in biopsies of masses or at necropsy. The most accurate technique to detect virus is by a procedure called "immunohistochemistry" and is performed on biopsy tissues.

Virtually every cat with FIP dies. The use of immunosuppressive drugs such as corticosteroids or cyclophosphamide may slow disease progression, but does not alter the outcome. Many veterinarians are using immunostimulants of various types (immunoregulin, interferon, acemannan, and so on) to treat cats with FIP, although this may be counterproductive given the immune-mediated pathogenesis of the disease. Cats should be rested and provided good nutrition, lack of stress, and broad-spectrum antibiotics for as long as they are comfortable. Once disease becomes debilitating and weight and appetite decline, the cat should be euthanized.

There is very little that can be done in the herd health sense to manage for FIP. Cats rarely acquire FIP directly from other cats; much more commonly, FECV is spread followed by the FIP-inducing mutation. Since FIPV lives in macrophages, it generally is in locations such as brain, kidney, or other sites without direct access to the outside world (or other cats). Most cats exposed to FIPV mutants orally eliminate the pathogen quickly. Cats that develop FIP may have underlying predisposing disorders that make it more difficult for them to eliminate the pathogen. If cats are exposed to FECVs, *there is always a risk that FIP may occur* and FECV can only be eradicated in very small groups of cats (less than 4 per building*).* In multiple-cat groups, 40–60 percent of the cats shed virus in their feces at any given time and *virtually all cats are FECV seropositive.* FECV-seropositive cats can be adopted unless they are sick; under no circumstances should cats be euthanized solely on the basis of positive titers (using any test, including those serological tests purported to be FIP-specific). The available FIP vaccine has low efficacy both against FIP and FECV but appears safe. Since FECV and FIPV are almost impossible to prevent, the shelter's focus should be on keeping cats as well as possible and efficiently diagnosing cases that do occur. See Table 16.6.

GENITOURINARY INFECTIOUS DISEASE IN SHELTERS

Leptospira Interrogans

Leptospirosis is a zoonotic disease caused by several different serovars of *L. interrogans* acquired through exposure to infected animals and contamination in the environment. The bacteria are small, filamentous spirochetes that persist in the environ-

ment only when protected in moist areas. The common serovars in dogs are Bratislava, Pomona, grippotyphosa, icterohemorrhagiae, and canicola. Preparations from the latter two have been available in canine vaccines and their prevalences have declined significantly. Rodents are primary reservoirs for Bratislava and icterohemorrhagiae. Reservoirs for Pomona include large domestic and wild species such as pigs and skunks. Reservoirs for grippotyphosa are numerous including rodents, skunks, and opossums. In parts of California, Pomona and Bratislava infections are common in wild coyotes and mountain lions.

Dogs acquire the infection through ingestion of contaminated water or occasionally prey. The bacteria travel across mucous membranes, into the blood, to kidneys and other tissues. Classically, icterohemorrhagiae causes liver and renal disease, although most recently diagnosed cases have been associated with acute renal failure. Signs of leptospirosis in dogs include vomiting, icterus, petechiae, fever, tachypnea, and poor capillary refill time. Serum biochemistry reveals elevated creatinine and urea nitrogen, and possibly elevated liver enzymes as well. The diagnosis is confirmed by PCR of blood or urine or serology. If a panel of serovars is evaluated serologically, infected dogs typically will be seropositive to several, with the highest titer documenting the serovars to which the dog was exposed. Four-fold titer increases over 2-4 weeks is retrospective confirmation of active infection.

Treatment of individual dogs typically must be begun before the diagnosis is confirmed, based on compatible clinical signs. Such dogs should be treated with antibiotics and medical management for the renal failure, including fluids, mannitol or other drugs to promote urine production, and possibly hemodialysis. Appropriate antibiotics include penicillin and tetracycline-class drugs, which rapidly terminate the active infection. However, recovery of severely affected kidneys may take weeks if it occurs at all. It is not known at what point following antibiotic administration dogs no longer shed infectious leptospires, although it is thought to be relatively soon (within a few days). General recommendations include using doxycycline to eliminate the carrier state. Any dogs with suspect leptospirosis should only be available to the public with full informed consent.

Table 16.6. Characteristics of Pathogens Associated with Canine and Feline Vector-borne, Bite-transmitted, and Systemic Diseases

Organism	Mode of Transmission	Incubation Period/ Duration of Shedding	Asymptomatic Carriers?	Clinical Presentation, Typical	Optimal Diagnostic Tests	Optimal Therapy [a]	Zoonotic/ Herd Risk?
FELV	Direct contact	Variable/lifelong	Yes	Lymphadenopathy, weakness, fever	Ag ELISA	None [b]	H
FIV	Bite	Variable/lifelong	Yes	Lymphadenopathy-AIDS	Serology [c]	None [b]	H
Bartonella spp.	Flea	NA/21+ mos	Yes	None	PCR	None	Z
Anaplasma phagocytophilum	Ticks	4–10d/14–21 d	Yes	Fever, anemia	PCR	Tetracycline	Z
Ehrlichia canis	Ticks	4–10 d/yrs [d]	Yes	Fever, anemia	PCR	Tetracycline	Z
Rickettsia rickettsii	Ticks	2-24 d/wks	Yes	Fever, lymphadenopathy, thrombocytopenia, severe dermatitis	IFA + PCR	Tetracycline	Z
Borrelia burgdorferi	Ticks	Wks/indefinite	Yes	Arthritis	Western blot	Tetracycline	Z
Rabies	Bite	2–14 wks + /until dead	No	Neurological	Necropsy	None [b]	Z, H
Toxoplasma gondii	Fecal-oral	Variable	Yes	None to CNS	Serology + PCR	Clindamycin	Z
Mycoplasma hemofelis	Not known	1–2 wks/mos	Yes	None to anemia	CBC	Doxycycline	
FIP	Fecal-oral [c]	Up to 2 yrs/ until dead	No	Effusion or organ failure	Multifactorial [e]	None [b]	

[a] These therapies include off-label therapies and drugs that may present significant risk to some or all patients. Before use, shelter veterinarians are advised to read all of the relevant text in this book, consult a small animal medical text, and use proper medical judgment.

[b] Euthanasia is a strong consideration if diagnosis is confirmed.

[c] Antibodies are cross-reactive with vaccine strain and must be interpreted appropriately.

[d] These ehrlichiae may be acquired by feeding ticks throughout duration of shedding but are not directly transmissible. The dog may or may not enter an asymptomatic latent phase but progress to a chronic phase.

[c] Direct infection with FIPV is highly unlikely; see text for details.

[e] Complex diagnosis—see text for details.

[f] Agent is environmentally persistent and contamination of the environment is a problem in herd management. None of the agents in this table have this characteristic.

H: important threat to herd in shelters

Z: zoonotic

Herd management for leptospirosis should include vaccination, appropriate facility decontamination, and management of potentially infectious dogs. Especially in areas where leptospirosis has been reported in dogs, vaccination should include all available serovars. Leptospires persist in moist areas in their environment, so appropriate use of bleach, reducing standing water, and preventing dogs access to possibly contaminated water sources near shelters can minimize risk. The exact timing and drug-dependence of cessation of *Leptospira* shedding are not known but common practice is to use doxycycline orally for 7-14 days after the dog has recovered to ensure eradication of a carrier state. Dogs can be adopted with informed consent of the owners when clinically stable.

Brucella canis

Brucella canis is an obligate intracellular Gram-negative pathogen of dogs. It is transmitted directly dog to dog via venereal or oral exposure, especially during estrus, breeding, and abortion. The bacterium also can be transferred transplacentally. Cats and humans are relatively resistant, although humans can acquire the infection as a zoonosis. Humans acquire the infection through exposure to urine and reproductive discharges of infected dogs. It can also be spread to humans via sexual contact with an infected animal and is thus a potential concern in cases of zoophilia or bestiality. Veterinarians who are involved in cruelty case investigations should be aware of this possibility.

It is more of a problem in the elderly and children. In dogs, infection may be chronic over weeks to years, especially residing in the prostate of male dogs. Infection is more common in poorly managed breeding populations.

Clinical disease in dogs often is subtle, with reduced fertility but normal estrous, abortion, permanent male infertility, testicular swelling, or scrotal dermatitis and atrophy. In infected testes, there is sperm leakage, the dog develops anti-sperm antibodies, and may develop delayed-type hypersensitivity. Other forms of canine brucellosis are vertebral osteomyelitis, diskospondylitis, lymphadenopathy, and immune complex disease in eyes, kidneys, and meninges.

In suspect dogs, serum biochemistry may reveal hyperglobulinemia. Rapid slide agglutination has decent sensitivity but low specificity (as do other serological tests such as complement fixation and agar gel immunodiffusion). False positive test results occur in animals infected with *Pseudomonas*, *Bordetella*, *Yersinia*, *Actinobacillus*, and in some breeds (for example, wolfhound). False negatives occur early in infection, and during chronic infection in females; serology is more likely to be positive during estrus. Blood culture is a much more precise way to evaluate possibly infected dogs and to evaluate their response to treatment. On cytology of suspected lesions, Kinyoun's acid-fast testing reveals red coccobacilli, and, in the testes, abnormal sperm. Finally, PCR testing is specific and sensitive. Any dogs with vertebral pain, swollen testicles, or a history of abortion should be tested (by blood culture) before adoption.

Treatment is most successful if the affected tissue is removed, often including neutering the dog using universal precautions. Antibiotics must penetrate the prostate and cells: possibilities include trimethoprim sulfonamide, minocycline, and tetracycline, although the rate of cure is only moderate. A confirmed-positive dog is a strong candidate for euthanasia because of the zoonotic risk and strong likelihood that the dog will be a permanent carrier.

Coxiella burnettii (Q fever)

C. burnettii is a rickettsial pathogen that causes Q fever most notably in sheep, goats, and cats. Infection is transmitted by tick, direct exposure to infectious fluids such as the vaginal discharge that accompanies abortions and live births, and via exposure to the environmentally resistant spores. More than 40 different tick species may participate in maintaining the infection in nature and transmitting it to domestic animals. Sheep and goats are particularly important in zoonotic disease because they achieve such high levels of bacteria in infectious material.

Once inoculated into a susceptible host, *C. burnettii* targets and reproduces in epithelia and endothelium, leading to vasculitis, necrotizing pneumonitis and necrotic vasculitis in other organs. Immune complexes are produced, possibly leading to immune-mediated problems associated with deposition in the joints, anterior chamber of the eye, and kidneys. Clinical disease ranges from no signs to pneumonia to abortion. After infection, the hosts may shed *C. burnettii* in urine, milk, feces, and especially in placental fluids/tissue; in cats, shedding may last for a month or more. People usually acquire Q fever by inhalation, and develop organ failure, vasculitis, chronic endocarditis, and other problems. It is one of the zoonotic diseases recognized by the government as a potential biological weapon.

Animals with Q fever may have lymphocytosis and thrombocytopenia. If Q fever is suspected, the diagnosis may be confirmed with a four-fold rise in titer (more than 4 weeks). Phase I antigens are those from the organism while in the host and are usually low in acutely ill patients and higher in chronic infection. Phase II antigens are present in the bacteria following repeated in vitro passage. Additionally, PCR will help diagnose acute infections. The treatments of choice for Q fever include tetracycline, chloramphenicol, or enrofloxacin. Trimethoprim-sulfonamide and erythromycin are variably effective. To decontaminate the environment, bleach, UV light, heat, and desiccation are not effective. Alcohol applied for 30 minutes and allowed to evaporate will kill the bacteria. Other important ways to prevent zoonotic disease are to eliminate ticks and to reduce exposure to infected hoofstock and cats, especially during parturition or abortion.

Canine Herpesvirus

Canine herpesvirus is an alpha-herpesvirus with only moderate (approximately 50 percent) genetic homology with feline herpesvirus. The only known hosts for canine herpesvirus are dogs and other members of the family Canidae. Transmission among dogs occurs in utero, during parturition, or via exposure to virus in oculonasal secretions. The course of disease depends upon the age and route of exposure. If the dog is greater than a month old, epithelial and lymphoid tissue in a number of locations may be infected but the dog often does not become severely ill. Genital vesicular lesions may contain herpesvirus, and some bitches may develop vaginal hyperemia. Herpesvirus is often recovered from respiratory secretions of dogs with kennel cough with unknown significance.

In utero infection may lead to abortion of the pups with no clinical signs in the bitch. If pups are born, they usually develop systemic disease within a week. Infection acquired at parturition also induces systemic fatal disease, often with disseminated intravascular coagulopathy. After prolifera-

tion in epithelium and viremia, renal and hepatic failure occur due to hemorrhagic necrosis. Other affected organs include lungs, trigeminal nerves, and brain. Occasionally, pups of seropositive bitches survive although often with permanent CNS lesions.

Herpesvirus present classically with pups dying between 1-3 weeks old. On physical examination, there may be serous or purulent rhinitis, petechiation on mucosa, vesicular lesions in the vulva, and depression. In older dogs, physical examination may not reveal disease, although infection becomes apparent if the bitch becomes pregnant. The diagnosis of herpesvirus depends on appropriate recognition of clinical syndromes followed by specific diagnostic testing. Gross necropsy may reveal diffuse ecchymotic hemorrhage on abdominal organs with grayish discoloration, serous abdominal fluid, splenomegaly, and lymphadenomegaly. Serology indicates previous exposure and is supportive evidence for a diagnosis with appropriate clinical disease. On culture of the virus on a variety of canine cell lines, there is a distinctive cytopathic effect. Good samples to submit are swabs of respiratory or genital discharge or spleen, kidney, or liver of dead puppies.

Given that very few dogs in shelters are breeding, the major management implications are for ensuring the well-being of neonates born to pregnant bitches in the shelter. Herpesvirus is particularly important in breeding kennels, where infection is maintained via infected dogs. The virus is susceptible to most disinfectants and is not persistent in the environment.

Individual dogs with herpesvirus rarely respond to therapy and may have permanent neurological or other impairments if they do survive. Possible treatment protocols include hyperimmune serum, elevating the temperature of the puppies, and acyclovir. Hyperimmune serum is harvested from bitches that had herpesvirus-infected litters over the last 6 months and is injected intraperitoneally into affected puppies. Elevation of body temperature is performed in order to inhibit viral replication, but is difficult to maintain. The effect should be measured by monitoring the puppy's rectal temperature and the goal should be 102-103°F. Acyclovir treatment is helpful according to anecdotes but only in conjunction with other supportive measures. See Table 16.7.

Table 16.7. Characteristics of Canine and Feline Genitourinary Pathogens

Organism	Mode of Transmission	Incubation Period/ Duration of Shedding	Asymp-tomatic Carriers?	Clinical Presentation, Typical	Optimal Diagnostic Tests	Optimal Therapy[a]	Zoonotic/ Herd Risk?
Leptospira interrogans	Urine and rodents	3–14 d/mos	Possibly	Renal failure	PCR	Ampicillin, doxycycline	Z
Brucella canis	Urine, sexual	1–8 wks/> 60 wks	Yes	Lymphadenopathy, orchitis, abortion	Culture	Tetracycline [b]	Z
Coxiella burnetii.	Vector and direct	4–30 d/30–70 d	Yes	Lymphadenopathy	Serology	Doxycycline [b]	Z
Canine herpesvirus	Direct, fomites	3–4 d/ indef recrudescence	Yes	None	PCR	Acyclovir, supportive	

[a] These therapies include off-label therapies and drugs that may present significant risk to some or all patients. Before use, shelter veterinarians are advised to read all of the relevant text in this book, consult a small animal medical text, and use proper medical judgment.

[b] Euthanasia is a strong consideration if diagnosis is confirmed.

[c] Agent is environmentally persistent, and contamination of the environment is a problem in herd management. None of the agents in this table have this characteristic.

H: important threat to herd in shelters

Z: zoonotic

ZOONOSIS

Zoonotic infections are transmissible to human beings from animals. These infections include directly transmissible infections such as rabies, in which the animal population is the reservoir, vector-borne infections such as Lyme disease and ehrlichiosis in which the animal or the vector functions as the reservoir, and infections in which the humans actually maintain the infection in nature (that is, humans function as reservoir) but animals may become infected, such as for *Mycobacterium tuberculosis*. This latter case generally is referred to as an anthroponosis.

A shelter veterinarian is more likely to see and diagnose zoonotic infectious diseases in dogs and cats than veterinarians in private practice. The most important reason is that shelter veterinarians typically see a very high volume of animals, especially in municipal (animal control) shelters. Additionally, animal shelter populations are characterized by turnover, with low prospects for herd immunity. Animals may have been roaming before entering a shelter and may have *sampled* diseases from many different locations, statistically increasing the likelihood of zoonotic diseases. Many times, animals entering shelters have compromised innate immune protection (reduced colonization resistance), because of previous poor care, poor standards of nutrition, high frequency of concurrent infection, lack of previous vaccination and medical treatment, and stress. Once in the shelter, animals may experience various different environmental factors that promote zoonotic diseases, including high animal density; structural features like crumbling paint, open drains, porous and concrete surfaces that make disinfection difficult or impossible; and iatrogenic activities such as vaccination and administration of antibiotic. The use of vaccines and antibiotics may modify the host's colonization resistance and, while treating or preventing some infections, increase the risk of others. Lastly, many previously untrained animals do not behave well in shelters. Bites and scratches are major risks, and untrained or nonvigilant staff and the public can dramatically increase the prospects of spread of zoonotic infections.

General measures may reduce the risk of zoonotic disease in shelters. Staff members and volunteers should know what universal precautions are and use them while in the shelter. The importance of frequent handwashing cannot be overemphasized. The staff should have adequate protective equipment and training to allow them to protect themselves, such as muzzles, jab sticks to administer medication or euthanasia solution, enough other staff to properly manage animals, properly placed and constructed feral cat cages to avoid direct contact, and so forth. The medical team can take the lead in protecting against zoonotic infections by adopting protocols that maximize herd and individual immunity among the animals. These include proper vaccination regimes (not over- or undervaccinating), appropriate use of antibiotics, management of animals to reduce stress, crowding, excessive contact among animals, and so forth. The shelter management staff can help protect against zoonoses through appropriate disinfection protocols, providing pre-exposure prophylaxis against rabies, and ensuring that staff have adequate health insurance.

Finally, shelter veterinarians have a responsibility, to the extent possible, to protect the public against zoonoses originating in shelter animals. Complete protection is not possible, for several reasons. Some zoonotic infections are not associated with clinical signs and, thus, nothing tips off medical professionals that the animal may present a zoonotic threat. Secondly, testing for some zoonoses is extremely difficult, expensive, or lacks sensitivity or specificity. Thirdly, some zoonotic risks are quite minimal and, thus, only become a significant problem in households where there is a person with immunocompromise. If a risk to the public is posed, the shelter has a duty to educate the public of the risks and to try to minimize those risks. Table 16.8 provides information that describes many of the zoonotic hazards in shelters and provides guidelines for testing and adoptability.

Table 16.8 Zoonotic Diseases

Taxonomic Group	Species of Pathogen	Route of Zoonosis	Testing[1]	Adoptability[2]
Virus	Rabies	Bite	A	DNA
Bacteria	*Anaplasma phagocytophila*	Tick		A
	Bartonella	Bite, scratch, flea	P	AWT
	Bordetella bronchiseptica	Aerosol	P	AWT
	Borrelia burgdorferi	Tick		A
	Brachyspira pilosicoli	Feces	P	AWT
	Brucella canis	Urine	A	DNA
	Campylobacter	Feces	P	AWR
	Capnocytophaga canimorsus	Bite		AWT
	Coxiella burnettii	Genital and placental tissue	A	AWR/DNA
	E. coli	Feces		AWT
	Francisella	Aerosol, tick	A	DNA
	Helicobacter	Feces		AWT
	Leptospira interrogans	Urine	A	AWR
	Pasteurella	Bite		A
	Plesiomonas	Feces, environment		A
	Rickettsia felis and rickettsii	Flea	A	AWT
	Salmonella	Feces	A	AWT
	Yersinia pestis, enterocolitica	Aerosol, flea	A	DNA
Fungi	Aspergillus	Environment		A
	Blastomyces	Environment		A
	Coccidiodes	Environment	A	A
	Cryptococcus	Environment	A	AWT
	Dermatophytes	Direct exposure	A	AWT
	Histoplasma	Environment		A
	Sporothrix schenkii	Environment, scratch	A	AWT
Protozoa	Cryptosporidium	Feces	P	AWT
	Giardia	Feces	A	AWT
	Toxoplasma gondii	Feces	P	AWT
Helminths	*Ancylostoma caninum*	Feces	A	AWT
	Tapeworms	Flea		AWT
	Toxocara	Feces	A	AWT
Arthropods	*Cheyletiella parasitovorax*	Direct	A	AWT
	Fleas	Direct	A	AWT
	Sarcoptes mites	Direct	A	AWT
	Ticks	Direct		A

[1]Recommendations for testing: Always (A), included in a profile when a client household has an immunocompromised member; (P), not necessary or recommended in most situations because tests are poor, unavailable, or risk to public very low.

[2]Recommendations for adoption: (A), adoptable with minimal or no risk; (AWT), adoptable if treated, pathogen eradicated *AND* this is feasible *OR* there is little risk *to immunocompetent owners* even if pathogen persists; (AWR), adoptable only with significant restrictions—new owner must understand nature of risk; (DNA), strongly advisable not to adopt, or adoption absolutely unacceptable.

REFERENCES

Appel, M. 1987. Canine adenovirus type 2 (infectious laryngotracheitis virus), in *Virus infections of carnivores*. M. Appel (ed.), Elsevier, Amsterdam, 45-51.

Axthelm, M. K., and S. Krakowka. 1998. Experimental old dog encephalitis (ODE) in a gnotobiotic dog. *Veterinary Pathology* (35): 527–34.

Barr, S. C. 1998. Enteric protozoal infections in *Infectious diseases of the dog and cat* C. Greene (ed.), Philadelphia, PA: Saunders, 9–22.

Baumgärtner, W. K., S. Krakowka, et al. 1982. Acute encephalitis and hydrocephalus in dogs caused by canine parainfluenza virus. *Veterinary Pathology* (19):79–92.

Bemis, D. A., H. A. Greisen, et al. 1977. Pathogenesis of canine bordetellosis. *Journal of Infectious Diseases* (135):753–62.

Binns, S. H., A. J. Speakman, et al. 1998. The use of pulsed-field gel electrophoresis to examine the epidemiology of *Bordetella bronchiseptica* isolated from cats and other species. *Epidemiology and Infection* (120):201–8.

Birkenheuer, A. J., M. G. Levy, et al. 1999. *Babesia gibsoni* infections in dogs from North Carolina. *Journal of the American Animal Hospital Association* (35):125–8.

Chomel, B., K. MacDonald, et al. 2001. Aortic valve endocarditis in a dog due to *Bartonella clarridgeiae*. *Journal of Clinical Microbiology* (39):3548–3554.

Chomel, B. B., M. T. Jay, et al. 1994. Serological surveillance of plague in dogs and cats, California, 1979–1991. *Comparative Immunology, Microbiology, and Infectious Disease* (17):111–23.

Coutts, A. J., S. Dawson, et al. 1996. Studies on natural transmission of *Bordetella bronchiseptica* in cats. *Veterinary Microbiology* (48):19–27.

Cross, R., and R. Claflin. 1962. *Bordetella bronchiseptica*-induced porcine atrophic rhinitis. *Journal of the American Veterinary Medical Association* (141):1467–1468.

Dambach, D. M., C. A. Smith, et al. 1997. Morphologic, immunohistochemical, and ultrastructural characterization of a distinctive renal lesion in dogs putatively associated with *Borrelia burgdorferi* infection: 49 cases (1987–1992). *Veterinary Pathology* (34):85–96.

Dawson, S., D. Jones, et al. 2000. *Bordetella bronchiseptica* infection in cats following contact with infected dogs. *Veterinary Record* (146):46–8.

Dorin, S., W. Miller, et al. 1993. Diagnosing and treating chlamydial conjunctivitis in cats. *Veterinary Medicine: Small Animal Clinics* (April):322–330.

Duhamel, G. E., D. J. Trott, et al. 1998. Canine intestinal spirochetes consist of *Serpulina pilosicoli* and a newly identified group provisionally designated "*Serpulina canis*" sp. nov. *Journal of Clinical Microbiology* (36):2264–70.

Dumler, S., K. Asanovich, et al. 1995. Serologic cross-reactions among *Ehrlichia equi, Ehrlichia phagocytophila*, and human granulocytic ehrlichia. *Journal of Clinical Microbiology* (33):1098–1103.

Fenwick, S. G., P. Madie, et al. 1994. Duration of carriage and transmission of *Yersinia enterocolitica* biotype 4, serotype 0:3 in dogs. *Epidemiology and Infection* (113):471–7.

Foley, J., S. Harrus, et al. 1998. Molecular, clinical, and pathological comparison of two distinct strains of *Hemobartonella felis* in domestic cats. *American Journal of Veterinary Research* (59):1581–1588.

Foley, J., C. Rand, et al. In press. Molecular epidemiology of feline bordetellosis in two animal shelters and the role of cats as a reservoir for canine kennel cough. *Preventive Veterinary Medicine*.

Foley, J. E., A. Poland, et al. 1997. Risk factors for feline infectious peritonitis among cats in multiple-cat environments with endemic feline enteric coronavirus. *Journal of the American Veterinary Medical Association* (210):1313–1318.

Goodnow, R. A. 1980. Biology of *Bordetella bronchiseptica*. *Microbiological Review* (44):722–38.

Gookin, J. L., E. B. Breitschwerdt, et al. 1999. Diarrhea associated with trichomonosis in cats. *Journal of the American Veterinary Medical Association* (215):1450–4.

Goossens, H., B. Giesendorf, et al. 1995. Investigation of an outbreak of *Campylobacter upsaliensis* in day care centers in Brussels: analysis of relationships among isolates by phenotypic and genotypic typing methods. *Journal of Infectious Diseases* (172):1298–1305.

Greene, C., and M. J. Appel. 1998. Canine distemper, in *Infectious diseases of the dog and cat*. C. Greene (ed.), Philadelphia, PA: Saunders, 9–22.

Gueirard, P., C. Weber, et al. 1995. Human *Bordetella bronchiseptica* infection related to contact with infected animals: Persistence of bacteria in host. *Journal of Clinical Microbiology* (33):2002–6.

Guillot, J., E. Malandain, et al. 2002. Evaluation of the efficacy of oral lufenuron combined with topical enilconazole for the management of dermatophytosis in catteries. *Veterinary Record* (150):714–8.

Haesebrouck, F., L. A. Devriese, et al. 1991. Incidence and significance of isolation of *Mycoplasma felis* from conjunctival swabs of cats. *Veterinary Microbiology* (26):95–101.

Hald, B., and M. Madsen. 1997. Healthy puppies and kittens as carriers of *Campylobacter* spp., with special reference to *Campylobacter upsaliensis*. *Journal of Clinical Microbiology* (35):3351–3352.

Hargis, A. M., and P. E. Ginn. 1999. Feline herpesvirus 1-associated facial and nasal dermatitis and stomatitis in domestic cats. *Veterinary Clinics of North America. Small Animal Practice* (29):1281–90.

Hnilica, K. A., and L. Medleau. 2002. Evaluation of topically applied enilconazole for the treatment of dermatophytosis in a Persian cattery. *Veterinary Dermatology* (13):23–8.

Jacobs, A. A., W. S. Chalmers, et al. 1993. Feline bordetellosis: Challenge and vaccine studies. *Veterinary Record* (133):260–3.

Macartney, L., H. Cornwell, et al. 1985. Isolation of a novel paramyxovirus from a dog with enteric disease. *Veterinary Record* (117):205–207.

Macintire, D. K., M. K. Boudreaux, et al. 2002. Babesia gibsoni infection among dogs in the southeastern United States. *Journal of the American Veterinary Medical Association* (220):325–9.

Maggs, D. J., M. R. Lappin, et al. 1999. Evaluation of serologic and viral detection methods for diagnosing feline herpesvirus-1 infection in cats with acute respiratory tract or chronic ocular disease. *Journal of the American Veterinary Medical Association* (214):502–7.

Magyar, T., N. Chanter, et al. 1988. The pathogenesis of turbinate atrophy in pigs caused by *Bordetella bronchiseptica*. *Veterinary Microbiology* (18):135–46.

Marks, S. L., A. Melli, et al. 1999. Evaluation of methods to diagnose *Clostridium perfringens*-associated diarrhea in dogs. *Journal of the American Veterinary Medical Association* (214):357–60.

Moise, N. S., J. W. Crissman, et al. 1983. *Mycoplasma gateae* arthritis and tenosynovitis in cats: case report and experimental reproduction of the disease. *American Journal of Veterinary Research* (44):16–21.

Neimark, H., K.E. Johansson, et al. 2001. Proposal to transfer some members of the genera Haemobartonella and Eperythrozoon to the genus Mycoplasma with descriptions of 'Candidatus Mycoplasma haemofelis,' 'Candidatus haemomuris,' 'Candidatus Mycoplasma haemosnis' and 'Candidatus Mycoplasma wenyonii'. *International Journal of Systematic and Evolutionary Microbiology* (51): 891–9.

Pedersen, N. 1995. The history and interpretation of feline coronavirus serology. *Feline Practice* (23):46–52.

Pedersen, N. C., J. W. Black, et al. 1983. Pathogenic differences between various feline coronavirus isolates. *Advances in Experimental Medicine and Biology* (173):365–380.

Pedersen, N. C., J. B. Elliott, et al. 2000. An isolated epizootic of hemorrhagic-like fever in cats caused by a novel and highly virulent strain of feline calicivirus. *Veterinary Microbiology* (73):281–300.

Perez, M., Y. Rikihisa, et al. 1996. Ehrlichia canis-like agent isolated from a man in Venezuela: Antigenic and genetic characterization. *Journal of Clinical Microbiology* (34):2133–2139.

Randall, R. E., D. F. Young, et al. 1987. Isolation and characterization of monoclonal antibodies to simian virus 5 and their use in revealing antigenic differences between human, canine and simian isolates. *Journal of General Virology* (68):2769–80.

Rima, B. K., K. Baczko, et al. 1987. Humoral immune response in dogs with old dog encephalitis and chronic distemper meningo-encephalitis. *Journal of General Virology* (68 [Pt 6]):1723–35.

Taboada, J., J. W. Harvey, et al. 1992. Seroprevalence of babesiosis in Greyhounds in Florida. *Journal of the American Veterinary Medical Association* (200): 47–50.

Tilley, L. and F. W.K. Smith Jr. 1997. *The Five Minute Veterinary Consult, Canine and Feline,* Baltimore, MD: Williams and Wilkins.

Vennema, H., A. Poland, et al. 1998. Feline infectious peritonitis viruses arise by mutation from endemic feline enteric coronaviruses. *Virology* (243):150–157.

Vieler, E., W. Herbst, et al. 1994. Isolation of a parainfluenzavirus type 2 from the prostatic fluid of a dog. *Veterinary Record* (135):384–5.

Welsh, R. D. 1996. *Bordetella bronchiseptica* infections in cats. *Journal of the American Animal Hospital Association* (32):153–8.

White-Weithers, N., and L. Medleau. 1995. Evaluation of topical therapies for the treatment of dermatophyte-infected hairs from dogs and cats. *Journal of the American Animal Hospital Association* (31):250–3.

Willoughby, K., S. Dawson, et al. 1991. Isolation of *B. bronchiseptica* from kittens with pneumonia in a breeding cattery. *Veterinary Record* (129):407–8.

Woolfrey, B. F., and J. A. Moody. 1991. Human infections associated with *Bordetella bronchiseptica*. *Clinical Microbiological Review* (4):243–55.

Wright, N. G., H. Thompson, et al. 1973. *Bordetella bronchiseptica*: A re-assessment of its role in canine respiratory disease. *Veterinary Record* (93):486–7.

17
Vaccination Strategies in the Animal Shelter Environment

Richard B. Ford

INTRODUCTION

The principles of infectious disease management (diagnosis, treatment, and prevention) are well known and routinely applied in companion animal practice today. And, in companion animal practice, they have proven highly effective. Yet, applying such time-honored principles of infection control, as anyone who has tried knows, can become ineffective and even inappropriate when attempting to do battle against the daily surge of infected, contagious dogs and cats presented to animal shelters throughout North America today. Companion animals residing in shelters, where overcrowding and incredibly high turnover rates are the norm, face the highest risk of exposure to infectious diseases. Infection rates soar despite implementation of expensive vaccination strategies, regimens of 'extreme' cleaning and disinfection, and euthanasia of all animals that screen positive on laboratory tests or just appear sick. Although it may be argued that we're doing the best we can with the technology available, the fact is, infectious disease management strategies in the shelter environment have not yet become the subject of sound scientific scrutiny. Overcrowding and high turnover rates are not going to change. But the ability to tailor diagnostic testing and disease prevention strategies within shelters, to maximize the impact of a health care program in shelter, and to do so on a cost-effective basis, are goals that demand immediate attention.

For those who are new to the challenges afforded by practicing veterinary medicine within the shelter environment, perhaps one of the most basic, if not important, lessons is the fundamental principles of vaccination, infection control, and health risk assessment routinely applied in clinical companion animal practice simply do not apply in the shelter environment. In companion animal practice, prevention of infectious diseases is well defined and somewhat procedural. The initial series of vaccines are administered somewhere between 6 and 16 weeks of age and then annually thereafter; puppies and kittens are empirically treated for intestinal parasites, and the usually life-long ritual of administering heartworm preventative to dogs, and some cats, begins around 3 to 4 months of age. And life is good. Such preventive care practices have proven to be incredibly effective at minimizing the occurrence of serious illness among millions of pet dogs and cats. Considering the relatively low risk of exposure most pets will face in a lifetime, why shouldn't they?

But all things are not necessarily as they should be . . . obviously, millions of dogs and cats don't have access to this level of health care early in life and, as such, face a substantially greater risk of exposure to infectious diseases and much higher incidence of infection. Companion animals residing in shelters throughout North America are certainly among those facing the highest risk. Overcrowding and incredibly high turnover rates are easily blamed for the high rates of infection and illness. However, another major contributor, not to be ignored, is the lack of sound infectious disease management strategies appropriate to high-risk environments. The fact is that we have really never studied infectious disease management strategies within the shelter environment. But, the dedication and commitment of veterinarians who do practice shelter medicine will have a substantial impact on meeting the health needs of this very unique population of companion animals.

To practice shelter medicine is to practice in an environment where eradication of infectious diseases is not an attainable goal. The challenge at hand, therefore, is to minimize the spread of diverse infections within a high-density, "high risk" patient population and maintain the health of those individuals that have not become the target of infectious agents. When the overall purpose is to place *healthy* pets into welcoming homes, the time and effort dedicated to controlling infectious disease is but one, of many, variables in the complex shelter-medicine equation. It's a variable for which there is a paucity of science needed to make rational, economically responsible decisions. What follows is an attempt to address some of the shelter-unique clinical strategies pertaining to control of infectious diseases that pose the greatest threat to animals residing within shelter populations. This is only a beginning. . . when it comes to advancing the practice of shelter medicine on a scientific basis, the 'brain-trust' is much less likely to be found among the faculty of veterinary schools than among those veterinarians who, on a daily basis, deal with the challenges of shelter medicine. Your comments and critique of the points made in this chapter are actively solicited as is your insight and experience.

SELECTION OF ANTIGENS

In small animal practice today, there is a general consensus that veterinarians are vaccinating too often, and with too many vaccines. In fact, the real issue surrounding dog and cat vaccination programs is to determine which vaccines are indicated, and which are not, in light of the risk of exposure and likelihood of infection. As expected, surveys of companion animal practitioners and veterinary teaching hospitals on vaccination protocols indicate that there is very little agreement within the profession on which vaccines should be administered and when (Mansfield, 1996). In shelters, there hasn't even been a survey!

Recently recommended vaccination guidelines for dogs and cats have focused on so-called **core** and **noncore** vaccines (American Association of Feline Practitioners [AAFP] 2000, American Animal Hospital Association [AAHA] 2003). **Core** vaccines are those recommended for administration to every dog/cat presented to the practice. Recom-

mendations for designating a particular vaccine as **core** are determined by 1) severity of disease, 2) transmissibility to other animals, and 3) the potential for a particular infection to be zoonotic. **Noncore** vaccines, on the other hand, would be recommended to clientele when a known or likely risk is anticipated or when an animal's lifestyle represents a reasonable risk of exposure to the infectious agent. Examples include feline leukemia virus (FeLV) and feline infectious peritonitis (FIP) virus and canine Lyme borreliosis vaccine.

Another issue pertaining to the selection of vaccines is the administration of modified-live virus (MLV) versus killed virus vaccine. Although recommendations against administration of multivalent, MLV vaccines were made several years ago (AVMA, 1989), most veterinarians continue to administer MLV biologicals. This is certainly justified since these products do provide a sustained immune response when compared to killed virus products. Furthermore, no data demonstrate that there are significant advantages to using killed virus vaccines over MLV vaccines. The suggestion that MLV vaccines pose an unreasonable safety risk is largely anecdotal and without scientific merit.

Implications for Shelter Medicine

There are no standardized formulae for absolute success with antigen selection in a shelter considering the numerous variables: shelter finances, euthanasia versus No-Kill policies, staff experience/ knowledge base with infectious disease (from cleaning to screening), census, concurrent illnesses, holding times, season of the year, construction, air exchange . . . to name a few. Therefore, in the absence of clear recommendations on which vaccines to use and when, the concept of **core** versus **noncore** vaccines seems especially applicable in the shelter setting. First, it offers an opportunity to provide broad-spectrum immunity against those pathogens most likely to be encountered in the shelter; second, defining and using only **core** vaccines supports cost control measures and budgeting efforts; and third, it's easy to communicate **core** vaccine protocols to minimally trained shelter personnel who may be responsible for administering vaccines. Tables 17.1 and 17.2 (canine) and 17.4 and 17.5 (feline) represent an attempt to define **core** and **noncore** vaccine administration schedules, respectively, appropriate for dogs and cats presented

Table 17.1. Canine **Core** Vaccine Administration Schedule Recommended for Use in Animal Shelters

Vaccine	Primary Vaccination for Puppies (≤ 16 weeks of age)	Primary Vaccination for Adults (≥ 16 weeks of age)	Comments
Canine Distemper Virus + Canine Adenovirus-2 + Parainfluenza Virus + Canine Parvovirus (MLV) Combination product administered SQ or IM.	Administer one dose on admission. **Repeat in** two weeks if still in the shelter.	Administer one dose on admission.	Ideally puppies should be vaccinated beginning at 6 weeks to eight weeks of age. Nursing history is not always available.
Rabies one-year (killed) Route of administration may *not* be optional See product literature for details.	Administer one dose as early as three months of age. Administer at the time of release from the shelter.	Administer one dose at the time of release from the shelter.	**Booster vaccination due in one year for all dogs.** Local statues apply. **There is no medical indication to vaccinate against rabies at the time of admission to the shelter** Separate regulations may apply to those dogs being held on rabies quarantine.
Rabies three-year (killed) Route of administration may *not* be optional See product literature for details.	*Note:* **Normally,** *rabies virus labeled as three-year would* **not** *be indicated in puppies. In selected situations, however, the three-year rabies vaccine may be used as an alternative to the one-year rabies vaccine for initial and subsequent doses. Local statutes apply.* Administer one dose as early as three months of age. Administer one dose at the time of release from the shelter.	*Note: In selected situations, the three-year rabies vaccine may be used as an alternative to the one-year rabies vaccine for initial and subsequent doses. Local statutes apply.* Administer at the time of release from the shelter.	**Booster vaccination due in one year for all dogs.** Local statues apply. **There is no medical indication to vaccinate against rabies at the time of admission to the shelter.** Separate rule may apply to those dogs being held on rabies quarantine.

NOTE: Route of administration is SQ or IM unless otherwise noted by the manufacturer.

287

Table 17.2. Administration Schedule for Canine **Noncore** or **Optional** Vaccines Selected for Use in Animal Shelters

Vaccine	Primary Vaccination for Puppies (≤ 16 weeks of age)	Primary Vaccination for Adults (≥ 16 weeks of age)	Comments
Canine Distemper-Measles Combination (MLV) **Intramuscular administration**	**One** dose between 4 and 12 weeks of age.	Not indicated. This vaccine should NOT be used in dogs over 12 weeks of age.	Vaccine is intended to provide temporary protection in puppies ≤ 12 weeks of age only. **Use only** in those environments where CDV is a recognized problem.
Bordetella bronchiseptica (killed bacterin-parenteral)	Administer 1 dose as early as 6 weeks of age at the time of admission. A second dose is required 2–4 weeks following the first dose	Not stipulated; however, two doses are recommended 2–4 weeks apart to maximize the immune response to the killed *B. bronchiseptica* bacterin.	With the possible exception of vaccinating puppies, topical vaccination is not necessarily superior to parenteral vaccination when administering parenteral vaccine to adult dogs. This is especially true when administering booster vaccination to adult dogs.
Bordetella bronchiseptica (killed bacterin-parenteral) + **Canine Parainfluenza Virus**	Administer 1 dose at the time of admission. A second dose is required 2–4 weeks following the first dose.	Not stipulated; however, 2 doses are recommended 2–4 weeks apart to maximize the immune response to the killed *B. bronchiseptica* bacterin.	With the possible exception of vaccinating puppies, topical vaccination is not necessarily superior to parenteral vaccination when administering parenteral vaccine to adult dogs. This is especially true when administering booster vaccination to adult dogs.
Bordetella bronchiseptica (live avirulent bacterin) + **Parainfluenza Virus** (MLV) + **Canine Adenovirus-2** (MLV) **Intranasal use only**	Administer a single dose as early as **three weeks of age.** (See product literature for specific age recommendations)	Not stipulated, although a single dose is recommended.	**Intranasal** vaccine is recommended in puppies **over** parenteral vaccine since the vaccine: 1) can be administered to puppies < 6 weeks of age; and 2) has a relatively rapid (48 to 72 hours?) onset of action.

Table 172. (*continued*)

Vaccine	Primary Vaccination for Puppies (≤ 16 weeks of age)	Primary Vaccination for Adults (≥ 16 weeks of age)	Comments
rLyme borreliosis *Borrelia burgdorferi* (recombinant-Outer Surface Protein A) Limited use in endemic regions	If an initial dose is given on admission, it should not be given earlier than 9 wks of age. A second dose is required in 2–3 wks	2 doses, 2–4 weeks apart are required.	Most shelters should not routinely administer Lyme borreliosis vaccine since risk of exposure/infection in the individual dog is best determined after placement.
• **Lyme borreliosis** *Borrelia burgdorferi* • (killed, whole cell bacterin) Limited use in endemic regions	Administer a single dose at 9 *or* 12 weeks of age (see manufacturer's recommendations. A second dose is required 2–4 weeks later	2 doses, 2–4 weeks are required.	Most shelters should not routinely administer Lyme borreliosis vaccine since risk of exposure/infection in the individual dog is best determined after placement.
Leptospirosis • (*L. canicola* combined with *L. icterohaemorrhagiae*) • (killed bacterin)	Not recommended for administration to dogs less than 12 weeks of age. IF administered, two doses must be administered 2–4 weeks apart.	IF administered, two doses are **required**, 2–4 weeks apart.	Cost: benefit value to shelters has not been determined. **Not generally recommended without knowledge that infection with either serovar is known to occur in the community**
•**Leptospirosis** • (*L. grippotyphosa* combined with *L. pomona*) (killed bacterin) • May be combined with: *L. canicola* & *L. icterohaemorrhagiae*)	Not recommended for administration to dogs less than 12 weeks of age. IF administered, two doses must be administered 2–4 weeks apart.	IF administered, two doses are **required**, 2–4 weeks apart.	Cost:benefit value to shelters has not been determined. **Not generally recommended without knowledge that infection with either serovar is known to occur in the community.**

NOTE: The letter "r" preceding the name of the antigen denotes the vaccine is recombinant.
NOTE: Route of administration is SQ or IM unless otherwise noted by the manufacturer.

to animal shelters. Tables 17.3 and 17.6 list vaccines that have little or no role in routine canine and feline immunization programs in shelters. These schedules are **not** intended to represent vaccination standards, only guidelines. They are, in effect, a proposed starting point from which a more tailored, refined vaccination protocol can be developed for the individual facility. One point, however, is worth emphasizing: Individual shelters should actively strive to establish and publish policies that define which vaccines will be administered to which age groups (puppies/kittens versus adult dogs/cats) and when (that is, on admission or following placement). Doing so sends a clear message to all personnel exactly what vaccination protocols are in place and how they should be implemented. Standardizing vaccination protocols within the shelter serves to provide a reasonable means for delivering consistent immunoprophylaxis, minimizing risk of transmission of serious infectious diseases, and minimizing economic losses associated with administering unnecessary vaccines.

ROUTE OF ADMINISTRATION

In veterinary medicine, there are three approved routes by which vaccine can be administered: intramuscular, subcutaneous, and topical (intranasal or intranasal/intraocular). Unless otherwise specified by the manufacturer, vaccines licensed for parenteral administration may be given by either the intramuscular or subcutaneous routes. Vaccines licensed for topical administration must be given in the manner outlined by the manufacturer, which with currently available vaccines means either intranasal or a combination of intranasal and intraocular. Parenteral vaccines must *not* be administered topically. Likewise, vaccines approved for topical use must not be administered parenterally. Considerable effort is currently under way to develop vaccines that can be administered by alternative delivery routes. In addition to mucosal vaccines (oral, intranasal, intraocular, and rectal), some unique methods under study today include the use of microneedles and nanoneedles for transdermal delivery. Considerable progress is being made in developing epicutaneous (needleless) vaccines. It is not known when or if these technologies will be available for use in veterinary medicine.

Topical Vaccines

The first vaccines for topical administration were licensed for cats in the 1970s. Since that time, several vaccines approved for topical administration have been licensed in the United States. More are expected in the future. For dogs, topical vaccines are available for *Bordetella bronchiseptica,* parain-

Table 17.3. Canine Vaccines **Not** Recommended for Use in Animal Shelters

Vaccine	Comments
rCanine Distemper Virus (recombinant)	The rCanine Distemper Virus vaccine provides excellent protection against virus challenge. However, two doses of vaccine administered 2–4 weeks apart are required to protect distemper-naïve dogs. The additional time needed to induce an immune response over conventional MLV vaccines precludes routine use in the shelter environment.
Canine Adenovirus-1 (MLV and killed)	Several products are still on the market. In several OTC products, CAV-1 will be combined with CAV-2.
Giardia (killed)	Vaccine does **not** prevent infection . . . only shedding. (Value of using this vaccine in the shelter environment is not known.)
Canine Coronavirus (killed and MLV)	Two reasons for **not being recommended:** 1) Diagnostic: there is no practical means for diagnosing infections and therefore no means of confirming that the disease poses any threat; 2) Medical: the clinical disease associated with canine coronavirus is **not** sufficiently severe to warrant routine vaccination.

Table 17.4. Feline **Core** Vaccine Administration Schedule Recommended for Use in Animal Shelters

Antigen	Primary Vaccination for Kittens (≤ 16 weeks of age)	Primary Vaccination for Adult (≥ 16 weeks of age)	Comments
Panleukopenia (MLV) (parenteral and topical forms available) Not Adjuvanted	Administer one dose on admission as early as 6 weeks of age. **Repeat** in two weeks if still in the shelter.	Administer 1 dose on admission. (MLV is recommended) two doses, three wks apart (if using killed)	**Caution**: Do **not** use **intranasal** [topical]panleukopenia vaccine.
Feline Viral Upper Respiratory Disease: Herpesvirus-1 + Calicivirus (MLV) Not Adjuvanted, Parenteral Vaccine	Administer one dose on admission as early as 6 weeks of age. **Repeat** in two weeks if still in the shelter.	Administer 1 dose on admission. (MLV is recommended) two doses, 2–3 wks apart (if using killed)	Parenteral vaccination may be recommended **over** topical vaccination (below)
Alternative: **Feline Viral Upper Respiratory Disease:** Herpesvirus-1 + Calicivirus (MLV) **Topical Use only** Not Adjuvanted	Administer one dose on admission. REPEAT in two weeks if still in the shelter.	Administer one dose on admission.	Post vaccinal sneezing can be severe; vaccine virus and associated signs may be transmitted to other cats. May make distinguishing infected cats from vaccinated cats difficult. Not generally recommended.
Alternative: **r-Rabies** (1 year vaccine)* (Recombinant vaccine) Not adjuvanted.	Administer first dose as early as three months of age. Administer at the time of release from the shelter.	Administer one dose at the time of release from the shelter.	**Note**: Local statutes apply to re-vaccination requirements. Although rabies is **not** required by law in all states, these guidelines recommend all cats be vaccinated at the time of release from the shelter.

(continues)

291

Table 174. (*continued*)

Antigen	Primary Vaccination for Kittens (≤ 16 weeks of age)	Primary Vaccination for Adult (≥ 16 weeks of age)	Comments
Rabies (one-year vaccine) (killed) **Route of administration may not be optional**—see Product literature for details. Adjuvanted	Administer first dose as early as three months of age. Administer at the time of release from the shelter.	Administer one dose at the time of release from the shelter.	*Note: Local statutes apply to revaccination requirements. Although rabies is **not** required in all states, these guidelines recommend all cats be vaccinated at the time of release from the shelter.*
Alternative: **Rabies (three-year vaccine)** (killed) **Route of administration may not be optional** See product literature for details.	*Note: In selected situations, the three-year rabies vaccine may be substituted for the 1-year Rabies vaccine for initial and subsequent doses.* Administer one dose as early as three months of age. Administer at the time of release from the shelter.	*Note: In selected situations, the three-year rabies vaccine may be substituted for the one-year Rabies vaccine for initial and subsequent doses.* Administer a single dose. Administer at the time of release from the shelter.	*Note: Local statutes apply to revaccination requirements. Although law in all states does not require rabies, these guidelines recommend all cats be vaccinated at the time of release from the shelter.*

NOTE: Route of administration is SQ or IM unless otherwise noted by the manufacturer.

*The manufacturer is currently pursuing a three-year label for the r-Rabies vaccine.

292

Table 175. Administration Schedule for Feline **Noncore** or **Optional** Vaccines Selected for Use in Animal Shelters

Antigen	Primary Vaccination (Kittens)	Primary Vaccination (Adult)	Comments
Feline Leukemia (killed) Adjuvanted & Non-adjuvanted products available	Two doses at 9 and 12 wks of age. (See comments)	Two doses required, 3–4 wks apart. (See comments)	**Not recommended for routine use** Generally, FeLV vaccination is only done in cats that are 1) placed and 2) tested negative for FeLV Ag (ELISA). Vaccine administered at the time of release.
Chlamydia psittaci bacterin Adjuvanted & Non-adjuvanted products available	9 and 12 wks of age	Two doses, 3–4 wks apart	**Not recommended for routine use** in shelters *unless* infections are confirmed.
Bordetella bronchiseptica (avirulent live bacterin) **Intranasal use only** (Limited Application: Read package insert carefully before using)	Administer 1 dose on admission. May be given as early as eight weeks of age. NOTE: manufacturer has advocated administration to kittens as early as four weeks of age. EARLY VACCINATION IS NOT RECOMMENDED IN SHELTERS.	Administer one dose on admission.	**Not recommended for routine use** Clinical signs of respiratory infection may develop subsequent to vaccination. Individual experience managing outbreaks of severe upper respiratory disease known to be associated with *B. bronchiseptica* should dictate the decision to incorporate this vaccine into a shelter protocol for cats.

NOTE: Route of administration is SQ or IM unless otherwise noted by the manufacturer.

*The manufacturer is currently pursuing a three-year label for the r-Rabies vaccine.

293

Table 17.6. Feline Vaccines **Not** Recommended for Routine Use in Animal Shelters

Antigen	Comments
Feline Giardia (killed) Adjuvanted	**Not recommended** Vaccine does NOT prevent infection . . . only shedding. *Also*, in the absence of reliable diagnostic testing, the need for this vaccine cannot be assessed. (Value of using this vaccine in the shelter environment is not known)
Feline Immunodeficiency Virus (killed) Adjuvanted	**Not recommended** Following administration of the 1st dose, all vaccinates will develop antibody that cross-react with every commercial FIV test on the market (ELISA and Western Blot). Commercial PCR testing for FIV is limited and expensive.
Feline Infectious Peritonitis (MLV) Topical (intranasal) use only Non-Adjuvanted	**Not recommended** Vaccine is safe, but it is not considered to be efficacious in protecting cats against FIP.

fluenza virus, and canine adenovirus-2. Currently, there are several vaccines approved for topical administration to cats: feline panleukopenia (a parvovirus), herpesvirus-1, calicivirus, feline infectious peritonitis virus (currently *not* a recommended vaccine), and feline *Bordetella bronchiseptica.* Note that the term "topical" has different meanings. Depending on the individual vaccine, topical may indicate administration via the intranasal route *only* . . . (for example, *Bordetella bronchiseptica* vaccine). On the other hand, topical may include intranasal administration as well as administration directly onto the conjunctiva (intraocular). The package insert should be carefully consulted prior to administering these products.

The introduction and relatively widespread use of topical vaccines in dogs and cats have resulted in a number of novel (unapproved) uses and expectations. Anecdotally, topical vaccines have been administered to cats and dogs with acute and chronic infections as a means of therapy. They have been administered to animals only a few weeks old as a means of preventing infections within endemic environments, and they have been administered concurrently with the same parenteral vaccine in hopes of enhancing the protective immune response derived from administering only one type of vaccine. Topical vaccines are often selected over parenteral vaccines when seeking rapid onset of protection. In the worst-case scenario, vaccines approved for par-

enteral administration have been administered intranasally . . . sometimes with disastrous results. Unfortunately, little or no substantive research is available to support any of these uses.

IMPLICATIONS FOR SHELTER MEDICINE

Having a choice of parenteral and topical vaccines raises important questions for shelters when attempting to develop the most effective vaccine protocol for dogs and cats. When both parenteral and topical vaccines are available, is one preferred over the other? When? Or, is it better to administer both vaccines to individual animals at the time of arrival? Faced with financial constraints, limited space for isolation, and daily influx of new animals, selecting the right vaccine at the right time can make a significant difference in the effectiveness, as well as the cost, of a vaccination program. Below, a number of key issues are presented for those respiratory infections for which both topical and parenteral vaccines are available.

CANINE *BORDETELLA BRONCHISEPTICA*

The efficacy of vaccination against *B. bronchiseptica,* administered by either the topical or the parenteral route, is well documented and, therefore, justifiably used as a **core** vaccine in the shelter environment. Vaccinated dogs experience substantially less coughing when compared to control dogs following challenge *regardless of the route of* *administration.* At issue, however, is whether or not topical vaccination is superior to parenteral vaccination in preventing infection and outbreaks of respiratory disease in the high-risk environment. Although that answer has never been specifically addressed, recently published studies do suggest that sequential vaccination (that is, administering a topical *B. bronchiseptica* vaccine *initially* followed by a booster vaccination administered by the parenteral route) may, in fact, provide a superior protective response in seronegative *puppies*. This is further supported by the fact that puppies may still derive local immunity in the face of maternal antibody following the administration of topical vaccine in young (3 to 6 weeks of age) dogs.

However, administration of an intranasal vaccine may not effectively boost the titer of *adult*, seropositive dogs, whereas subcutaneously administered vaccine will. In effect, perhaps the best protocol to use when administering *B. bronchiseptica* vaccine to dogs in shelters would be to administer intranasal vaccine to all puppies and young dogs with an unknown vaccination history. All adult dogs, and those with presumed or known prior exposure, should receive parenteral vaccine.

It has been suggested that seronegative puppies *may* derive the greatest degree of protection from the simultaneous (that is, both vaccines administered at the same time) administration of parenteral and topical *B. bronchiseptica* vaccine. However, the cost:benefit ratio for routine simultaneous administration of parenteral and topical *B. bronchiseptica* vaccine to all puppies in shelters probably does not justify the additional cost. There appears to be no benefit in administering parenteral and topical vaccine simultaneously to adult, seropositive dogs. Duration of immunity studies on *B. bronchiseptica* vaccines have not been reported but is assumed to be no longer than 10–12 months.

Despite previously published recommendations that topically administered vaccine provides the most rapid onset of immunity, it is likely that this may be true only when vaccinating puppies. It is not known if intranasally administered vaccine will immunize a susceptible dog in less than five days.

Several commercially licensed canine vaccines for protection against *B. bronchiseptica* are combined with CPiV or with CPiV and CAV-2 and are available for topical (intranasal only) as well as parenteral administration. There are no published studies that suggest one route of administration or that one combination is superior to another when administering combination products.

FELINE *BORDETELLA BRONCHISEPTICA*

At this time, there is only one vaccine licensed for protection against feline *B. bronchiseptica* infection. The feline *B. bronchiseptica* vaccine is approved for topical (intranasal) administration only. Recommendations outlined by the American Association of Feline Practitioners/Academy of Feline Medicine indicate that *B. bronchiseptica* vaccination is not required in all cats. Use of the vaccine is generally limited to cluster households and shelters where *B. bronchiseptica* is known to be associated with respiratory infections. The value of *B. bronchiseptica* vaccine in reducing either the occurrence or the severity of respiratory disease in shelters has not been established.

Anecdotal reports have suggested that shelter outbreaks of upper respiratory infections in dogs and cats can be managed through administration of topical *B. bronchiseptica* vaccine. In our experience, doing so does not appear to shorten the course of infection in individual animals, lessen the duration of intensity of the outbreak, or limit the spread of infection to susceptible animals.

FELINE VIRAL UPPER RESPIRATORY INFECTION

The availability of both parenteral and topical (conjunctival and intranasal) vaccines for feline herpesvirus-1 and calicivirus has raised questions regarding the routine use of such vaccines in shelter medicine. Topical herpesvirus-calicivirus vaccines are uncommonly used in private practice today. However, the prospect that these vaccines might induce a rapid onset local immune response, can be administered to young (as early as three weeks of age) kittens, and can be divided without compromising the protective response has considerable appeal in shelter medicine.

The use of topical respiratory virus vaccines for kittens and cats, however, is not universally embraced. Perhaps the most significant drawback to the use of topical respiratory vaccines in shelters is the occurrence of post-vaccinal respiratory signs, sneezing and nasal discharge, especially in kittens.

The inability to distinguish post-vaccinal sneezing from that associated with actual infection is a significant restriction for some facilities. However, it must be acknowledged that some shelters do use topical respiratory vaccines routinely and have appreciated a significant decline in the incidence of respiratory infections among cats and kittens.

Unfortunately, no studies advocate one route of administration over the other. Early studies support the ability of a topical vaccine to induce a protective response (following challenge) within 48 hours post-vaccination in immunologically naive cats. Additional studies have shown a significant advantage to early vaccination. Administering the first dose of topical vaccine to kittens at three weeks of age and every three weeks thereafter until 12 weeks of age in endemic households was associated with a significant decrease in respiratory disease within defined households of cats. In shelters, the high rates of new cat/kitten introduction and the difficulty associated with isolating new arrivals conceivably would make similar results difficult to achieve. Those shelters that do elect to vaccinate kittens against viral upper respiratory infection with a topical vaccine can economize by dividing the dose. Typically, one 0.5 ml dose can be divided among two to three kittens. Although a topical feline panleukopenia vaccine is still available in combination with herpesvirus-1 and calicivirus, topical administration of panleukopenia vaccine is not recommended.

Administering a topical respiratory virus vaccine has been advocated as a means of mitigating clinical signs of adult cats with chronic sneezing and nasal discharge associated with a chronic virus carrier state. Virtually 100 percent of kittens recovering from acute herpesvirus-1 infection become chronic virus carriers for life . . . respiratory tract shedding is intermittent. It is estimated that up to 80–85 percent of kittens recovering from acute calicivirus infection become chronic virus carriers for months to years . . . respiratory tract shedding is continuous. A single 0.5 ml dose, administered as recommended by the manufacturer, can be expected to result in resolution of clinical signs within about 10 to 14 days *in some cats.* If time permits, a second dose may be administered three to four weeks later in cats that fail to respond to the initial dose. However, topical vaccination neither eliminates virus from the upper respiratory tract nor prevents infection in cats/kittens vaccinated prior to natural exposure.

ANNUAL VACCINATION VERSUS DURATION OF IMMUNITY (DOI)

In 1989 the AVMA Council on Biologic and Therapeutic Agents published immunization guidelines for dogs and cats (AVMA, 1989). In their report, booster vaccinations for all canine and feline vaccines were recommended annually (vaccines for canine Lyme disease, canine coronavirus, canine giardiasis, feline infectious peritonitis, feline Bordetella bronchiseptica, feline giardiasis, and Feline Immunodeficiency Virus vaccines were not available at the time these recommendations were made). As recently as 1996, a survey of vaccination practices conducted in veterinary schools throughout North American indicated that annual revaccination of adult dogs and cats was routinely performed (Mansfield, 1996). It is reasonable to assume, therefore, that most practicing veterinarians still recommend *annual* booster vaccinations to their companion animal clientele. Various publications (Philips and Schultz, 1996; Smith, 1995; Bowlin, 1996; Larson and Bradley, 1996) along with the December 2000 Guidelines on Feline Vaccination (AAFP, 2000) and the March/April 2003 Guidelines on Canine Vaccination (AAHA, 2003) suggest that current recommendations fail to address realistic duration of immunity (DOI). At issue is the fact that a protective immune response (that is, the Duration of Immunity or DOI) is likely to persist for several years following administration of *some* vaccines. On the other hand, administration of annual booster vaccines to all dogs and cats does not necessarily guarantee protection over the 12 months following vaccination. Despite the absence of comprehensive DOI studies, a growing body of data supports recommendations for booster vaccination that include administering core vaccines (for example, feline panleukopenia, herpesvirus-1, calicivirus, canine distemper, canine parvovirus, canine adenovirus-2, and rabies) at three-year intervals in adult animals. It also has been suggested that several vaccines routinely used in companion animal practice, such as *Bordetella bronchiseptica,* and Leptospira serotypes, and feline chlamydia, fail to provide protective immunity for 12 months (Mansfield, 1996).

Among the most significant changes outlined in the current vaccination guidelines for dogs and cats are recommendations that selected booster vaccinations recommended for *adult* dogs (distemper virus, parvovirus, and adenovirus-2) and *adult* cats (panleukopenia, feline herpesvirus-1 and calicivirus) be administered every three years rather than annually. The incidence of canine distemper, canine parvovirus, and feline panleukopenia among vaccinated adult (> 1 year of age) animals is virtually zero. The correlation between vaccination, the development of a positive antibody titer and protection from exposure to virulent virus is excellent. Furthermore, protection derived from immunization against these virus infections is expected to last for five to six years or longer. The implication for shelter medicine is an economic one . . . *adult* dogs and cats entering a shelter have likely been vaccinated or have developed natural immunity to high-risk infections (such as feline panleukopenia, canine distemper, canine parvovirus) and will probably do well whether or not they are vaccinated on admission.

However, vaccines intended to protect against diseases such as *B. bronchiseptica* are not known to provide protection against challenge for more than one year. In fact, the DOI may be less than one year. In private practice, annual boosters are likely to continue to be recommended for those animals considered at risk of exposure to diseases caused by these organisms.

Implications for Shelter Medicine

In shelters, the decision to vaccinate dogs and cats at the time of admission is commonly employed. However, the decision about which vaccine(s) should be administered varies significantly from facility to facility. The question of administering annual versus triennial boosters may seem to be a nonissue for shelters unless, perhaps, they operate under a no kill policy. After all, animals seldom remain in the facility one month, much less two or three years, so why worry about booster vaccination? But . . . to address this issue in a *Shelter-Unique* context, it is important to understand that triennial booster recommendations for adult dogs/cats evolved from knowledge that the minimum duration of immunity for the core vaccines has been documented to be from five to six years. We don't know what the maximum DOI is. This information has at least some impact on developing vaccination policies within an animal shelter.

Shelters maintaining a policy that all dogs and all cats, at the time of admission, receive a "booster" vaccination may not be enjoying the best cost-ben-

efit ratio from their vaccine program. A *booster vaccination* can be defined as any vaccine administered to a dog or cat at some designated time following completion of the *primary* vaccine series or administration of vaccine following recovery from prior infection. (The term "primary vaccination" is preferred over "Puppy or Kitten shots" since vaccine obviously can be administered to an adult dog or cat that may never have received a prior vaccination.) Many *adult* animals admitted to shelters are already effectively immunized (either naturally or from previous vaccination) and, therefore, may not actually benefit from booster vaccination. It's just that the shelter personnel simply do not consistently have access to reliable information on when or if an individual *adult* ever received a primary vaccination. Certainly there's no means for determining whether an individual animal had prior exposure to a specific infectious agent. The policy decision to administer booster vaccines to adult dogs and cats on entry to the shelter, therefore, is more complex than it might seem:

A. *Economical*—if it is feasible to *assume* preexisting immunity exists in adults presented to the shelter, then it's feasible not to vaccinate adults . . . (this saves money)
B. *Immunological*—if existing policy stipulates that all dogs and cats will be vaccinated on entering the shelter, is protective immunity conferred or even boosted? The fact is, if an adult dog or cat has had prior vaccination or prior exposure/infection, then vaccinating at the time of admission will result in
   1. A rapid (within 24–72 hours) anamnestic antibody response if existing antibody levels are low (that's good)
   2. No additional immunity if the dog or cat is already immune (that's expensive)

Consider the other side of this equation: In truly susceptible (never vaccinated; never exposed) animals, vaccination at the time of entry is, in effect, a *primary vaccination*, regardless of the animal's age. The effective time from inoculation to immunization can be two weeks or longer . . . so why bother administering vaccine since that individual animal, whether placed or euthanitized, is not likely to remain in the facility long enough to derive benefit from the vaccine? In the no-kill shelter environment, considering the concentration of animals and risk of exposure to infectious disease, administering an annual booster vaccination for core vaccines seems prudent. The consequences of extrapolating triennial recommendations intended for adult household pets into vaccination protocols in no-kill facilities are unknown.

TITERS VERSUS VACCINATION

What is the feasibility of performing annual antibody titers in dogs and cats residing in or admitted to shelters? In shelter medicine, cost and time factors virtually preclude determining serum antibody titers to establish 'immunity' in the individual dog or cat. Despite the fact that a growing number of laboratories are beginning to offer selected canine and feline antibody titers to veterinarians, a number of significant factors that (in this author's opinion) do not justify routinely offering this service within a private practice, much less within a shelter.

In addition to the fact that antibody concentration does not necessarily correlate with protection against disease, there are other compelling reasons that widespread acceptance and use of antibody determinations in the individual dog or cat will not likely happen in clinical practice. First, national standards or methods for determining serum antibody levels to the various vaccine antigens have not been achieved. The risk lies in the fact that a single serum sample, divided three times, and sent to three different laboratories, could yield three different titers or, quite possibly, three different interpretations. What may be deemed protective by one laboratory might be labeled susceptible by another.

Furthermore, it is important to note that an individual dog or cat that does not have a significant concentration of antibody may, in fact, have protective immunity. A negative antibody titer does not necessarily correlate with susceptibility to infection. Likewise, the presence of antibody, even at very high levels, does not guarantee immunity subsequent to exposure.

Implications for Shelter Medicine

In private small animal practice there continues to be much deliberation and debate over the value of drawing blood for antibody titers . . . some confusion exists over how to interpret test results. In the context of this text, it would be prudent to recommend that shelters avoid using antibody titers in an attempt to assess immunity in individual animals. Time and cost are at least two factors that justify not performing titers within the shelter environment.

Scientifically speaking, however, there may be another side to this coin. In other words, there actually may be value in looking at trends related to antibody levels within a population of dogs or cats entering an individual shelter. Consider this . . . in the event funds were actually available, applying knowledge gained from determining antibody levels on hundreds of dogs and cats as they enter the shelter could actually be a cost effective strategy in the long run. *For example*, at the time of admission to the shelter, measure serum antibody concentrations for the major infectious diseases in several dogs (distemper and parvovirus) and cats (panleukopenia, herpesvirus, and calicivirus) and do so according to defined age groups (Group A: < 6 months; Group B: > 6 months < geriatric; and Group C: geriatric). Assessment of the titers could provide insight on the susceptibility (that is, lack of prior exposure or vaccination) of animals entering the shelter and the need (or lack thereof) to administer the core vaccines on admission. Conceivably, substantial savings could be realized if it were found that virtually 100 percent of adult and geriatric dogs and cats had significant levels of antibody to respective pathogens. Vaccination of adults on admission to the shelter, therefore, would not necessarily be required. The resulting savings in vaccine costs alone could be substantial.

HEALTH RISK ASSESSMENT

Developing a rational vaccination protocol for the shelter population certainly does not mandate that all cats and all dogs presented to the shelter be inoculated with each of the antigens for which a vaccine is currently licensed. Several factors should be considered when establishing vaccine recommendations within the individual facility. The decision to vaccinate a cat or dog with a vaccine that is not core should be based on an assessment of the health risk profile among animals presented to the shelter and takes into consideration information about the 1) individual animal (host factors), 2) the animal's environment (environmental factors), and 3) awareness of the spectrum of infectious agents (agent factors) within the environment.

Host Factors

Suboptimal response to vaccination is possible among cats that are malnourished, have concurrent infection or illness, or are receiving regular doses of immune suppressive drugs. Additional intrinsic factors considered to influence the outcome of infection include heritable resistance (and possible susceptibility) factors and stress. Age at the time of exposure is an important, independent variable in assessing an individual's risk to an infectious agent. Although no age-group can be considered entirely free of risk, kittens (less than 6 months of age) are generally more susceptible to infection than adult cats following exposure and, therefore, represent the principal target population for feline vaccination protocols.

The presence of maternal antibody is an intrinsic host factor known to protect a puppy or kitten following exposure to an infectious agent. However, interference of vaccine antigen by maternal antibody is the single most common cause of vaccination failure. Failure to vaccinate a kitten at an age when maternal antibody has declined sufficiently (approximately 12 weeks of age) will increase an animal's risk.

Environmental Factors

Population density, cleaning techniques, air exchange, construction/floor plan, and rates of turnover are perhaps among the most critical environmental issues affecting the risk of exposure to an infectious agent within a shelter. Cats and kittens clustered within a defined area of the shelter, for example, are at substantial risk of exposure to herpesvirus and calicivirus. Furthermore, the frequent and direct introduction (that is, no quarantine) of new animals into the facility poses a potential risk to the entire population. Geographic distribution of various infectious agents may represent significantly different risk profiles to animals living in different parts of the United States and should be considered when determining which noncore vaccines would be appropriate. Sustained high ambient temperatures and humidity, in addition to housing environments with fewer than 12 air exchanges per hour, significantly increase the risk of animals' exposure to respiratory pathogens. In kennels, a single puppy with parvovirus could put a large percentage of the canine population at risk for a month because of the long survival time of the virus in the environment.

Agent Factors

Independent agent-associated variables, such as virulence, dose, and mutation (often related to population density and rate of virus replication) do influence the outcome of infection but are difficult to objectively assess in the shelter setting. However, in the domain of risk assessment, it is the *interaction* between the agent, the host, and the environment that dictates the outcome following exposure and infection. The severity of an infection, particularly a viral infection, is highly variable within a population of animals with similar exposure to the same agent. Clinical illness in susceptible animals exposed to the exact same pathogen can range from inapparent or mild to severe acute illness to chronic or latent infection. Predicting the health impact of numerous variables on animals at high risk of exposure is among the most significant challenges facing veterinarians who practice shelter medicine.

IMPLICATIONS FOR SHELTER MEDICINE

The reason for presenting risk factor assessment in the context of shelter medicine is important from the standpoint of mitigating the consequence of exposure . . . not *eliminating* the risk of exposure. The effectiveness of any vaccination program employed within a shelter is going to be influenced by the interaction of various host, agent, and environmental factors. In developing a vaccination program for an animal shelter, the following must be taken into consideration:

- Assume infectious disease exposure has already occurred.
- Assume that puppies and kittens are at considerably more risk than adults are.
- Assume that littermates and healthy-appearing adults are the critical reservoir of infection for puppies and kittens.
- Assume that vaccination will not preclude outbreaks of infectious disease.

VACCINE SAFETY

Among the most important vaccine issues facing practitioners today is that of safety. For most vaccines on the market today, it must still be assumed that the benefits of vaccination, when performed in accordance with currently published standards far outweigh the risk of vaccine-induced illness or disease. However, recent reports have raised serious concerns within the profession over the relationship between vaccination and delayed adverse events, specifically vaccine-associated fibrosarcoma in cats (Hendrick and Goldschmidt, 1991; Hendrick et al., 1994; Kass et al., 1993) and immune-mediated hemolytic anemia in dogs (Duval and Giger, 1996). Determining which vaccines pose a risk to which animals, and when, simply cannot be determined with the information available today. However, it is still the practitioner who assumes responsibility for not only recommending a particular vaccination protocol but for any consequences that might arise as a result of administering a vaccine (see "Liability"later in this chapter).

Concern over the risks associated with the use of attenuated (modified-live) vaccines, disease caused by residual virulence, or disease attributed to contamination during manufacture, has sustained the market for inactivated products (Tizard, 1990). However, significant advantages are associated with using attenuated vaccines, such as rapid-onset, sustained protection, the ability to stimulate cell-mediated immunity, and the ability to immunize by way of natural routes, that may not justify the decision to offer only killed vaccines to companion animal patients.

The Adverse Event

Information on the behavior of individual vaccines used under everyday field conditions is maintained by the manufacturers and reported to the U.S. Department of Agriculture (USDA) Center for Veterinary Biologics (Animal Immunobiologic Vigilance, 1996). Such post marketing surveillance also serves as an alert system for the rapid detection of vaccine-related events that appear to be unusual in nature or frequency. However, the single most significant factor that serves to compromise the effectiveness of the post marketing surveillance program is the lack of *adverse event* reporting by practitioners. In many instances, not even deaths associated with vaccine administration are reported.

An adverse event is any undesirable occurrence following the use of immunobiological product, including illness or reaction, whether or not the product caused the event. Anecdotal surveys suggest that adverse event reports from veterinarians dramatically under-represent the number of reactions observed and regarded to be vaccine-associated. Despite efforts to categorize adverse events as Type-1, -2, -3, and so on, there are still no uniform standards used by practitioners, or manufacturers, to classify frequency and type of event. However, the USDA has developed adverse event reporting guidelines that practitioners should use when addressing known or suspected adverse events associated with administration of any vaccine (see Appendix 17.1).

Although only a few reports specifically address various causes of adverse events, reactions have been attributed to: preservatives, purity, contamination, virulence of attenuated agents, adjuvant, route of administration, concurrent administration of other vaccines, and the ordinal number of the vaccine are reported. Neither the cause nor the exact frequency of delayed reactions, such as tumor formation or immune-mediated hemolytic anemia, is known.

Reporting of adverse events remains the responsibility of the practitioner who administers the vaccine and observes the reaction. Reports should be made directly to the vaccine manufacturer, usually to the technical service section. The information to include in an adverse event report is the same as that outlined in Appendix 17.1.

IMPLICATIONS FOR SHELTER MEDICINE

Observing and reporting adverse events in the shelter environment is of considerable importance. Not only do shelter personnel vaccinate more animals on a daily basis than most private practices, but they have the distinct advantage of maintaining vaccinates within the facility post vaccination, for several days at least. This conceivably would allow accurate observation of both acute and a limited number of chronic (delayed) reactions. Shelter veterinarians are an untapped source of critical information on vaccine safety. A cooperative effort among shelters to identify and report vaccine adverse events would be of considerable interest and importance to the entire profession.

LIABILITY

Generally, the use of a biologic product by a veterinarian is left to the individual's professional judgment. The latitude afforded practitioners is broad, but there are boundaries. The analysis of the law governing use is complicated. The USDA's Center for Veterinary Biologics (CVB) regulates the licensure and preparation of most veterinary biologics. The Virus–Serum–Toxin Act (VST) empowers CVB to stop the sale, barter or exchange of "any worthless, contaminated, dangerous, or harmful virus, serum, toxin, or analogous product." In the event discretionary use of a CVB regulated product was viewed as unsafe, and so on . . . it could initiate an enforcement action. However, unless a safety issue is implicated, USDA has historically not considered such enforcement to be a priority. On the other hand, some vaccines are licensed with specific restrictions, noted on the label, regarding their use (Flemming, 2001).

The Food and Drug Administration's (FDA) Center for Veterinary Medicine (CVM) also regulates some products that most practitioners would consider biologics. The jurisdictional gray zone between the two agencies is confusing, constantly blurred and evolving. Products regulated by CVM are covered by the Animal Medicinal Drug Use Clarification Act (AMDUCA), which established specific rules for "extra-label" drug use (Flemming, 2001).

Discussions with vaccine manufacturers, practicing veterinarians, attorneys, as well as representatives from the AVMA Liability Trust suggest that there is considerable confusion among practicing veterinarians over 1) the use of vaccines in a manner not specifically recommended by the manufacturer (as published in the package insert), and 2) the liability assumed when a vaccine causes, or is presumed to cause, a serious and/or expensive injury to the patient.

Vaccination protocols for companion animals vary considerably throughout North America. Furthermore, it is the veterinarian who, after assessing the various risk factors unique to the individual patient, makes recommendations as to which type of vaccine and which choice of antigens are to be administered, which product is used, when the vaccine is administered, and how often. Veterinarians are *not* obligated to follow the recommendation outlined in the package insert for a specific product. Administering vaccines in accordance with hospital or shelter policy that differs from the manufacturers recommendations is acceptable as long as that policy is consistent with the "standard of care" in that

community. In clinical practice, the "standard of care" for administering vaccines is generally dictated by the manufacturers' recommendations as published in the vaccine package insert (label) or as outlined in the context of the AAFP Feline Vaccination Guidelines (AAFP, 2000) and the recently published AAHA Canine Vaccine Guidelines (AAHA, 2003). Liability issues surrounding administration of vaccines in a shelter environment are unclear. Obviously, decisions over which vaccine products to purchase as well as when and how to administer vaccines is oftentimes the responsibility of nonveterinarian employees of the shelter. Such decisions are often based on economical factors rather than immunological factors. In the absence of defined standards or guidelines for administering vaccines in shelters, vaccination protocols employed in shelters are expected to be remarkably diverse if not impractical.

Implications for Shelter Medicine

Veterinarians who vaccinate, or oversee the vaccination of, dogs and cats in animal shelters are extended no special consideration nor are they exempt from any liability associated with vaccination-associated injury to an animal. It's also appropriate to point out that litigation against veterinarians (in private practice or in shelters) for malpractice/injury associated with the administration of a vaccine is rare! A veterinarian's liability exposure associated with canine and feline vaccination programs in animals shelters must be considered minimal. However, if there is any exposure, it is more likely to center on one of three areas: failing to provide adequate supervision/training to individuals designated to administer vaccines; failing to define (in writing) and implement a vaccination policy for the facility, and failure to maintain adequate records on individuals vaccinated.

RECOMBINANT VACCINE TECHNOLOGY

Recombinant vaccines are among the newest products in the rapidly emerging biotechnology/ vaccine market (Van Kampen, 2001). The technologic advance behind these products is the ability to isolate and splice (or recombine) gene-size fragments of DNA from one organism and transferring them to another by way of a vector virus or plasmid DNA. It has already been demonstrated that the hybrid organism resulting from the in-vitro exchange of genetic material has tremendous potential to deliver safe and immunogenic DNA into the host animal and, as such, represents a truly new generation of vaccine development for the veterinary profession. The recombinant vaccines currently being introduced into companion animal practice are exceptionally safe, although efficacy and duration of immunity will still have to be established for each product.

The technology behind recombinant vaccines is quite sophisticated and has quickly moved routine vaccination of dogs and cats from the level of the whole organism to the subcellular level. The practice of administering attenuated, live agents, or whole killed products will surely change in the near future (Adams et al., 1997). As we enter the twenty-first century, it is anticipated that even newer technologies will be introduced that will give rise to veterinary-label vaccines that are safer, have exceptional efficacy, and a duration of immunity that persists for several years, if not for the life of the patient. Veterinarians are encouraged to become familiar with recombinant vaccines, to understand the basic technology behind their development, and to become familiar with the potential advantages and disadvantages of each new product as it is introduced. Then the clinician, considering both conventional and recombinant vaccines, will be able to administer the most appropriate product only as often and necessary to prevent significant disease.

Implications for Shelter Medicine

It should be noted that over the next 5–10 years recombinant (genetically engineered) vaccines are likely to become the predominant type of biological (vaccine) introduced into the companion animal market. Veterinarians who practice shelter medicine or who advise shelters on which vaccines to purchase need to be aware of certain issues pertaining to the use of recombinant vaccines.

First, measurable antibody titers are expected to be associated with administration of some recombinant vaccines, but not all. This is particularly true of vaccines for viral infections. The ability of recombinant vaccines to provoke immunity through cell-mediated immune (CMI) mechanisms is clearly an immunologic advantage. However, shelters that elect to routinely perform antibody titers on dogs and/or cats may find this impractical. Measuring CMI responses to vaccination is complex, and availability is limited to specialized laboratories

(usually research laboratories) assessing responses in individual animals.

Second, recombinant vaccines bring at least one unique (albeit limited) and important advantage to infection control efforts within animal shelters. Since recombinant vaccines are capable of targeting a highly defined immunologic response against a particular infection, at least some recombinant products are known to immunize in the presence of maternal antibody. At least for canine distemper, the recombinant vaccine (Recombitek rDistemper, Merial Ltd, Duluth, GA) has been shown to immunize 6-week-old puppies in the face of measurable quantities of maternal antibody. In the shelter environment, this might seem to be an important means of controlling canine distemper among a population of young, susceptible dogs with an unknown nursing history. However, the immunogenic properties of the recombinant distemper virus are such that the manufacturer has recommended two initial doses of vaccine, 2–4 weeks apart, to provide immunity against canine distemper virus infection. Use of recombinant canine distemper vaccine would be impractical in the shelter setting because of the extended time required to develop a protective immune response. On the other hand, the recombinant canine distemper vaccine is a suitable alternative to the modified-live canine distemper vaccine in boosting dogs previously immunized.

Rabies vaccine should be a core vaccine in all shelters for both dogs and cats. Today, there is no licensed recombinant rabies vaccine for use in dogs. However, a nonadjuvanted, recombinant rabies vaccine (PurVax Feline Rabies Vaccine, Merial Ltd., Duluth, GA) for cats is currently on the market and is in widespread use throughout the United States today. At issue for shelters is the decision over whether to select an adjuvanted, killed virus vaccine for rabies or the recombinant vaccine. Perhaps the single most important consideration is that related to fibrosarcoma risk associated with the use of adjuvanted vaccine in cats. All killed virus rabies vaccines licensed in the United States today contain an adjuvant; the recombinant feline rabies vaccine does not. At least one long-term (five-year) study of cats has shown a five–times significantly greater occurrence of fibrosarcoma in cats receiving an adjuvanted FeLV vaccine compared to cats having only received nonadjuvanted, modified-live virus vaccines (Veterinary Products Committee, 2002).

OVER-THE-COUNTER SALES OF VACCINES

The percentage of companion animals in the United States that are vaccinated each year with vaccine purchased through over-the-counter (OTC) sources, such as catalogues and various Web sites, is largely unknown. However, estimates that from 10–20 percent of pet dogs and cats are vaccinated by non-veterinarians administering OTC vaccines suggests this is a significant and growing market. Discounts for bulk sales may actually be an incentive for some shelters to purchase and use OTC vaccines within the dog and cat population.

Caution: Although it may be possible to purchase vaccine through commercial OTC channels at a lower price than that offered by distributors, *not all vaccines are the same!* Many of the OTC canine vaccines, for example, contain canine adenovirus-1 (previously called the infectious canine hepatitis virus), known to cause corneal injury and permanent blindness (hepatitis "blue eye") in some dogs. Some products even contain a combination of canine adenovirus-1 *and* canine adenovirus-2 . . . a completely unnecessary, and potentially harmful, combination.

Although many of the vaccines sold through OTC sources are produced by the major vaccine manufacturers, many other products are not. This raises important questions regarding safety and efficacy studies of at least some of products on the market. Rabies vaccine can be, and is, sold to nonveterinarians through catalogue sales in 23 states (Omaha Vaccine Co., Omaha, NE). In effect, rabies vaccine can be sold and administered by nonveterinarians *throughout* the United States. The implications are not insignificant when, for example, a dog or cat vaccinated by a nonveterinarian bites a person. The lack of documentation regarding which rabies vaccine was administered and when it was administered could have serious implications for the bite victim.

Although vaccination protocols among individual veterinary practices do vary, the protocols recommended by at least some companies offering catalogue sales of vaccine is, quite simply, wrong. For example, at least two pet catalogues offering canine vaccines advise customers to administer the first dose of a combination vaccine to puppies at five weeks of age with a second dose at six weeks of age. Such practice is simply not in accordance with either the canine vaccination guidelines or current practice standards in the US. There is no immunologic rationale behind the recommendation to vaccinate puppies or kittens at intervals of less than two weeks. Yet, the resources to monitor and address these standards do not exist and the companies that make these recommendations are under no legal obligation to change.

Implications for Shelter Medicine

It can only be assumed that animal shelters in the United States preferentially purchase companion animal vaccines through ethical channels rather than through catalogues or a pet-oriented Web site. However, for shelters, cost of the product can become the single most important determining factor when purchasing vaccine. It should be noted, however, that OTC biologicals for dogs and cats are a predominant source of vaccines *not* recommended for dogs and cats, such as CAV-1 and FIP. Buyer beware!

An additional issue of concern for shelters that elect to purchase vaccines through OTC sources relates to safety and the occurrence of adverse reactions to a particular vaccine or lot of vaccine. In the event that there are widespread complications or adverse reactions associated with administration of a vaccine purchased through OTC channels, medical and financial support is unlikely to be provided by the retailer.

NOSODES

That pet owners are concerned about vaccination recommendations traditionally offered by veterinarians is apparent from the proliferation of antivaccination Web sites in which animal owners, breeders, and veterinarians offer alternative approaches, largely homeopathic, to protecting pets against infectious diseases. Their concerns center predominantly on immune-system overload and vaccine-induced disease. One of the proposed alternative approaches to vaccination of dogs and cats involves the administration of nosodes, products prepared from infected tissues, infected discharges, or the actual pathogenic organism that cause the disease one is attempting to immunize against. All nosodes are administered orally but, according to various Web site resources, do not need to be swallowed. What prevents the nosode from actually infecting the animal and causing illness is the fact that the final product is subjected to homeopathic dilution and *potentization*. Apparently, infectious material is subjected to multiple dilutions such that the quantity of infectious material remaining is insignificant to cause disease. There are no known standards in place to ensure dosing standards or product safety. Dosing recommendations seem to vary but generally entail administering either a three-drop dose (small animals) or a six-drop dose (large animals) orally. A dose is given on three days of the first week (of life?); once weekly for the next three weeks; once monthly for the next six months; and once every six months thereafter. To the author's knowledge, only one controlled study on the efficacy of a canine parvovirus nosode has been conducted. Subsequent to administration of the parvovirus nosode, dogs were orally challenged with virulent parvovirus. Results showed that 100 percent of the control dogs and 100 percent of the inoculates became infected with parvovirus.

Implications for Shelter Medicine

There is virtually no data to support the role of nosodes in providing a protective immune response in dogs and cats. In the shelter environment, nosodes should *not* be used.

REFERENCES

Adams, L.G., Ford, R.B., et al. 1997. Recombinant vaccine technology. Veterinary Exchange. *Compendium on Continuing Education, Pract Vet (Supplement)* 19:5–16.

American Animal Hospital Association (AAHA), 2003. Report of the Canine Vaccine Task Force: Executive Summary and 2003 Canine Vaccine Guidelines and Recommendations. *JAAHA.* 39:119–131.

American Association of Feline Practitioners, 2000. Report of the American Association of Feline Practitioners and Academy of Feline Medicine Advisory Panel on Feline Vaccines Nashville, TN.

Animal Immunobiologic Vigilance, 1996. Brochure published by the United States Department of Agriculture, Center for Veterinary Biologics, 223 S. Walnut Ave, Ames, IA 50010. November.

AVMA Council on Biologic and Therapeutic Agents, 1989. Canine and feline immunization guidelines *Journal of the American Veterinary Medical Association (JAVMA)* 195:314–317.

Bowlin, C.L. 1996. Proceedings from *Perspectives on Vaccines in Feline Practice*, Eight Annual Feline Practitioners Seminar. Columbus, OH. July.

Duval, D., and Giger, U. 1996. Vaccine-associated immune-mediated hemolytic anemia in the dog, *Journal of Veterinary Internal Medicine* 10:290–295.

Flemming, D. 2001. The potential for liability in the use and misuse of veterinary vaccines. *Veterinary Clinics of North America: Small Animal Practice* 31:515–523.

Hendrick, M.J., and Goldschmidt, M.H. 1991. Do injection site reactions induce fibrosarcomas in cats? *JAVMA.* 199:968.

Hendrick, M.J., Kass, P.H., et al. 1994. Postvaccinal sarcomas in cats. *Journal National Cancer Institute* 86:341–343.

Kass, P.H., Barnes, W.G., et al. 1993. Epidemiologic evidence for a causal relation between vaccination and fibrosarcoma tumorigenesis in cats *JAVMA.* 203:396–405.

Larson, R.L., and Bradley, J.S. 1996. Immunologic principles and immunization strategy *Compendium of Continuing Education Pract Vet* 18: 963–971.

Mansfield, P.D. 1996. Vaccination of dogs and cats in veterinary teaching hospitals in North America *JAVMA* 208:1242–1247.

Phillips, T.R., and Schultz, R.D. 1992. Canine and feline vaccines in Kirk, R.W. (ed.): *Current Veterinary Therapy XI.* Philadelphia, PA: W.B. Saunders, 202–206.

Smith, C.A. 1995. Are we vaccinating too much? *JAVMA.* 207:421–425.

Tizard, I. 1990. Risks associated with use of live vaccines. *JAVMA.* 196:1851.

Van Kampen, K.R. 2001. Recombinant vaccine technology in veterinary medicine. *Veterinary Clinics of North America* Small *Animal Practice* 31:535–538.

Veterinary Products Committee (VPC), 2002. Working Group on Feline and Canine Vaccination Final Report Department for Environmental, Food & Rural Affairs. DEFRA Publications, London.

Appendix 17.1
Adverse Event Reporting Criteria to Be Reported to the Vaccine Manufacturer

PATIENT INFORMATION

- Patient Signalment (Age, Breed, Sex)
- Pertinent History
- Case identification number (if applicable)
- Concurrent Illnesses

ADVERSE EVENT

- A description of the event (for example, onset of signs following inoculation; clinical signs/ lesions)
- Supporting laboratory data-include normal and abnormal findings (if applicable)
- Date of inoculation
- Date signs were first noticed
- Outcome
- A list of *all* immunobiological products administered[1] that might be associated with the adverse event, to include
  – Product brand name
  – Serial or Lot number
  – Product code number

- Administration information (each vaccine administered):
  – Dose
  – Route
  – Site
  – Needle size
  – Administration of concurrent (nonbiological) drugs
  – Date vaccine was reconstituted

PERSONA INFORMATION

- Name, address, and phone number of the shelter
- Name, address, and phone number of owner/agent (if known)
  – Needle size
  – Administration of concurrent (nonbiological) drugs
  – Date vaccine was reconstituted

Notes

[1] For combination products, list the product code and serial number of each vial, as well as the product code of the combination package.

Disease Recognition and Diagnostic Testing

Kate F. Hurley

INTRODUCTION

In order to segregate animals appropriately and protect adopters from taking home an unexpected veterinary bill along with their new pet, systems must be in place for the prompt recognition and reporting of disease. The most basic level of disease recognition is observation for overt symptoms by all staff and volunteers that have any animal contact. The next level is a formal intake or pre-adoption exam by trained staff. This allows for detection of more subtle signs. Finally, specific diagnostic testing can be performed to determine the cause of symptoms or screen for asymptomatic but potentially serious conditions.

DISEASE RECOGNITION: MONITORING FOR OVERT SYMPTOMS

Before handling any animal, all staff and volunteers should be trained to go through the following three-point health check:

1. **Look for any paperwork** on kennel indicating that there is a disease or handling concern with the animal.
2. **Look at animal** for signs of disease (e.g., attitude, eyes, nose, coughing/sneezing).
3. **Look in kennel** for signs of disease (e.g., diarrhea, vomit, sneeze marks on kennel wall).

Clear oral and written directions should be provided and prominently posted detailing what to do if a disease problem is observed (i.e., do not take animal out of cage, notify designated staff). This three-point check should also be performed as part of a daily shelter walk-through by animal care or medical staff.

DISEASE RECOGNITION: ADMITTING AND PRE-ADOPTION EXAM

In an ideal world, every shelter animal would receive a full physical exam by a veterinarian. This is impractical in many shelters. A reasonable next choice is to train designated staff to perform a screening exam either at the time of intake or prior to placing an animal up for adoption (or both). Abnormal findings can then be brought to the attention of a veterinarian for further assessment. Performance of the screening exams is an ideal job for a registered veterinary technician in a shelter. Benefits of routine screening exams on all shelter animals include the following:

- Quick recognition of infectious conditions, allowing for the appropriate segregation and treatment (i.e., ringworm, upper respiratory infection).
- Recognition of non-infectious conditions that would benefit from prompt treatment in the shelter (i.e., wounds, abscesses).
- Recognition of conditions that are not treatable in the shelter but may affect adoptability, or of which adopters should be advised (i.e., heart murmur, tumor, dental disease).
- Detection of identifying features that help accurately describe the animal and speed up reclaim (i.e., spay scars, tattoos).
- Documentation of pre-existing conditions at the time of shelter entry (may be important for liability reasons).

Accurate assessment of animal health, identification, and spay/neuter status can decrease turnover time as well as improve animal care. A 10-minute exam can reduce an animal's stay in the shelter by several days if an identifying feature is recognized that speeds reclaim, or a medical condition is noted, assessed, and dealt with promptly.

As with all medical procedures, documentation is important. A sample health check form is shown in Appendix 18.1. This particular form was designed to progress from the least invasive aspects of a physical exam to more "personal" and potentially risky areas such as examination of eyes, teeth, and genitals. This allows at least minimal assessment of temperament as the exam progresses, and staff can discontinue the exam or get help if an animal appears likely to bite at any point. Many other models are available for physical exam forms that may suit your particular shelter's needs. Whatever form is used should flow logically and be quick and simple for busy staff to fill out.

DISEASE RECOGNITION: USING DIAGNOSTIC TESTING

Any procedure used to determine whether or not a disease or other condition is present can be considered a diagnostic test. This includes blood and fecal tests, cultures, skin scrapings, observation of physical symptoms, and tests designed to detect potential behavioral concerns. Diagnostic testing in a shelter may serve multiple purposes, including the following:

- Population protection
- Identification and segregation or removal of infectious animals
- Adopter protection
- Recognition of zoonotic conditions
- Recognition of serious and/or expensive conditions that could lead to heartbreak
- Recognition of potentially dangerous or problematic behaviors
- Early recognition and treatment of disease
- Risk assessment prior to investment in an individual animal (i.e., FeLV/FIV testing cats prior to sending out to foster care or treatment for upper respiratory infection)
- Periodic surveillance for the identification of prevailing causes of common syndromes (i.e., diarrhea, upper respiratory infection) to evaluate management and treatment strategies

A well-thought out diagnostic testing strategy is a key component of a preventive medicine plan in a shelter. This section will cover the general considerations for testing in shelters. Details on testing for specific diseases can be found in chapter 16.

General Considerations for Diagnostic Testing in a Shelter

The stakes are high when performing diagnostic testing in a shelter. False negative test results can lead to a false sense of security and devastating outbreaks, while a false positive can needlessly cost an animal its life. It is crucial that tests be chosen, administered, and interpreted in a way that maximizes the benefit while minimizing the cost, both for the population and individual animals. No single recipe for diagnostic testing is appropriate for all shelters. Questions to consider when developing a testing program include the following:

- Should you test at all? (cost/benefit analysis)
- What are the factors that influence the test's accuracy?
- Which tests should you use?
- Which animals should you test?
  - All animals at risk (screening test)
  - Certain asymptomatic animals at increased risk
  - Only symptomatic animals (diagnostic test)
- What actions will be taken based on the test results?
  - Confirmatory testing
  - Isolation
  - Treatment
  - Euthanasia

To test or not to test?

The answer to this question is not always immediately obvious. Testing should only be performed when the benefits of doing so outweigh the risks. In addition to the cost of the test itself, the accuracy of available tests must be considered. Virtually all diagnostic tests result in some false positive and negative results. The risks of *not testing* or accepting a *false negative* result include the following:

- Failure to detect an infectious disease that can spread within the population and/or cause zoonotic disease
- Failure to identify a condition requiring immediate treatment

• Failure to identify a sick animal that then gets adopted out, causing heartbreak, angry phone calls, lawsuits, and so on

For a disease or condition where these risks are high, testing is a high priority, and a test that is unlikely to give false negative results is preferred (high negative predictive value). Conditions in this category include serious infectious and zoonotic diseases, behavioral conditions such as aggression towards humans, and diseases where early intervention is key to a good prognosis.

The risk of *testing* or accepting a *false positive* result includes the following:

• Euthanasia or rejection of an animal that is not really ill (including stigma of disease that may discourage adopters)
• Cost and possible complications of treatment
• Cost and staff time required for testing takes resources away from other needed programs

For a disease that poses a low population and human health risk, the risk of testing at all may outweigh the risk of not testing, particularly if the disease in question is uncommon, or if the only available test is error prone and/or expensive. If the decision is made to test, a test that is very unlikely to give a false positive result is preferred.

Factors Influencing Test Accuracy

Whenever testing is performed, inaccurate results will occur some percentage of the time. False results occur due to the characteristics of the test itself, frequency of disease in the tested population, an assortment of biological factors, and of course mishandling of the test or sample (Barr, 1996). Test accuracy influences choice of test(s), choice of test population, and interpretation of the test results.

Measuring Test Accuracy: Sensitivity, Specificity, and Predictive Value

A test may result in one of four outcomes: true positive, true negative, false positive, or false negative. Some terms used to describe the likelihood of various test outcomes are as follows:

Sensitivity: The probability that an animal that *does* have the disease in question will test *positive* for the disease. A very sensitive test recognizes almost all animals that have the disease as positive. For example, an FIV test that is 90 percent sensitive

will call 90/100 truly infected cats positive, but 10 will test false negative using this test. The higher the sensitivity, the fewer false negatives.

Specificity: The probability that an animal that *does not* have the disease in question will test *negative*. A very specific test means very few animals that don't have the disease will test positive. For example, an FIV test that is 95 percent specific would call 95 truly uninfected cats negative, and five would test false positive. The better the specificity, the fewer false positives.

Positive predictive value (PPV): The probability that a positive test result is true (the animal actually has the disease in question). PPV is high when a test is very *specific* (few false positives) and the *disease is common* in the population being tested. Calculation of the predictive value requires knowledge of the test sensitivity, specificity, and disease frequency in the test population.

PPV = true test positives/total test positives

Negative predictive value (NPV): The probability that a negative test result is true (the animal really doesn't have the disease in question). NPV is high when a test is very *sensitive* (few false negatives) and the *disease is rare* in the population being tested.

NPV = true test negatives/total test negatives

Example 1, found in Appendix 18.1, demonstrates the calculation of PPV and NPV for a hypothetical FIV test. In this example, even though the sensitivity and specificity of the test are quite good, a positive test result is correct only 15 percent of the time, although a negative result is correct over 99 percent of the time. The poor positive predictive value of the test is mainly due to the low frequency of disease in the tested population. This is discussed further in the section on disease frequency.

EVALUATING SENSITIVITY AND SPECIFICITY

An ideal test is both very sensitive and specific, leading to accurate prediction of true disease status. Often, however, a trade-off is required. A very sensitive test is frequently less specific (results in more false positives) and vice versa. Some of the tests commonly used in shelters have been evaluated by independent studies for sensitivity and specificity (Brunner, Hendrix, et al., 1988; Swango, 1991; Hoskins, Mirza, et al., 1996; Maggs, Lappin, et al.,

1999). If independent studies can't be found for that test, experts in the field may be able to give an idea of the test's accuracy. Test manufacturers can also be asked for data regarding test sensitivity and specificity, keeping in mind that conditions under which tests are used will influence how well the laboratory results carry over into field situations.

The testing strategy and an interpretation of the results can be used to manipulate sensitivity and specificity to some extent. This is especially helpful when no single test has the desired characteristics. *Specificity* of testing can be increased by using two tests, and by requiring that *both* tests be positive to call an animal infected. For instance, one could require that a cat test positive on both an ELISA and Western Blot test for FIV before being considered infected. *Sensitivity* is increased by using two tests, and by calling an animal positive if it is positive on *either* test. An example would be considering a dog parvo-positive if it tests positive on a fecal ELISA *or* if it has symptoms and decreased white blood cells on a blood smear. Another example would be in testing for possible aggression; because the consequences of failing to detect an aggression problem are potentially severe, the shelter may require that the dog be negative on several different assessment criteria (such as handling, food guarding, and toy or resource possession), in order to call the overall test results negative for signs of aggression.

UNDERSTANDING THE EFFECT OF
DISEASE FREQUENCY

No matter how sensitive or specific the test, positive predictive value is decreased when the disease is uncommon in the population being tested and vice versa. This can be a concern when using a screening test on a healthy population, as was demonstrated in example 1. Sometimes estimates of disease frequency are available in the literature, and true disease prevalence can also be estimated from test results by a simple formula described in example 3 in Appendix 18.2.

Although the numbers given in example 1 are used for demonstration purposes only, the effect of disease frequency on predictive value is not simply a hypothetical concern. In one study, for example, it was estimated that as many as 69 percent of positive results from FeLV ELISA tests in veterinary hospitals were incorrect (Hardy and Zuckerman, 1991). This may make the shelter practitioner think twice

about the utility of using these tests in shelters. In addition to medical reasons for testing, however, it is important to consider the political and emotional costs of adopting out animals that go on to test positive for serious illness at veterinary clinics soon afterwards.

IMPROVING PREDICTIVE VALUE

Although sensitivity and specificity are useful measures, predictive value is the most important in practice because it indicates the level of confidence that should be placed in a given test result. As discussed previously, if the consequences of a false positive test result are very severe (such as euthanasia of the individual), a test with a high positive predictive value is desired. If the consequences of a false negative test result are potentially devastating (such as the spread of parvo to the entire shelter population), a high negative predictive value is crucial. PPV can be improved by selecting a test population in which the disease is more likely, as shown in example 2 in Appendix 18.2, where the positive predictive value of an FIV test is improved by testing only adult intact male cats. This does not mean that testing need actually be restricted to this population, only that more confidence should be placed in a positive result in an animal with consistent signalment (high risk age, breed, sex, and so on) and clinical signs suggestive of the disease in question.

Predictive value can also be manipulated by choosing tests (or test combinations) with greater sensitivity or specificity, as discussed previously. This is the best way to improve NPV (applying the test to a population in which the disease is infrequent would also work, but it makes little sense). Choosing a more sensitive test or considering an animal positive if it meets any of several test criteria will improve NPV, while choosing a more specific test or requiring more than one test criteria to make the diagnosis will lead to an improved PPV.

Beyond Sensitivity and Specificity: Other Factors Influencing Test Accuracy

Apart from the characteristics of the test itself and the frequency of disease in the test population, biological factors influence whether the test results can be accurately interpreted. Commonly used tests detect either antibodies to disease, some component of the disease-causing agent (i.e., antigen), or the agent itself. To understand what can interfere with test interpretation, it is necessary to know what the test detects. FIV and distemper are two common diseases in shelters for which an antibody test may be used. Parvo, panleukopenia, FeLV, and most heartworm snap tests look for antigen. Considerations for individual tests are discussed in chapter 16. False negative results occur when the test sample does not contain the antigen or antibody the test is designed to detect, even though the animal is infected. Reasons for this include the following:

• Antibodies not being produced
  – Immune incompetence due to age (puppies and kittens), concurrent or overwhelming disease
  – Recent infection
  – For example, FIV ELISA can be a false negative in kittens less than six months old and in adult cats with a recent infection
• Antigen no longer being shed late in infection, or not yet being shed early in infection
  – For example, a parvo test results in a false negative after day five to seven of clinical disease (Greene, 1998)
• Antigen not present in test sample even though animal is systemically infected
  – For example, the saliva/tear test for FeLV is prone to false negatives (Hawkins, 1991)
• Antigen not yet present due to the organism's life stage
  – For example, heartworm tests can detect adult worms that take six months to develop in infected animals. Puppies under six months of age and recently infected dogs also test false negative.
• Antigen all bound by an antibody
  – For example, all parvo antigen may be bound by an antibody in an immune competent animal around day five

False positive results occur when the test sample contains the antigen or antibody detected by the test, but not because the animal is infected. Reasons for this include the following:

•Antibodies exist due to vaccination.
  – Both killed and modified live vaccines produce antibodies that can interfere with the interpretation of antibody-based testing.
  – For example, vaccination for FIV will cause false positive results on the FIV snap test.

• Modified live vaccines can cause antigen shedding for a short period after vaccination, leading to false positive results on antigen-based tests.
  – For example, an antigen from modified live vaccine for parvo or panleukopenia can cause false positive for 5–12 days after vaccination, possibly more for "high antigen mass" vaccines (usually a weak positive).
• Maternal antibody is present.
  – For example, kittens under six months of age may test positive for FIV due to the presence of maternal antibodies.
• Environmental contamination occurs.
  – For example, a positive ringworm culture occurs due to coat contamination in an uninfected cat.

False positive results can also occur with some tests because the test is unable to differentiate between the disease agent in question and another closely related but benign agent. In addition, testing for some diseases is further complicated by the natural history of the disease. For instance, cats may test positive and be truly infected with FeLV, but some go on to recover from the infection. Feline infectious peritonitis (FIP) can't be accurately detected by any single blood test currently available because it is indistinguishable from infection with the feline enteric corona virus (FeCV) from which it is derived. Finally, a positive result may reflect an animal's true infection status, but still not identify the cause of its symptoms. For instance, *Bordetella bronchiseptica* may be cultured from the oropharynx of a cat, but its disease may be caused by a viral infection (or vice versa). All of these factors must be considered when deciding who to test and what to conclude from the results.

Choice of Test Population

Careful selection of the animals to test increases the likelihood of accurate results, and minimizes the cost of unnecessary testing. Before testing any animal, consider whether the results can be meaningfully interpreted. Obviously, puppies should not be tested for heartworm, and the value of testing kittens for FIV is minimal. Testing recently vaccinated animals for parvo or panleukopenia can be valuable if a negative test result is obtained—this can certainly help rule out the disease. However, a positive test result is of limited value during the period when fecal antigen shedding is possible due to vaccination. In such a situation, other factors such as symptoms, probability of disease based on age and breed risk, and results of other tests also must be considered. As discussed previously, the PPV of a test is improved by administering it only to those animals at relatively high infection risk.

To further limit the number of animals that need to be tested, consider the purpose of testing. If adopter protection is the main reason for testing, only those animals that are very likely to be adopted should be tested. On the other hand, if population protection is the goal, all animals at risk for spreading the disease in question should be tested.

Risk Assessment and Decision Making

When interpreting a test result, there are two choices: The initial result can be taken at face value, or further confirmatory testing can be performed. This decision depends on the likelihood that the initial result is correct; the availability, cost, and practicality of confirmatory testing; and the ramifications of accepting an inaccurate result (as discussed previously). Most commonly, when screening for disease in a healthy population, negative results are accepted at face value. This is generally appropriate; recall that NPV is high when the likelihood of disease is low in the test population. On the other hand, when the consequences of accepting a false negative are severe and the sensitivity of the test is low, confirmation may be indicated, especially in an animal at high risk for disease. For example, a negative result from Woods lamp screening for ringworm might be acceptable before adding a healthy adult cat to a group housing area, but the same results in a kitten with characteristic signs of ringworm infection must be viewed with suspicion.

In deciding what do with animals testing positive for infectious disease, shelters must also consider the current fate of healthy animals in their shelter and community. For instance, false positive test results for FeLV may be common, due to the low prevalence in the healthy population and the natural history of the disease. Various confirmatory tests are available, which involve additional cost and the logistical difficulties of holding the animal while awaiting results. The risk of euthanizing the cat is that it *may* be perfectly healthy. Sadly, however, many shelters are overwhelmed by large numbers of cats that are FeLV negative and also seem perfectly healthy. A cat testing positive even on a test

with relatively poor predictive value is still much more likely to be ill than one testing negative. When choosing between euthanizing FeLV-positive and FeLV-negative cats that are otherwise of similar adoptability, it makes sense to choose the FeLV-positive cats, leaving more resources available for the rest of the population. On the other hand, for a shelter that must choose between euthanizing an unconfirmed FeLV-positive cat and not euthanizing any cat at all, investing in additional testing is indicated. The same logic applies to a limited admission shelter in deciding whether to admit or turn away test positive animals without confirmation.

Training and Documentation

As mentioned at the start of this section, stakes are high when performing diagnostic testing in a shelter, and incorrect handling of the tests or samples will undermine the accuracy of even the best test. Therefore testing should be performed only by designated and trained staff. All staff responsible for this testing should be trained directly by a veterinary or registered veterinarian technician (RVT). Sample handling must be meticulous and the manufacturer's instructions followed exactly. In addition to noting the test's results on each animal's permanent record, a log also should be kept for each type of test used. This makes it possible to calculate the percentage of positive, negative, and inconclusive results over time, thus allowing you to track patterns of increasing or decreasing diagnosis of disease in the tested population. Testing logs also help monitor the usefulness of a given test. If you find animals only test positive a tiny percentage of the time, the benefit of testing should be carefully considered.

CONCLUSION

A successful disease recognition program in a shelter involves all staff and volunteers monitoring and reporting signs of illness; screening exams for all shelter animals performed by trained staff; and a diagnostic testing plan that makes rational use of the available tests and the shelter's resources. A well designed program protects the shelter population from disease spread; protects adopters from zoonotic disease, unexpected vet bills, or the heartbreak of serious disease in their new companion; and ensures that individual animals receive the care they need.

REFERENCES

Barr, M. C. 1996. FIV, FeLV, and FIPV: Interpretation and misinterpretation of serological test results. *Seminars in Veterinary Medicine and Surgery (Small Animal)* 11 (3): 144 –153.

Brunner, C. J., Hendrix, C.M., et al. 1988 Comparison of serologic tests for detection of antigen in canine heartworm infections. *Journal of the American Veterinary Medical Association* 192 (10): 1423–1427.

Greene, C. E. 1998. *Infectious Diseases of the Dog and Cat*. Philadelphia, PA: W.B. Saunders.

Hardy, W. D., Jr., and Zuckerman, E. E.. 1991. Ten-year study comparing enzyme-linked immunosorbent assay with the immunofluorescent antibody test for detection of feline leukemia virus infection in cats. *Journal of the American Veterinary Medical Association* 199 (10): 1365–1373.

Hawkins, E. C. 1991. Saliva and tear tests for feline leukemia virus. *Journal of the American Veterinary Medical Association* 199 (10): 1382 –1385.

Hoskins, J. D., Mirza, T., et al. 1996. Evaluation of a fecal antigen test for the diagnosis of canine parvovirus. *Journal of the American College of Veterinary Internal Medicine* 10: 159.

Maggs, D. J., Lappin, M. R., et al. 1999. Evaluation of serologic and viral detection methods for diagnosing feline herpesvirus-1 infection in cats with acute respiratory tract or chronic ocular disease. *Journal of the American Veterinary Medical Association* 214 (4): 502–507.

Swango, L. J. 1991. Evaluation of feline leukemia virus diagnostic tests available for in-office use by veterinarians. *Journal of the American Veterinary Medical Association* 199 (10): 1386–1389.

Appendix 18.1
Sample Animal Health Check Form

Animal Health Check   Evaluator: _____

Date: _____   **Animal ID #:** _____   **Kennel:**_____

1. **Temperature:** _____ **Weight:**_____ kgs/lbs (circle one)
2. **Approximate age:** _____ **mo**   Young adult ___   Adult ___   Older ___
3. **Overall appearance:**   Bright, alert, responsive ___   See below ___
4. **Temperament:**   Initial assessment: Social, friendly ___   See below ___
5. **Hydration:**   No sign of dehydration: ___   See below ___
6. **Muscoloskeletal:**   Lameness or asymmetry? No ___   Yes/See below ___
7. **Body Condition Score:** _____/9
8. **Skin:**   Fleas/ticks?   No ___   Yes: _____
   Hair loss/itching?   No ___   Yes: _____
   Masses/sores?   No ___   Yes: _____
9. **Ears:**   Clean and free of inflammation or discharge ___   See below ___
10. **Eyes:**   Clear, no discharge, white sclera: ___   See below ___
11. **Nose:**   Clear, no discharge ___   See below ___
12. **Mouth: Teeth:** Clean ___   Moderate dental disease ___   Severe dental disease ___
    Broken, missing or very worn teeth?_____
      Gums: Pink and healthy ___   See below ___
      Oral pain, ulcers or masses? _____
13. **Trachea:** Cough present with mild tracheal stimulation? No ___   Yes ___
14. **Heart and lungs:** Heart murmur heard? No ___   See below ___
    Lungs sound clear? Yes ___   See below ___
15. **Abdomen**:   Pain or masses felt on palpation? No ___   See below ___
16. **Urogenital:**   Double check sex/presence of both testicles/check for spay scar:
    Male ___   Female ___   Neutered male ___   Spay scar ___   See below ___

Abnormal findings: _____

_____

_____

Appendix 18.2
Examples

NOTE: Values for sensitivity, specificity, and frequency used in this and all other examples in this chapter are intended for demonstration purposes only and do not necessarily reflect actual test accuracy or disease frequency.

Example 1: Sensitivity, Specificity, Frequency, and Predictive Value

A hypothetical FIV test with a sensitivity and specificity of 90 percent and 95 percent, respectively, is applied to a test population of 1000 shelter cats of unknown disease status, with an estimated frequency of FIV infection at 1 percent.

Frequency of 1 percent means that out of 1000 cats, 10 will be infected with FIV, and 990 will be free of the disease. Sensitivity of 90 percent means of the 10 true positives, 90 percent will test positive: $.90 \times 10 = 9$. Specificity of 95 percent means 95 percent of the truly negative cats will test negative: $.95 \times 990 = 940.5$ (round off to 940 for simplicity). That leaves 990 - 940 = 50 of the truly negative cats test positive:

	FIV +	FIV –	Total
Test +	9	50	59
Test –	1	940	941
Total	10	990	1000

Positive Predictive Value (PPV) = true positives/total positives = 9/59 = .15 (15 percent).
Negative Predictive Value (NPV) = true negatives/total negatives = 940/941 = .9989 (99.89 percent)

Example 2: Increasing Frequency Improves Positive Predictive Value.

Return to the scenario described in Example 1, but this time test only adult, intact male cats, with an estimated disease frequency of 10 percent (as opposed to 1 percent in Example 1).

Frequency = 10% × 1000 cats = 100 infected with FIV, and 900 free of the disease. Sensitivity = 90% × 100 truly infected = 90 true positives and 100-90 = 10 false negatives.

Specificity = 95% × 900 truly uninfected = 855 true negatives, and 900-855 = 45 false positives:

	FIV +	FIV –	Total
Test +	90	45	135
Test –	10	855	865
Total	100	900	1000

PPV = true positives/total positives = 90/135 = .666 (66.6 percent) .
NPV = true negatives/total negatives = 855/865 = .988 (98.8 percent)

So by choosing a test population in which disease is more likely, a positive result is more than four times more likely to be correct compared to the preceding example, and negative predictive value is still quite good.

Example 3: Estimating True Disease Prevalence from Apparent Prevalence

Knowing that a proportion of positive test results are inaccurate, it is sometimes helpful to be able to estimate the true frequency of disease in the test population. In order to calculate this for your shelter population, you will need to keep records of test results until you have a reasonable number of samples (more samples the less common positive results are) and obtain an estimate of the sensitivity (SE) and specificity (SP) of the test used. The formula to calculate true prevalence (TP, the total actually diseased out of the total population tested) from the apparent prevalence (AP, the total positive results out of the total population tested) is

$$TP = AP + (SP – 1)/ (SE + SP – 1)$$

Use the same numbers as in Example 1, but assume this time that we don't know the true frequency but are working backward from the test results:

SE = .9 (90 percent)
SP = .95 (95 percent)
AP = 59/1000 = .059 (total test positives out of total population tested)
TP = .059 + (.95-1)/ (.9 + .95 – 1) = .009/.85 = .01, or 1 percent, which was the true frequency we assumed when we set up the exercise—so it worked! Go ahead . . . try it on some of the test data you have collected over the last six months in your shelter.

Section 4:
Shelter and Community Programs

INTRODUCTION

In order for shelters to deal effectively with pet overpopulation and promote the health and welfare of animals in both shelters and the community, a variety of programs have come into existence. Many of these innovative programs have been very controversial, dividing both veterinarians and the humane community. Some of these programs were created to address specific issues of concern identified by the community, while others were the result of needs identified by the shelter that are not always understood by the general public. Some needs have changed with time. In some shelters, shortages of puppies and kittens have been accompanied by the arrival of a rising number of adolescent animals with behavior problems. This has caused a shift in focus from neutering to behavior programs to not only evaluate the animals in the shelter, but to help prevent relinquishment. Reid, Goldman, and Zawistowski discuss current knowledge and trends in shelter behavior programs in chapter 19, while Marder and Posage provides a brief look at the use of drugs to treat behavior problems in chapter 20. Sinclair provides an in-depth examination of foster care in chapter 21. These programs should be considered essential for any shelter trying to reduce its euthanasia numbers and raise staff morale. The opportunity for the public to become involved in the life of the shelter and save lives by providing temporary, alternative humane environments for marginal but adoptable animals should not be ignored.

Humane societies have clashed for years with professional veterinary associations over the provision of low-cost neutering services for the public. While it might seem that a chapter dedicated to spaying/neu-

tering is not necessary in a textbook on shelter medicine, veterinarians will find that chapter 22 by Appel is a thoughtful consideration of the normal and special situations encountered when performing multiple surgeries in the shelter environment. The author sets realistic standards that reflect efficiency as well as safety. Levy tackles the controversial topic of feral cat management in chapter 23 by providing the latest data about feral cats and guidelines for setting up trap neuter release programs.

Even as shelters struggle to reduce their euthanasia rates, it is critical to establish and maintain high standards to ensure that when it must be performed, it is with dignity, humane care, and concern for both the animals and staff. Sinclair provides valuable and detailed information for designing safe and compassionate euthanasia protocols in chapter 24, which includes a section on animal handling.

While it is hoped that most shelter veterinarians never find themselves confronted with natural or manmade disasters, it is important to be prepared. Lloyd gives basic information in chapter 25 on disaster preparedness, with guidelines based largely on his own personal experiences. Hopefully this information will help veterinarians be an effective member of any management team facing the challenge of providing care for animals affected by disasters.

There is insufficient space to cover all the other shelter programs that veterinarians may be asked to design and participate in, such as humane education programs, dog bite prevention, media events, responsible pet care seminars, and so on. All these programs contribute to the health and welfare of animals and help strengthen the human animal bond, and veterinarians are encouraged to participate in them.

19
Animal Shelter Behavior Programs

Pamela Reid, Jill Goldman, and Stephen Zawistowski

INTRODUCTION

For most of the 20th century, animal shelters confronted an animal population problem perpetuated by the seemingly unending production of puppies and kittens by unaltered pets. As humane groups and others began to implement programs that advocated legislation, education, and sterilization (see Zawistowski and Morris, chapter 1 in this volume) in the later half of the century, a slow but steady decline in the numbers of unwanted companion animals was realized. In studies by Salman et al. (1998), Patronek et al. (1996a, 1996b) and others, it became clear that adolescent and adult animals now constitute the most significant proportion of dogs and cats relinquished to animal shelters. Additional analyses by Salman et al. (2000) and Patronek et al. (1996a and 1996b) indicate that behavior problems with companion animals constitute one of the most significant reasons for these relinquishments. In addition, surveys of pet owners who still have their pets indicate that while they "claim" that their dogs and cats are well-behaved, further probing reveals that many of them have problems with housetraining, aggression, and other issues (Ralston-Purina, 2000). Given the context that many shelters are receiving fewer animals than they have in the past, and that those animals they do have are likely to have behavior problems, there has been a trend to develop programs that evaluate the problems animals may present, provide enrichment and rehabilitation when possible, determine which animals may not be appropriate for placement in new homes, and provide support services following placement in new homes.

This chapter will cover topics related to the evaluation of animals upon intake, the relative validity and utility of available temperament tests, the use of enrichment programs to provide a more humane environment for dogs and cats, and the provision of support services for new companion animal guardians following adoption.

EVALUATING THE BEHAVIOR OF SHELTER ANIMALS

One of the most daunting challenges faced by shelter workers is to assess the temperament of an animal entering the system. Temperament or "personality" is assumed to be the result of an interaction between genetic influences and environmental persuasions (Goodloe, 1996). Temperament, therefore, can only be assessed through an examination of the animal's behavioral characteristics. A behavioral profile is critical in a shelter environment for a variety of reasons: (a) first and foremost, to provide an indication of the adoptability of the animal; (b) to suggest suitable housing and enrichment for the animal; (c) to allow for safe handling of the animal by workers; (d) to best match the animal to a prospective adopter; and (e) to guide any behavioral intervention that might be undertaken with the animal during the shelter stay and/or following adoption. Despite the tremendous value of behavioral descriptions, surprisingly little scientific effort has been directed toward designing a reliable, valid, and precise measurement tool.

Some shelters rely solely on intake information, where available, and observations of the animal's behavior by staff. Other shelters also require that the animal undergo a series of standardized tests designed to simulate common everyday events that might be experienced by the animal following adoption. A summary of the animal's temperament is generated from the animal's reactions during testing. Some shelters only evaluate dogs; others evaluate both dogs and cats. A variety of evaluations for dogs exist in the shelter community, transmitted via word of mouth, and through presentations, instructional books, and videotapes by respected authorities (i.e., American Humane, 2002; Sternberg, 2002). Current evaluations vary tremendously in complexity. The SAFER (Safety Assessment for Evaluating Rehoming) evaluation is probably the simplest, as it consists of five items and requires approximately 10 minutes to administer. The ASPCA evaluation developed by Amy Marder is significantly more intensive, as it consists of 142 items and requires between one and a half to two hours to administer (Marder 2002). The value of the information generated from these evaluation procedures is perpetuated by a self-fulfilling prophecy. The dogs that do well after adoption that were predicted to do well substantiate the test. The dogs that do poorly after adoption, despite predictions to the contrary can be explained away. Maybe the evaluation didn't address the type of behavior problem that arose; maybe contingencies in the new home prompted development of the problem.

A Behavior Evaluation Validation Study

The first evaluation instrument for shelter dogs appearing in the scientific literature (van der Borg, et al., 1991) included 21 subtests, incorporating set-ups the authors felt were most likely to elicit aggression, fear, separation anxiety, and behaviors stemming from a lack of training. Short descriptions of a sample of the subtests are as follows:

1. Friendly approach by a stranger while the dog is in its cage
2. Basic obedience commands: "sit", "down", "stay", and "come"
3. Play tug-of-war with handler
4. Mock veterinary examination by stranger in a white coat
5. Approach by a doll mounted on wheels, representing a two- to three-year old child, while the dog is tied in a corner
6. Approach by a threatening man, staring and making striking movements at the dog, while the dog is tied in a corner

7. Five-minute trip in a car, then left alone in the car for 10 minutes
8. Removal of food bowl while the dog is eating
9. Pass by a jogger
10. Unfold an umbrella.

Van der Borg et al. (1991) tested 81 dogs (strays and owner-surrenders) from five animal shelters and, one to two months following adoption, interviewed 72 owners about their dog's behavior. The objective was to measure the predictive validity of the evaluation procedure. They also asked each animal's attendant to complete a questionnaire on the dog's behavioral characteristics. Only 26 dogs showed no signs of aggression in all 21 subtests, and over half of the dogs reacted fearfully in response to the threatening stranger. Thirty-two dogs showed indications of anxiety when left alone, and 30 dogs failed to respond to at least one basic obedience command. When interviewed, 65 of the 72 owners reported a whopping 190 problem behaviors displayed by their adopted dogs. Forty-three of these owners conveyed that the problems were substantial. The problems most frequently reported were pulling on a leash, aggression toward people, general disobedience, anxiety when left alone, aggression toward dogs, and car-related problems. Interestingly, *none* of the owners who adopted dogs that displayed aggression when food or a bone was removed during the evaluation considered this aggression a problem. This was the case, despite the fact that only 25 percent of owners did not try to take items away from the dog.

The behavioral evaluation predicted almost 75 percent of the problem behaviors reported by the new owners, whereas shelter staff predicted only 33 percent. In general, the tests were better at correctly predicting the presence of problem behavior than at correctly predicting the *absence* of problem behavior. In fact, the test generated many false positives, saying that dogs would exhibit a variety of problem behaviors when, in fact, they did not. On the other hand, shelter staff was better at correctly predicting the absence of problem behaviors than they were at predicting the presence of problem behaviors. They generated more false negatives, prophesying that dogs would not exhibit problem behaviors when, indeed, they did.

Thus, the van der Borg et al. (1991) behavior assessment instrument, which includes many of the same subtests as other shelter evaluations, is not a precise tool for describing dog temperament. In fact, it could prove to be an even poorer assessment because the dogs tested were not selected randomly. These dogs had already been prescreened, via the shelters' usual processes, and only those considered candidates for adoption were subsequently tested. Furthermore, it cannot be discerned if weaknesses lay in the subtests used, in the interpretation of the behaviors displayed, and/or in the way the problem behaviors were measured post-adoption. Subsequent attempts to validate behavior assessment tools have been similarly unimpressive (American Humane, 2002; Netto and Planta, 1997).

Psychometric Theory

Instruments designed to measure aspects of human personality are subjected to rigorous reliability and validity testing to ensure that the tools do what test developers claim they do. If we hope to design a useful evaluation test for shelter dogs, we would be wise to adopt psychometric theory rather than work toward our goal intuitively and haphazardly. Psychometricians painstakingly analyze test content, administration procedures, reliability coefficients, scoring methods, and finally, validity assessments before applying a stamp of approval to a human personality test (Nunnally and Bernstein, 1994).

CONTENT VALIDITY

Content validity refers to the actual design of the instrument to ensure that the sampling is reflective of the animal's behavior. Each item must be scrutinized to ensure it provides useful information. In the case of behavioral assessment tools for shelter animals, most subtests consist of actual exposure to the stimuli of interest. For instance, how does the dog respond to being handled, to having food removed, to being verbally admonished? We simply don't know if it is accurate to surmise that if the dog reacted in one manner during the test, the dog is likely to react in the same manner in other similar situations. Other subtests demand far greater leaps of extrapolation: For instance, if the dog chases, grabs, and shakes a moving furry toy, does this accurately reflect how the dog will behave toward a cat or rabbit? Likewise, if the dog barks and lunges at a lifelike doll in the test, does this mean that the dog will act the same toward an infant? We do, in fact, know that this is not true. Reid et al. (2002, in preparation) demonstrated that dogs with a history

of displaying aggressive behavior toward children are no more likely to react aggressively to a lifelike doll than are dogs with a history of displaying friendly behavior toward children. Child-aggressive dogs do, however, take more time to approach and investigate any of a variety of novel objects presented to them than child-friendly dogs.

An internally valid behavioral tool will generate similar patterns of behavior from different subtests meant to measure the same aspects of temperament. For instance, some evaluations include the presentation of a variety of loud noises. You would expect that a noise-sensitive dog would respond in a similar fashion to all of the sounds. Similarly, a dog that snaps at a person manipulating its feet would also be expected to react unfavorably to having its nails clipped during the mock veterinary examination.

Also related to validity are questions of how the tool should be administered. How should test items be ordered? Can one order elicit a different pattern of behavioral reactions than a different order? For instance, if the dog reacts fearfully or aggressively to one subtest, does this influence its reactions to subsequent tests? It may be sufficient to allow a set amount of time between items. Alternatively, some type of neutral experience may need to be inserted between each item to "reset" the dog before the next subtest.

When should a dog be tested? Some shelters run the dog through the behavioral evaluation upon presentation of the animal by the owner, as a means for determining whether the animal should be accepted. However, Hennessy et al. (1997) revealed that dogs experience elevated levels of the stress-related adrenal hormone cortisol during their first three days in an animal shelter. On the first day, cortisol levels in the shelter dogs were nearly three times those of pet dogs sampled in their homes. Presumably stress influences a dog's reactivity to events so this suggests that shelters should delay evaluations until the dog has been in the shelter for at least three days. As more and more shelters go "no kill" in their philosophy, there is need for an evaluation tool that can be administered and interpreted easily and quickly so only highly adoptable animals are accepted into their facilities.

RELIABILITY

Test-retest reliability should, in general, be expected from an evaluation tool because temperament is expressed through consistent patterns of behavior. In certain subtests, however, the point is to assess the dog's reaction to novel stimuli. Netto and Planta (1997) tested 112 dogs on their aggression evaluation instrument and then retested 37 dogs. They established that aggressive displays toward people were significantly correlated in the test and retest. They were not able to demonstrate good test-retest reliability in the subtests that measured aggression toward dogs. The stimulus dog behaved more aggressively during the second testing, and they felt this caused the test dogs to be more inhibited.

Interobserver reliability is another important measure of the test's worth. A good evaluation should be designed such that multiple people watching the same dog will score its behavior the same way. Not surprising, the more objective the scoring system, the higher the interobserver reliability coefficient (Burch et al., 2002).

PREDICTIVE VALIDITY

Predictive validity refers to how well the instrument actually predicts behavior in situations of interest. Does the test predict how the dog behaves in the shelter and/or in its new home? You might expect certain patterns of behavior to be less flexible across time and situations than others. Furthermore, some problem behavior is highly owner-dependent, such as dominance aggression and attachment disorder, or being spatially dependent, such as territorial aggression.

There are two procedures by which predictive validity can be measured. One possibility is to test two populations of animals with known behavioral histories, with one group displaying no significant behavior problems and the other displaying significant behavior problems. If the evaluation is valid, it should differentiate clearly between these two populations. This was the procedure adopted in Netto and Planta's (1997) study of evaluating aggressive behavior in dogs.

A second option is to validate the test on shelter animals. However, it is critical that the test's results play no part in determining the nature of the home into which the animal is adopted. Extensive follow-up on the animals once they are placed into homes is required, with the follow-up consisting of owner reports (obtained through interviews or questionnaires), retesting of the animals in their home environments, or both. Researchers who did not evaluate the animals should conduct the follow-ups, so

that animals' performance on the evaluation will not inadvertently bias data collection. The ideal duration of the follow-up is unknown, although it is reasonable to assume that after a time, influences from the new environment will play a substantial role in determining the animal's behavior. Once follow-up data are collected, the final step is to statistically link the results on the evaluation with behavior manifested in the home. Some items on the test will hopefully prove to be good predictors of specific behavior patterns, while other items may prove to be uninformative or redundant and can be eliminated.

Decision Criteria

The use of behavioral evaluations to classify a subset of shelter animals as unadoptable is a controversial issue. Life-and-death decisions are made on the output of instruments that may not be predictive of behaviors at other times or in other circumstances. Some shelters have liberal decision criteria, while others have conservative criteria. It may be that our existing evaluation tools are only valuable for identifying animals at the extreme ends of the behavioral continuum: Dogs that are highly sociable, confident, and nonreactive are identified for adoption, and dogs that are asocial, fearful, and aggressive are identified for euthanasia. Alternatively, our tools may not even do that adequately. There are so many unknowns that quality scientific research is sorely needed. In the meantime, we recommend that when behavior evaluations are used at animal shelters, they are used as part of an overall shelter management process. Rarely should the results be used as a stand-alone tool for determining whether an animal should be made available for placement. Much like the use of medical diagnostic tests discussed elsewhere in this text, placement and euthanasia decisions reflect the resources and experience of shelters, the demographics and volume of animals received, and the policies adhered to by individual shelters.

Dangerous Dogs

The evaluation of dangerous dogs, those presented to the shelter following a serious or fatal attack on either humans or conspecifics, or those seized from dog fighting activities, can be a difficult and controversial endeavor. Concern for the safety of those involved often makes it difficult to conduct the evaluation in a way that would clearly reveal the likelihood of the dog engaging in a similar attack again, or identifying the crucial stimuli that may have precipitated the attack. In many cases, the purpose of the evaluation is to assess whether the owner was aware or even contributed to the animal's aggressive proclivities. Shelter veterinarians and staff asked to conduct evaluations of dangerous dogs should contact professionals in animal behavior for guidance, as often it will usually be necessary to develop a procedure specific to the individual dog and suspected circumstances of the attack.

ENRICHMENT

When animals are housed in unnaturally restricted environments (such as in zoos, laboratories, and shelters), the physical and behavioral welfare of those animals is a serious concern. According to the National Research Council's guide for the care and use of laboratory animals (1996, p.22): "Animals should be housed with the goal of maximizing species-specific behaviors and minimizing stress-induced behavior. For social species, this normally requires housing in compatible pairs or groups." We believe that shelter animals deserve no less than animals housed in laboratories. Creating an environment that stimulates and allows for the expression of normal patterns of behavior promotes a behaviorally healthy and therefore, more adoptable, shelter animal. Shelters often work within tight budgetary and personnel constraints, which limit efforts to do more than the bare minimum for the animals in their care. Nevertheless, shelters should place a priority on enrichment programs that reduce stress and promote the physical and psychological well-being of their animals.

Restrictions on Species-Typical Behavior

Free-ranging animals live in environments with enough space, stimulation, and social contact to nurture the expression of their species-typical behavioral repertoire. Behaviors include play, rest, foraging, mating, communicating, rearing of offspring, and territorial investigation and defense. For instance, dogs travel substantial distances, engage in territorial disputes with other dogs, and scavenge for food. Cats hunt, urine mark along regular routes, groom, and sleep. The life of free-ranging animals is not without challenges, such as the scarcity of, and competition for, resources, including food, mates, and shelter.

Shelter animals, in contrast, live in environments with significant physical and social restrictions that usually limit and prevent the expression of their normal range of behaviors. There is no need to search for food or water, there is no territory to patrol or defend, investigation is limited to a small sterile cage or run, and interaction with their conspecifics is typically nonexistent or severely restricted. We contend that an enriched environment for confined animals should stimulate a diverse and flexible repertoire of species-typical behaviors.

In addition to the frustration associated with the inability to engage in species-typical activities, shelter animals experience various psychogenic stressors, such as a lack of control over external events, exposure to novel or frightening surroundings, and separation from social attachment figures (Hennessy et al., 1997). A critical difference between the lives of free-ranging versus shelter animals is not exposure to stress and unpredictability per se, but rather the ability to react to challenging circumstances (Wiepkema & Koolhaas, 1993). Shelter animals usually cannot escape situations that induce stress; they can neither remedy nor rectify potential problems.

Is there a "recipe" for providing the physical and social environment that promotes a healthy expression of the shelter animal's species-typical behavior? There are considerable behavioral differences between dogs and cats, and, within a species, between breeds, ages, and individuals (see Coppinger and Coppinger, 1998; Hart, 1995; Manteca and Deag, 1993; Scott and Fuller, 1965; Serpell, 2000; Sonderegger and Turner, 1996; Turner and Bateson, 2000; Wells and Hepper, 1999). Consequently, individual animals have different environmental requisites for "normal" behavior, and the effects of shelter living will vary with each animal and the amount of time it has been in the shelter.

Quantification of Shelter Animal Welfare

Assessing the welfare of animals is a complex endeavor. Generally, researchers assume that compromised welfare in animals is reflected as higher than normal levels of stress (Wiepkema and Koolhaas, 1993). Poor welfare is typically inferred by measuring 1) behavioral indicators of stress, such as the uniform repetition and distortion of motor patterns or vocalizations (i.e., stereotypies, compulsive behaviors) (Luescher, 2000); and 2) physiological indicators of stress, such as the activation of the body's stress-responsive neuroendocrine system (i.e., hypothalamic-pituitary-adrenal axis [HPA]) and elevated cortisol levels (Wiepkema and Koolhaas, 1993).

Several studies have examined the impact of acute stress (Beerda et al., 1998; Hennessy et al., 1997) and chronic stress in dogs (Beerda et al., 2000; Beerda, Schilder, Bernadina et al., 1999; Beerda, Schilder, van Hooff et al., 1999). For example, Beerda et al. (1998) measured dogs' salivary cortisol and heart rate in response to various aversive stimuli, including sound blasts, shocks from an electronic collar, and a paper bag falling from above. Certain behaviors were also correlated with the physiological responses to these distressing events, such as cowering (a rapid and pronounced lowering of the body), oral behaviors such as tongue flicking and yawning, restlessness, and low body postures (low tail carriage, ears flattened back, and bent legs). Salivary cortisol levels remained elevated for up to 30 minutes after stimulus presentation.

Beerda, Schilder, van Hooff et al. (1999) and Beerda, Schilder, Bernadina et al. (1999) examined behavioral and physiological indicators of chronic stress by transferring dogs from spacious, enriched, outdoor group housing to small, indoor, single-animal kennels. When housed alone, dogs exhibited lower body postures and higher frequencies of auto grooming, paw lifting, vocalizing, coprophagy, and repetitive behavior than when group housed. In addition, male dogs behaved more dominantly and aggressively in the presence of conspecifics (e.g., piloerection, growling, and standing over) when they were housed individually compared to when they were housed in groups.

Elevated HPA hormone levels are also associated with psychogenic stressors in shelter dogs, such as exposure to novel surroundings (Hennessy et al., 1997; Tuber et al., 1996). As mentioned earlier in this chapter, dogs arriving at a shelter experience an increase in cortisol, with levels returning to normal approximately three days later (Hennessey et al., 1997). Similarly, research has shown that laboratory cats, when deprived of human contact and exposed to sudden and unpredictable events such as noise, experience a rise in urinary cortisol and suppress exploratory and play behavior (Carlstead et al., 1993).

There is consensus that housing animals alone, isolation, lack of physical exercise, and under-stimulation are detrimental to the welfare of dogs and promote the development of behavior problems (Hetts et al., 1992; Hubrecht et al., 1992; Hubrecht, 1995). Cats, on the other hand, are more of a conundrum. Free-ranging cats spend a good portion of their time alone and so, housing cats singly may not inflict the same level of social deprivation as it does for dogs. DeMonte and Le Pape (1997) failed to observe behavioral indicators of stress, such as stereotypies or distress vocalizations, in individually housed cats. This is not surprising, however, as evidence suggests that cats react to stress by inhibiting normal behavior rather than exhibiting abnormal behavior (Carlstead et al., 1993; Rochlitz, 2000).

Forms of Enrichment

Shelters can consider a variety of interventions designed to enrich and improve the quality of the animals' lives. Coppinger and Zuccotti (1999, p. 285) contend that, "Agents of enrichment should be goal oriented, in the sense that they allow the animal to develop normally, both physically and behaviorally." With this objective in mind, we present information on housing, object play, physical exercise, foraging activities, training, and social contact with humans and conspecifics.

HOUSING

Dogs require a species-specific social environment to maintain mental health (Coppinger and Zuccotti, 1999). For shelter dogs, group housing satisfies their predisposition to live in social groups. Housing varies between shelters, but, generally, shelters tend toward easy-to-clean facilities and small cages, in order to house as many animals as possible (Hubrecht, 1995). For hygienic reasons, animals are usually housed singly. Dog kennels are often barren because shelter dogs eliminate in their kennels and place heavy wear and tear on toys and bedding. In comparison, shelter cats live in more comfortable cages, primarily because they eliminate in litter boxes and are less destructive than dogs.

There is overwhelming evidence that behavioral, and possibly neurological, disorders develop in a range of species when housed singly in impoverished cages (e.g., feather-picking in parrots [Meehan et al., 2003]; self-biting in macaque monkeys [Reinhardt and Rossell, 2001]; and body rocking in chimpanzees [Spijkerman et al., 1994]). These disorders can be prevented and, in some cases, arrested and even reversed when the animal's environment is enriched to support a healthy, diverse, and flexible behavioral repertoire (Meehan et al., 2003). In social species, the best behavioral option is to house animals in pairs or groups. Shelters may find paired housing more manageable, while still providing dogs with the necessary social stimulation (Hubrecht, 1993). Loveridge (1998a) recommends housing adult dogs in pairs and, when possible, puppies in groups of three. Interestingly, the Waltham Centre for Pet Nutrition houses retired stud dogs with puppies to help the puppies develop inter-dog social skills (Loveridge, 1998a).

Wells and Hepper (1992) believe it is the physical exercise and psychological stimulation (i.e., play, intra-specific communication and interaction, and so forth) animals experience, when housed in groups, that produces fewer inappropriate and compulsive behaviors. The communicative value of olfactory cues, such as scent marking, glandular secretions, and other signals, provide additional sources of environmental enrichment (Bekoff, 2001; Bradshaw and Cameron-Beaumont, 2000; Pal, 2003).

Although group housing may not be as vital for cats as it is for dogs, it is a cost-efficient way to provide an enriched environment. Many shelters, including the American Society for the Prevention of Cruelty to Animals (ASPCA), maintain groups of unrelated cats in cat habitats. The keys to successful cohabitation are to (a) select social cats; (b) provide sufficient space for cats to avoid each other; (c) provide room for solitary play; (d) make food, water and litter boxes easily accessible; and (e) offer ample comfortable locations for rest and sleep (Loveridge, 1998b). We recommend large beds to accommodate cats that like to sleep together, and small boxes for cats that prefer to sleep alone.

Despite the tremendous benefits from housing shelter animals in groups, there are considerable drawbacks. The main concerns are the increased risks of disease and injury (Hubrecht, 1995; Rochlitz, 2000; Wells and Hepper, 1992, and chapters 8 and 16 of this text). Dogs are at risk for kennel cough and parvovirus; cats are vulnerable to upper respiratory infections, ringworm, and pan-leukopenia, to name but a few. Social play and aggressive encounters can result in injuries. Housing animals singly while still allowing visual, olfactory, and acoustic access to conspecifics can mitigate these risks. According to Wells and Hepper (1998), allowing dogs to see other dogs increases

stimulation and encourages adoptions, because the dogs spend more time at the front of the runs than at the back. Podberseck et al. (1991) recommend providing cats with the opportunity to see other cats, to compensate for the lack of social contact resulting from individual housing. Communication among singly housed cats can be accommodated by replacing steel walls with glass or Plexiglass and drilling strategically placed holes at ear and nose level (Loveridge, 1998b). These allow for the transmission of visual, olfactory, and acoustic signals.

Another concern associated with group housing is the stress experienced by new animals being introduced to the group. Provided a careful integration process is implemented, stress experienced by cats gradually decreases (Kessler and Turner, 1999) and social behavior of dogs gradually increases (Sonderegger and Turner, 1996). To improve the likelihood of successful integration, shelter workers can select dogs that appear to be friendly and playful with other dogs, supervise body postures during introductions, and keep initial introductions short and pleasant. It may be helpful to first establish a friendship between the new dog and an existing group member outside the enclosure, and then introduce both individuals into the group together. Young playful cats, and cats that previously lived harmoniously with other cats, are more likely to benefit from group housing than solitary cats. However, formerly solitary cats may become comfortable in the presence of other cats, provided there are ample hiding places. Temporarily segregating the new cat from the group with a barrier, while providing sensory contact, is the safest means of introduction (Hetts, 1999). Group enclosures for dogs and cats should be furnished with multiple sleeping/resting sites so that individuals can control the amount of social interaction they receive.

Some animals display behaviors that make them inappropriate or unsafe to house in groups, such as aggression, fear, and overly exuberant play. Other forms of enrichment are even more important for single-housed animals because of their greater susceptibility to boredom and deprivation.

Ideally, all kennels, whether for groups or individual animals, should be furnished with platforms. Platforms add complexity to the cage, thereby creating additional living space. Both cats and dogs prefer elevated structures (e.g., vertical shelving) for resting and vantage points. Cat cages can be fitted with kitty condos and climbing posts to encourage exercise. Animals also appreciate enclosed or covered areas for hiding (Carlstead et al., 1993; Ibanez et al., 2001; Rochlitz, 2000). If possible, natural lighting is desirable because it creates a pleasant atmosphere and maintains the animal's normal circadian rhythms.

Bedding can be a contentious issue for shelter workers because, while animals appear to enjoy bedding, it often becomes soiled, destroyed, or pushed out of the cage. Cats like to sleep on or hide under bedding, and dogs like to lie on or rest their heads on soft substrates. Animals that destroy bedding may be less appealing for adoption because the public may assume, possibly correctly, that the pet would similarly destroy household belongings. The tendency to chew and rip bedding can be reduced by offering dogs more desirable items on which to gnaw, such as rope toys and safe chew bones.

Cats have the additional need of an elimination site and scratching substrates. Litter trays should be kept clean, with at least two inches of litter, to encourage the cat's use of the box and the burying of urine and feces. Scratching posts made of wood, carpeting, Hessian (coarse cloth used for bags), or rope, can be fixed to the floor or walls to help cats wear their claws.

Finally, animals appreciate access to interesting visual stimuli. Cats can be housed near a window (ideally with bird activity), a safely located aquarium, and/or a television (Parry, 1998). Maddie's Center at the San Francisco Society for the Prevention of Cruelty to Animals (SFSPCA) furnishes their group cat cages with trees, couches, and televisions. The group dog cages are also "real-life rooms" that boast couches, chairs, and televisions. Many of the furnishings most effective as enrichment tools pose hygienic risks. The use of these materials must be considered within the overall health care program of the shelter and current disease loads.

COMMUNICATION

Cats and dogs send and receive communication signals through their visual, olfactory, acoustic, and tactile sensory systems. In addition, both species possess an accessory olfactory organ, the vomeronasal, or Jacobson's, organ that receives odor molecules. The vomeronasal organ is used particularly when animals investigate scent marks left by others. When dogs and cats mark, they release chemicals called

pheromones that are presumed to have powerful effects on the emotional state of animals receiving the signal. Recently, synthesized cat facial pheromones (Feliway™ and Felifriend™) and dog appeasing pheromone (D.A.P.™) have appeared on the commercial market. These products are purported to reduce anxiety-related behaviors in pet and shelter animals, such as house soiling, excessive vocalizing, and urine spraying (Gautier and Pageat, 2002; Griffith et al., 2000; Sheppard and Mills, in press). The claim that these pheromones can reduce stress in shelter animals has prompted a number of investigations (Goldman and Reid, 2003; Kakuma and Bradshaw, 2001; Marder to Goldman personal communication, June 24, 2003). To date, the impact of synthesized pheromones on shelter animals is inconclusive, and further research is warranted.

Shelter workers will attest to the fact that animals express themselves through acoustic signals. Although cats and dogs are capable of a variety of vocalizations (Bradshaw and Cameron-Beaumont, 2000; Bradshaw and Nott, 1995), the most commonly heard are meows and barks, respectively. Barking contributes heavily to the excessive amount of noise in dog kennels (65–125 dB; Sales et al., 1997). Sales et al. (1997) measured the decibel (dB) level in dog kennels and showed that levels exceeded those known to cause auditory damage in humans. Both dogs and cats have wider audible ranges and more sensitive auditory systems than humans (Fay, 1988), and it is unknown if continual exposure to high dB noise causes auditory damage or chronic stress in shelter animals.

The negative impact of barking on both dogs and shelter workers can be mitigated with sound-absorbent material in the kennels. Wells et al. (2002) revealed the effectiveness of a less expensive option: Playing classical music in dog kennels increased resting behavior and decreased barking. In contrast, playing heavy metal music increased the amount of time dogs spent standing and increased rates of barking. Neither pop music nor human conversation had a measurable effect on behavior.

HUMAN CONTACT

For many shelter dogs and cats, the lack of contact with people may be more devastating than the lack of interaction with conspecifics (Gacsi et al., 2001; Topal et al., 1998). Although, evolutionarily speaking, dogs have been companions to people for longer (Leonard et al., 2002) than have cats (Serpell, 2000), individuals of both species, which are socialized to humans, are highly motivated to seek human contact and attention (Podberseck et al., 1991). The tendency for dogs, in particular, to form strong bonds with people may explain why Tuber et al. (1996) observed that dogs, placed in a novel environment, were more inclined to seek contact from a human caretaker than from their kennel mate. In addition, shelter dogs seem especially vulnerable to forming quick and strong attachments with staff (Gacsi et al., 2001).

Studies have revealed that stroking shelter dogs has the effect of reducing stress (Hennessy et al., 1997; Hennessy et al., 1998). For example, massaging/stroking a dog for the 20 minutes following a stressful event (i.e., venipuncture procedure) prevented an increase in blood cortisol levels when compared to dogs that were not stroked (Hennessy et al., 1998). It is interesting to note that the massaging action of long firm strokes, accompanied by a soft voice, was most effective in reducing stress (Hennessy et al., 1997; Tuber, 1999).

The benefits of human contact, especially handling, are particularly evident for young animals. During the sensitive "socialization" period of development, puppies and kittens need exposure to people (as well as places and things) in order to mature into animals that cope with novelty and interact appropriately with people. This period falls roughly between six to 12 weeks of age for puppies and between two to seven weeks for kittens (Hetts, 1999). Scott and Fuller (1965) recommend puppies receive a minimum of 40 minutes of human handling per week to prevent the development of problematic fearful behavior, including fear of people, handling, restraint, inanimate objects, and unfamiliar environments. Karsh and Turner (1988) demonstrated that kittens handled by people before seven weeks of age were more likely to approach and stay near people than kittens that were not handled. Cats handled for 40 minutes a day were more friendly to people than those handled for only 15 minutes a day. Cats handled regularly by multiple people were less afraid of strangers than cats handled by only one person.

The ASPCA utilizes office and home foster programs for shelter dogs and cats that appear to have been denied vital human contact during the socialization phase of development. Data on the effects of remedial socialization on adolescent and mature dogs are inconclusive; some studies report the acquisition of near-normal social behavior (Stanley and Elliot, 1962), while other studies note little change in behavior (McBryde and Murphree, 1974).

Social play with people is also a valuable form of enrichment for shelter animals. In addition to the gains of physical exercise and mental stimulation, dog-human play is qualitatively different from dog-dog play (Rooney et al., 2001; Rooney & Bradshaw, 2002). Dogs destined to be adopted, as companion animals, need to learn the "rules" of play with people. Cats also enjoy play with humans, sometimes to the detriment of the cat-owner bond. Young cats, in particular, are notorious for climbing up legs, ambushing passersby, and latching onto wriggling feet. Engaging cats in play with toys (e.g., balls, cat dancers, and so on) is an excellent means for reducing play aggression directed toward humans.

EXERCISE AND SOCIALIZATION

Animals in shelters rarely receive adequate physical exercise. The adage "a tired dog is a good dog" is, without question, true and "good dogs" are perceived as more adoptable by the public. Furthermore, regular exercise and interaction with conspecifics are considered essential for canine mental and physical health (Coppinger and Zuccotti, 1999; Loveridge, 1998a). Shelters can provide exercise through the use of treadmills, swimming pools, large outdoor runs, and regular walks. Incorporating daily exercise and/or play sessions into the shelter schedule helps alleviate the shortcomings of single housing.

Social play among groups of dogs is a time-efficient way to provide both interaction and exercise. Shelters, such as the ASPCA and the SFSPCA, have regularly scheduled sessions for shelter dogs to play, off-leash, in enclosed areas. The ASPCA forged a relationship with a community group that manages the neighborhood dog run, and the shelter dogs have exclusive use of the fenced run for two 1-hour periods each week.

Conspecific play is especially important for puppies and kittens (see Guyot et al., 1980; Mendle, 1988). As previously mentioned, research has established that there is a sensitive "socialization" period during which appropriate social behavior develops, provided the youngsters are able to interact with conspecifics. If deprived of opportunities to interact with conspecifics during this period, animals often behave inappropriately as adults. They may lack the skills to recognize certain species-specific signals, such as the "play bow" in dogs (Bekoff & Allen, 1998) or low-level threat displays in cats, or, worse, they may act overly fearful or aggressive with conspecifics (Estep, 1996). Dunbar (2001) purports that puppies learn "bite inhibition", in other words, they learn to modulate the strength of their bites, during play with conspecifics. Shelters with puppies can hold daily kindergarten classes that include play, training, and handling sessions. Volunteers can easily be motivated to serve as puppy handlers. Ideally, puppies from the same litter should be distributed across different classes so the puppies learn to cope with new experiences on their own, rather than always functioning as a group.

TRAINING

Basic training can enhance the lives of animals, especially dogs, during their stay in the shelter and has the added benefit of improving adoptability. A dog that is trained to come to the front of the cage and sit when people approach is more likely to encourage adoption than overactive, noisy, aggressive, or reclusive animals (Wells & Hepper, 2000). Training exercises need not be time consuming, and can be often accomplished "on the go" during routine shelter activities. In various programs, volunteers have effectively trained shelter dogs in basic manners, such as sit, stay, and quiet, with minimal guidance from shelter staff (McLeroy, 2003; Pryor, 2003). Pryor (2003) touts the benefits of clicker training for shelter animals and volunteers. Her shelter volunteers use clicker training to encourage withdrawn cats to approach and target an object held near the front of their cages. Volunteers also use clicker training to establish quiet behavior in caged dogs.

Walking programs and training classes provide excellent opportunities for shelter dogs to be stimulated psychologically and better prepared for their future adoptive homes. Walks and training provide one-on-one interaction with people and the opportunity to learn basic manners. Regularly scheduled walks for dogs housed in indoor kennels also makes housetraining possible.

More advanced husbandry training can reduce the stress experienced by shelter animals that undergo routine or specialized care. Animals can be trained to remain still for weighing and grooming, to stand for injections, to have pills placed in their mouths, and to present their paws for nail clipping.

This type of training has proved invaluable for animals in zoos and laboratories, obviating the need for frightening and sometimes painful restraint procedures (Laule, 1993; Reinhardt & Cowley, 1990).

FEEDING

Providing captive animals with opportunities to forage for food is a simple and effective procedure for reducing boredom, inactivity, and stereotypic behaviors (Bayne et al., 1992; Ings et al., 1997; Kessel and Brent, 1998; Meehan et al., 2003; Reinhardt, 1993). Cats are hunters, so simulating predator-prey interactions may be more stimulating for a shelter cat than eating from a bowl. One option is to feed cats in containers with holes so the cat must move the container around to release the food, one kibble at a time (Rochlitz, 2000). A variation of this is to hang a container from the top of the cage so the cat has to bat at the object to obtain food. There are also a variety of commercially available enrichment devices for cats, including feeders equipped with timers so food appears and disappears intermittently.

Free-ranging dogs spend a considerable amount of their day hunting and scavenging for food. Hubrecht (1993) showed that providing laboratory dogs with chew bones significantly increased activity. In addition to providing chew bones, shelter workers can simulate foraging activities by presenting dogs with food in puzzle boxes (e.g., Buster Cube™), rubber toys (e.g., Kong™ and Goodie Ship™) and/or plastic bottles with holes. These food dispensers require the dogs to manipulate them with their paws, nose, and mouth to obtain the food. Soft food can be packed tightly, or even frozen, inside some of these toys so that feeding is more challenging and time consuming. The repetitive licking motion required to remove the food from the toy is hypothesized to reduce stress, much the same as compulsive licking (acral lick dermatitis) (Spijkerman et al., 1994).

OBJECT PLAY

Shelter animals should have toys in their cages so they can engage in object play. This is especially important for individually housed animals that lack the opportunity for social play. Cats engage in object play with balls and various other toys (Loveridge, 1998b). DeMonte and Le Pape (1997) showed that a log and a suspended ball sparked increased activity, play, and investigation in caged cats. Cats played with the ball more than the log, presumably because of the movement. Toys bearing complex textures and mimicking characteristics of prey, such as rapid and erratic movement, stimulate play in cats (Rochlitz, 2000).

Dogs also enjoy object play and show clear preferences for certain types of toys, such as rawhide chews (DeLuca and Kranda, 1992; Hubrecht, 1995). Dogs are more likely to play for longer periods of time with toys that make noise (DeLuca and Kranda, 1992), and puppies are more likely to play with objects on which they can chew and tug (Hubrecht, 1995). In both studies, novel toys sparked longer bouts of play than familiar toys. With these findings in mind, shelter dogs should be provided with frequently rotated chew, tug, and squeaky toys.

Enrichment Summary

Enrichment programs pay big dividends for shelters. Animals that are behaviorally healthy are more appealing to the public and are more likely to remain in their adoptive homes. There remains a dearth of quality research on behavioral enrichment of shelter animals. Such research would not only function as an additional form of enrichment for the subject animals, but would greatly contribute to our understanding of companion animal behavior and animal welfare.

POST-ADOPTION PROGRAMS

Information on companion animals following placement in a new home is notoriously difficult to acquire (Patronek and Zawistowski, 2002). Even when available, these data may be difficult to interpret because there is no clear picture on whether those adopters you are able to contact differ in some significant way from those you are unable to contact. Neidhart and Boyd (2002) conducted a fairly large study contacting new adopters to determine if they still had the dog or cat they had adopted. Their primary focus was to determine whether or not the success of an adoption was affected by the animal placement format. As part of their study, they also asked for information on the satisfaction of adopters with their new companion animals. It is sobering to note that of 2,042 individual adopters, just 1,178 were successfully contacted two weeks after adoption (58 percent), and just 667 (33 percent) were willing to participate (Patronek and Zawistowski, 2002), and by the end of

the 12 months post-adoption, data were available on just 315 of the placements (15 percent). In those cases where the data were available, most of the dog adopters (77 percent) and nearly all cat adopters (90 percent) indicated that their pets were well behaved. When people did indicate a problem with their pets, about half cited behavior problems as an issue, including housebreaking, chewing, and some forms of household destruction.

In a study conducted by Marder (2002) that specifically addressed behavior issues of dogs following adoption from the ASPCA, data were available for 43 of 62 dogs (69 percent) six to 12 months after placement. People who adopted dogs were contacted by telephone and were asked to respond to a 60-item questionnaire. Similar to the study conducted by Ralston-Purina (2000), while owners tend to say they do not have problems with their pets, further probing reveals a variety of problem behaviors. Those most commonly cited were house soiling, household destruction, barking, and aggression to people. This is not surprising, as previous work conducted at the ASPCA (Zawistowski et. al., 1996) identified these concerns as primary problems managed through a free animal behavior help-line service. It is important to note that in Marder's study, most of the problem behaviors declined in frequency over time. The critical exception to this observation was that aggression to individuals outside the adopting household increased during the course of the study. This observed increase in aggression to people outside the household is a significant concern and deserves further detailed study.

While the studies mentioned previously have been limited in scope and size, they have generated observations of the need to provide proactive support for adopters in the first several months following the placement of a dog or cat in the home. Many shelters are already providing a variety of post-adoption support programs including behavior help-lines and dog obedience classes (Lawson, 2000a and 200b). In many cases, these programs can be crafted to meet the particular needs of the community, the adopters, and the animals placed. An important consideration, however, is that it may require persistence because experience (Zawistowski personal communication from M. Salman, 1998) suggests that it may take effort to interest people in the programs you have to offer (Zawistowski and Marder, 2000).

CONCLUSION

Given the changing demographics of the animals received by animal shelters, combined with an increasing demand in services and programs offered by shelters, behavior programs may become an ever more important part of the shelter environment. Continued development in this area will require cooperation and ongoing skill development among a variety of professionals. Behaviorists, veterinarians, dog trainers, shelter professionals, and others will need to work together to develop appropriate programs. Most important will be continued efforts to document the success, or failing of particular efforts to allocate resources and efforts in the most effective manner.

REFERENCES

American Humane. (2002). *American Humane's SAFER: The Safety Assessment for Evaluating Rehoming.* Englewood, CO: American Humane.

Bayne, K., S. Dexter, H. Mainzer, C. McCully, G. Campbell, and F. Yamada. 1992. The use of artificial turf as foraging substrate for individually housed rhesus monkeys (*Macaca mulatta*). *Animal Welfare* 1: 39–53.

Beerda, B., M. B. H. Schilder, J. A. van Hooff, H. W. de Vries, and J. A. Mol. 1998. Behavioural, saliva cortisol and heart rate responses to different types of stimuli in dogs. *Applied Animal Behaviour Science* 58: 365–381.

Beerda, B., M. B. H. Schilder, J. A. van Hooff, H. W. de Vries, and J. A. Mol. 1999. Chronic stress in dogs subjected to social and spatial restriction. I. Behavioral Responses. *Physiology and Behavior* 66 (2): 233–242.

Beerda, B., M. B. H. Schilder, W. Bernadina, J. A. van Hooff, H. W. de Vries., and J. A. Mol. 1999. Chronic stress in dogs subjected to social and spatial restriction: II. Hormonal and immunological responses. *Physiology and Behavior* 66 (2): 243–254.

Beerda, B., M. B. H. Schilder, J. A van Hooff, H. W. de Vries, and J. A. Mol. 2000. Behavioural and hormonal indicators of enduring environmental stress in dogs. *Animal Welfare* 9: 49–62.

Bekoff, M. 2001. Observations of scent-marking and discriminating self from others by a domestic dog (*Canis familiaris*): Tales of displaced yellow snow. *Behavioral Processes* 55: 75–79.

Bekoff, M., and C. Allen. 1998. Intentional communication and social play: How and why animals negotiate and agree to play. In M. Bekoff and J. A. Myers (eds.), *Animal Play: Evolutionary Comparative and Ecological Perspectives.* Cambridge, UK: Cambridge University Press, pp. 97–114.

Bradshaw, J., and C. Cameron-Beaumont. 2000. The signalling repertoire of the domestic cat and its undomesticated relatives. In D. C. Turner and P. Bateson (eds.), *The Domestic Cat: The Biology of Its Behaviour*, 2nd edition, Cambridge, UK: Cambridge University Press, pp. 68–93.

Bradshaw, J. W. S., and H. M. R. Nott. 1995. Social and communication behaviour of companion dogs. In J. A. Serpell (ed.), *The Domestic Dog: Its evolution, behaviour and interactions with people.* Cambridge, UK: Cambridge University Press, pp.115–130.

Burch, M. R., S. Davidson, and G. Meloche. 2002. The A.D.O.P.T.: A research based assessment for shelter dogs. Paper presented at the 3rd Annual Tufts Animal Expo, September 12, 2002, Boston, MA.

Carlstead, K., J. L. Brown, and W. Stawn. 1993. Behavioral and physiological correlates of stress in laboratory cats. *Applied Animal Behaviour Science* 38: 143–158.

Coppinger, R., and L. Coppinger. 1998. Differences in the behavior of dog breeds. In T. Grandin (ed.), *Genetics and the Behavior of Domestic Animals.* New York: Academic Press, pp. 167–202.

Coppinger, R., and J. Zuccotti. 1999. Kennel enrichment: Exercise and socialization of dogs. *Journal of Applied Animal Welfare Science* 2 (4): 281–296.

De Monte, M., and G. Le Pape. 1997. Behavioral effects of cage enrichment in single-caged adult cats. *Animal Welfare* 6: 53–66.

DeLuca, A. M., and K. C. Kranda. 1992. Environmental enrichment in a large animal facility. *Laboratory Animals* 21: 38–44.

Dunbar, I. 2001. *After You Get Your Puppy.* Berkeley CA: James & Kenneth Publishers.

Estep, D. Q. 1996. The ontogeny of behavior. In V. L. Voith and P. L. Borchelt (eds.), *Readings in Companion Animal Behavior.* Trenton, NJ: Veterinary Learning Systems, pp. 19–31.

Fay, R. 1988. *Hearing in Vertebrates. A Psychophysics Databook.* Winnetka, IL: Hill-Fay Associates.

Gacsi, M., J. Topal, A. Miklosi, A. Doka, and V. Csanyi. 2001. Attachment behavior of adult dogs (*Canis familiaris*) living at rescue centers: Forming new bonds. *Journal of Comparative Psychology* 115 (4): 423–431.

Gautier, E., and P. Pageat. 2002. Treatment of separation-related anxiety in dogs with a synthetic dog appeasing pheromone-preliminary results. Meeting Proceedings of the Annual Symposium of Animal Behavior Research. July 14, 2002, Nashville, TN.

Goldman, J., and P. Reid. 2003. The sweet smell of D.A.P. Presented at the 7th Annual Meeting of the

Interdisciplinary Forum for Applied Animal Behavior, February, 2003, Austin, TX. [Abstract]

Goodloe, L. P. 1996. Issues in description and measurement of temperament in companion dogs. In V. L. Voith and P. L. Borchelt (eds.), *Readings in companion animal behavior*. Trenton, NJ: Veterinary Learning Systems.

Griffith, C. A., E. Steigerwald, and C. A. T. Buffington. 2000. Effects of a synthetic facial pheromone on behavior in cats. *Journal of the American Veterinary Medical Association* 217: 1154–1156.

Guyot, G. W., T. L. Bennet, and H. Cross H. 1980. The effect of social isolation on the behavior of juvenile domestic cats. *Developmental Psychobiology*, 13: 317–329.

Hart, B. L. 1995. Analysing breed and gender differences in behaviour. In J. A. Serpell (ed.), *The Domestic Dog: Its evolution, behaviour and interactions with people*, Cambridge, UK: Cambridge University Press, pp. 65–77.

Hennessy, M. B., M. T. Williams, D. D. Miller, C. W. Douglas, and V. L. Voith. 1998. Influence of male and female petters on plasma cortisol and behaviour: Can human interaction reduce the stress of dogs in a public animal shelter? *Applied Animal Behaviour Science* 61: 63–77.

Hennessy, M. B., H. N. Davis, M. T. Williams, C. Mellot, and C. W. Douglas. 1997. Plasma cortisol levels of dogs at county animal shelter. *Physiological Behaviour* 21: 295–297.

Hetts, S. 1999. Problem prevention for kittens and new adult cats. In S. Hetts (ed.), *Pet Behavior Protocols: What to say, what to do, when to refer*. Lakewood, CO: AAHA, pp.63–80.

Hetts, S., J. D. Clark, J. P. Calpin, C. E. Arnold, and J. M. Mateo. 1992. Influence of housing conditions on beagle behaviour. *Applied Animal Behaviour Science* 34: 137–155.

Hubrecht, R. C. 1993. A comparison of social and environmental enrichment methods for laboratory housed dogs. *Applied Animal Behaviour Science* 37: 345–361.

Hubrecht, R. C. 1995. The welfare of dogs in human care. In J. A. Serpell (ed.), *The domestic dog: Its evolution, behaviour and interactions with people*. Cambridge, UK: Cambridge University Press, pp.179–198.

Hubrecht, R. C., J. A. Serpell, and T. B. Poole. 1992. Correlates of pen size and housing conditions on the behaviour of kenneled dogs. *Applied Animal Behaviour Science* 34: 365–383.

Ibanez, M., C. Y. Dominguez, and M. A. Martin. 2001. Cats showing comfort or well-being in cages with an enriched and controlled environment, In K. L. Overall, D. S. Mills, S. E. Heath, and D. Horwitz (eds.), Proceedings of the Third International Congress on Veterinary Behavioural Medicine, pp. 50–52.

Ings, R., N. K. Waran, and R. J. Young. 1997. Effect of wood-pile feeders on the behaviour of captive bush dogs (*Speothos venaticus*). *Animal Welfare* 6: 145–152.

Kakuma, Y., and J. W. S. Bradshaw. 2001. Effects of feline facial pheromone analogue on stress in shelter cats. In K. L. Overall, D. S. Mills, S. E. Heath, and D. Horwitz (eds.), Proceedings of the Third International Congress on Veterinary Behavioural Medicine, pp. 218–220.

Karsh, E. B., and Turder, D. C. 1988. The human-cat relationship. In D. C. Turner and P. B. Bateson (eds.), *The domestic cat: the biology of it's behavior*. Cambridge, UK: Cambridge University Press, 159–177.

Kessel, A. L., and L. Brent. 1998. Cage toys reduce abnormal behavior in individually housed pigtail macaques. *Journal of Applied Animal Welfare Science* 1 (3): 227–234.

Kessler, M. R., and D. C. Turner. 1999. Socialization and stress in cats (*Felis silvestris catus*) housed singly and in groups in animal shelters. *Animal Welfare* 8: 15–26.

Laule, G. 1993. Using training to enhance animal care and welfare. *Animal Welfare Information Centre Newsletter* 4 (1): 8–9.

Lawson, N. 2000a. Minding their manners: Training shelter animals. *Animal Sheltering*, January–February, 1–4.

Lawson, N. 2000b. Minding their manners: Teaching people and their pets. *Animal Sheltering*, March–April, 1–4.

Leonard, J. A., R. K. Wayne, J. Wheeler., R. Valadez, S. Guillen, and C. Vila. 2002. Ancient DNA evidence for Old World origin of New World dogs. *Science* 298: 1613–1616.

Loveridge, G. G. 1998a. Environmentally enriched dogs housing. *Applied Animal Behaviour Science* 59: 101–113.

Loveridge, G. G. 1998b. Comfortable environmentally enriched housing for domestic cats. In V. Reinhart (ed.), *Comfortable Quarters for Laboratory Animals*. Washington, DC: Animal Welfare Institute.

Luescher, A. 2000. Compulsive behavior in companion animals. In K. A. Houpt (ed.), *Recent Advances in Companion Animal Behavior Problems*. Ithaca, NY: International Veterinary Information Service.

Manteca, X., and J. M. Deag. 1993. Individual difference in temperament of domestic animals: A review of methodology. *Animal Welfare* 2: 247–268.

Marder, A. R. 2002. The animal shelter as an educational and research institution for applied animal behavior. Paper presented at the Animal Behavior Society meeting, July, Bloomington, IN.

McBryde, W. C., and Murphree, O. D. 1974. The rehabilitation of genetically nervous dogs. *Pavlovian
Journal of Biological Science* 9: 76–84.

McLeroy, M. 2003. Head Start. Presented at the 7th
Annual Meeting of the Interdisciplinary Forum for
Applied Animal Behavior, February, 2003, Austin,
TX.

Meehan, C. L., J. R. Milliam,, and J. A. Mench. 2003.
Foraging opportunity and increased physical complexity both prevent and reduce psychogenic feather
picking by young Amazon parrots. *Applied Animal
Behaviour Science* 80: 71–85.

Mendl, M. 1988. The effect of litter size variation on the
development of play behaviour in the domestic cat:
litters of one and two. *Animal Behaviour* 36: 20–34.

National Research Council. 1996. *Guide for the care
and use of laboratory animals,* 7th ed. Washington,
DC: National Academy Press.

Neidhart, L., and R. Boyd. 2002. Companion animal
adoption study. *Journal of Applied Animal Welfare
Science* 5 (3): 175–192.

Netto, W. J., and D. J. U. Planta. 1997. Behavioural
testing for aggression in the domestic dog. *Applied
Animal Behaviour Science* 52: 243–263.

Nunnally, J. C., and I. H. Bernstein. 1994. *Psychometric Theory,* 3rd ed.. New York: McGraw-Hill.

Pal, S. K. 2003. Urine marking by free-ranging dogs
(*Canis familiaris*) in relation to sex, season, place,
and posture. *Applied Animal Behaviour Science* 80:
45–59.

Parry, D. 1998. Shelter cats: The behavioral implications of long-term stay, and methods for alleviating
stress. Prepared for Maddies' Pet Adoption Center
(http://www.sfspca.org).

Patronek, G. J., L. T. Glickman, A. M. Beck, G. P.
McCabe, and C. Ecker. 1996a. Risk factors for
relinquishment of dogs to an animal shelter. *Journal
of the American Veterinary Medical Association* 209
(3): 572–581.

Patronek, G. J., L. T. Glickman, A. M. Beck, G. P.
McCabe, and C. Ecker. 1996b. Risk factors for
relinquishment of cats to an animal shelter. *Journal
of the American Veterinary Medical Association* 209
(3): 582–588.

Patronek, G. J., and S. Zawistowski. 2002. The value
of data. *Journal of Applied Animal Welfare Science*
5 (3): 171–174.

Podberscek, A. L., J. K. Blackshaw, and A. W. Beatties.
1991. The behavior of laboratory colony cats and their
reactions to a familiar and unfamiliar person. *Applied
Animal Behaviour Science* 31, 119–130.

Pryor, K. 2003. Clicking with cats: A proven, positive
intervention that benefits cats and owners too. Presented at the 7th Annual Meeting of the Interdisci-

plinary Forum for Applied Animal Behavior, February 2003, Austin, TX.

Ralston-Purina. 2000. The State of the American Pet: A
study among pet owners. Available at http://www.
purina.com/images/articles/pdf/TheStateofthe.pdf

Reid, P. J., S. Calvin, and N. Penny. 2002. Reactions to
life-like dolls by child-friendly and child-aggressive
dogs. Manuscript in preparation. University of
Guelph, Ontario.

Reinhardt, V. 1993. Using the mesh ceiling as a food
puzzle to encourage foraging behaviour in caged
rhesus macaques (*Macaca mulatta*). *Animal Welfare*
2: 165–4 172.

Reinhardt, V., and D. Cowley. 1990. Training stump-
tailed monkeys (*Macaca arctoides*) to cooperate
during in-home cage treatment. *Laboratory Primate
Newsletter* 29 (4): 9–10.

Reinhardt, V., and M. Rossell, M. 2001. Self-biting in
caged macaques: Cause, effect, and treatment.
Journal of Applied Animal Welfare Science 4 (4):
285–294.

Rochlitz, I., A. L. Podberseck, and D. M. Broom.
1998. The welfare of cats in a quarantine cattery.
Veterinary Record 143: 181–185.

Rooney, N. J., and J. W. S. Bradshaw. 2002. An experimental study on the effects of play upon the dog-
human relationship. *Applied Animal Behaviour Science* 75: 161–176.

Rooney, N. J., J. W. S. Bradshaw, and I. Robinson.
2001. Do dogs respond to play signals given by
humans? *Animal Behaviour* 61: 715–722.

Sales, G., R. Hubrecht, A. Peyvandi, S. Milligan, and
B. Shield. 1997. Noise in dog kenneling: Is barking
a welfare problem for dogs? *Applied Animal Behaviour Science* 52 (3–4): 321–329.

Salman, M. D., J. G. New, J. M. Scarlett, P. H. Kass,
R. Ruch-Gallie, and S. Hetts, S. 1998. Human and
animal factors related to the relinquishment of dogs
and cats in 12 selected animal shelters in the United
States. *Journal of Applied Animal Welfare Science* 1
(3): 207–226.

Salman, M. D., J. Hutchinson, R. Ruch-Gallie, L.
Kogan, J. C. New, P. H. Kass, and J. Scarlett. 2000.
Behavioral reasons for relinquishment of dogs and
cats to 12 shelters. *Journal of Applied Animal Welfare Science* 3 (2): 93–106.

Scott, J. P., and J. L. Fuller. 1965. *Genetics and the
Social Behavior of the Dog.* Chicago: The University of Chicago Press.

Sheppard, G., and D. S. Mills. (in press). Evaluation of
dog appeasing pheromone as a treatment for fear of
fireworks by dogs. *Veterinary Record.*

Serpell, J. A. 2000. Domestication and history of the
cat. In D. C. Turner and P. Bateson (eds), *The*

Domestic Cat: The biology of its behaviour, 2nd edition. Cambridge, UK: Cambridge University Press, pp.180–192.

Sonderegger, S. M., and D. C. Turner. 1996. Introducing dogs into kennels: Prediction of social tendencies to facilitate integration. *Animal Welfare* 5: 391–404.

Spijkerman, R. P., H. Dienske, J. A. R. A. M van Hooff, and W. Jens. 1994. Causes of body rocking in chimpanzees (*Pan troglodytes*). *Animal Welfare* 3: 193–211.

Stanley, W. C., and Elliot, U. 1962. Differential human handling as reinforcing events as treatments influencing later behavior in basenji puppies. *Psychological Reports 10*: 775–788.

Sternberg, S. 2002. *Great Dog Adoptions: A Guide for Shelters*. Alameda, CA: The Latham Foundation.

Topal, J., A. Miklosi, V. Csanyi, and A. Doka. 1998. Attachment behavior in dogs (*Canis familiaris*): A new application of Ainsworth's (1969) Strange Situation Test. *Journal of Comparative Psychology* 112 (3): 219–229.

Tuber, D. 1999. Teaching Rover to relax: The Soft Exercise. *Animal Behavior, Society Newsletter* 16(1).

Tuber, D. S., M. B. Hennessy, S. Sanders, and J. A. Miller. 1996. Behavioral and glucocorticoid responses of adult domestic dogs (*Canis familiaris*) to companionship and social separation. *Journal of Comparative Psychology* 110: 103–108.

Turner, D. C., and P. Bateson. 2000. *The Domestic Cat: The biology of its behaviour*. Cambridge, UK: Cambridge University Press.

Van der Borg, J. A. M., W. J. Netto, and D. J. U. Planta. 1991. Behavioural testing of dogs in animal shelters to predict problem behaviour. *Applied Animal Behaviour Science* 32: 237–251.

Wells, D .L., and P. G. Hepper. 1992. The behaviour of dogs in a rescue shelter. *Animal Welfare* 1: 171–186.

Wells, D. L., and P. G. Hepper. 1998. A note on the influence of visual conspecific contact on the behaviour of sheltered dogs. *Applied Animal Behaviour Science* 60: 83–88.

Wells, D. L., and P. G. Hepper. 1999. Male and female dogs respond differently to men and women. *Applied Animal Behaviour Science* 61: 341–349.

Wells, D. L., and P. G. Hepper. 2000. The influence of environmental change on behaviour of sheltered dogs. *Applied Animal Behaviour Science* 68 (2): 151–162.

Wells, D. L., L. Graham, and P. G. Hepper. 2002. The influence of auditory stimulation on the behaviour of dogs housed in a rescue shelter. *Animal Welfare* 11: 385–393.

Wiepkema, P. R., and J. M. Koolhaas. 1993. Stress and animal welfare. *Animal Welfare* 2: 195–218.

Zawistowski, S., J. Schultz, D. Ryan-Rivas, and J. Kopelman. 1996. Animal behavior helpline: Calls, critters and crises. Poster presented at the Animal Behavior Society meetings, August 1996, Flagstaff, AZ.

Zawistowski, S., and A. Marder. 2000. Center for Behavioral Therapy. *ISAZ Newsletter*, November 2000, no. 20.

20
Behavioral Pharmacotherapy in the Animal Shelter

Amy Marder and Michelle Posage

INTRODUCTION

Behavioral pharmacotherapy (the use of drugs to treat behavior problems) is now commonly prescribed as part of veterinary behavioral therapy programs. Recent developments over the past decade have allowed practitioners to rationally use psychotropic drugs to aid in the treatment and management of difficult behavioral problems in dogs and cats. Unfortunately, drug therapy is rarely feasible for the treatment of behavioral problems in shelter animals because of limitations inherent in the shelter environment. However, when an animal's well-being is compromised by long-term housing and enrichment techniques have proved to be ineffective, drug therapy should be considered. Pheromone therapy may also be effective to reduce the stress associated with shelter housing. Shelter veterinarians should be familiar with the commonly prescribed psychotropic drugs, their indications, side effects, and contraindications because behavior problems are a common cause of relinquishment and the return of animals after adoption.

WHY DRUG THERAPY IN SHELTERS IS NOT PRACTICAL

As with any disease, in order to choose the most effective treatment, a veterinarian must make a diagnosis. To make a behavioral diagnosis, the veterinarian must obtain a thorough behavioral history. This is a relatively easy task when dealing with owned animals but is usually not possible when working with animals in most shelters. The intake information given by surrendering owners is often inaccurate, and for stray animals no information is available.

Drug therapy is most effective when used as part of a behavioral therapy program. Permanent staff members who can implement consistent behavioral therapy programs are often in short supply in most animal shelters.

Most drugs require daily or twice daily dosing, and some are unpalatable, making administration difficult. Many shelters do not have staff members able to administer the drugs at the required frequency.

All drugs have potential side-effects. Daily health monitoring of animals is required to prevent serious problems. Many shelters do not have qualified staff to monitor side-effects.

Many drugs require one month or more of treatment to reach stable therapeutic blood levels. Many shelters do not have sufficient space to keep animals for this length of time.

Psychotropic drugs are expensive. Even those that are available in generic forms can still cost one to two dollars a dose, depending upon the size of the animal.

Most psychotherapeutic drugs are not approved for use in dogs and cats. In order to enhance the safe use of these drugs, a baseline CBC and blood chemistry panel is required. This is an additional expense.

Animals who are placed on drug therapy while in the shelter will most likely need to be sent home on drug therapy. Drug therapy, due to cost and responsibility, makes an animal less adoptable.

Many behavior problems do not appear while animals are housed in the shelter. Therefore, the effectiveness of drug therapy cannot be determined while the animal is in the shelter. Problems, such as separation anxiety, which contribute to relinquishment, do not occur while the dog is in the shelter and may or may not reappear after the dog is rehomed.

The results of treatment of a behavior problem while the animal is housed in the shelter, whether by behavior modification or drug therapy, may not persist after the animal is in a home. Both a home environment and attachment to new caretakers have a significant impact on an animal's behavior.

WHEN DRUG THERAPY SHOULD BE CONSIDERED

Compulsive Behaviors

The conflict and frustration experienced by shelter animals due to confinement, lack of consistency, lack of social interactions, and inability to perform species-typical behaviors may result in the appearance of compulsive behaviors. Compulsive behaviors are repetitive, sustained, and out of context. Common compulsive behaviors seen in dogs housed in shelters are tail-chasing, pacing, jumping, weaving, self-licking, leg or foot chewing, self-directed aggression, cage licking, and persistent barking. In cats, tail chasing, tail chewing, and over grooming may be observed. There appears to be a genetic predisposition for compulsive disorders. German Shepherds and American Pit Bull Terriers tend to tail chase, while Doberman Pinschers flank suck (Luescher, 2003). Compulsive behaviors are more likely to appear when animals are housed in confinement for longer periods of time. Therefore, when long-term confinement is anticipated (law enforcement cases), preventative behavior modification programs should be implemented as soon as possible.

Treatment for Compulsive Disorder

Treatment for compulsive disorders must always begin with the identification and removal of causes of the animal's conflict, frustration, and stress. Although a difficult task in the shelter environment, every attempt should be made to increase consistency and reduce unpredictability. A regular schedule of feeding and walking with one or two caretakers should be implemented. Social interactions through play groups with the same dogs may also be helpful. A food-reward training program can be used by staff to support the consistent use of commands. Food-dispensing toys can be placed with animals to help them feel more in control of their

environment. Many similar techniques can be used for cats. Moving the cat to a less stressful location is often warranted. Petting and play can replace walking, and clicker training can be used to teach commands (Leuscher, 2003).

In many cases, drug therapy is necessary to facilitate a behavior modification program. Serotonin reuptake inhibitors have been shown to be the most effective in controlling compulsive behaviors. Clomipramine (Hewson, 1998) and Fluoxetine (Rapoport, 1992) have been subjected to clinical trials. As it may take four weeks or longer to see an effect, it is imperative that a behavior modification program be implemented at the onset of drug therapy. Drug therapy should be continued for at least three weeks after a satisfactory reduction has been seen. The drug then is gradually weaned over 3 to 4 weeks (Leuscher, 2003).

Fears

Some animals exhibit an extreme fear response when introduced to the shelter environment. Some are afraid of the environment, and some are afraid of people. Most acclimate within days, and others fail to do so. If alternative housing, such as foster care, is not available, anti-anxiety medication may be considered. Anti-anxiety medication (for example, benzodiazepines or buspirone) is sometimes helpful to facilitate adjustment. However, as some anti-anxiety medication may disinhibit aggression (Simpson, 2003), close monitoring is required to ensure the safety of the shelter staff.

PHEROMONE THERAPY

Recently, the use of synthetic pheromone preparations has been promoted for the treatment of some behavioral problems. Investigators believe that their effect on individual behaviors could be explained by a generalized effect on stress reduction (Paget, 2003). If this is true, they are promising candidates for use in animal shelters. Unlike drug therapy, synthetic pheromones have no toxicity or side-effects. Administration is external, either through an environmental spray or diffuser, making dispensing simple. Although expensive, many animals are treated at the same time. Feliway® (Veterinary Products Laboratories), a mixture of synthetic feline facial pheromones, has been shown to be effective in reducing urine marking and anxiety in cats when transported, having intravenous catheterization, and while being hospitalized. Dog Appeasing Pheromone® (Veterinary Products Laboratories), a synthetic analogue of the appeasing pheromone secreted by nursing bitches, has been shown to reduce signs of separation anxiety and noise phobia (Paget, 2003).

Although several anecdotal reports of pheromones reducing stress in shelter animals exist, no controlled studies of their effectiveness have been published at this time.

CONCLUSION

When clients seek help for behavior problems before surrender and after adoption, drug therapy in conjunction with behavior modification should be considered. Pharmacotherapy should never be prescribed without seeing the patient. A physical examination and appropriate laboratory tests are required to rule out medical etiologies and a thorough behavioral history is necessary to make an accurate behavioral diagnosis. If a practitioner is uncomfortable or unfamiliar with the use of psychotropic drugs, the client should be referred to a qualified animal behavior consultant.

REFERENCES

Hewson, C. 1998. Efficacy of clomipramine in the treatment of canine compulsive disorder: A randomized, placebo-controlled, double blind clinical trial. *Journal of the American Veterinary Medical Association* 213, 1760–1766.

Luescher, A. 2003. Diagnosis and management of compulsive disorders in dogs and cats. *Veterinary Clinics of North America, Small Animal Practice* 33 (2) 253–267.

Paget, P., and Gaultier, E. 2003. Current research in canine and feline pheromones. *Veterinary Clinics of North America, Small Animal Practice* 33(2) 201–208.

Rapaport, J. 1992. Drug treatment of canine acral lick: An animal model of obsessive compulsive disorder. *Archives of General Psychiatry* 49, 517–521.

Simpson, B., and Papich, M. 2003. Pharamacologic management in veterinary behavioral medicine. *Veterinary Clinics of North America, Small Animal Practice* 33 (2) 377–382.

Table 20.1. Behavior Pharmacology

Drug	Canine Dose	Feline Dose	Uses	Relative Cost	Side Effects
Acepromazine	0.55–2.2 mg/kg[1]	1.1–2.2 mg/kg[1]	Chemical restraint	$	Hypotension, CNS stimulation, contradictory responses, use with caution in boxers and greyhounds
Alprazolam	0.02–0.1 mg/kg PO q 8-12h[2]	.125–.25 mg/cat q 12h[3]	Anxiety, noise phobias, canine submissive urination, feline urine marking	$	Sedation, ataxia, increased appetite, paradoxical excitation
Amitriptyline HCl	2.2–4.4 mg/kg q 12–24h[4,5]	5–10 mg/cat q 24[3,6] 2.5–5.0 mg/cat q 12–24h[7]	Anxiety, canine/feline fear aggression, feline urine marking, feline displacement grooming, canine stereotypy	$	Sedation, gastrointestinal effects, dry mouth, increased thirst, urinary retention
Buspirone HCl	2.5–10 mg/dog q 12–24h or 1.0–2.0 mg/kg q 12h[6] 1.0 mg/kg q 8–12h[8]	2.5–7.5 mg/cat q 12h[8] 2.5–5.0 mg/cat q 8–12h[3]	Phobia, anxiety, feline urine marking	$$$$	Uncommon, not sedating
Chlorpheniramine Maleate	0.22 mg/kg q 8h[9]	1–4 mg/cat q 12–24h[9]	Sedation	$	Sedation, anticholinergic effects, GI effects
Clomipramine HCl	2–4 mg/kg q 24h or divided q12h[10]	0.5–1 mg/kg q24h[11]	Canine separation anxiety, feline urine marking, compulsive disorder, feline hyperesthesia syndrome, feline psychogenic alopecia, canine acral lick dermatitis, phobia	$$	Sedation, GI effects, anticholinergic effects, cardiac effects
Clorazepate Dipotassium	2 mg/kg q12h[6] 0.55–2.2 mg/kg q 4h[12]	0.5–1.0 mg/kg q 12–24h[12]	Anxiety, noise phobias, canine submissive urination, feline urine marking	$$	Sedation, ataxia
Cyproheptadine HCl		2 mg/cat q12h[13]	Feline urine marking	$	Anticholinergic effects, sedation
Diazepam	.55–2.2 mg/kg prn[8]	1–4 mg/cat q 12–24h[6]	Phobia (canine or feline), feline urine marking	$	Rare cases of acute liver failure in cats, sedation, paradoxical

336

Drug	Dosage (dog)	Dosage (cat)	Indications	Cost	Side Effects
		0.2–0.4 mg/kg q 12–24 h[14]			excitation, muscle relaxation, increased appetite
Doxepin HCl	3–5 mg/kg q 12h (max dose 150 mg/dog q12h)[15]		Compulsive disorders resulting in self mutilation, feline psychogenic alopecia	$$	Hyperexcitability, GI effects, lethargy
Fluoxetine HCl	1.0–1.5 mg/kg q 24h[15]		Aggression, canine separation anxiety, compulsive disorders, feline urine marking	$$$	Lethargy, inappetence, anorexia, GI effects
Hydrocodone Bitartrate	0.25–1.0 mg/kg q 8–12h[16]	1.25–5.0 mg/cat q 12–24h[16]	Compulsive disorders resulting in self mutilation	$	Sedation, constipation, GI effects
Imipramine HCl	2–4 mg/kg q 12–24[6]	0.5–1.0 mg/kg q 12–24[8]	Canine submissive urination	$	Sedation, anticholinergic effects
Medroxyprogesterone Acetate	5–10 mg/kg SQ, IM; do not exceed 3 treatments per year[17]	10–20 mg/kg SQ[17]	Treatment of last resort for aggression and feline urine marking	$	Polyphagia, polydipsia, sedation, diabetes mellitus, pyometra, mammary hyperplasia, endometrial hyperplasia, carcinoma
Megestrol Acetate	1.1–2.2 mg/kg q24 for 2 wks, then 0.5–1.1 mg/kg q24 for 2 wks[17]	5 mg/cat q 24h × for 2 months[18]	Treatment of last resort for aggression and urine marking	$	Same as medroxyprogesterone acetate
Melatonin	0.1 mg/kg q8–12h (with amitriptyline)[19]		Canine fear, phobia	$	Side effects appear to be minimal, but not well studied
Methylphenidate HCl	5 mg (small dog)–20 mg (large dog) q 8–12h; do not give near bedtime[8]	2–4 mg/kg q 12–24h[16]	Canine hyperkinesis	$$$$	CNS arousal, GI effects, inappetence, cardiac effects, hypertension, stranguria
Naltrexone HCl	2.2 mg/kg q 12h[6]	25–50 mg/cat q 24h[8]	Canine acral lick dermatitis, canine stereotypic behavior, compulsive disorders	$$$$	GI effects, insomnia, nervousness
Paroxetine HCl	0.5–1.0 mg/kg q24[6]	0.5–1.0 mg/kg q 24h[8]	Aggression, canine separation anxiety, compulsive disorders,	$$$	Lethargy, GI effects, inappetence, constipation

(*continues*)

Table 20.1. (*continued*)

		1.25–2.5 mg/cat q 24h[20] 2–3 mg/kg prn[9]	feline urine marking		
Phenobarbital	2–8 mg/kg q 12h[6] 1.5–2.0 mg/kg q 12[21]		Canine/feline compulsive tail chasing, unprovoked canine rage aggression	$	Lethargy, ataxia, polyuria, polydipsia, polyphagia,
Phenylpropanolamine HCl	1.1 mg/kg q 8h[22]		Canine submissive/excitement urination	$	Restlessness, hypertension, anorexia
Propranolol HCl	5–40 mg/dog q 8h[15]	0.25 mg/kg prn[15]	Canine fear aggression, noise phobia	$	Bradycardia, lethargy, hypotension, syncope
Selegiline HCl	0.5–1.0 mg/kg q 24h in am[23]		Canine cognitive dysfunction syndrome	$$$$	GI effects, restlessness or lethargy, anorexia
Sertraline	0.5–4.0 mg/kg q 24[8]	0.5–1.0 mg/kg q 24[8]	Anxiety, fear, aggression	$$$	Sedation, GI effects

All doses are per os unless otherwise indicated.
Abbreviations: prn, as needed; h, hours.

Notes

[1] Package Insert, Prom Ace®, Fort Dodge.
[2] Landsberg, G., Hunthausen, W., Ackerman, L. 1997. *Handbook of behavior problems of the dog and cat.* Oxford: Butterworth Heinemann Publishers.
[3] Marder, A.R. 1991. Psychotropic drugs and behavioral therapy. *Vet Clin North Am Small Anim Pract;* 21:329–42.
[4] Juarbe-Diaz, S.V. 1997a. Social dynamics and behavior problems in multiple dog households. *Vet Clin North Am Small Anim Pract;* 27:497–514.
[5] Juarbe-Diaz, S.V. 1997b. Assessment and treatment of excessive barking in the domestic dog. *Vet Clin North Am Small Anim Pract;* 27:515–32.
[6] Papich, M.G. 2002. *Saunders handbook of veterinary drugs.* Philadelphia: WB Saunders.
[7] Sawyer, L.S., Moon-Fanelli, A.A., et al. 1999. Psychogenic alopecia in cats: 11 cases (1993–1996). JAVMA; 214:71–4.
[8] Crowell-Davis, S.L., Curtis, T., et al. 2001. Pharmacology for veterinarians: Knowing which drug to use and when to use it. Lecture Notes, College of Veterinary Medicine, University of Georgia .
[9] Overall, K.L. 2000. Behavioral Pharmacology. American Animal Hospital Association 67th Annual Meeting, Toronto.
[10] Package Insert, Clomicalm®, Novartis.
[11] Reisner, I., Houpt, K. 2000. Behavioral disorders. In: Ettinger, S., Feldman, E., eds. *Textbook of Veterinary Internal Medicine: Diseases of the Dog and Cat.* Philadelphia: WB Saunders.
[12] Overall, K.L. 1997. *Clinical Behavioral Medicine for Small Animals.* St. Louis: Mosby.
[13] Schwartz, S. 1999. Use of cyproheptadine to control urine spraying and masturbation in a cat. JAVMA; 214:369–371.

338

14 Cooper, L., Hart, B.L. 1992. Comparison of diazepam with progestin for effectiveness in suppression of urine spraying behavior in cats. JAVMA. 200:797–801.

15 Crowell-Davis, S. 1999. Behavior Psychopharmacology. Central Veterinary Conference, Kansas City.

16 Marder, A.R., Bergman, L. 1999. Guidelines for the use of psychotropic drugs for behavior problems. In: Hetts, S. *Pet Behavior Protocols*. Lakewood, CO: AAHA Press.

17 Voith, V.L., Marder, A.R. 1998. Canine Behavioral Disorders. In: Morgan, R.V., ed. *Handbook of Small Animal Practice*. New York: Churchill Livingstone.

18 Hart, B.L., Eckstein, R.A. 1998. Progestins: Indications for male-typical behavior problems. In: Dodman, N.H., Shuster, L., eds. *Psychopharmacology of Animal Behavior Disorders*. Boston, MA: Blackwell Science, 255–263.

19 Aronson, L. 1999. Animal behavior case of the month: extreme fear in a dog. JAVMA; 215:22–4.

20 Mills, D.S., Simpson, B.S. 2002. Psychotropic agents. In: Horwitz, D.F., Mills, D.S., Heath, S., eds. *BSAVA manual of canine and feline behavioral medicine*. Gloucester, UK: BSAVA Press, 237–48.

21 Dodman, N.H., Miczed, K.A., et al. 1992. Phenobarbital-responsive compulsive tail chasing in a dog. JAVMA; 201:1580–3.

22 Plumb, D.C. 1988. Veterinary Pharmacy Formulary. 2nd ed. St. Paul: Minnesota: Veterinary Teaching Hosp.

23 Package Insert; Anipryl®; Pfizer.

21
Foster Care in the Animal Shelter

Leslie Sinclair

INTRODUCTION

Foster care programs can play a crucial supplemental role to the mission of an animal sheltering agency. For those agencies that do not have a physical facility, a foster care program often forms the core of services provided. Most animal sheltering agencies create a foster care program to increase the likelihood of adoption of some of the animals they shelter. Few animal sheltering agencies have adequate isolation facilities, and a foster care program can be used to address this deficiency by removing animals with mild infectious diseases to minimize transmission, as well as isolating young, orphaned, injured, and otherwise immunostressed animals from the shelter environment to one in which the potential for infection is much less likely. Some animal sheltering agencies also use a foster care program specifically to provide a steady supply of puppies and kittens during a seasonal shortage, knowing that those animals have a greater chance of adoption than adult animals.

Other types of foster care programs provide a haven for pets of domestic violence victims (Ascione, 2000) and/or of pet owners who are no longer capable of providing care (such as those who are elderly, hospitalized, or who have severe or terminal illness). Some agencies also provide care for pets of families undergoing such turmoil as divorce or homelessness. This chapter will focus on foster care programs for animals intended for adoption, but many aspects of such programs are applicable to the other types of foster care programs.

The role of the veterinarian in a foster care program depends on the role of the veterinarian in the particular sheltering agency. Later in this chapter, we will discuss different methods of providing vet-erinary care for animals in foster care programs, including offering in-house care with a staff veterinarian, contracting with a private practitioner to provide care for the program's animals, and allowing foster caregivers to seek veterinary care from the private practitioner of their choice. Obviously, the method chosen will determine what role the veterinarian providing the care plays, and how much control he or she has over the animal's care. Regardless of the method and of the veterinarian's role, he or she should strive to view the foster animal holistically, in the context of not only the foster animal's best interests but also that of the caregiver, the foster care program, the entire sheltering program, and the animal's future adopter.

Foster care programs often form "spontaneously" at animal sheltering agencies, as a natural outgrowth of the desire of shelter employees and volunteers to do more as individuals for specific animals than the shelter as an entity is capable of doing. It is possible for an informal program to be successful, but too often the result is poor monitoring of animals, lack of support—both financial and emotional—for foster caregivers, and "burnout" of foster caregivers. Animals suffer under these circumstances, and so does the enthusiasm and morale of staff and volunteers, as does public support.

The benefits of a well-administered foster care program are numerous. A good program supports employee and volunteer morale, improves the agency's relationship with the general public, allows the agency to offer animals who are healthier and more thoroughly screened to the adopting public, and may improve the overall health of the shelter's population by isolating those who are sick or particularly susceptible to illness.

Ideally, an agency carefully considers the ramifications of administering a foster care program before one is created. Time, money, and staff and volunteer hours are required, and the agency must first determine whether a foster care program is the best use of those resources. The agency should review their stated mission, and determine whether a foster care program fits well within that mission. The input of a veterinarian should play a significant part in this decision, as he or she can provide the agency with detailed information about what resources will be necessary to provide health and behavioral care to foster animals, as well as what the zoonotic and other risks are to foster caregivers.

It is important for an agency to realize that the public will, rightfully, expect that greater care has been provided to a foster care animal than to the general population of the shelter, including thorough veterinary care. While many agencies do not employ veterinarians and instead require that adopters have animals examined by their own veterinarians shortly after adoption, adopters will expect that an animal that has been in the agency's care for several weeks will have received a veterinary examination and proper veterinary care. To create a foster care program without the resources or intention to provide veterinary care for the program's animals is ill-advised and often leads to public relations problems, as well as to possible significant setbacks (such as a disease outbreak) to the program. Medical protocols for foster animals should also be tailored to the individual animal's specific needs; simply creating a "standard protocol" for treating sick foster animals should not be thought to constitute appropriate veterinary care.

Once an agency decides to create (or formalize) a foster care program, primary considerations include who will administer the program, what services the agency will offer to foster care candidates and their caretakers, and who will be the program's participants (foster caregivers).

A foster care program needs a dedicated coordinator—someone who is knowledgeable about the shelter's operation and policies, willing to support and guide caregivers, is meticulous about record keeping, and has strong public relations skills. Because most foster care animals have significant and ongoing health and behavioral issues, it is desirable that the foster care program coordinator have a working knowledge of animal health and

behavior. He or she can be the shelter's operations director, volunteer director, veterinary technician, veterinarian, or someone else involved with the agency who has the skills and abilities previously listed and is capable of and willing to work with the rest of the shelter staff.

There are several different (and sometimes overlapping) types of foster caregivers, including shelter employees, shelter volunteers, foster-specific volunteers (those whose only, or primary, interaction with the shelter is participation in the foster care program), and breed-specific foster caregivers. Employees are often the most knowledgeable foster caregivers. Some wish to provide foster care on an ongoing basis, while others occasionally identify an animal whose needs they can address. New employees, as they come to terms with the innate frustrations and realities of animal sheltering, often express interest in providing foster care, sometimes because they truly wish to expand their ability to help animals, but more often because they are attempting to deal with the grief and stress that being inducted into shelter culture creates (White and Shawhan, 1996; Arluke, 1991; Kirkwood, 1999). In shelters where euthanasia is performed, new (and seasoned) employees may seek to provide foster care as a method of dealing with their euthanasia-related stress. While it is appropriate to use a foster care program to support employee morale by offering enhanced services for some animals (who might otherwise be euthanized), the program should not be used as a crutch for those in need of counseling or support to deal with the work stress associated with animal sheltering or with euthanasia-related stress.

Volunteers usually are the core of a shelter's foster care program, allowing the program to become a community-wide effort. Some volunteers will be foster-specific volunteers, or those who provide foster care but no other volunteer services to the agency. In this way, a foster care program allows people who find on-site work inconvenient or emotionally difficult to support the work of the shelter with hands-on services. Nonetheless, foster-specific volunteers should receive an orientation to and ongoing education about the shelter's day-to-day operations and limitations so that they understand the opportunities and resources that may—or may not—be available for their foster animals. Breed-specific foster caregivers are a subset of foster-specific volunteers. These may be members of "breed rescue groups" who wish to work through the shelter's foster care program (as opposed to receiving the animal from the sheltering agency and providing all subsequent care, including adoption), or just people who are particularly fond of one or a few specific breeds and wish to work only with those. Breed-specific foster caregivers can be a valuable resource for some animals, bringing expertise and enthusiasm about the breed to the program, as well as a network of potential adopters. Breed-specific foster caregivers should receive the same orientation as all other foster caregivers. Breed-specific foster caregivers may find it difficult to understand why a member of "their" breed is not a good candidate for foster care or adoption; thorough orientation and clear foster candidate selection policies, applied in a fair and consistent manner, can ease this situation.

SELECTING FOSTER CAREGIVERS

Applying to become a foster caregiver should be somewhat like being considered for a job, as indeed it is. The caregiver candidate should complete a formal application to the program, providing a permanent address and identifying information such as a driver's license number. If the candidate rents or lives in someone else's home, he or she should provide verification in writing that permission has been obtained to house animals there for a specified period of time. The foster caregiver's residence should provide adequate facilities for the type of animal(s) the candidate has applied to foster. Ideally, the foster care program coordinator should conduct a home visit, and the candidate should agree in writing to allow future visits on a regular basis, or as deemed necessary by the program coordinator. Foster care candidates should be 18 years of age, as they must be able to enter into a legally binding contract. Minors who wish to participate in the foster care program should be allowed to do so only in partnership with a responsible adult.

Every foster caregiver candidate should submit to an assessment of their own animal companions. The candidate's veterinarian (at the candidate's expense) should perform an evaluation of the general health, temperament, and well being of any animals that reside in the foster caregiver's home, including those who belong to someone other than the foster caregiver candidate. The candidate and

their veterinarian should thoroughly discuss and apply health care measures that are meant to protect the resident animal as well as potential foster animals, such as testing for feline leukemia virus and feline immunodeficiency virus; application of flea, tick, and heartworm preventatives; and vaccination against diseases to which a foster animal might provide exposure. Compliance with rabies vaccination and licensing ordinances also should be verified. Potential foster caregivers should be thoroughly advised of the risks a foster animal may pose to their own pets, including, but not limited to, transmission of viral, bacterial, and fungal diseases, parasitic infestation, and behavioral conflicts. They should understand that exposure to a foster animal will require their animal to receive vaccines and other treatments they might not otherwise require.

Foster caregiver candidates should be carefully advised of the zoonotic potential of foster animals. Scabies, ringworm, rabies, and *Giardia* sp. are only a few of the zoonotic agents to which they, other persons in their household, or visitors to their home may be exposed by participating in a foster care program. They should understand both direct and fomite transmission of disease agents. Resources for educating them about these risks include the Centers for Disease Control and Prevention (www.cdc.gov) and articles published in the scientific literature, particularly the *Journal of the American Veterinary Medical Association* and Chapter 16 in this text on infectious diseases and zoonosis.

TRAINING FOSTER CAREGIVERS

Once potential foster caregivers have been approved, they should participate in a foster caregiver training program. This program should consist of the same orientation that other shelter volunteers receive, as well as specific orientation to the foster care program. The caregiver should be advised of the resources that are available to him or her. Creating a manual for foster caregivers that lists contact information for program administrators and key shelter personnel, emergency procedures, and caregiver responsibilities (financial and other) is a good practice. A veterinarian should participate in the training, either directly or in the preparation of the training manual. Potential caregivers should be advised about what disease and behavioral conditions are to be expected in foster animals, and what the usual course of treatment and the prognosis for those conditions is. While much of fostering is on-the-job training, a review of many common questions and scenarios is helpful for new caregivers. There are many available books about caring for a newly adopted pet that can provide valuable information to be applied to foster care animals and that will be particularly useful for a novice foster caregiver (Benjamin, 1988; Benjamin, 1990; Carroll and Zawistowski, 2001; Christensen and HSUS, 2002; Jankowski, 1993; Lane, Irwin, and Milani, 2001). Creating a list of these books, or building a lending library for the foster care program, is recommended.

The sheltering agency may wish to give foster caregivers a list of suggested vaccines and tests or other health procedures to be performed on the caregiver's own pets, based on health problems commonly seen in the shelter's population.

Once the foster caregiver has completed their orientation, they should be matched with a foster animal that fits their interest, abilities, and housing capabilities. The caregiver should sign a legally binding contract that clearly spells out the responsibilities of the sheltering agency and of the caregiver (see sample contracts in Appendices 21.1 and 21.2). The contract should state that the animal remains the property of the sheltering agency at all times, and designate the date on which the animal must be returned. The contract should include a detailed description of the animal, as well as the address at which the animal will be kept at all times. The contract should also make clear that the caregiver must provide adequate medical care for the animal, as determined by the sheltering agency, and that the animal may legally be seized and returned to the agency's possession if such care is not provided.

SELECTING FOSTER CARE CANDIDATES

Much of the success of a foster care program depends on choosing the right animal candidates. In all cases, the question must be not only whether the animal can be provided with an appropriate foster home, but whether the animal can ultimately be provided with an appropriate adoptive home. A chronic illness or long-term behavioral issue that can be successfully managed by an experienced foster caregiver might still prevent the animal from assimilating into a permanent home.

Ideally, the foster care program coordinator will select the animal candidates in cooperation with the shelter's veterinarian and key shelter personnel, and then match them to available foster homes. Allowing caregivers to pick and choose animals from among the shelter population is a process likely to create ill will within the program and among staff and volunteers. A veterinarian should examine all foster care candidates before they are placed with a caregiver, so that all existing medical problems may be diagnosed and not just those that are obvious.

Foster care should usually be a short-term process; the animals themselves should not become so entrenched in their "foster life" and attached to their foster caregiver that rehoming will be significantly difficult for them. Likewise, foster caregivers can easily become "burnt out" by an animal whose needs are extensive and long term. Frequent turnover of animals in the program also allows a greater number of animals to be provided with care, and it provides a greater resource for removing unhealthy animals from the shelter.

Puppies and kittens who are nearly old enough for adoption, or who have minor and easily treated illnesses (such as intestinal worm infestation), are good candidates, although future admission trends should be carefully considered. It may not be appropriate to put a litter of kittens in a foster home if, when they become ready six weeks hence, the shelter will be overflowing with healthy, highly adoptable kittens. Pregnant females, or females with neonatal offspring may also be good candidates, although the program and the caregiver must be willing and able to adequately address any problems (such as dystocia or maternal neglect) that might arise. Foster caregivers who are interested in animal "families" must be carefully advised of the (potentially extensive) amount of time and effort necessary to properly care for them, especially for dogs and their puppies. The mother animal should be thoroughly assessed for adoptability before it is determined that she and her litter should be placed into foster care. For sheltering agencies that limit or prohibit adoption of specific breed-types of dogs, whether by choice or in compliance with laws or ordinances, determining whether unborn or newborn puppies are of those breed-types is a significant concern and one that is not easily addressed. Allowing the puppies to mature until it becomes apparent what breed-type they are, and then deciding to euthanize them, is an onerous task for the foster program coordinator and the foster caregiver, one that is likely to defeat the intention of using a foster care program to support the morale of all involved with the shelter.

While hand rearing orphaned puppies and kittens is an enjoyable task that many foster caregivers will volunteer for, evidence exists that hand-reared kittens may become overly attached, timid or aggressive toward humans due to improper intra- and inter-species socialization (Beaver, 1992) and that these behaviors may prevent them from becoming acceptable pets. The same may be true of puppies. When deciding whether to provide foster care to orphaned pups and kittens, the long-term consequences to the neonate must be the primary consideration. Multiple puppies or kittens raised together without a mother frequently mutilate each other by nursing one another's genitals, causing bruising, dermatitis, and urinary tract infections. A better solution for both species is to introduce them into the litter of another lactating female, a feat that can often be successfully accomplished.

Some disease transmission potential exists when placing orphaned animals with a new mother and/or litter, and the degree of potential can be difficult to assess. Most puppies and kittens under eight weeks of age are protected from highly contagious diseases (such as canine and feline parvoviruses) by maternal antibodies, if they received them. Orphaned newborn kittens and puppies can be artificially provided with maternal antibodies: A blood sample from any healthy, well-vaccinated adult animal of the same species (either male or female) is centrifuged and the serum is mixed 1:1 with milk replacer and fed to the neonate for the first two feedings (Schultz, 1993). Alternately, newborn kittens can obtain maternal antibodies from queen's milk at any stage of lactation; the immunoglobulin content of a queen's milk does not decrease significantly after the first few days of lactation, as it does in other species (Casal, Jezyk, and Giger, 1996). Therefore, newborn kittens can be placed with a queen whose litter is much older, and still be expected to receive adequate maternal antibody protection.

Potential infection with feline leukemia virus (FeLV) and/or feline immunodeficiency virus (FIV) is a concern when placing neonatal kittens with a foster queen. Because FeLV tests detect antigen rather than antibody, maternally derived antibodies do not influence test results, and kittens may be tested at any age. However, infection in newborn kittens may not be detected until weeks to months after birth (American Association of Feline Practitioners, 2001). Maternally derived antibodies to FIV in kittens confound the interpretation of positive test results. Kittens born to infected queens may test positive for antibody, yet most will not be infected. The recent availability of a vaccine against FIV will further complicate the evaluation of the FIV status of orphaned foster kittens. Cats administered the vaccine develop antibodies to the inactivated virus present in the vaccine. Currently available antibody-based FIV diagnostic tests cannot distinguish vaccinated cats from FIV-infected cats or from cats that are both vaccinated and infected. Negative FIV-antibody test results remain reliable, but until tests that differentiate vaccinated cats from infected cats become readily available, it will be impossible to assess the significance of positive test results in cats of all ages. Kittens born to vaccinated queens will likely test positive for passively acquired FIV antibody. According to studies conducted by the vaccine's manufacturer, antibody levels drop to levels that won't interfere with the test results by the time kittens reach eight weeks of age, however, this is long after the decision to place the kittens with a foster queen must be made. Both FeLV and FIV are rare diseases, affecting only two to three percent and one and a half to three percent of healthy cats, respectively (Barr, 2000a,b). The risk of transmission of FeLV and/or FIV between a foster queen and her kittens and orphaned kittens added to the litter is present, but it can be argued that all of the kittens share that risk equally (all are possibly infected, all are possibly susceptible) and that their risk of having either viral infection is no greater than that of the entire shelter's feline population.

Another virus of concern when mixing populations of neonatal kittens is feline infectious peritonitis (FIP). Because of the difficulty of diagnosing, controlling, and preventing this disease, the risk for it to spread between commingled litters is difficult to assess, but it must be weighed against the many known benefits of attempting to transfer orphaned kittens to a foster queen.

Foster caregivers who take on the task of hand rearing orphaned pups and kittens should be thoroughly advised of the work involved, and be knowledgeable about how to feed them, clean them, stimulate defecation and urination, and closely monitor their health, as neonatal animals can quickly fade or simply fail to thrive. References that describe the care and behavior of neonatal puppies and kittens (Hoskins, 2001a; Beaver, 1992; Beaver, 1999; Johnston et al., 2001) should be made available to these caregivers.

Highly adoptable types of dogs are good candidates for foster care. Most sheltering agencies are able to easily place well-socialized and small breed dogs, such as terriers and small poodles. All of a dog's attributes must be considered, however, including his health, behavior, and rehabilitation potential. For example, a terrier with a mild case of kennel cough might be easily treated, but if he has a history of significant aggression, he's not a good candidate. Purebred animals may be good candidates, especially if the agency has a matching program for people who wish to adopt animals of specific breeds, and also if there are interested breed-specific foster caregivers. Again, all of the animal's traits must be considered, not just his purebred status.

Animals who need behavioral rehabilitation are often poor candidates for a foster care program. An adult animal that was not adequately socialized to human contact (as well as to other species with whom he might be expected to live once adopted) may not be able to live comfortably as an animal companion, particularly if a home with a person sensitive to his needs and willing to provide necessary behavioral therapy is not available. A fearful or fractious animal that adjusts well to her foster caregiver's home and presence may not be able to adjust similarly to a new home and adopter. Like all animals considered for adoption by an animal sheltering agency, animals placed in foster care programs who have a history of aggression, or who show aggression while in the foster caregiver's possession, carry with them significant liability for adoption. Ideally, any animal considered for placement in foster care that has a significant behavioral problem—whether or not that is the primary reason for foster care—should be evaluated by a veterinary behaviorist, certified applied animal behaviorist, or other experienced and qualified individuals to determine a treatment plan and a prognosis for the animal's behavioral issues.

Animals with physical disabilities differ in their potential for rehabilitation and adoption. The underlying reason for their disability must also be carefully considered. For example, a dog who is blind but otherwise healthy and behaviorally sound, might be a good candidate for foster care, if he has an additional condition that necessitates it. If his blindness is the result of diabetes or glaucoma, however, finding an adopter willing and financially able to provide the extensive medical care he needs might be a difficult task, no matter how well a foster caregiver is able to manage his disability and illness. Deaf and blind animals can be temporarily placed in the care of an experienced foster caregiver, who can assess their ability to adjust to a new environment and their response to training to determine whether they will be able to be adopted. Most cats and small- to medium-sized dogs deal very well with the amputation of a limb; assuming the animal is otherwise a good candidate for adoption, amputation of a permanently injured limb, followed by recovery and rehabilitation in a foster home, often results in successful adoption.

MONITORING FOSTER ANIMALS

Regular examination and monitoring of foster animals are crucial to a program's success. The myriad of disastrous consequences of an unmonitored foster care program cannot be underestimated. The purpose of monitoring is to verify that the animal is still in the foster caregiver's possession, to determine whether appropriate care is being provided for the animal, and whether the condition for which he is being treated is progressively improving. Ideally, the animal is examined during each visit by the shelter veterinarian so that the veterinarian can estimate the date on which the animal will be healthy enough for adoption. Most animals should be presented to the sheltering agency for examination at least every two weeks; it should occur more often for special cases such as animals recovering from significant disease or for very young puppies and kittens. The animals assigned to novice foster caregivers may need to be examined more often than those of experienced program participants, who will be more skillful at providing care and more adept at recognizing developing problems. A medical record should be kept for each individual animal, and body weight and physical examination findings, as well as the results of any tests and administration of any vaccines, anthelmintics, or medications should be recorded for each visit. Any behavioral issues should be discussed and addressed. A date and appointment for the next visit can be agreed upon at this time.

If the sheltering agency does not provide medical care for the animals in its foster care program, but instead requires foster caregivers to acquire veterinary care themselves, a biweekly visit to the sheltering agency is still recommended. The animal should be weighed by shelter personnel, and the foster caregiver should provide records of any examination or treatment provided by their veterinarian since the previous visit. A written record of the events of each visit should be kept for each animal by the agency.

PROVIDING VETERINARY CARE FOR FOSTER CARE PROGRAM ANIMALS

Providing in-house veterinary care for foster care program animals is the best option of those available. It allows the sheltering agency to keep close tabs on each animal and their progress, requires less emotional and financial investment on the part of the foster caregiver, and results in less foster caregiver burnout. The total financial investment for the animal's care is reduced, because the sheltering agency's overhead covers many of the costs that a private practitioner must pass on to the foster caregiver or to the sheltering agency. Offering in-house veterinary care for the foster care program also results in more standardized procedures and less confusion about what each animal requires.

Understandably, however, not every sheltering agency has a staff veterinarian, either full-time or part-time. In such cases, private practitioners must be used. The sheltering agency can contract with a specific veterinarian or veterinary hospital to provide care for the foster program, or can allow each foster caregiver to use the veterinarian of their choice. If outside veterinarians are used, the sheltering agency should provide those veterinarians with information about what the shelter's health care protocols are, and about what procedures are expected to be provided for foster care program animals. It may be helpful for the shelter to contact or establish a relationship beforehand with the private practitioners who are working with foster caregivers to avoid misunderstandings or hard feelings if animals they have provided medical care for are ultimately rejected for placement.

Provisions for emergency care for foster animals also must be a part of the program. Like any other animal, a foster animal may unexpectedly exhibit an emergency condition. For example, a puppy undergoing routine care for an upper respiratory infection may exhibit his first epileptic seizure in the middle of the night. Emergency care needs can be anticipated for pregnant foster animals. Foster caregivers should be given instructions about who to call and where to go in such a case, what degree of intensive care should be sought, and who will pay for costs.

The list of medical disorders encountered in the course of administering a shelter foster care program is, of course, endless. There is a relatively smaller list of conditions commonly dealt with during foster care, including those primary conditions for which animals require foster care, and those that arise secondary to them. Demodectic, sarcoptic, and notoedric mange, other external and internal parasites, dermatophytosis, malnutrition, and upper respiratory infection head the list. Dogs with parvovirus and cats with panleukopenia are rarely good candidates for foster care because those conditions require extensive and expensive treatment and often have a poor prognosis. However, animals may show clinical signs after the decision has already been made to place them in foster care and the decision may be made to pursue treatment at that time. While selected information is presented here, it is not possible to review thoroughly diagnosis, treatment, and prognosis for all of these conditions; more information can be found elsewhere in this text and in numerous other references.

Foster care of animals infected with demodectic mange is often rewarding because many animals develop demodicosis secondary to an immunostressor, such as malnutrition, weaning, pregnancy, environmental exposure, and infestation with other parasites. Once these other problems are addressed, the animal's immune system is able to overcome demodicosis in response to treatment. Foster care program administrators and caregivers must keep in mind, however, that a cure may not be achieved with a small percentage of animals, and lifelong treatment may be necessary. It should also be kept in mind that adult-onset demodicosis can be associated with internal disease or malignant neoplasia (Rhodes, 2000).

Foster care of animals with sarcoptic and notoedric mange is similarly rewarding because multiple effective treatments are available (Medleau and Hnilica, 2000), and the prognosis for a cure within a few weeks is good. Caregivers must be carefully advised of the zoonotic potential of these conditions, as well as the potential for the infection of other animals in the home and infestation of the environment in which the foster animal is kept.

Upper respiratory infections are the bane of shelter animal health. Infectious tracheobronchitis of dogs is usually a mild and self-limiting disease that responds well to treatment, and in most cases requires no treatment other than good nursing care (a clean, warm home and nutritious food) and a few days' time. Foster caregivers should be warned that any dogs residing in their home are susceptible, even if they have received a "kennel cough" (*Bordetella bronchiseptica* bacterin-parainfluenza virus) vaccine.

The outcome of treatment for cats with upper respiratory disease that are placed in foster care is less predictable. Many cats respond well to isolation from the shelter environment and supportive treatment, only to exhibit symptoms once again when they are placed back in the shelter. Clinical signs of feline upper respiratory disease (i.e., sneezing, ocular and nasal discharges) can also become chronic, and some cats may take months to recover sufficiently for symptoms to diminish. Foster caregivers must understand the possible outcomes of providing care for cats with upper respiratory disease, as well as the risk for infection of their own cats, even if properly vaccinated. It must be remembered that cats who have recovered from upper respiratory infections are viral carriers and—in most cases—shedders. When they are returned to the shelter, consideration should be given to housing them individually rather than in communal or group housing, if those forms of housing are used.

Ringworm also is commonly encountered in foster care programs, usually secondary to another condition. In this author's experience, hand-reared kittens seem particularly susceptible as they begin to eat formula-moistened cat food from a bowl and spend a great deal of time with moist milk and food on their faces, an ideal climate for fungal growth. Most cases are caused by *Microsporum canis*, *M. gypseum*, or *Trichophyton mentagrophytes*; longhaired kittens are especially susceptible to *M. canis* (Hoskins, 2001b). Puppies, kittens, and immunocompromised animals are at greatest risk. Treatment usually consists of application of a topical antifungal preparation; lime sulfur dips and miconazole and ketoconazole shampoos are popular and effective choices. Systemic treatment is usually reserved for persistent cases, and may consist of griseofulvin, itraconazole, or lufenuron. Spontaneous remission within a few months of the appearance of clinical signs is common, but treatment should be instituted to speed the process and minimize environmental contamination. A dermatophyte culture is the only reliable method for monitoring the recovery of an infected animal. Once the clinical signs of infection have resolved, a culture of a sample obtained by thoroughly brushing the animal's hair coat with a sterile toothbrush should be performed on a weekly basis while treatment is continued until two to three consecutive negative culture results are obtained (Gram 2002). Foster caregivers should be advised that a small number of animals may take an excessively long time to recover from ringworm, that the condition is potentially zoonotic, and that the environment in which the animals are kept may remain contaminated for a significant time period—posing a risk to both humans and animals who enter the environment long after the foster animal is gone. Adoption of animals recovered from ringworm can be difficult, because the potential adopters of animals must be advised that the animal may be capable of transmitting the fungus even after the clinical signs have resolved. The sheltering agency must carefully consider and accept the liability of providing foster care and adoption for an animal infected with ringworm, due to the significant zoonotic risk.

In addition to treating the condition for which the animal is placed in foster care, general health and behavioral care also should be provided. This includes routine vaccination, disease testing, and treatment for internal and external parasites (including heartworms in adult dogs). Heartworm preventative should be administered throughout the foster care period, as well as flea and tick preventatives as needed. All animals should be vaccinated against rabies once they are old enough and healthy enough to respond to the vaccine. Spaying and neutering of both adults and kittens and puppies should be performed while the animals are still in foster care, allowing them to recover in a somewhat familiar environment before being offered for adoption. Allowing puppies and kittens to recover from spay and neuter surgery while still with their littermates decreases any stress the procedure may induce.

Routine training should also be provided. To the greatest extent possible, all animals should be socialized to human handling, including restraint for examination and other procedures such as having their nails clipped, ears cleaned, and teeth brushed. Dogs and puppies should be housetrained and crate-trained, and be taught basic requests such as how to sit, stay, and walk on a leash. Kittens and cats should be trained to use a litter box and scratching post. Teaching a foster animal basic pet "etiquette" increases their chances of adoption and the possibility that they will be successfully and permanently rehomed.

PROVIDING LONG-TERM FOSTER CARE

The foster care situations described in this chapter are meant to be short-term, lasting a few weeks to months at the longest. Longer-term situations are characteristic of some of the other types of foster care programs mentioned in the introduction. One additional form of long-term foster care is hospice care, a relatively new but growing trend in veterinary care. Hospice, or palliative, care is meant to ease the end of life for an animal with a terminal condition. Treatment for pain and discomfort is provided, as well as palliative care for any clinical signs. Euthanasia may play a part in hospice care, but does not take the place of it. Foster care programs that wish to provide hospice care for animals should take advantage of the growing number of information resources regarding this form of care, including the proceedings from veterinary scientific meetings at which the concept has been presented and discussed, and a number of Internet sites that address the subject.

Some shelters are involved with legal cases (such as cruelty cases) that result in animals being held for lengthy time periods until the case is resolved. Permission should be sought from the court to determine if foster care is an acceptable option because the shelter does not "own" the animal. If the court permits the animal to be placed in foster care, in addition to ensuring the animal's medical and behavioral well-being, guidelines and safeguards must be in place to ensure that the animal cannot escape from the foster home and that no invasive procedures (such as neutering) are performed unless the animal's life is in jeopardy and the court is notified first. Caregivers must be carefully screened and counseled so they understand and accept that they must surrender the animal even if they disagree with the final court decision. Some shelters restrict foster caregiving in these circumstances to employees only. In criminal cases, consideration must also be given to issues of confidentiality and safety, making certain that the foster home is not in close proximity to the home of the accused.

Not all foster care relationships come to a successful resolution. Foster caregivers often become, understandably, attached to their foster animals, and then choose to adopt them. This is a happy ending for the animal but may eliminate the foster caregiver from the program, especially in those cases where a foster caregiver adopts more than one animal at a time or repeatedly adopts successive foster animals. Foster caregivers should go through the same process and meet the same criteria for adoption as any other adopter, and care must be taken to prevent a foster caregiver from acquiring more animals than he or she is able to provide adequate care for or legally allowed to own. Some foster caregivers return the animal to be placed for adoption, but become overly involved in the adoption process, disapproving of an adopter who has been approved by the sheltering agency, and attempting to thwart the adoption and/or harboring ill feelings toward the agency for completing the adoption. It should be made clear to potential caregivers, when they apply to participate in the program and during their program's orientation, that adoption decisions are made entirely at the discretion of the sheltering agency. Such information should be stated in the contract that the caregiver signs when agreeing to provide foster care for a specific animal.

Another difficult scenario is one in which the foster animal's rehabilitation is not successful. Death or euthanasia can be the outcome of foster care. A medical or behavioral condition may not respond to treatment, or a new problem may be identified during the foster care period that is not amenable to treatment. Most foster caregivers are able to deal successfully with this scenario if they have received well-structured orientation to the program (including this possible outcome) and if the sheltering agency deals with the situation objectively but compassionately.

CONCLUSION

Being a foster caregiver can be a rewarding experience, but it can also be difficult, frustrating, and disheartening. Foster caregiver "burnout" is common, especially when a foster care program is poorly structured and/or poorly managed. Frequent monitoring of foster care animals is an important tool for preventing caregiver burnout. It not only ensures that the animals are safe and sound, but also that foster caregivers have an opportunity to obtain support in the form of written materials, the chance to ask questions and receive timely answers, and reassurance that their efforts to care for the animal are having a beneficial effect. It gives the foster caregiver an opportunity to admit, if necessary, that they need assistance or possibly that they can no longer properly care for the animal. Veterinarians can often be very effective in helping foster caregivers cope with or avoid burnout by being particularly sensitive and receptive to their needs and concerns when it comes to the health of their foster animals.

The frequency and intensity of foster care services provided by a caregiver also plays a part in burnout. Some foster caregivers will need to take a break after an animal is returned, particularly if that animal had need for fairly intensive care. As eager as the sheltering agency may be to "fill the void" when a foster care home becomes available, allowing the foster caregiver to take a break if they wish will allow them to provide better care for the next animal when they are ready. Another technique is to vary the number and type of foster animals a particular caregiver receives, and therefore the intensity of care they must provide. For example, a caregiver who has just finished caring for a mother dog and her eight puppies, from birth to weaning, may want to provide care for an adult cat with short-term needs next.

Administering a foster care program in a manner that is strict but fair, consistent, well planned, and supportive ensures that the program is successful and a popular endeavor for employees and volunteers. These efforts allow everyone involved to clearly see the positive results a foster care program can have for any sheltering agency.

REFERENCES

American Association of Feline Practitioners. 2001. *Report on Feline Retrovirus Testing and Management.* Nashville, TN: American Association of Feline Practitioners.

Ascione, F. R. 2000. Safe *Havens for Pets: Guidelines for Programs Sheltering Pets for Women Who Are Battered.* Logan, UT: Ascione.

Arluke, A. 1991. Coping with euthanasia: A case study of shelter culture. *Journal of the American Veterinary Medical Association* 198: 1176 – 1180.

Barr, M. C. 2000a. Feline Immunodeficiency Virus (FIV). *The 5-Minute Veterinary Consult: Canine and Feline,* 2d edition. Edited by Larry P. Tilley and Francis W. K. Smith, Jr. Baltimore: Lippincott Williams & Wilkins, pp. 694 – 695.

Barr, M. C. 2000b. Feline Leukemia Virus (FeLV). *The 5-Minute Veterinary Consult: Canine and Feline,* 2d edition. Edited by Larry P. Tilley and Francis W. K. Smith, Jr. Baltimore: Lippincott Williams & Wilkins, pp. 698 – 699.

Beaver, B. V. 1992. *Feline Behavior: A Guide for Veterinarians.* Philadelphia, PA: W.B. Saunders Co.

Beaver, B. V. 1999. *Canine Behavior: A Guide for Veterinarians.* Philadelphia, PA: W.B. Saunders Co.

Benjamin, C. Lea. 1988. *Second-Hand Dog: How to Turn Yours Into a First-Rate Pet.* New York: Howell Book House.

Benjamin, C. Lea. 1990. *The Chosen Puppy: How to Select and Raise a Great Puppy from an Animal Shelter.* New York: Howell Book House.

Carroll, D. L., and Zawistowski, S. 2001. *The ASPCA Complete Guide to Pet Care.* New York: Plume.

Casal, M. L., Jezyk, P. F., et al. 1996. Transfer of colostral antibodies from queens to their kittens. *American Journal of Veterinary Research* 57: 1653 – 1658.

Christensen, W. and the staff of the Humane Society of the United States. 2002. *The Humane Society of the United States Complete Guide to Cat Care.* New York: St. Martin's Press.

Gram, W. D. 2002. *The 5-Minute Veterinary Consult Clinical Companion—Small Animal Dermatology.* Karen Helton-Rhodes (ed.) Baltimore, MD: Lippincott, Williams, and Wilkins, 324.

Hoskins, J. D. 2001a. *Veterinary Pediatrics: Dogs and Cats from Birth to Six Months.* Philadelphia, PA: W.B. Saunders Co.

Hoskins, J. D. 2001b. Protect yourself from dermatophytosis. *DVM Newsmagazine,* November, 2S – 4S.

Jankowski, C. 1993. *Adopting Cats and Kittens: A Care and Training Guide.* New York: Howell Book.

Johnston, S. D., Root-Kustritz, M., et al. 2001. *Canine and Feline Theriogenology.* Philadelphia, PA: WB Saunders.

Kirkwood, S. 1999. When stress turns into distress. *Animal Sheltering,* March – April.

Lane, M. S., Irwin, P. G., et al. 2001. *The Humane Society of the United States Complete Guide to Dog Care: Everything You Need to Know to Keep Your Dog Healthy and Happy.* New York: Little Brown & Company.

Medleau, L., and Hnilica, K. A. 2000. Sarcoptic mange. *The 5-Minute Veterinary Consult: Canine and Feline,* 2d edition. Edited by Larry P. Tilley and

Francis W. K. Smith, Jr. Baltimore: Lippincott Williams & Wilkins, p. 1184.

Rhodes, K. H. 2000. Demodicosis. *The 5-Minute Veterinary Consult: Canine and Feline,* 2d edition. Edited by Larry P. Tilley and Francis W. K. Smith, Jr. Baltimore: Lippincott Williams & Wilkins, pp. 608 – 609.

Schultz, R. W. 1993. Speaker, Shelter Veterinarian Conference, American Humane Association. San Diego, CA.

White, D. J., and Shawhan, R. 1996. Emotional responses of animal shelter workers to euthanasia. *Journal of the American Veterinary Medical Association* 208: 846 – 849.

Appendix 21.1:
Sample Foster Care Agreement

ALL FOSTER PLACEMENTS ARE SUBJECT TO APPROVAL AND ARE AT THE SOLE DISCRETION OF FOSTER CARE MANAGEMENT

"Your shelter here" FOSTER CARE AGREEMENT

The parties hereto agree as follows: The Foster Caretaker signing below hereby acknowledges receipt from the "your shelter here," of the animal(s) described below for foster care: and in accepting this (these) animal(s), and in consideration for being entrusted with the care, custody, and possession of the animal(s), agrees to be bound by the covenants and conditions stated below.

Foster Care Personal Information

Name: _____

Address: _____ Apt. #:_____

City:_____ State:_____ Zip:_____

Daytime Phone: _____ Evening Phone: _____

Animal(s) Received

Intake # and Name	Intake Date	Breed/Sex/Age	Medical Condition

The parties agree that:

a) The Foster Caretaker shall provide the animal(s) with good care, including, but not limited, to food, water, shelter, grooming, training and medication when required.

b) As between the Foster Caretaker and the "your shelter here", the animal(s) shall remain the sole property of the "your shelter here".

c) The animal(s) shall be returned to the "your shelter here" upon request by the "your shelter here", or if the Foster Caretaker is no longer able to adequately care for the animals(s), of if the Foster Caretaker is relocating outside of the xxxxx metropolitan area.

d) Agents of the "your shelter here" will be allowed to inspect the premises in which the animal(s) will be maintained or are maintained, from time to time, for the purpose of determining the suitability of those premises for the care and maintenance of the animal(s).

e) The Foster Caretaker understands and acknowledges that she/he does not have any right or authority to keep the foster animal(s) or to place foster animal(s) in other homes or places with other individuals unless permission is given in writing by "your shelter here" Foster Caretaker Management Personnel.

f) The Foster Caretaker understands and acknowledges that she/he is responsible for all expenses incurred as a result of fostering an animal. The sole exception to this is that the "your shelter here" will provide, at no charge, initial vaccination and medication for minor existing ailments. All other expenses will be at the Foster Caretaker's expense.

g) The Foster Caretaker agrees that should the animal(s) require extensive medical treatment the "your shelter here" may request immediate return of the animal(s) and may euthanize the animal(s) for humane reasons.

h) In the unfortunate event that the animal(s) becomes so ill during foster care as to warrant humane euthanasia, the Foster Caretaker will notify the "your shelter here" before having the animal(s) euthanized and supply the "your shelter here" with medical documentation from her/his veterinarian verifying euthanasia and the reasons for euthanasia.

i) The Foster Caretaker agrees to defend, indemnify and hold the "your shelter here" harmless from any direct or remote and consequential damages arising out of this foster care arrangement.

The Foster Caretaker agrees to return said animal to the "your shelter here" no later than _____ (subject to change if authorized by Foster Care Management Personnel).

This contract represents the entire agreement between the parties and any modifications will be made in writing and signed by both the Foster Caretaker and a representative of the Foster Care Management Personnel.

Foster Caretaker:
Executed this _____ day of _____

Signed:_____

For the "Your shelter here":
Executed this _____ day of _____

Signed (Foster Care Management ONLY):_____

Appendix 21.2:
Sample Foster Care Application

Name:	
Address: apt#	Employer:
City: State: Zip:	Address:
Phone: e-mail address:	City: State: Zip:

Living Accommodations: Rent Own Home Other:	Does your lease allow pets? yes no
Describe area where foster animals will stay:	Do you have a fenced-in-yard? yes no
	Do you have screens on windows? yes no
How many children at home? ___ Age? _____	

Do you currently have other pets? yes no How many?_____ Breeds:_____ Sexes:_____ Ages:_____ Are they neutered/spayed? yes no Any behavioral concerns or chronic illnesses? Name & address of your current vet: How can you keep them separated? _____ Have you had pets in the past? yes no dogs cats Where are they now?	How much time can you devote to foster care: Do you: work school home Is it: F/T P/T What is your schedule/availability like? How many days/weeks can you foster an animal? How often would you like to foster? What are the care arrangements when you are not home? If you live with other people are they interested in helping? What is their schedule/availability like?

What kind of animal(s) would you like to foster?

Injured Adult Cat   Ill Adult Cat   Injured Young Cat   Ill Young Cat   Mother with Kittens   Litter of Orphaned Kittens   Pregnant Cat   Injured Adult Dog   Ill Adult Dog   Injured Young Dog   Ill Young Dog   Mother with Puppies   Litter of Orphaned Puppies   Pregnant Dog   **Anything**

How did you hear about the Foster Care Program? Why do you want to Foster? When would you like to start?	Does anyone in the household have allergies? How will you cope? What pet supplies do you have? _____ Have you taken other training classes?

22
Spay and Neuter Surgical Techniques for the Animal Shelter

Leslie D. Appel and Robert C. Hart

INTRODUCTION

Pet overpopulation in this country is an enormous problem. Estimates suggest that millions of dogs and cats are euthanitized each year because there are not enough adoptive homes for these animals (Patronek and Rowan, 1995). The reproductive potential of cats and dogs is significant; a single pair of cats can be the progenitors of 174,760 offspring in just 7 years (Root-Kustritz, 1999). A critical step in trying to alleviate this tragic overpopulation problem is achieved through providing surgical spay and neuter services for animals in shelters. Therefore, the most common, and perhaps the most important, surgical procedures performed in shelter veterinary practice are canine and feline ovariohysterectomies and castrations.

If possible, all animals should be spayed or neutered prior to being adopted from the shelter. Despite spay/neuter contracts requiring these procedures for shelter obtained dogs and cats, studies have shown less than a 60 percent compliance rate after adoption of these animals (Howe, 2001). Although the majority of family pets are spayed or neutered, an estimated 16 percent of pets have had one litter prior to receiving sterilization surgery (National Pet Alliance, 1993). Furthermore, spaying/neutering an animal prior to adoption from the shelter not only aids in decreasing pet overpopulation, but also reduces medical problems in the animal's future, and gives that animal a greater chance of being successfully adopted.

This chapter focuses on the standard and complex ovario-hysterectomies and castrations of dogs and cats. Standard anesthetic and surgical principles

and techniques will be detailed. In addition, an overview of some of the controversial medical and surgical issues surrounding these procedures in a shelter environment has been included. Surgical complications will be reviewed with an emphasis on prevention of these problems. Finally, mobile spay/neuter services and special Spay Day projects will be described. With an understanding of the principles and techniques described in this chapter, safe and effective spay/neuter procedures can be performed on adoptable shelter animals. There are special considerations for surgery in the shelter situation that are still safe and effective. Also, shelter veterinarians are often involved in high volume neuter situations unlike the private practice setting, and this accounts, in part, for the need for this chapter. Safe shelter standards are a reflection of shelter reality without compromising the safety of the patients. Speed is accomplished as surgeons develop greater proficiency by performing several procedures each day (not by taking unsafe "shortcuts"), and by training technical staff to be very efficient in anesthetizing and prepping surgery patients. Shelters must strive to provide the best standard of care for the safety of the patients. The standards for surgery in shelters are not minimal standards, but rather are standards that reflect the circumstances and needs of shelter animals.

STANDARD SPAY/NEUTER

The term 'spay' refers to the surgical procedure of ovariohysterectomy. The term 'neuter' refers to either the surgical procedures of ovariohysterectomy or orchidectomy; although most of the time this term is used to refer to the surgical procedure of castration. In this chapter, the term neuter will refer to castration. A "standard" spay/neuter can be performed on any healthy young adult animal. A young adult animal refers to animals between 6 months and 6 years of age. For all cases, a complete medical and surgical record should be completed and maintained as for all medical records in veterinary practice.

Patient Selection

Healthy, adoptable, sexually intact, adult and pediatric animals can undergo sterilization surgery. Any animal with a serious medical condition or behavioral problem that is therefore not a good candidate for adoption should not be sterilized unless a home has been secured. An exception to this is a potentially aggressive animal that may benefit from being neutered. However, the surgery alone rarely solves aggressive tendencies (behavior modification training is usually necessary). Pregnant females or females with litters may show aggression in an attempt to protect the puppies or kittens, and surgical sterilization and/or weaning the litter may help to better evaluate the temperament of these animals. If possible, all animals should be spayed or neutered prior to adoption.

Preoperative Evaluation

In private practice the gold standard for the preoperative evaluation of a healthy young adult surgical patient is a physical examination and basic blood work commonly referred to as a Quick Assessment Test or QATs. These tests include packed cell volume (PCV), total serum protein (TP), blood urea nitrogen (BUN) and blood glucose concentration (GLU). However, thousands of animals are safely spayed and neutered in both shelter settings and private practices without benefit of QATs. Any shelter that has the ability to perform QATs is certainly encouraged to do so, but no shelter should view their inability to perform such tests on healthy young animals as sufficient reason to not spay and neuter the shelter animals. In any situation, the physical examination should be performed on the day of surgery. More in-depth blood work, such as complete blood count (CBC) and serum biochemistry analysis (CHEM), should be strongly considered for animals with clinical signs of systemic illness. Viral testing for FeLV/FIV infections in cats remains controversial in shelter settings

because of limitations of the tests, yet should be considered in accordance with the recommendations of the Association of Feline Practitioners that all cats be tested for the diseases. No healthy cat should be diagnosed and euthanized for either disease based on the results of a single positive test. (See chapters 16 and 18 on infectious diseases and diagnostic testing, respectively, for more information on this topic.) Heartworm tests in dogs (and cats) should be performed in endemic areas. If the heartworm test is positive, but the dog is asymptomatic (Class I heartworm infection), and the dog is to be adopted out, then spay or neuter should be performed prior to adoption. The PE and blood work will screen for unhealthy animals in order to minimize anesthetic and surgical complications. Screening blood work also identifies healthy animals and increases their chances for adoption. An animal's adoptability is often directly related to the animal's health status.

As part of the physical examination, all female patients (dogs and cats) should be shaved along the ventrum to check for a spay scar prior to anesthesia and surgery. The shaved spot must be large enough to include the umbilicus cranially and should extend to the distal third of the abdomen. A surgery light or other bright light will help in identifying any surgical scar. The external genitalia and mammary glands should also be examined. The adult female dog or cat that has already had an ovariohysterectomy will usually have a small or juvenile vulva. There is usually no development of mammary tissue (unless the animal has had previous litters), and the nipples are often very small. If an animal has a scar, but also has a prominent vulva, prominent mammary tissue and nipples, an abdominal exploratory should be performed. However, if the animal was in heat, pregnant, or recently nursing at the time of surgery the vulva, mammary glands and nipples may remain enlarged for several weeks. If an animal was spayed as a pediatric patient and has now entered the shelter as an adult, a scar may or may not be seen. In these patients, the external genitalia and mammary tissue should be examined for characteristics described above. Additionally, the linea should be palpated in cases that have a questionable surgical scar. If an animal has had a previous abdominal incision, the linea may feel roughened or thickened. Suture material may also be palpated if the surgery was recent, or if non-absorbable sutures were used. If the physical examination or palpation is not conclusive as to whether or not the animal was spayed previously, an abdominal exploratory may be necessary. This is better than leaving an animal intact, not only to stem the overpopulation problem, but also to prevent mammary tumors and pyometra in the patient later in life. If possible, a LH (Luteinizing Hormone) test can be performed to distinguish between the intact animal and the ovariectomized animal (Lofstedt and Vanleeuwen, 2000). A positive result (high LH value) is a strong predictor of a spayed animal (or an animal in anestrous), while a negative result (low LH) indicates an intact animal, and therefore the need for surgery. The LH test comes in a commercially available test kit from Synbiotics, or samples can be sent to a local laboratory. A progesterone assay is not as reliable as the LH test to determine if a dog is intact. The presence of progesterone indicates an intact dog. However, as the intact bitch's ovaries only contain corpora lutea for 60–80 days after ovulation, any blood sample taken outside of this window will fail to detect progesterone and hence the presence of ovaries.

In the male dog or cat, palpation of both testicles must be done to rule out cryptorchidism (retained testicle). Bilateral cryptorchidism, although very rare, presents a diagnostic challenge when the animal has an unknown medical history. Removing fur from the prescrotal (dog) and scrotal (cat) regions may facilitate observation of previous surgical incisions in those areas. Furthermore, secondary sex characteristics are generally absent in neutered animals, and a neutered male dog can have a juvenile prepuce and penis.

The surgeon should confirm that the animal has been fasted for the appropriate length of time prior to surgery. Finally, the surgeon, prior to surgery, must confirm the sex of the patient. Unfortunately, there are occasional incidents of an abdominal exploratory being performed on a male cat during a busy surgery day because the sex was not determined correctly prior to surgery. The veterinarian should bear in mind that, regardless of the procedural set-up, the ultimate responsibility for these surgical errors rests with them. This error can always be avoided with a thorough preoperative physical exam.

Special Considerations

UPPER RESPIRATORY INFECTIONS
Certain common shelter medical problems should not prevent the animal from being spayed/neutered.

One of the most common medical problems in the shelter environment is Upper Respiratory Infection (URI). URIs are more common in cats than dogs, but can occur in both species. In cats, URIs are primarily caused by viruses, including herpes virus, calicivirus, and *Chlamydia*. In dogs, kennel cough is common with the predominant causative bacteria being *Bordetella bronchispetica*. Unlike the client owned animal that can be sent home and treated for the URI prior to anesthesia and surgery, this is not often an option for shelter animals. Although it is not ideal to anesthetize and perform surgery on an animal with a URI, it can be done safely and is a necessity in the shelter situation.

Cats with URIs should be treated with supportive care during the perioperative period. This treatment can consist of subcutaneous (SQ) fluid administration, antibiotic therapy (if necessary to treat secondary bacterial invasion) and adequate nutrition. Amoxicillin/clavulinate combination (Clavamox®) is an appropriate antibiotic for these cases. Antibiotics should be used in patients that exhibit severe pyrexia, purulent nasal and/or ocular discharge, or the worsening of clinical signs. URIs in shelter cats are so common that antibiotics should be reserved for treatment of severe cases in order to try and prevent the development of bacterial antibiotic resistance. Cats with fevers as high as 106°F have been successfully spayed/neutered while providing supportive care (personal experience). These cats most often recover well from both surgery and the URI and ultimately are more adoptable than an unaltered cat with a URI.

THE SURGICAL SUITE
The shelter should designate a room to be the "surgery suite." This room must be kept clean, and have as little traffic as possible to help maintain sterility. Ideally, this room should be maintained for surgery only. No other medical or shelter procedures should be done in this room. The door should be kept shut at all times. Different shelters will have different abilities to maintain an ideal surgical environment. If conditions are at all questionable, perioperative antibiotics should be used. Cefazolin (22mg/kg IV) or ampicillin trihydrate (Polyflex, 22mg/kg SQ) are good choices for preoperative antibiotic administration. The shelter should also have on hand monitoring equipment, resuscitative and emergency drugs, and equipment as would be found in any typical surgery setup.

Anesthetic Considerations

Once the patient has been selected and the preoperative evaluation has been completed, an anesthetic protocol should be considered. There are many acceptable anesthetic protocols. As spay and neuter procedures are painful, analgesics should be included in the anesthetic plan. Premedications are typically analgesics, anticholinergics that support cardiac function during anesthesia, and occasionally tranquilizers. Postoperative analgesia is appropriate for ovariohysterectomy, but not usually necessary for most routine castrations as the procedure is short and the analgesia administered in the preoperative period should still be effective. The author commonly uses the anesthetic protocols found in Table 22.1 for routine spay/neuter of both dogs and cats.

If the ketamine/valium combination is not available, thiopental (12mg/kg thiopental IV) can also be used as the induction agent. A low dose of acepromazine is usually effective to sedate the very excited patient. The dose range for acepromazine is 0.02–0.04mg/kg SQ, not to exceed a maximum of 3 mg per animal. Acepromazine is safe in healthy young adult animals, but should be avoided in patients with a known seizure history, liver disease, heart disease, geriatric or pediatric patients, any dehydrated animal, and Boxers. As a true history is not usually known for shelter animals, acepromazine should generally be used only when needed in the nontractable patient.

Some shelters may not have access to gas anesthesia. Cat spays and castrations can easily be done under injectable anesthesia. An injectable anesthesia protocol is listed in the Special Spay Day Projects section at the end of this chapter. Although dog castrations can also be done under injectable anesthesia, it is generally recommended to use inhalant maintenance anesthesia for dog spays and castrations.

Intravenous fluid support is not necessary in the healthy, young adult dog or cat during spay or cas-

tration. Intravenous (IV) catheterization is ideal in case of emergency, but not absolutely necessary in these patients either. Protective eye lubricant should always be placed in both eyes at the time of anesthetic induction to prevent corneal injury. Patient monitoring devices such an ECG, pulse oximetry or doppler blood pressure monitor should be used during anesthesia/surgery if available. As is often the case in shelters, there is little technical support to assist the veterinarian. If the surgeon is alone in the operating room with the patient, monitoring equipment with an auditory component should be considered. For example, an ECG machine can provide both a visual and auditory means of monitoring the patient as does a pulse oximeter. A doppler blood pressure monitor also provides auditory information about patient status during anesthesia. An esophageal stethoscope with an auditory component is another good option when finances are limited for monitoring devices.

Patient Preparation

After the patient is anesthetized, the urinary bladder should be completely emptied by gentle manual expression. The fur should be carefully clipped to avoid skin irritation. If the skin is nicked or cut, the animal is much more likely to bother the incision, and extra care must be taken during the postoperative period to prevent problems. The skin is then aseptically prepared in a standard manner. For ovariohysterectomies in dogs and cats, a wide surgical preparation is recommended, extending from just above the xiphoid cranially to the pubis caudally. The site should be wide on the lateral margins as well. This large cranial extension is done in case a vascular pedicle is dropped in surgery, and the incision site needs to be extended. If this occurs, the surgeon can extend the incision as necessary without worrying about hair contamination of the surgical field. Some surgeons may elect to spay a feral

Table 22.1. Anesthetic Protocol for Routine Spay/Neuter of Young Adult Dogs and Cats

Premedication	0.02mg/kg atropine SQ or 0.01 mg/kg glycopyrrolate SQ
	0.2mg/kg butorphanol SQ
Induction	1ml/10kg ketamine:valium IV (in a 1:1 ratio)
Maintenance	Isoflurane inhalant anesthesia in 100 percent oxygen delivered via an inflatable cuff
	endotracheal tube
Postoperative	0.2mg/kg butorphanol SQ
Analgesia	(To be given at time of extubation, directly after the endotracheal tube is removed)

cat through a flank incision. This approach is acceptable and is the surgeon's preference. (This procedure is described in chapter 24 on trap neuter release programs.)

For dog castrations the prescrotal region from the mid-portion of the prepuce to the scrotum is clipped and prepared. The fur on the scrotum should also be carefully clipped to prevent contamination of the surgery site. For cat castrations the fur on the scrotum can be gently "plucked" or removed with clippers and the skin aseptically prepared. After the patient is positioned on the surgery table, the skin can be cleansed and prepared for sterile surgery with products containing chlorhexidine or povidone iodine and applied with gauze sponges in a standard manner (Fossum et al., 2002).

While the patient is being prepped for surgery, the surgeon should perform a surgical scrub of the hands and forearms with antimicrobial soaps such as povidone-iodine or chlorhexidine. The first surgical scrub of the day for the surgeon should be at least 5 minutes in duration, followed by subsequent 3-minute surgical scrubs as needed to maintain sterility for surgeries that day. Surgical cap and masks plus sterile surgical attire are recommended. The patient is draped with sterile quarter towels and/or a large barrier drape for all surgeries with exception of cat castrations.

Surgical Technique

There are many variations of the ovariohysterectomy and castration surgeries. The surgical technique that the surgeon is most comfortable performing should be used. Sterility must be maintained, and new surgical gloves and a new surgical pack should be used for each patient. There are several standard techniques to perform ovariohysterectomies and castrations. The following descriptions are the surgical techniques used by this author.

Dog Ovariohysterectomy

The surgeon should stand at the surgery table according to dexterity. Some veterinarians performing high volume spay/neuter surgery report back problems and other repetitive motion injuries, so they should make certain they are comfortable while performing the surgery and standing on the appropriate side of the surgery table. The table should be adjusted to the appropriate height. A rubber mat can be used to stand on to help reduce back and leg prob-

lems. A standard 4-corner draping procedure is used. A midline skin incision is made with a scalpel blade starting at the umbilicus and extending one third of the way caudally to the pubis. The length of the midline skin incision is based on the size of the dog (Stone et al., 1993) and the skill and experience of the surgeon. Incisions heal from side to side, not end to end. Therefore, the incision length should be adequate to perform the ovariohysterectomy. An approach is made to the linea alba using sharp dissection with a scalpel blade. Metzenbaum scissors may also be used to dissect the subcutaneous tissue, but an approach with a blade typically creates less tissue trauma and dead space than an approach with Metzenbaum scissors. Dead space can lead to seroma or hematoma formation, which can subsequently lead to infection and dehiscence. A stab incision is made through the linea with an inverted scalpel blade. The linea incision is extended caudally and then cranially using the blade and Adson tissue forceps as a guide. Once inside the abdomen, the uterus is identified dorsal to the bladder and ventral to the colon. Although the use of a spay hook is common and acceptable, it must be remembered that there are some dangers associated with its use, and therefore it must be used with care. For example, a spay hook may inadvertently damage mesentery, mesometrium, or abdominal vasculature. Once the uterus is identified, the left uterine horn is traced cranially to the left ovary.

The ovary of the dog is inside the ovarian bursa. As animals age, fat accumulates in the bursa and the ovary cannot be completely visualized. The entire extent of the ovary must be palpated to ensure complete removal of the ovary. Failure to remove the ovary in its entirety can result in stump pyometra. Failure to remove the entire ovary can also lead to poor client relations, as the animal can continue to show signs of estrus. Also, by spaying a female dog or cat before the first heat cycle, mammary neoplasia will be drastically reduced. This benefit will not be gained if the complete ovary is not removed. The left ovary is removed before the right ovary because it has a more caudal position within the abdomen and is therefore easier to exteriorize through the incision. The removal of the left ovary first also facilitates locating the right ovary by tracing the uterus from its bifurcation proximal along the right uterine horn to the ovary. The left and right ovarian pedicles are triple clamped and double ligated using a standard triple clamp and flash technique to reduce the risk of hemorrhage. If the pedicles are small, a modified double clamp and single ligature may be used. The clamp most distal from the ovary is removed, and the ligature is placed in the groove created by the clamp. The clamp above the ligature is flashed (opened) to release tension on the pedicle and tighten the ligature. Then a third clamp is placed across the proper ligament to prevent back bleeding as the pedicle is transected proximal to the clamp remaining below the ovary. This ensures the ovarian vascular pedicle is crushed as well as ligated. If the pedicle is large and contains a large amount of fat, triple clamps will be used and the ligatures will be placed in the crushed marks left by the two most distal clamps.

The same triple clamp and flash technique is used to ligate and transect the uterine pedicle. The uterine pedicle is transected as close to the cervix as possible or the cervix may also be resected. A dog in heat will have a greatly enlarged cervix and therefore the pedicle should be ligated where the cervix begins to taper into the uterus to ensure security of the ligature. The point of ligation of the uterine pedicle depends on the surgeon's preference, the size of the cervix, and the age of the dog. If the dog is young, there is no evidence to promote ovariohysterectomy versus ovariectomy. This will depend on the surgeon's preference. However, if the dog is older and has experienced many estrus cycles, the uterus will be predisposed to Cystic Endometrial Hyperplasia (CEH), which will then predispose the patient to stump pyometra. Therefore, in older dogs, a complete ovariohysterectomy is recommended. Many theriogenologists recommend complete removal of the uterus in all cases, because then there is no chance of stump pyometra in the future.

Absorbable suture material is recommended. The size of the suture is determined by the size of the pedicle and not by the size of the dog. Polydioxanone (PDS®) is the author's suture material of choice. The most common sizes of suture used for ovarian and uterine pedicles in the dog are 2–0 and 0. The left paravertebral space is checked for hemorrhage by retracting the descending colon and using its mesentery as a sling for the other abdominal structures. The right paravertebral space is checked for hemorrhage by retracting the duodenum and its mesentery (Stone et al., 1993).

The linea alba is closed in a routine manner. Care must be used to ensure full thickness bites through the linea alba or external rectus sheath in order to prevent dehiscence. A surgeon's knot and continuous pattern are generally used in suturing the linea. In animals less than 10 lbs, 3–0 suture can be used. In animals 10 lbs to 45 lbs, 2–0 suture can be used. 0 suture should be used in animals weighing greater than 45 lbs. Monofilament absorbable suture on a taper needle is recommended. PDS® is a good choice of suture to close the linea alba. The choice of suture is the surgeon's preference. This author does not recommend the use of chromic gut because it loses the tensile strength required for holding too rapidly. The subcutaneous tissue is closed with 3–0 or 2–0 interrupted absorbable sutures to close any dead space created with the incision. A continuous subcuticular pattern is done to appose the skin. Absorbable suture, size 3-0 on a cutting needle is typically used. No skin sutures are placed because suture removal may not be possible in shelter animals. Skin adhesive (glue) can be used if necessary, but should be used minimally and should not be used along the entire length of the incision. The surgeon should closely appose the skin edges, and avoid getting excessive glue inside the incision as this can lead to granulomas and potentially draining tracts.

Cat Ovariohysterectomy

The ovariohysterectomy in the cat is performed in a similar manner to the procedure in the dog. The skin incision in the cat is made further caudal than that of the dog as the ovaries are easier to remove in the cat because of the lack of tight suspensory ligaments. Also, due to its close association with the urinary bladder, the uterine body in the cat is more difficult to retract through the abdominal incision than in the dog. The skin incision is made in the distal two-thirds of the distance between the umbilicus and the pubis. The ovarian pedicles usually contain very little fat tissue so 3-0 or 2-0 suture material can be used. In the cat, the ovaries are not inside a bursa, so the extent of the ovary can be easily identified and completely removed. The infundibulum often surrounds the cat ovary and should be completely removed as well when possible. The uterine pedicle is closely associated with the bladder in the cat, so complete bladder expression is strongly recommended in the cat prior to ovariohysterectomy. 3–0 or 2–0 suture can be used for the uterine pedicle. If the cat is in heat, the uterine pedicle is friable, so gentle tissue handling must be used. If the cat is less than 10 lbs, 3–0 absorbable suture can be used to close the linea. If the cat is more than 10 lbs 2–0 absorbable suture can be used. The remainder of the closure is similar to the dog with adjustments made for suture sizes, such as 4–0 for the subcutaneous tissue and for the subcuticular pattern.

Dog Castration

Some surgeons do not clip the hair from the scrotum when preparing the dog for castration. If care is taken, the scrotal hair can be shaved off without cutting or irritating the scrotal skin. Clipping the hair is recommended to avoid contamination of the incision during the procedure. Closed castration technique is preferred to the open castration technique. In a closed castration, there is no direct access into the abdominal cavity, thus eliminating the possibility of peritonitis if contamination occurs. The closed castration procedure is also faster and easier to perform and appears to cause less postoperative swelling for the dog. A closed castration can be performed in any size dog. If the spermatic cord is large, a closed castration may still be performed with the utilization of transfixation ligatures instead of circumferential ligatures.

A prescrotal incision in the adult dog is preferable to a scrotal incision, as the scrotal skin is more fragile and sensitive in the mature dog. A scrotal incision makes the dog more likely to lick the incision, which can make the incision susceptible to infection and slower to heal. Either testicle can be removed first. To begin the procedure, one testicle is pushed cranially out of the scrotum into the pre-scrotal area. The testicle is stabilized in the pre-scrotal position and a midline skin incision is made over the testicle using a scalpel blade. The incision is extended sharply through the subcutaneous tissue and spermatic fascia to expose the parietal vaginal tunic (Boothe, 1993). The testis is exteriorized through the incision and freed from the scrotal attachment by manually breaking down the ligament of the tail of the epididymus. Fat and fascia are reflected off the spermatic cord using a gauze sponge (Boothe, 1993). Once the testicle and spermatic cord have been maximally exteriorized a standard triple, or double clamp and flash technique is used to ligate the cord. The pedicle is transected proximal to the remaining clamp and the testicle removed. Double ligatures of 0 or 2–0 absorbable suture are recommended for large spermatic cords. Single ligatures can be used for small spermatic cords. The second testis is removed in the same manner.

The subcutaneous tissue is closed with two simple interrupted sutures of 3–0 absorbable suture material, and a subcuticular pattern is performed with 3–0 absorbable suture on a cutting needle. If fascial bleeders were encountered while making the incisions, an ice pack applied to the area for 15 minutes after surgery will reduce swelling. In addition to helping reduce pet overpopulation, castration also prevents benign prostatic hyperplasia (BPH), which can occur in as high as 99 percent of male dogs over 8 years of age. If BPH occurs, the ideal treatment is castration.

Cat Castration

The cat castration procedure is a clean but not sterile procedure and can be done under injectable anesthesia. The anesthetic protocol recommended for tractable cats is found in Table 22.2.

A closed castration technique is preferred over an open castration for similar reasons to the dog castration. A separate longitudinal scrotal skin incision is made over each testis (Boothe, 1993). The spermatic fascia is incised to expose the parietal vaginal tunic. The testis is exteriorized through the incision using steady traction. Manual reflection of fat and fascia is done using a gauze sponge. Once the testis and spermatic cord are completely exteriorized, the spermatic cord is tied using a hemostat technique to tie an overhand knot. (Some surgeons prefer to use sutures or hemoclips to ligate the pedicle.) Once the testicle is removed and the knot is tightened, the pedicle is replaced into the scrotum. The procedure is repeated on the second testicle. No glue, subcutaneous or skin sutures are used.

Postoperative Considerations

Tattooing and Ear Notching

If possible, all animals should be tattooed at the time of surgery. There is no standard manner in

Table 22.2. Anesthetic Protocol for Young Adult Cat Castrations

Premedication	0.02mg/kg atropine SQ
	0.2mg/kg butorphanol SQ
Induction	1ml/10kg ketamine:valium IV
	(in a 1:1 ratio)

which to tattoo an animal to indicate that the animal has been spayed/neutered. If a tattoo unit is available, it is recommended to mark OVH directly next to the incision line. If later in its life the animal is evaluated for surgery, the letters will be noticed when the abdomen is shaved prior to surgery. An alternative to writing out OVH is to make the symbol for female with a line through it. These techniques can be done in the male patient as well. If a tattoo unit is not available, another option is to put the tattoo ink along the incision, so the incision will "appear" easily if the animal presents for spay/neuter later in life.

Additionally, if feral cats are spayed or neutered, ear notching should be done so cats already spayed/neutered can be identified at a distance and will not be re-trapped and re-anesthetized. The goal is to make a surgically altered change to the ear, such as a notch or cutting the tip straight off. This can be differentiated from injury, such as the cat losing part of the ear from frostbite, which would leave irregular borders.

POSTOPERATIVE INSTRUCTIONS

All patients should be fed and offered water once they are alert and in the evening of the surgery day. Most patients can also be discharged the same day as the surgery, once they are fully alert. Regardless of whether they are sent to a home or returned to the shelter, standard post-operative orders should include the following directions:

1. Monitor incision for signs of heat, pain, swelling, discharge, or odor. Contact a veterinarian if these signs occur.
2. Keep the animal quiet for 10–14 days (for abdominal surgery) or 7 days (for castration surgery).
3. There are no sutures to remove.

POSTOPERATIVE ANALGESIA

During the immediate postoperative period, patients should be monitored for signs of pain such as an increased heart and respiratory rates, restlessness/agitation, and vocalization. Additional analgesics should be administered if pain is suspected, using the same analgesic and dosage given as a pre-medication. Antibiotics are generally not administered after surgery unless a break in sterile technique occurred during surgery. Under usual circumstances, animals do not need to be released with oral analgesics. Controversy surrounds the decision as to whether or not to provide patients with anti-inflammatory/analgesic medications. Some surgeons believe that the animals will recover more quickly if they receive anti-inflammatory medications, while others believe that mild discomfort reminds the patient to remain quiet. Too much activity in the immediate post-op period can lead to dehiscence of the linea alba. Depending on the shelter, post-op patients may not be monitored as closely as patients that are sent home, but they will at least be confined to a cage and less active. On the other hand, owners who work are unable to monitor the patient during the day and these animals are likely to be more active. Postoperative analgesic decisions must be tailored by the surgeon to the animal's responses and the conditions into which the animal is released. Animals should be fully recovered from anesthesia prior to discharge and should not be discharged until they are alert, able to ambulate and urinate on their own.

PEDIATRIC SPAY/NEUTER IN THE SHELTER

Performing pediatric spay/neuter is safe for all patients and highly recommended for shelter animals. The pediatric patient is 6-16 weeks of age, although some extend that definition to up to 24 weeks of age, the earliest age when dogs may generally reach puberty. In order to make certain that the surgery is performed prepubertally in cats, the surgery must be performed before 16 weeks of age. The procedures are safe and effective, and allow every animal to be spayed or neutered before leaving the shelter. As long as specific anesthetic and surgical guidelines are followed, pediatric patients as young as 6 weeks can safely be spayed and neutered.

Many controversies and concerns have surrounded the issue of pediatric spay/neuter. However, most of these concerns have not been verified by scientific research. The concept of pediatric spay/neuter is currently supported by the American Veterinary Medical Association (AVMA). Spay/neuter surgeries have been performed on very young animals as early as the 1970's, and some reports go back to the early 1900's (Salmeri, Olsen, et al., 1991). An important concept to remember is that many veterinarians spay and neuter animals before they reach puberty, so any long-term health risk that is present at 10 weeks is also present at 6 months, as both ages are usually prepubertal. In addition to helping stem the pet over-population problem, there are definite advantages to spaying and neutering pediatric patients. The surgery is faster, easier, less expensive, and there are fewer perioperative complications, Additionally, the recovery and healing times are typically shorter in pediatric patients.

Concerns About Pediatric Spay/Neuter

Critics of pediatric spay/neuter techniques have raised concern that obesity will develop in the patients who undergo these procedures. A published study has indicated that dogs did not develop obesity when spayed/neutered either pre- or post-pubertal (Salmeri, Bloomberg, et al., 1991). Cats, however, can gain weight after gonadectomy is performed at both the traditional age and pre-pubertal (Stubbs et al., 1996). Obesity is a multifactorial problem, and an animal that will be obese after being spayed or neutered at 10 weeks may also be obese after being spayed/neutered at 6 months. Even intact animals can become obese if a healthy diet and exercise regimen is not followed.

Another concern about pediatric spay/neuter procedures is that these patients would have stunted growth and be of smaller than normal physical stature. This concern has been refuted by multiple scientific studies and stunted growth has not been demonstrated to occur in animals spayed/neutered pre-pubertal (Root-Kustritz, 1999). Ultimate skeletal size depends on normal physiologic function of physeal growth plates. Closure of the growth plates is dependent on gonadal hormones and may therefore be delayed in animals that are spayed/neutered at an early age. In contrast to intact dogs, puppies spayed or neutered at 7 weeks and male puppies neutered at 7 months had greater final radius and ulna lengths (Salmeri, Bloomberg, et al., 1991). Similar results were seen in cats, where cats spayed/neutered at 7 weeks and 7 months had delayed physeal closure compared to intact cats (Stubbs et al., 1996). The delayed closure of growth plates in cats did not lead to clinically significant differences in the final length of the long bones. Therefore, pediatric spay/neuter likely results in normal or greater stature (Stubbs et al., 1995). Some concern has been expressed that the delayed physeal closure will result in an increased incidence

of Salter type fractures, but this has not been demonstrated or found clinically in any setting.

Development of perivulvar dermatitis is another issue thought to be associated with ovariohysterectomy performed in the pediatric patient. At 15 months of age, puppies spayed at 7 weeks and 7 months had immature vulvar development compared with intact puppies, but no increased predisposition to perivulvar dermatitis was noted (Salmeri, Bloomberg, et al., 1991). Older female dogs can also undergo vulvar atrophy following ovariohysterectomy (Root-Kustritz, 1999). Perivulvar dermatitis can occur in any ovariohysterectomized dog, but is most often more a function of obesity rather than a function of a pediatric spay. If the female dog has urinary incontinence as well, the incidence of perivulvar dermatitis increases (Root-Kustritz, 1999).

Normal function of the urinary tract is another concern. Spayed female dogs may develop urinary incontinence secondary to a lack of circulating estrogen levels (Root-Kustritz, 1999). A long-term study with a four year follow-up indicated that dogs that undergo pediatric spay are not more likely to develop urinary incontinence than dogs that undergo ovariohysterectomy at the traditional age (Howe et al., 2001). Puppy vaginitis is another concern, but was not seen more in puppies neutered prepubertally as compared to those spayed at the traditional age in this study. Feline lower urinary tract disease has also been cited as a concern in pediatric neutering. Refuting studies have shown that neutered male cats do not have a higher incidence of feline lower urinary tract disease than intact male cats, and that the diameter of the penile urethra of castrated male cats is not smaller than that of intact male cats (Root-Kustritz, 1999). Concerns that cats would have a higher incidence of lower urinary tract disease and urethral obstruction were not supported by a long-term study with a follow-up period of 3 years (Howe et al., 2000).

The possibility that pediatric spay/neuter may lead to behavioral problems is another area of concern. However, pediatric spay/neuter has not been shown to produce negative behavioral effects. In one study, all neutered dogs, whether neutered at the age of 7 weeks or 7 months, were scored as more active than intact dogs (Salmeri, Bloomberg, et al., 1991). In that same study, the group of male dogs neutered at 7 weeks was also judged as more excitable, but this was not assessed as a negative behavior. In a study comparing kittens spayed and neutered at 7 weeks, 7 months, and intact kittens, all groups were similar with respect to behavior except that the cats in the intact group showed more intraspecies aggression and fewer displays of affection toward the observer (Stubbs et al., 1996). Concerns exist regarding performing these surgical procedures during the animal's fear imprinting period, which is 6 to 8 weeks in the dog and cat (Theran, 1993), but the significance of this is unknown (Root-Kustritz, 1999) and has not been seen to be detrimental in the clinical setting. To prevent distress during this period of the animal's life, the use of pre-anesthetic medication may be important to ensure a smooth and gentle anesthetic induction (Theran, 1993).

Some questions have also been raised regarding the failure of development of secondary sex characteristics in animals that undergo pediatric spay/neuter. Animals that are spayed/neutered, whether it is done at 7 weeks or 7 months, will have juvenile genitalia. However, there is no clinical significance to this. Some studies (Root-Kustritz, 1999) have shown that male cats may have a decrease in the inability to completely extrude the penis from the prepuce if they were neutered prepubertally, while another study did not document this difference (Stubbs, 1996). This does not appear to be clinically significant.

Infectious disease in dogs, most notably parvovirus, has been reported as a potential concern of spaying and neutering the pediatric shelter patient (Howe et al., 2001). In the shelter environment, young puppies are susceptible to parvovirus, regardless of being spayed or neutered. Therefore, pediatric spay/neuter is not contraindicated in this environment. Some shelter veterinarians will also work with client owned animals. In these animals, neutering is recommended after the last parvovirus vaccine is given, which is often administered by 16 weeks of age. In this way, client-owned animals can also be spayed/neutered younger than the traditional age while limiting their exposure to infectious diseases.

Long term studies and clinical experience have supported results of earlier short-term studies indicating the safety and efficacy of pediatric spay/neuter. Prepubertal ovariohysterectomy and castration has been performed safely in cats without causing physical or behavioral problems for at least

a 3-year follow-up period (Howe et al., 2001). Prepubertal ovariohysterectomy and castration has been performed safely in dogs without any demonstration of physical or behavioral problems for at least a 4-year follow-up period, with the exception of the possibility of an increased risk of infectious disease (Howe et al., 2000). In summary, performing pediatric spay/neuter is safe and helps shelters and humane societies ensure that every animal is spayed or neutered prior to being adopted from the shelter.

Techniques for Pediatric Spay/Neuter

There are many reported anesthetic protocols and surgical techniques for performing pediatric spay/neuter. This text will only describe the methods preferred by the author. The reader is advised to consult the references at the end of the chapter for other anesthetic and surgical protocols. Pediatric spay/neuter is well within the ability of any veterinarian who performs routine spay/neuter on young adult patients. The surgery is shorter and easier, has minimal hemorrhage, and the patients recover rapidly.

PREOPERATIVE EVALUATION

As for the young adult patient, a complete PE should be performed. If pre-surgical blood work is performed, it should consist of QATs, if possible. The PCV of a puppy or kitten is normally lower than that of the adult animal, ranging from 28-35 percent in the pediatric patient. In accordance with the recommendations of the Association of Feline Practitioners that all cats be tested, the FeLV/FIV test is suggested in the pediatric feline patient. (It must be remembered that there are limitations to the use of the test in a shelter environment, and no healthy animal should be euthanized based on the results of a single positive test. See chapters 8 and 16.) Once the puppy or kitten is assessed as healthy, an anesthetic protocol can be determined.

ANESTHETIC CONSIDERATIONS

Performing anesthesia on pediatric animals is safe and effective, as long as some of their special physiologic considerations are understood. Pediatric patients have immature hepatic enzyme systems, decreased protein binding of drugs, and a decreased glomerular filtration rate (Root-Kustritz, 1999). These factors can lead to altered drug metabolism and excretion, and anesthetic protocols should be chosen carefully. Due to decreased glycogen stores secondary to a small liver size and small skeletal muscle mass, the pediatric animal is prone to hypoglycemia, and steps should be made to maintain euglycemia (Root-Kustritz, 1999). Pediatric patients also are at risk for hypothermia during anesthesia, as they have a larger surface area to volume ratio, a lower percentage of body fat, and a decreased ability to shiver (Grandy and Dunlop, 1991). Further, these young animals have a higher rate of oxygen consumption than the adult animal and, subsequently, higher respiratory rates. The pediatric cardiovascular system is also different from that of the adult, as cardiac output is mostly dependent on heart rate, so bradycardia should be prevented (Grandy and Dunlop, 1991). Hypotension is also a greater problem in anesthetized pediatric patients and anesthetic agents that can cause hypotension should be avoided. Intravenous administration of fluid may help correct hypotension, but the cardiac ventricles in the pediatric patient are less compliant and therefore the puppy or kitten has a limited ability to increase cardiac output in response to volume loading (Grandy and Dunlop, 1991).

The following anesthetic guidelines should be followed to account for the concerns mentioned previously. Prior to anesthesia, the pediatric patient should be housed with littermates and kept in a quiet environment with minimal handling, because preanesthetic disposition has a significant effect on response to anesthetic drugs (Aronsohn and Faggella, 1993; Theran, 1993). Fasting should only be done for 3 to 4 hours in animals less than 10 weeks of age and no more than for 8 hours in older pediatric patients to aid in preventing hypoglycemia (Root-Kustritz, 1999). Hypothermia can be minimized by providing a supplemental heating source such as a circulating warm water blanket, by clipping the minimal amount of hair from the surgical site, and by using warmed surgical scrub (Root-Kustritz, 1999). The use of alcohol should be avoided in the surgical prep because of its cooling effects on the skin.

The use of acepromazine is not recommended as a pre-medication because of its hypotensive effects. Tranquilization is usually not needed as these animals are typically calm when kept in the quiet environment mentioned above. Barbiturates such as thiopental should also not be used because of the immature hepatorenal system in the pediatric patient. Isoflurane is the gas anesthetic agent of choice. If propofol is used, the patient should be pre-oxygenated.

The author uses the anesthetic protocols in Table 22.3 and Table 22.4. Induction via an IV injection of Ketamine: Valium is the author's preferred method (see Figure 22.1), but it may occasionally be necessary to mask patients down with isofluorane (Figure 22.2).

Intraoperative intravenous or subcutaneous fluid administration is seldom necessary because the pro-

Table 22.3. Pediatric Canine and Feline Ovariohysterectomy Anesthetic Protocols

Premedication	0.02 mg/kg atropine SQ	OR	0.01 mg/kg glycopyrrolate SQ
	0.20 mg/kg butorphanol SQ	OR	0.05 mg/kg oxymorphone SQ
Induction	ketamine/valium IV	OR	Propofol
	1.0ml/10 kg		6.0mg/kg IV
	1:1 ratio		Give slowly
Maintenance	Isoflurane		

Table 22.4. Pediatric Canine and Feline Castration

Premedication			
	0.02 mg/kg atropine SQ	OR	0.01 mg/kg glycopyrrolate SQ
	0.20 mg/kg butorphanol SQ	OR	0.05 mg/kg oxymorphone SQ
Induction			
	ketamine/valium IV	OR	propofol
	1.0 ml/10 kg		6.0mg/kg IV
	1:1 ratio		Give slowly

Mask with isofluorane if necessary.

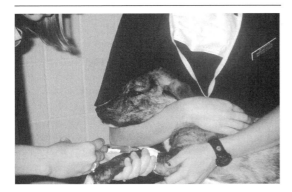

Figure 22.1. Four-month-old female pediatric patient receiving an IV injection. Photo credit to Lila Miller.

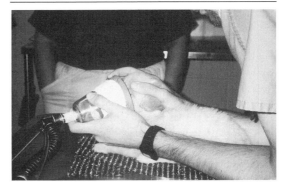

Figure 22.2. Two-month-old male puppy being masked down before intubation for castration. Photo credit to Lila Miller.

cedure is so short. A fluid administration rate of 10 ml/kg/hr IV can be used if needed. Intubation is best for pediatric spays, and a non-rebreathing circuit should be used for delivering anesthetic gas and oxygen for patients weighing less than 10 lbs. Postoperative analgesia is generally not necessary for either pediatric spays or castrations, as the procedures are so short; therefore, the preoperative analgesia is still effective. Recovery from anesthesia is rapid for both male and female puppies and kittens. All pediatric patients should be fed within the first hour from anesthesia recovery. If recovery is slow, and hypoglycemia is suspected or diagnosed, 50 percent dextrose or corn syrup can be given orally. Pediatric patients should be kept warm in recovery as well, and can be recovered on a circulating hot water blanket, with multiple towels to cover the patient.

SURGICAL CONSIDERATIONS

The surgical procedures of ovariohysterectomy and castration in the pediatric patient are faster and easier than in the adult. The basic principles of pediatric surgery are to minimize surgery time, perform careful tissue handling, and implement meticulous hemostasis. No significant changes in the surgical techniques used for the young adult animal are necessary, but a few adjustments must be made for the pediatric patient.

PEDIATRIC CANINE AND FELINE
OVARIOHYSTERECTOMY

The procedure of ovariohysterectomy is nearly identical for the puppy and kitten. The abdominal

incision is made caudal to the umbilicus in both species. This positioning of the incision is different in the canine pediatric patient when compared to the adult patient. The incision does not have to start at the umbilicus, because pediatric patients do not have tight suspensory ligaments and the ovaries are therefore easy to exteriorize. In the very young animal, visualization of the reproductive tract is very good, as there is minimal abdominal fat. These structures are fragile in the pediatric patient. Gentle tissue handling must be used and excessive traction avoided to prevent tearing. Also different than the adult patient, there is an increased amount of free abdominal fluid present. The uterus is very small, and the ovaries are large relative to the size of the uterus. See Figure 22.3. As in the adult, care must

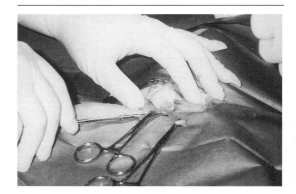

Figure 22.3. Ovariohysterectomy in a two-month-old pediatric patient. Photo credit to Lila Miller.

be taken to remove the entire ovary on each side. Double ligatures are not necessary on any pedicle, as the pedicles are small and contain very little fat. Most often, only a single clamp is placed on the pedicle, and the vessels are ligated below the clamp. Two clamps can be used in the larger pediatric patients if necessary, to create a crush mark for the placement of the suture ligature. Before the ovarian pedicle is cut proximal to the clamp, another clamp should be placed across the proper ligament to prevent back bleeding of the uterine artery. As with adult patients hemorrhage should be avoided. Meticulous hemostasis is even more important in the pediatric patient, as they have a smaller blood volume than the adult patient, so even minimal hemorrhage can be significant. Also, pediatric patients are prone to hypotension as previously discussed, so blood loss must be minimized. The same procedure is followed for the uterine pedicle. The use of absorbable suture (usually 3–0 PDS®) on all the pedicles and especially on the uterine pedicle is preferred. Hemoclips have been used successfully (Faggella and Aronsohn, 1994; Aronsohn and Faggella, 1993), but are unlikely to be used in the shelter due to their expense.

During closure of the abdomen, the linea can be apposed in a simple continuous suture pattern using absorbable suture material of 3–0 size if the animal is less than 10 lbs (2–0 can be used in a larger puppy). In the subcutaneous tissue, a few simple interrupted absorbable sutures of 3–0 or 4–0 size are placed to close dead space. Then, the skin is apposed with a continuous subcuticular pattern, using absorbable suture on a cutting needle. Polyglactin 910 (Vicryl®) in 4–0 size is excellent closing for this layer. Skin sutures should be avoided as the pups and kittens often chew these out. There have been reports that PDS® suture may be associated with calcinosis circumscripta in young dogs (Davidson et al., 1998; Kirby et al., 1989) and although a direct cause and effect relationship has not yet been proven, PDS® should be avoided in the subcutaneous and subcuticular layers to eliminate this potential complication.

PEDIATRIC CANINE AND FELINE CASTRATION

The pediatric castration in the dog and cat is similar to the procedure done for the adult cat castration. A scrotal approach and incision is used in both species. This is different than the prescrotal approach used for the adult dog castration. In the puppy, a sterile aseptic surgical procedure is performed. It is possible to prepare the surgical site with minimal restraint. One technique that works well is to administer the anesthetic pre-medication, and then wait 15–20 minutes before getting the puppy out of the cage. Usually the puppy is sedate enough at this stage to be supported on his back, while the scrotal area is clipped and scrubbed before giving the induction agent intravenously. Then, chlorhexidine soaked gauze is placed over the site, and the puppy is given the induction agent without changing the position of the puppy. Once the puppy is induced, the chlorhexidine soaked gauze is removed, a final chlorhexidine spray is applied, and the surgeon can immediately drape the patient and start the procedure. The puppy can be masked with isoflurane if the injectable anesthesia is not enough to provide a surgical plane of anesthesia. A puppy can be castrated from a single small scrotal incision. A closed castration is recommended. One testicle is held in place, and a 1-2 cm scrotal incision is made over the testicle. The testicle is removed from the incision, and the spermatic cord stripped with a gauze sponge as described for the adult dog. The pedicle is then ligated using the technique of tying the cord in a knot on itself. Instead of using mosquito hemostats, a larger clamp such as a Kelly or Crile clamp or a Carmalt can be used if necessary, because of the increased size of the cord. Sutures or hemoclips are other options for pedicle ligation. The second testicle is removed through the same scrotal incision (this incision does not have to be on the median raphe, it can be just to one side of the midline) and tied off in the same manner. No subcuticular or skin sutures are used, and the incision will heal by second intention. Tissue glue is not recommended or needed.

The pediatric feline castration is clean but not a sterile procedure, done in a similar manner to the adult cat. After the animal is induced, the fur is plucked from the scrotum, and chlorhexidine scrub is used to prepare the site. Each testicle is removed via a separate scrotal incision. The technique of tying the cord in a knot on itself can be safely and successfully used, although some surgeons do not recommend this because of the small size and fragility of the spermatic cord. As long as careful tissue handling is performed, there should be little problem. Suture or hemoclips may also be used alternatively. The scrotal incisions are not sutured.

The pediatric castration should not be performed unless both testicles can be palpated and removed. An animal is not truly considered cryptorchid until 6 months of age, but if only one testicle is palpated in the scrotum, castration should be delayed until the second testicle descends into the scrotum, or until 6 months of age, when a cryptorchid neuter can be done. Sometimes an inguinal or prescrotal testicle can be found, and can be easily pushed down into the scrotum for castration.

Postoperative Considerations

Postoperative complications are rare in pediatric spay/neuter. As previously stated, the pediatric patient should be fed a small meal within the first hour after anesthetic recovery (Faggella and Aronsohn, 1993). Animals with prolonged recovery may be hypoglycemic, and can be given 50 percent dextrose or corn syrup orally in the early postoperative period (Root-Kustritz, 1999). Generally, puppies and kittens can be fed within 20–30 minutes of extubation.

Animals can be released on the same day that surgery is performed. Pediatric patients not only recover quickly from anesthesia, but they heal rapidly as well. Tattooing of pediatric patients is especially important. When animals are spayed/neutered as puppies and kittens, scars may be difficult to see or feel later in life. Similar tattooing techniques as described previously for the routine spay/neuter patients can be applied.

Conclusions About Pediatric Spay/Neuter

Puppies and kittens can safely and effectively be spayed and neutered as long as special anesthetic and surgical considerations are followed. Both short term and long term studies have not shown any detrimental effects to the patients. Pediatric spay/neuter is essential for shelters in an effort to make sure all animals are spayed/neutered before leaving the shelter. These procedures are also safe for client-owned animals, and will help prevent accidental breeding in this population as well. Pediatric spaying and neutering of dogs and cats is safe, effective, easy to perform, and is a highly recommended way to aid in controlling the animal overpopulation problem.

COMPLEX SPAY/NEUTER

Estrus

In shelter animal medicine and surgery, some patients will require complex gonadectomy. The most common example of this is spaying dogs and cats while they are in estrus. In the shelter setting, it is strongly recommended that animals in heat be spayed. The actual surgical procedure for ovariohysterectomy of a dog or cat that is in estrus is similar to the routine ovariohysterectomy. The difference is that during estrus, the uterine and ovarian vessels are enlarged, and the tissue is fragile. For this reason, some surgeons prefer not to spay dogs at this time. For surgeons who feel this way, it is important that extra care be taken when examining female dogs to check for a bloody vaginal discharge, enlarged vulva or other signs of estrus. Even so, some dogs in estrus will slip through undetected until the surgery has begun and the uterus and ovaries are exposed. Meticulous tissue handling should be used, and each pedicle should be double ligated in the dog. The cervix in the dog also becomes greatly enlarged and thickened, and the ligatures of the uterine pedicle cannot usually be placed across the cervix, but need to be placed where the cervix starts to taper towards the uterus. In this case, larger suture size must be used. Depending on the size of the pedicle, either 2–0 or 0 suture material is appropriate. Transfixation ligatures are rarely necessary, unless the uterine arteries and size of the cervix indicate the need for this technique.

In the cat, one ligature is still adequate for the ovarian pedicles, but the uterine pedicle should be double ligated. The uterus of a cat in estrus is turgid and friable, and care should be taken not to put excessive traction on the uterine pedicle. Clamps for the triple clamp technique should be large enough to surround the pedicle without tearing the uterine or cervical tissue. Because of the potential for intraoperative blood loss, intravenous fluid should be readily available for administration during the ovariohysterectomy of a dog in estrus. If intravenous fluid is not available, subcutaneous fluid can be used. Cats spayed while they are in heat rarely require fluid administration unless they are debilitated with a chronic URI or poor nutrition.

Pregnant Animals

Pregnant animals are also often spayed in the shelter situation. Dogs and cats can safely undergo ovariohysterectomies up until the time they start parturition. The surgical procedure is based on the routine ovariohysterectomy with minor changes in procedure to compensate for the gravid uterus and enlarged vessels. In both the dog and cat, ovarian pedicles should be double ligated. In the late-term pregnant dog, two transfixation ligatures should be used on the uterine pedicle. In the late term pregnant cat, the uterine pedicle does not usually need transfixation ligatures because it still tapers in at the cervix and can be adequately ligated with two circumferential ligatures. Depending on the size of the ovarian and uterine pedicles in pregnant dogs and cats either 2-0 or 0 absorbable suture material should be used. In the case of late term pregnancies in both dogs and cats, intravenous or subcutaneous fluids should be administered.

The length of gestation and the length of the surgery will determine whether or not the individual fetuses need to be humanely euthanitized. Most of the time the embryos or fetuses will expire as the uterus is being removed because their blood supply is cut off once all pedicles are clamped. In late term pregnancy, some fetuses will not die from hypoxia, and should be humanely euthanitized with euthanasia solution.

Pyometra

Pyometra is encountered in shelter animals and usually requires emergency surgery. Pyometra is more common in dogs, but can happen in cats as well. An animal with closed cervix pyometra is often more clinically debilitated than an animal with an open cervix pyometra. Both should be stabilized and surgery performed as soon as possible. Intravenous fluid and antibiotics are administered (such as Cefazolin at 22mg/kg IV) prior to the spay surgery. The patient's medical condition should be carefully assessed to determine how long it is necessary to continue the intravenous fluids whenever possible. The intravenous antibiotics should be repeated in two hours and then every six to eight hours when possible. The patient should be started on oral antibiotics the day following surgery. If intravenous antibiotics are not available, subcutaneous or intramuscular antibiotics can be used, and followed with a course of oral antibiotics. The ovariohysterectomy for a dog or cat with pyometra is the same as a routine ovariohysterectomy with minor changes. It may be necessary to make a longer abdominal incision to safely remove uterus if it is greatly enlarged. Special care must be taken not to puncture or rupture a friable uterus, as leakage of the uterine contents into the abdomen can result in peritonitis. Lap sponges should be available in case this occurs. The ovarian and uterine pedicles should be double lig-

ated. The uterine pedicle should not be transfixed. If necessary the uterine arteries can be individually ligated, but this is rarely the case. Two circumferential ligatures are usually adequate for the uterine pedicle. Depending on the size of the pedicles, 2-0 or 0 suture material should be used. If possible, the abdomen should be lavaged with warm saline at the end of the procedure.

Mammary Gland Tumors

Older intact female dogs should be carefully palpated for the presence of mammary gland tumors. If identified, these tumors should be removed at the time of the spay. If possible, chest radiographs to check for metastasis are recommended. If chest radiographs are not possible, the excisional biopsy of the mammary gland tumor should still be performed, as mammary gland tumors in the dog are usually benign and slow to metastasize. Histopathology should be performed on the excised tissues and new owners should be told to monitor the animal for tumor regrowth in the mammary glands. Often, removal of mammary neoplasia in dogs results in a favorable prognosis. In cats, mammary tumors are often malignant, and a full metastasis work-up should be performed prior to surgery and potential adoption.

Uncertain Sexual Status

On occasion, an abdominal exploratory may be indicated when it is uncertain if the animal has been previously spayed or when signs of estrus are present despite evidence of prior abdominal surgery. All three pedicles must be identified in animals that are explored. Using the mesocolon and mesoduodenum to retract abdominal structures aids in visualizing and identifying of the ovarian pedicles. The uterine pedicle can be identified by retracting the urinary bladder and looking between the bladder and the colon. Remaining ovarian and uterine tissue should be resected if encountered. The exploratory is best performed when the animal is showing signs of estrus, as this is when remnant ovarian tissue is easiest to identify.

Cryptorchidism

Cryptorchidism will also be found in shelter animals. The testicles descend in most cats by 6-8 weeks of age, but it can be much later in dogs. Usually just one testicle is retained, but bilateral cryptorchidism has been reported. If a stray dog or cat has no palpable testicles, it is more likely that the animal is neutered rather than having bilateral cryptorchidism. Dogs are more commonly cryptorchid than cats. In the dog, the retained testicle is more commonly the right testicle, and the most common location for this testicle is in the abdomen, near the bladder and the inguinal ring. In the cat the right testicle is also the more commonly retained testicle, but unlike the dog, the cryptorchid testicle in the cat is usually in the inguinal region, and sometimes is found in the inguinal ring itself.

If an inguinal testicle is not palpated, a caudal ventral midline approach should be made to the abdomen. The testicle can usually be located next to the urinary bladder on the right side of the caudal abdomen. If the surgeon has trouble locating the testicle, the ductus deferens can be traced from its prostatic termination to the testicle (Boothe, 1993). If an inguinal testicle is clearly palpated, a skin incision should be made in the inguinal area over the testicle. In some cases, the testicle will be in the prescrotal position, and can be pushed into the scrotum and removed in a routine manner. In either species, the retained testicle must be identified and removed to prevent the future development of testicular cancer and also to prevent objectionable male behavior.

Scrotal Ablation

Occasionally, a scrotal ablation will have to be performed at the time of castration. The indication for scrotal ablation is trauma or irritation to the skin of the scrotum. In the shelter situation, dogs can develop chemical burns on the scrotum if cleaning agents are not completely rinsed when the cages are cleaned. The fragile scrotal skin can be easily traumatized or injured. A large pendulous scrotum of an older male dog may also need to be ablated, but even pendulous scrotums will become smaller over time, making scrotal ablation rarely needed for this reason. The scrotal ablation is done using a curvilinear skin incision around the scrotum. Adequate skin should be left for closure. The testicles are removed through this incision in a routine manner. The traumatized scrotum may be more vascular than normal, and care should be taken to provide good hemostasis and to obliterate tissue dead space.

Postoperative Considerations

The basic post-op considerations and instructions used for routine spay/neuter should be applied to

the complex spay/neuter. The care and discharge instructions should be modified accordingly for each situation. A patient with pyometra should be sent home with a course of oral antibiotics. Cryptorchid dogs that undergo abdominal procedures should be kept quiet for 10-14 days instead of 7 days. Fluid and nutritional supportive care should be given as indicated, and the patient should be adopted when recovered and stable.

RABBIT SPAY/NEUTER

Species other than dogs and cats will present to animal shelters. The types of species will depend on the area of the shelter. In rural areas rabbits are commonly surrendered at local shelters. Rabbits, like cats and dogs, should be spayed/neutered prior to being adopted from the shelter. Anesthetic and surgical techniques differ for this species from those of cats and dogs. Rabbits have different behavioral characteristics and different anatomy and physiology. As a submissive prey species, rabbits are easily stressed with pain or fear and can become anorectic following a surgical procedure if frightened or in pain. Therefore, rabbits must be kept in a quiet, comfortable environment and be given adequate pain medication. Proper handling and restraint are also important for the rabbit as vertebral fractures can occur with struggling. Rabbits are hindgut fermenters, and therefore if antibiotics are indicated, the choice of antibiotic should minimize disturbance of the gastrointestinal microflora. Rabbits commonly have an upper respiratory infection, referred to as "snuffles", caused by the *Pasteurella sp*. Rabbits with a known history of this infection should be started on antibiotics prior to surgery because the infection can be dormant and become clinical if the rabbit is stressed. A fluoroquinolone is a good choice for "snuffles" in rabbits, and can be given subcutaneously before surgery. Finally, food and water should be withheld for no more than 1 to 2 hours during the preoperative period (Jenkins, 2000).

Preoperative Evaluation and Anesthetic Considerations

A complete PE (with or without QATs as discussed previously) should be performed prior to creating an anesthetic plan. Normal values for rabbits are shown in Table 22.5 (Carpenter et al., 2001).

The rabbit should be weighed accurately and drug calculations performed carefully. Parenteral

Table 22.5. Normal Rabbit Values

Heart rate: 130–325 beats/minute	TS 5.4–7.5
Respiratory rate: 30–60 breaths/minute	Glucose 75–150
Temperature 101.3–104.0°F	PCV 30–50
	BUN 15–30

Table 22.6. Anesthetic Protocols for Rabbits

Premedication	0.50mg/kg butorphanol SQ and
	0.50mg/kg midazolam SQ and
	0.01mg/kg glycopyrrolate SQ
Induction	Isoflurane in oxygen via facemask using a nonrebreathing system
Maintenance	Isoflurane inhalant anesthesia
Postoperative Analgesia	0.20mg/kg butorphanol SQ q4hrs

fluids are usually not needed for the spay/neuter of healthy rabbits. If intravenous fluid administration is indicated by conditions such as debilitation or pregnancy, a cephalic or ear vein catheter can be placed. Fluid with balanced electrolytes is given at a rate of 10ml/kg/hr IV (Cantwell, 2001). Subcutaneous administration of fluid can be done if necessary, but intravenous administration is preferred. An anesthetic protocol for healthy adult rabbits is recommended in Table 22.6.

Pre-oxygenation of the patient should be performed prior to anesthetic induction (Cantwell, 2001). Rabbits can be difficult to intubate because their mouths cannot be opened widely, so anesthesia can be induced and maintained via a facemask. For patient monitoring, a Doppler blood pressure monitor can be used with the probe positioned on the foot, on the ear, or on the ventral thorax directly over the heart. If the probe is placed on the thorax, care must be taken not to restrict ventilation. An ECG is another option for patient monitoring during anesthesia. Body temperature can be rapidly lost in small patients because of their large surface area to body weight ratio (Cantwell, 2001). Body temperature must be maintained during the entire perioperative period. Circulating hot water blankets are useful. Hot water bottles can be used as long as their temperature is closely monitored. Patient monitoring is challenging because of the small size of the patient and potential lack of accessibility during the procedure. Monitoring during anesthesia is often minimal and done by visually observing the animal (Cantwell, 2001). Rabbit's corneas are traumatized easily, so protective eye lubricant should be used.

Patient Preparation

Rabbits have thin skin and dense fur, both of which make clipping the hair difficult without cutting the skin. Care should be taken to minimize nicks and cuts by using a No. 40 clipper blade and keeping the skin spread flat while slowly clipping the fur (Jenkins, 2000). A minimal amount of fur should be clipped from the surgical field, and warm surgical scrub should be used.

Surgical Techniques

As in the surgical sterilization procedures for dogs and cats, there are several accepted techniques. Meticulous tissue handling should be performed, as rabbits are prone to forming adhesions following abdominal surgery. The following techniques are those employed by the author.

OVARIOHYSTERECTOMY IN THE RABBIT

The rabbit uterus is bicornate, each uterine horn has a separate cervix, and there is no uterine body (Jenkins, 2000). The mesometrium of a healthy rabbit is a major fat storage site in this species (Jenkins, 2000). The uterine vessels are not closely adjacent to the uterus as in the dog and cat; instead they are in the mesometrium and must be ligated separately from the uterine pedicle. The oviduct and infundibulum are much larger than those of the dog and cat. Care must be taken to remove the entire oviduct (Jenkins, 2000). Rabbit tissue is more fragile than that of cats and dogs, therefore delicate tissue handling techniques must be employed.

Adhesive drapes can be useful to keep the thick hair from entering the surgical field and prevent the need for towel clamps in thin rabbit skin. The ventral midline skin incision is centered midway between the umbilicus and the pelvis. The linea is entered via a small stab incision. Care is made to control entry into the abdominal cavity as the linea is thin, and abdominal organs are positioned close to the linea (Jenkins, 2000). The uterus is easy to identify cranial to the bladder, and is easily removed from the abdomen. Clamps are used on each pedicle, but the flashing technique is not necessary. The mesometrial fat is more friable than in the cat or dog, and the suture easily cuts through the fat and encircles the vessels. A single clamp is placed below the oviduct and infundibulum, which is also below the small ovary embedded in the mesovarium, and a single ligature is placed below this clamp. If the pedicle is large, two clamps can be used to create a crush mark in which to place the suture. Typically, 2–0 or 3–0 suture size is needed and absorbable suture such as PDS® is used. Rabbits can have a caseous, suppurative response to foreign material, and a proclivity to form adhesions. Therefore, an absorbable, monofilament, less reactive suture absorbed by hydrolytic degradation is recommended (Jenkins, 2000). After ligating the ovarian pedicle, the mesometrium on that side is also ligated. The uterine vessels are well within the mesometrium, and therefore the mesometrium itself is ligated separately from the uterine pedicle. After a second "window" is created in the mesometrium between the uterine vessel and the uterus, a single clamp is placed in the mesometrium, and a suture is placed below that clamp. A clamp is placed above the first clamp to prevent back bleeding as the mesometrium is cut proximal to the first clamp. The procedure is repeated on the opposite side for the other ovary and mesometrium. Then the uterine pedicle is removed. Two clamps are placed in the distal vaginal vault, which is very large in a rabbit, just proximal to the double cervices. The ligature is placed in the crush mark of the most distal clamp, and the pedicle is transected proximal to the remaining clamp, with removal of the cervices with the uterus. The linea is closed in a simple continuous pattern using 3-0 PDS®. One or two subcutaneous simple-interrupted sutures are placed with 4-0 absorbable suture material, followed by a subcuticular pattern with 4–0 absorbable suture material. Skin sutures should be avoided as the rabbit will most likely remove them.

CASTRATION IN THE RABBIT

A closed castration technique is recommended in the rabbit. Rabbits have testes that can move freely through open inguinal canals (Jenkins, 2000). During surgical preparation of the patient, care must be taken not to push the testicles back into the abdomen. An adhesive drape is again recommended to keep the incision area clean, especially as this area is close to the animal's scent glands. An incision is made over each scrotum. The testicle in the rabbit is closely associated with the scrotum, and gentle blunt dissection with a Metzenbaum scissor should be done to remove the testicle from the scrotal incision. The spermatic cord is gently stripped with gauze in a similar manner to a cat castration. Once the cord is extended and isolated, a triple clamp and double ligature technique should be done. In small male rabbits, a double clamp and single ligature can be used. Typically, 2–0 or 3–0 PDS® is used for this procedure. Once the cord is ligated and transected, it is replaced through the scrotal incision. The procedure is repeated on the opposite testicle. No sutures are necessary in the incisions; healing is achieved by second intention. The technique of tying the cord in an overhand knot with a mosquito hemostat has not been successful in the rabbit, as the tissue is not pliable enough and will tear when this is attempted.

POSTOPERATIVE CONSIDERATIONS

Both the male and female rabbits should be kept quiet for the week following surgery. Close monitoring should be performed to ensure the rabbit is not in pain and resumes eating right away. Pain medication as previously described can be used when necessary to make the rabbit comfortable. Antibiotics are indicated if the stress of anesthesia and surgery cause clinical signs of a respiratory infection. Most rabbits do well and can be adopted from the shelter a day or two after surgery.

SURGICAL COMPLICATIONS

All surgical procedures have the potential for complications. Adherence to good surgical principles, including aseptic techniques, short surgery times, gentle tissue handling, careful vessel ligation and suture placement, and adequate exposure will greatly reduce the number of complications.

The most frequently encountered post-operative problem following ovariohysterectomy is hemorrhage. Bleeding is typically a result of an error in pedicle ligation. This can be a concern with overweight, older dogs. Affected animals show typical signs of blood loss including tachycardia, pale mucous membranes, lethargy, weak pulse, and, in some instances, hemorrhage from the incision. Laboratory valves may not change initially, but eventually will show a decrease in PCV and TS.

Conservative therapy consisting of patient monitoring, intravenous fluids, and application of an external abdominal bandage should be considered. If the PCV decreases consistently or the tachycardia persists, an abdominal exploratory should be considered.

The original incision should be reopened and extended both craniad and caudad to permit necessary exposure. The right ovarian pedicle can be quickly identified by using the mesoduodenum to gain exposure to the pedicle, as previously described in this chapter. The left ovarian pedicle can be found by using the mesocolon in the same manner. The uterine pedicle can be located by retracing the urinary bladder. Once the bleeding pedicle is identified, care should be used to exteriorize only the tissue of the pedicle that includes the bleeding vessel. Once the bleeding pedicle has been identified and exteriorized, a new ligature should be applied before gently releasing the pedicle back into the abdomen. The ureter is close to these tissues and should be avoided. Adequate exposure will help prevent inadvertent ureter ligation.

Dehiscence of the abdominal incision can be avoided by using good surgical technique and by taking deep bites in the linea alba. Careful selection of the appropriate suture material to close the linea alba is important, as it is the layer that has the holding strength. Muscle, subcutaneous tissue and skin have no holding strength. If the skin has been irritated when the hair was clipped, or the animal is seen licking at the incision, an Elizabethan collar should be used to prevent further damage to the incision site. It is particularly important that shelter animals be monitored carefully to ensure that they can eat and drink while wearing the collar.

Recurrent estrus can result from incomplete removal of the left and/or right ovaries. The right ovary is more likely to be incompletely resected, as the right ovarian pedicle is farther cranial and usually harder to exteriorize than the left ovary. When signs of estrus recur, an abdominal exploratory is indicated to remove any remaining ovarian tissue. This is best done when the dog or cat is showing signs of heat, as this is the easiest time to find the ovarian tissue remnant. Recurring estrus can be prevented by good surgical technique, and making sure the entire left and right ovaries are removed during the initial ovariohysterectomy.

Stump pyometra is another surgical complication that can occur when the ovaries and the uterus are not completely resected. Clinical signs are similar to any pyometra including lethargy, vomiting, polyuria, polydipsia, fever, and anorexia. The development of pyometra is usually secondary to the influence of progesterone from residual ovarian tissue on the endometrium. Stump pyometra can be prevented by complete removal of both ovaries, uterine horns, and uterine body (Kyles et al., 1996). The treatment for stump pyometra is to stabilize the patient with IV fluid and broad-spectrum antibiotics followed by surgical excision of the infected tissue.

Inadvertent ligation of a ureter can be another complication of an ovariohysterectomy. In the cat, the distal portion of a ureter is more commonly traumatized because the uterine pedicle and the urinary bladder are closely associated. In the dog, the proximal portion of the ureter is more at risk. Adequate surgical exposure and clear identification of the ovarian and uterine pedicles help to prevent this complication. The urinary bladder should be expressed prior to surgery to help prevent iatrogenic damage to the urogenital tract. The options for surgical treatment for inadvertent ligation of a ureter include ureteral resection and anastomosis, ureteroneocystostomy or complete nephrectomy (Kyles et al., 1996). These cases are usually best referred to a specialist. Simple removal of the ligature will not be effective.

Vaginal bleeding can follow ovariohysterectomy. A small amount of blood-tinged, mucoid vaginal discharge can occur normally for a few days post ovariohysterectomy. Significant frank blood from the vagina several days to weeks after surgery is not normal. Contamination at the time of surgery can result in a localized infection and erosion of a uterine vessel (Kyles et al., 1996). An exploratory laparotomy should be done to re-ligate the uterine pedicle (Kyles et al., 1996). Some authors suggest that single ligatures around the uterine pedicle are more likely to lead to erosion of the uterine vessels (Stone et al., 1993); however, single ligatures are routinely used around uterine pedicles without incidence.

Uterine stump granuloma and inflammation can be caused by poor aseptic technique, using ligatures of non-absorbable braided suture material, or excessive remaining devitalized uterine tissue (Stone et al., 1993). Ovarian stump granulomas can also occur for similar reasons (Kyles et al., 1993). The stump granulomas can be treated with antibiotics and surgical excision.

Urinary incontinence caused by adhesions or granulomas of the uterine pedicle that interfere with the urinary bladder can occur following ovariohysterectomy (Stone et al., 1993). However, the most common cause of urinary incontinence following ovariohysterectomy is urethral sphincter laxity, which is most likely secondary to a lack of circulating estrogen levels. The mechanism for sphincter incompetence is poorly understood (Kyles et al., 1996). This type of incontinence is not caused by surgical technique, and can be treated with medication such as phenylpropanolamine to increase the competence of the urethral sphincter.

Finally, obesity has been reported as a complication following ovariohysterectomy. However, obesity is a multifactorial problem, and can be managed with proper diet and exercise.

The most common complications following castration are scrotal swelling and bruising (Boothe, 1993). Scrotal swelling can be minimized by using atraumatic surgical technique and proper hemostasis (Kyles et al., 1996). Closed castration techniques usually lead to less scrotal swelling than open castration techniques. Closing the subcutaneous layer of the incision will also reduce potential swelling. In older male dogs the spermatic fascia may contain more vasculature, and if post-operative swelling is expected, an ice pack can be placed on the scrotum for the first 10-15 minutes after surgery. If scrotal swelling develops, it is usually transitory but the patient should have strict rest. Antibiotics are only used if indicated. If the patient licks the incision, a protective Elizabethan collar should be put in place. In the shelter situation, patients should be monitored to make sure they can still eat and drink while wearing this collar.

Hemorrhage can occur following castration, usually from fascial tissues. However, significant bleeding can result from a bleeding pedicle. If the patient is tachycardic and deteriorating, the bleeding pedicle should be identified and re-ligated. This may require an abdominal incision and exploratory to locate the bleeding pedicle. Infection can also occur if proper aseptic technique is not followed. Treatment consists of local drainage and systemic antibiotics (Kyles et al., 1996).

Complications of cryptorchid castration are similar to those described above. Prostatectomy secondary to a cryptorchid castration has been reported. This can be prevented by using adequate surgical exposure and proper identification of the cryptorchid testicle.

MOBILE UNIT CONSIDERATIONS

Mobile units that provide veterinary care are becoming more popular, especially where humane society organizations are trying to provide wide-reaching spay/neuter services. The advantage of using a mobile unit is the ability to bring spay/neuter services to rural areas where stray animals, farm dogs and cats, and cat colonies are often problems. The standard of care provided on a mobile unit should be equal to that provided at the shelter, or in a traditional hospital. All of the guidelines, techniques, and protocols described in this chapter also apply to spay/neuter surgery in a mobile unit. The size of the mobile unit will determine the number of animals that can be done per day. In addition to the recovery and holding cages inside the unit, additional cages can be set up outside under the cover of an attachable awning if weather permits. Another option is for the mobile clinic to use the parking lot of a facility that can be rented to set up more recovery cages, such as a 4-H, or shelter facility. Animals that have been spayed or neutered can be discharged the same day, once they have recovered from anesthesia. The surgery schedule should be planned for more extensive procedures to be done earlier in the day, in order to allow adequate recovery for the animals undergoing these longer procedures. For example, the dog spays should go first, followed by cat spays, dog castrations, and cat castrations. Pediatric spay/neuter surgeries can also be performed following the same guidelines and recommendations previously described in this chapter. Because they recover more quickly from anesthesia, they may be done toward the latter part of the day, keeping in mind that they should not be fasted for more than 4 hours.

Arrangements should be made for follow up or emergency care with the shelter veterinarians or local veterinarians in case of complications. Surgical and anesthetic records should be kept as with any other patient. Patient selection is critical, as patients cannot be kept overnight in case of problems. Careful consideration should be given before performing surgery on very old or obese animals who might take longer to wake up from anesthesia, and therefore should be done first, early in the day. Mobile units can be effectively used to deliver spay/neuter services.

SPAY DAY PROJECTS

Special spay/neuter projects can be organized to enhance spay/neuter efforts already done through the shelter. The scale of these projects will be determined by the availability of both veterinary and non-veterinary volunteers. If there is a College of Veterinary Medicine close to the shelter, a good working relationship can often be established which will benefit both the veterinary students and the shelter animals. For example, at Cornell University College of Veterinary Medicine, a program called the Cornell Animal Sterilization Assistance Program (C-ASAP) was developed. Through this program, veterinarians, technicians and students worked with the shelters of several local counties to perform monthly spay/neuter clinics. Each month the program rotated counties, and the local SPCA from the given county scheduled the animals for the clinic. Eligible animals included feral cats, stray cats, barn cats, farm dogs, dogs and cats belonging to people with low income, and shelter animals. Each month, the clinic was either a dog or cat clinic depending on what the county needed most at that time. The local shelter was responsible for scheduling the animals, assuring that the animals were eligible for the free clinic, providing volunteers to help at admission, discharge, and recovery, supplying clean towels and clean holding cages, and supplying food for all volunteers. The C-ASAP program was responsible for organizing veterinarians (both volunteers from the Cornell University College of Veterinary Medicine and private practitioners), technicians (from both the veterinary college and from private practice), and student volunteers. The C-ASAP program provided all of the equipment to perform the physical examinations, rabies vaccines, spay/neuter anesthesia and surgery, ear notching, and post-operative monitoring. All volunteers worked together to set up and clean up the facility. The clinics were held at the Cornell College of Veterinary Medicine. On average, 100 cats or 50 dogs were spayed/neutered in one day. For projects similar to this one, the number of surgeries per day is determined by the number of available veterinarians and technicians, and by the number of surgical packs available. Grants can be written to secure funding for the clinics, as well as letters soliciting funds from large pharmaceutical or pet food companies.

The anesthetic protocol used for injectable anesthesia for cats is found in Table 22.7. The protocols for dogs are the same as those listed in the routine spay/neuter section of this chapter, as inhalant anesthesia is recommended for dogs.

Animal shelters not in close proximity to veterinary colleges can also set up special Spay Day Projects by utilizing the local veterinarians in their area. The scale of the project may be smaller, but the support for animal shelters will still be advanced.

REFERENCES

Aronsohn, Michael G., and Alicia M. Faggella. 1993. Surgical techniques for neutering 6- to 14-week-old kittens. *Journal of the American Veterinary Medical Association* 202(1): 53–55.

Boothe, Harry W. 1993. Testes and epididymides. In *Textbook of Small Animal Surgery*, 2nd ed., vol. 2, edited by Douglas Slatter. Philadelphia, PA: W.B. Saunders Company, 1325–1336.

Cantwell, Shauna L. 2001. Ferret, rabbit, and rodent anesthesia. *Veterinary Clinics of North America: Exotic Animal Practice* 4(1): 169–191.

Carpenter, James W., Mashima, Ted Y., and Rupiper, David J. 2001. *Exotic Animal Formulary*, 2nd ed. Philadelphia, PA: W.B. Saunders Company, 320–321.

Davidson, Ellen B., Schulz, Kurt S., Wisner, Erik R., and Schwartz, Julie A. 1998. Calcinosis circumscripta of the thoracic wall in a German shepherd dog. *Journal of the American Animal Hospital Association* 34:153–156.

Table 22.7. Injectable Anesthesia for Spaying/Neutering Cats

0.02mg/kg atropine SQ
and
1.0ml/10kg of ketamine/xylazine mixture
(ket/xyl mixture: 2 mls of 100mg/ml Xylazine into bottle [10 ml] of Ketamine)

Faggella, Alicia M., and Aronsohn, Michael G. 1993. Anesthetic techniques for neutering 6- to 14-week-old kittens. *Journal of the American Veterinary Medical Association* 202(1): 56–62.

Faggella, Alicia M., and Aronsohn, Michael G. 1994. Evaluation of anesthetic protocols for neutering 6- to 14-week-old pups. *Journal of the American Veterinary Medical Association* 205(2): 308–314.

Fossum, Theresa Welch (ed.). 2002. *Small Animal Surgery*, 2nd ed. St. Louis: Mosby, Inc.

Grandy, Jacqueline L., and Dunlop, Colin I. 1991. Anesthesia of pups and kittens. *Journal of the American Veterinary Medical Association* 198(7): 1244–1249.

Howe, Lisa M., Slater, Margaret R., Boothe, Harry W., Hobson, H. Phil, Fossum, Theresa W., Spann, Angela C., and Wilkie, W. Scott. 2000. Long-term outcome of gonadectomy performed at an early age or traditional age in cats. *Journal of the American Veterinary Medical Association* 217(11): 1661–1665.

Howe, Lisa M., Slater, Margaret R., Boothe, Harry W., Hobson, H. Phil, Holcom, Jennifer L., and Spann, Angela C. 2001. Long-term outcome of gonadectomy performed at an early age or traditional age in dogs. *Journal of the American Veterinary Medical Association* 218(2): 217–221.

Jenkins, Jeffrey R. 2000. Surgical sterilization in small mammals: Spay and castration. *Veterinary Clinics of North America: Exotic Animal Practice* 3(3): 617–627.

Kirby, Barbara M., Knoll, Joyce S., Manley, Paul A., and Miller, Lisa M. 1989. Calcinosis circumscripta associated with polydioxanone suture in two young dogs. *Veterinary Surgery* 18(3): 216–220.

Kyles, Andrew E., Aronsohn, Michael, and Stone, Elizabeth Arnold. 1996. Urogenital surgery. In *Complications in Small Animal Surgery: Diagnosis, Management, Prevention*, edited by Alan J. Lipowitz, Dennis D. Caywood, Charles D. Newton, and Anthony Schwartz. Baltimore, MD: Williams & Wilkins, 496–511.

Lofstedt, Robert M., and Vanleeuwen, John A. 2002. Evaluation of a commercially available luteinizing hormone test for its ability to distinguish between ovariectomized and sexually intact bitches. *Journal of the American Veterinary Medical Association* 220(9): 1331–5.

National Pet Alliance. 1993. S*urvey Report: Santa Clara County's Pet Population*. Available at www.fanciers.com/npa/santaclara.html. Accessed July 11, 2002.

Patronek, Gary J., and Rowan, Andrew N. 1995. Determining dog and cat numbers and population dynamics. *Anthrozoös* 8(4): 199–205.

Root-Kustritz, Margaret V. 1999. Early spay-neuter in the dog and cat. *Veterinary Clinics of North America: Small Animal Practice* 29(4): 935–943.

Salmeri, Katharine R., Bloomberg, Mark S., Scruggs, Sherry L., and Shille, Victor. 1991. Gonadectomy in immature dogs: Effects on skeletal, physical, and behavioral development. *Journal of the American Veterinary Medical Association* 198(7): 1193–1203.

Salmeri, Katharine R., Olson, Patricia N., and Bloomberg, Mark S. 1991. Elective gonadectomy in dogs: A review. *Journal of the American Veterinary Medical Association* 198(7): 1183–1192.

Stone, Elizabeth Arnold, Cantrell, Charles G., and Sharp, Nicholaus J. H. 1993. Ovary and Uterus. In *Textbook of Small Animal Surgery*, 2nd ed., vol. 2, edited by Douglas Slatter. Philadelphia, PA: W.B. Saunders Company, 1293–1308.

Stubbs, W. Preston, Bloomberg, Mark S., Scruggs, Sherry L., Shille, Victor M., and Lane, Thomas J. 1996. Effects of prepuberal gonadectomy on physical and behavioral development in cats. *Journal of the American Veterinary Medical Association* 209(11): 1864–1871.

Stubbs, W. Preston, Salmeri, Katharine R., and Bloomberg, Mark S. 1995. Early neutering of the dog and cat. In *Kirk's Current Veterinary Therapy XII*, edited by John D. Bonagura. Philadelphia, PA: W. B. Saunders Company, 1037–1040.

Theran, Peter. 1993. Early-age neutering of dogs and cats. *Journal of the American Veterinary Medical Association* 202(6):914–917.

23
Feral Cat Management

Julie Levy

INTRODUCTION

The domestic cat has increased in popularity as a household pet in recent decades, surpassing the dog to become America's most numerous pet. However, despite the enhanced status of cats as human companions, millions of unwanted cats are admitted to animal shelters each year, and the vast majority of these are euthanized because homes cannot be found. Debate about the true impact of free-roaming cats on the environment, on feline health, and as a reservoir of both feline and zoonotic diseases is ongoing, often emotional, and fueled largely by a lack of sound scientific data on which to form credible conclusions. It is also difficult to separate the impacts of owned cats from those of unowned ones. Of primary concern is the welfare of the cats themselves.

Definitions of various cat populations defy universal acceptance, focusing variably on ownership status, lifestyle, and level of socialization. Cats may be defined as "free-roaming" if they are not confined to a yard or house, a definition based on confinement of the animal, rather than ownership or socialization status. Strictly speaking, feral cats are defined as untamed and evasive. They are either born in the wild and lack socialization or are returned to the wild and become untrusting of humans. Although feral kittens can be tamed into acceptable pets if captured at a very young age, enormous effort is often required to tame older feral cats. Stray cats may be defined as homeless cats that remain socialized and friendly toward humans. The lines between loosely owned outdoor cats, stray cats, and feral cats are often blurred. Owned outdoor cats that wander or become lost may become stray cats. Stray cats that have lived in the wild for

an extended time may become feral. Thus, individual cats may be included in different categories at various stages of their lives. For the purposes of this discussion, the term "feral cat" will be used to denote any unconfined, unowned cat, regardless of its socialization status.

CHARACTERISTICS OF FERAL CATS

Interactions with Humans

The number of feral cats in the United States is unknown, but is suspected to rival that of pet cats (73 million in 2000) and to contribute substantially to cat overpopulation (Levy et al. 2003b). Feeding of homeless cats is a common activity practiced by both pet owners and those without pets of their own. In the suburban southern community of Alachua County, Florida, 1 in 8 households acknowledged feeding an average of 3.6 cats they did not own, or approximately 36,000 feral cats (Levy et al. 2003b). County residents also owned an estimated 45,000 pet cats. This indicates that feral cats comprise at least 46 percent of the local cat population, but does not include feral cats that are not fed by residents. These findings are similar to studies performed in Santa Clara County, where 10 percent of households fed an average of 3.4 cats each (Johnson et al., 1994), in San Diego County, where 8.9 percent of households fed an average of 2.6 cats each (Johnson et al., 2002), and in Massachusetts, where 7.9 percent of households fed an average of 3.7 cats each (Manning and Rowan, 1992). These studies also concluded that feral cats comprised at least 36–41 percent of the total cat population. Feeding of feral cats is a widespread activity that crosses many socioeconomic strata. Almost half of cat feeders do not own pets, implying that attempts to involve cat feeders in control strategies should extend beyond the pet-owning public typically served by veterinarians, animal control agencies, and animal welfare organizations (Levy et al. 2003b). For purposes of estimating the size of a community's feral cat population, it is reasonable to estimate 0.5 cats per household. County household data are available at www.census.gov.

Although provision of food for unowned cats is a common activity, few cat feeders take further action to have the cats sterilized. Sterilization of pet cats owned by feeders of feral cats was common (90.1 percent) in Alachua County, indicating high compliance with veterinary and animal welfare recommendations for neutering of pets not intended for breeding (Levy et al., 2003b). This is consistent with previous reports that 82–91 percent of pet cats were sterilized, although not always before producing a litter of kittens (Johnson et al. 1994, Johnson et al. accessed 2002, Manning et al. 1992). Given the high rate of sterilization among pet cats, unowned cats may represent the single most important source of cat overpopulation.

In Alachua County, most (61 percent) cat colonies consist of a small group of 3–10 cats, and are usually described as a female with kittens and an occasional wandering male (Centonze and Levy 2002). This is consistent with results of a national survey (Clifton 1992) that reported a mean colony size of 4–12 cats, and a Hawaii study (Zasloff and Hart 1998), which reported that 65 percent of the colonies consisted of 1–10 cats. In most cases, cat colonies are located on private property, particularly at the feeder's residence or workplace. Although large cat colonies on public property, such as parks and institutions, often comprise the most visible and controversial cat populations, it appears that the vast majority of feral cats associated with humans live in small groups near their feeder's homes.

Caretakers report a strong bond with the feral cats they care for, even though they do not consider these cats to be their pets (Centonze and Levy 2002). This is different than the traditional image of the human-animal bond, as many of the cats cannot be touched or held and do not live indoors with the caretaker. Nevertheless, the cooperation of caretakers is imperative if cat population control programs are to be effective.

Physical Characteristics

Data collected from feral cats undergoing sterilization provide information about their physical condition, but might not accurately reflect all groups of feral cats, such as young kittens or cats not associated with caretakers. In Florida and California, approximately 57 percent of more than 20,000 cats admitted for sterilization were females (Scott, Levy, Crawford 2002). This contrasts with findings of feral cats in the field. Cats caught on Marion Island (n = 857) near South Africa were equally distributed between males and females, and those caught on Macquarie Island (n = 246) near Australia included more males than females (56 vs. 44 percent, respectively). Cats in central Rome (n = 301) included fewer males than females (44 vs. 56 percent, respectively), whereas 55 percent of feral cats on an urban Florida university campus (n = 155) were males (Scott, Levy, Crawford 2002). The frequent finding of equal to higher numbers of males in populations observed in the field versus the predominance of females referred for neutering suggests that females may be easier to capture or that caretakers may preferentially select females for neutering.

In Florida, the first pregnancies of the breeding season appear in January (Scott, Levy, Crawford 2002). This is consistent with the first occurrence of the minimum day length required to induce estrus in cats at this latitude. Later in the spring, almost half of the female cats evaluated are pregnant. A second smaller peak in the summer suggests second pregnancies during the same breeding season for some females, or first pregnancies for late-born kittens from the previous year. A similar pattern was observed in cats in southern California (Figure 23.1). On the basis of a mean gestation period of 65 days and the pregnancy rate of 19 percent found in Florida cats, each adult female cat is projected to produce a mean of 1.1 litters per year. This estimate assumes that pregnant cats are no more or less likely to be trapped than nonpregnant cats, and is consistent with previous findings that feral cats can produce multiple litters during each breeding season. Depending on geographic location, annual pregnancy rates in feral cats have been reported to range from 0.98 to 2.0 and to produce 4 to 5 fetuses per litter (Scott, Levy, Crawford 2002). Pyometra is diagnosed in 0.4 percent of female cats presented for spaying in Florida (Scott, Levy, Crawford 2002).

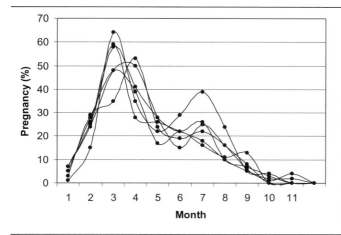

Figure 23.1. Pregnancy is highly seasonal in cats and is correlated with day length. Data collected from more than 12,000 feral cats presented for sterilization in San Diego, California, during 1995—2000 demonstrate synchronization of pregnancies early each year, followed by a second, smaller peak of pregnancies in the summer.

The frequency (2 percent) and clinical findings of cryptorchid cats are similar to those reported for pet cats undergoing castration (Scott, Levy, Crawford 2002). Most cats have unilaterally retained testicles that occur with equal frequency on the left and right sides, and equally in inguinal and abdominal locations. Bilaterally retained testicles were more likely to be found in the abdomen than in the inguinal region. The scrotum of bilaterally cryptorchid males may resemble that of castrated cats, so procedures should be established for confirmation of the true reproductive status, such as examination for penile barbs or exploratory laparotomy. Although retained testicles are usually infertile, they are still capable of secreting testosterone, which contributes to objectionable territorial behavior, aggression, and urine odor. Thus, it is inappropriate to leave retained testicles in place.

A study of adult feral cats found that the cats were generally lean, but not emaciated at the time of sterilization (Scott, Levy, Gorman, Newell 2002). One year later cats were significantly fatter than they were at the time of neutering, indicating that feral cats, like their tame counterparts experience enhanced fat accumulation following neutering. Only 0.4 percent of feral cats presented for sterilization were euthanatized for humane reasons in Florida (Scott, Levy, Crawford 2002).

Infectious Diseases

The threat that feral cats pose to both feline and human public health is a topic of much debate. Rabies is of particular concern to public health officials. Although the dog is the primary vector of rabies world-wide, widespread vaccination of dogs and reduction of the stray dog population since the 1940s have greatly reduced the number of canine cases in the United States. Today, more than 90 percent of rabies cases occur in wildlife, primarily in raccoons, skunks, coyotes, foxes, and bats. Since 1981, rabid cats have outnumbered rabid dogs in the United States, with 249 feline cases reported in 2000 (Jenkins et al., 2002). Although dogs account for three-quarters of reported animal bites to humans, rabies post-exposure prophylaxis is more commonly administered as a result of cat bites (Moore et al., 2000, Hensley 1998). Most cat bites are reported to be provoked from stray cats, with adult women more likely to be bitten than children and men (Hensley 1998, Patrick and O'Rourke 1998, Wright 1990). This is in contrast to dog bites, which are more likely to occur when unprovoked pet dogs bite children. This suggests that human exposure to rabies can be limited by reducing and immunizing the stray cat population and by avoiding direct handling of stray cats. Despite continued concern about the role of cats in human rabies exposure, no human cases have been associated with cats since 1975 in the United States (Veterinary Public Health Notes 1975). Even when rabies is not involved, cat bite wounds are often serious. They most frequently occur on the hands, and risk of infection is highest when puncture wounds occur (Dire 1992). Public health recommendations include immediate cleansing of the wound, medical attention, and prophylactic treatment with amoxicillin-clavulanate.

The American Association of Feline Practitioners (AAFP) recommends FeLV and FIV testing of all cats, but that a positive test result should not be used as the sole criteria for euthanasia (Levy et al. 2001). The AAFP further recommends that all positive screening test results undergo confirmation. Large epidemiological studies indicate that FeLV and FIV are present in approximately 4 percent of feral cats, which is not substantially different that the infection rate reported for pet cats (Lee et al. 2002). As expected, male cats are four times more likely to carry FIV than female cats, due to biting as the primary mode of transmission. FeLV, which is most commonly spread from infected queens to their kittens, occurs at approximately the same rate in males and females. Testing recommendations for pet cats are difficult to apply to feral cats for several reasons. Of primary importance is the cost-benefit ratio of testing a large number of cats in order to detect the small percentage of seroreactors. Resources for treating feral cats are limited, and many programs have decided to focus on mass sterilization as the primary goal. Because the accuracy of positive test results decreases when prevalence is low, as is the case for FeLV and FIV, more than 50 percent of positive test results in feral cats would be expected to be false-positives. Confirmatory testing is often impractical, since recommended confirmatory tests require use of a reference laboratory and it may be several days before results are available. The recent advent of FIV vaccination has added an additional complication to testing, due to false-positive results in the currently available tests for FIV antibodies induced by the vaccine. For these reasons, and because sterilization reduces the behaviors most associated with viral transmission, most large sterilization programs for feral cats do not routinely test for FeLV and FIV.

Parasitism is the most common infectious problem of feral cats. In Florida during the summer, 92 percent of cats presented for sterilization were infested with fleas, and 37 percent had ear mites (Akucewuch et al. 2002). A study of 80 feral cats in California revealed that 54 percent carried intestinal ascarids, compared with only 4 percent of 70 pet cats (Levy et al. 1999). Tapeworms and coccidia were found in 26 percent and 13 percent of feral cats, compared with 4 percent and 0 percent of pet cats, respectively. The same study identified a higher rate of seropositivity for *Toxoplasma gondii*

in feral cats (20 percent) compared with pet cats (3 percent), which may represent exposure via hunting in feral cats. Interestingly, feral cats were significantly less likely to have antibodies against coronavirus, the source of feline infectious peritonitis, (4 percent) than were pet cats (59 percent). Coronavirus is primarily transmitted via a fecal-oral route. The behavior of feral cats of burying their feces may reduce the risk of transmission compared to pet cats sharing a litter box in a multi-cat household. FeLV (0–1 percent) and FIV (3–5 percent) were uncommon in both groups of cats. *Bartonella henselae* (34 percent) was the most common infection identified in 553 feral cats in Florida (Luria et al. 2003). Two organisms formerly grouped under the classification of *Haemobartonella felis*, *Mycoplasma hemominutum* and *M. hemofelis*, were present in 12 percent and 8 percent of cats, respectively. Other infections included coronavirus (18 percent), *T. gondii* (10 percent), FIV (5 percent), and FeLV (3 percent). Male cats were significantly more likely to be infected with FIV and mycoplasmas than were female cats. Similar infection prevalences have been reported for pet pats.

Control of Feral Cats

The control of feral cats has emerged as one of the most controversial issues in animal control and welfare. Historically, feral cats have been largely ignored by both governmental and humane agencies. Specific cats that are declared a nuisance may be removed, but few agencies have comprehensive programs designed to decrease the number of feral cats in their communities.

Although the humane movement has yet to establish minimum acceptable standards of living for pet cats or cats in shelters, some believe that feral lifestyle is too fraught with risk and discomfort to be acceptable. Others believe that the quality of life of feral cats should be judged no differently than those of other species existing in a "wild" state. The growth of the "No Kill" movement has caused some animal welfare leaders to re-examine traditional beliefs that killing large numbers of healthy animals to prevent *potential* suffering or as a method of population control can be compatible with the values of a humane society.

Feral cats have been extirpated from several small uninhabited islands as a result of decades of intensive control measures including poisoning, hunting, trapping, and introduction of infectious feline diseases (Levy et al. 2003b). Despite the success of eradication campaigns on geographically isolated islands, logistic barriers and opposition from resident citizens would likely make application of such lethal strategies in populated mainland areas unfeasible. Cat control programs in populated areas must incorporate safety considerations for nontarget animals and humans, be affordable for participating municipal agencies or charitable organizations, include plans to curtail continuous cat immigration and reproduction, and be aesthetically acceptable to the public. Clearly, any realistic plan to control feral cats must recognize the magnitude of the feral cat population, the need to engage in continuous control efforts, and the significance of the public's affection for feral cats. The most successful examples of enduring community-wide animal control have incorporated high-profile nonlethal feral cat control programs into integrated plans to reduce animal overpopulation.

TRAP-NEUTER-RETURN

A growing grass roots movement has promoted control of feral cat populations through sterilization. Trap-Neuter-Return (TNR) seeks to sterilize large numbers of cats and return them to their colonies. Some programs are quite elaborate, including extensive veterinary care, colony registration, monitoring, and adoption of tame cats, whereas others focus solely on sterilization. Whereas most programs are small, privately run volunteer groups dependent on donations for operating costs, a few are operated with public funds by municipal animal control agencies on the premise that sterilization is ultimately more efficient and cost-effective than extermination. The Animal Services Department of Orange County, Florida, reported decreased complaints about cats, decreased cat admissions to the shelter, and decreased operating costs following development of a free sterilization program for feral cats funded by the county. Alley Cat Allies, a national organization advocating TNR for control of feral cats, counts more than 8,000 programs and individuals in its database. Accompanying growing awareness of feral cats is increased controversy about their impacts, welfare, and place in society.

Increasingly, veterinarians are asked to participate in nonlethal control of feral cats, frequently by providing free and low-cost veterinary services. The concept of TNR as a method for cat population control is described by the American Veterinary Medical Association (AVMA 1996), and endorsed by many humane organizations (Centonze and Levy 2002). More than 1,000 members of the California Veterinary Medical Association sterilized approximately 168,000 cats between July 1999 and May 2002 in a $12 million project funded by Maddie's Fund.

A TNR program at a Florida university was highly successful in reducing the feral cat population during an 11–year period (Levy et al. 2003a). Before the initiation of the program, feral cats were considered by campus authorities to constitute a nuisance. Periodic trap and removal efforts were made when excessive cat numbers prompted complaints about on-site noise and odor, but employees and students openly violated policies against feeding the cats and interfered with trapping efforts by university officials during removal campaigns. The TNR program instituted in 1991 incorporated neutering, euthanasia of sick animals, and adoption of socialized cats and feral cats that eventually became tame enough to become pets. With the exception of 1 male cat, all original study cats were neutered between 1991 and 1995, and no kittens were known to be born on campus after 1995. As a result of deaths, disappearances, and adoptions, the known maximum cat population (68 cats in 1996) gradually decreased to 23 cats, the lowest number for the entire recording period. A majority of the cats were found as kittens, and most of those were feral cats born on site. Adoptions accounted for 47 percent of the decrease in the cat population, even among feral cats. It has been reported that feral cats become less aggressive toward each other and more friendly toward their feeders following neutering, and this may have encouraged adoption of previously feral cats. Cats were often transferred to private homes only after several years of feral status. Despite widespread concern about the welfare of feral cats, many of the animals survived for a number of years. Most cats (83 percent) still remaining on site at the end of the observation period had been present for > 6 years. This compares favorably with the mean lifespan of 7.1 years reported for pet cats, particularly as almost half of the cats were first observed as adults of unknown age (Nassar 1984). Most cats (61 percent) that disappeared, died, or were euthanatized for debilitating conditions had been present for at least 3 years. In general, the cats were in adequate physical condition and only 4 percent were euthanatized for humane reasons. Newly arriving sexually intact socialized cats, apparently abandoned, periodically joined the colonies; their presence could have undermined the control program had they not been promptly captured and neutered. Migration of cats between colonies was common, and resident cats did not always prevent the immigration of new members.

These results indicate that long-term reduction of feral cat numbers is feasible by TNR. However, the extended survival of feral cats following sterilization indicates that natural attrition would be expected to result in a slow rate of population decline. Adoption of socialized cats accelerates population reduction. These results also refuted an oft-cited claim that an established colony of cats will defend its territory and prevent the immigration of new arrivals. Immigration or abandonment of new cats in sterilized colonies may be a frequent event, and feral cats do not appear to have sufficient territorial activity to prevent new arrivals from permanently joining colonies. These new arrivals could substantially limit the success of TNR if an ongoing surveillance and maintenance program is not effective.

Failures of TNR to control cat colonies also exist. A 1–year study of TNR programs in 2 southern Florida parks revealed that the presence of well-fed cat colonies encouraged illegal abandonment of additional cats (Castillo 2001). While the original population of 81 cats declined 20 percent during 1 year, the arrival of new cats prevented reduction of the colonies and 88 cats were present at the end of the study. Minimal territorial activity by the cats was observed and aggressive encounters between cats were usually limited to enforcement of feeding order.

Veterinary Procedures for Feral Cats

There are many approaches to delivering veterinary care to feral cats. This discussion focuses on techniques for large-scale sterilization with the goal of reducing the feral cat population (Fig. 23.2).

SAFETY FIRST

One of the dominant concerns about working with feral cats is safety. Feral cats have an uncanny abil-

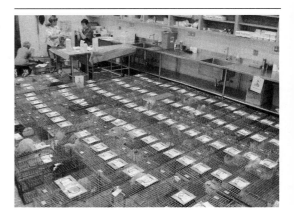

Figure 23.2. Some large-scale clinics specializing in feral cat surgery are capable of sterilizing more than 150 cats in a single day. Photo by Julie Levy.

ity to escape during handling, and can inflict serious injury during recapture attempts. A loose cat can thoroughly damage a clinic in its frantic efforts to escape. It is recommended that anyone who works with stray animals, including feral cats, receive prophylactic rabies immunizations. Gloves should be worn at all times to reduce exposure to body secretions from cats. The most common health risks for individuals working with feral cats are bites and scratches. Even semi-tame cats may bite defensively if they are startled, as in the attempt to place a cat in a carrier for transportation. For these reasons, it is imperative that safe cat handling techniques be developed and enforced. Not only does this guarantee the safety of personnel, but it also prevents the unfortunate situation in which public health officials require the euthanasia of biting cats for rabies examination. The safest method for handling feral cats is to admit them only in wire humane traps. The traps are escape-proof, and anesthetic is easily injected through the wire mesh. The traps should not be opened until the cats are recumbent. At the completion of surgery, the cats are returned to their traps before awakening. With this system, cats are never handled awake. Handling systems that involve transferring cats from one container to another or opening a container to restrain a cat only invite escapes and injuries. If cats must be housed for several days, they may be released into a secure cage. Special feral cat boxes can be purchased which have "portholes" that may be latched closed after the cat has hidden in the box. These boxes allow safe movement of the cat to other areas. If a feral cat escapes from its cage, the safest method of capture is with a net on a pole. Attempts to catch a feral cat by hand, or with a blanket are extremely dangerous for personnel. Rabies poles are very dangerous for cats and only serve to cause more panic.

ADMISSIONS

Caretakers of feral cats should be informed in advance where to obtain a trap and how to safely capture and transport a cat. It is advisable to accept all cats, even friendly ones, in traps exclusively, because confinement and transport can frighten any cat, leading to escape or injury. Release forms should be used to assure that the cats are believed to be unowned and that the caretakers are aware of the risks of anesthesia and surgery in cats of unknown health conditions. An agreement should be reached at the time of admission about how to proceed if unanticipated health problems are detected once the cat is anesthetized. Caretakers should be advised not to leave food in the traps, but it must be recognized that food is required to bait the traps, and that some cats may have eaten within a few hours of surgery. A practical system for identifying the cats is to place 2 identical numbered stickers on the trap at admission. One of the stickers is placed on the cat when it is removed from the trap. This allows cats to be matched back to their traps following surgery.

ANESTHESIA

Injectable anesthetics are preferred for feral cats because they can be administered to cats still in their traps and there are no waste gases (Figure 23.3). A cocktail of tiletamine and zolazepam (Telazol) (1 500-mg vial) reconstituted with ketamine (100 mg/ml, 4 ml) and large animal xylazine (100 mg/ml, 1 ml) instead of water is just one of many that have been used in feral cats (Williams et al. 2002). "TKX" has several advantages for large-scale cat anesthesia. A small injection volume (0.25 ml for average adult cats, 0.15 ml for kittens) can be administered "intracat" through the wire of the trap, eliminating the need to handle conscious cats. Time to recumbency is generally 3–5 minutes, and vomiting is uncommon. General anesthesia is adequate for abdominal surgery. The xylazine component of

the cocktail is reversed with yohimbine administered intravenously at the same volume as the TKX. The major disadvantages of TKX include hypothermia, prolonged recovery time, and poor postoperative analgesia. Cats generally return to sternal position within two hours, but frequently are not fully recovered from anesthesia until the following morning. Faster recovery times may be achieved by using a lower dose of TKX for immobilization and then using gas anesthesia by mask to obtain a surgical plane. TKX has been used on more than 15,000 feral cats with a remarkable safety record. Considering that these are often unthrifty, parasitized animals of unknown background, highly stressed, and unsuited for preanesthetic examination, the observed rate of 3 deaths per 1,000 cats compares favorably with reports of anesthetic death rates of pet animals in private practices (Williams et al. 2002). A cocktail of medetomidine, ketamine, and buprenorphine has also been used in feral cats (Cistola et al. 2002). "MKB" offers the advantages of improved blood pressure and oxygenation compared to TKX, rapid recovery following reversal with atipamezole, and good analgesia, but some cats experience rough recoveries and marked hyperthermia with this combination.

SURGICAL PREPARATION AND SURGERY

Upon recumbency, cats are removed from their traps and identified. If antibiotics are used, they

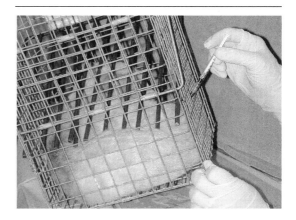

Figure 23.3. Commercially available humane traps accompanied by a metal comb facilitate safe hands-free restraint of feral cats during injection of anesthetic drugs. Photo by Karen Scott.

should be administered prior to surgery for the optimal prophylactic effect. The eyes should be lubricated with plain ophthalmic ointment. Cats have been reported to suffer anaphylaxis associated with ophthalmic ointment containing antibiotic as an uncommon idiosyncratic reaction. Since anaphylaxis would be difficult to recognize and treat in anesthetized cats, it is recommended to avoid antibiotic-containing eye lubricants. Tying females to "spay boards" facilitates preparation and moving of cats between stations (Fig. 23.4). Routine preparation for aseptic surgery is performed. Ideally, the pace of the clinic should be controlled so that there is always a cat ready to be spayed, and veterinarians never have a lull in surgery.

Cats may be spayed by either a midline or left flank approach (Dorn 1975, Krzaczynski 1974). The flank approach offers slightly increased surgical efficiency and reduced risk of evisceration should an incisional complication occur following release. It is ideal for lactating cats, but cats with

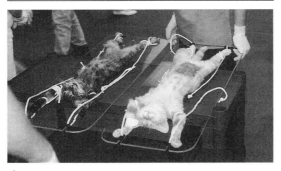

A

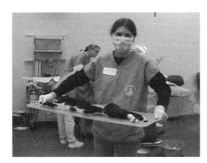

B

Figure 23.4. Cats can be tied to Plexiglas spay boards for (a) surgical preparation and (b) movement around the clinic. Photos by Julie Levy

advanced pregnancy are more easily spayed via a midline approach. The flank incision can also be monitored easily by the caretaker following release to the colony. Flank incisions have been described from both the left and right approaches. An area approximately 8 cm square is aseptically prepared, using the greater trochanter as the landmark for the dorsocaudal corner of the square. Following draping of the area, the surgical site is identified lying approximately midway between the dorsum and the ventrum and approximately 3–4 cm cranial to the greater trochanter. A 1–2 cm skin incision is made either vertically or horizontally. The body wall is tented with forceps and entered using blunt dissection with scissors or forceps. Sharp dissection of the muscle wall should be minimized to avoid bleeding. The spleen may underlie the incision on the left side, and care should be taken to avoid laceration of the organ when the abdomen is entered from the left. The uterine horn lies just beneath the body wall and is retrieved with a spay hook. From this point forward, the spay is performed similarly to the midline approach. If the incision is properly placed, it is possible to remove both ovaries and as much of the body of the uterus as with the standard procedure. The body wall is closed with a single absorbable suture, as is the subcutaneous tissue. In feral cats, the skin is best closed with a buried suture. The major disadvantage of the flank spay is the inability to explore the abdomen in the event of intra-operative complications or to confirm previous ovariohysterectomy.

Because of the sheer number of feral cats and the high euthanasia rate of cats at shelters, it is difficult to rationalize not sterilizing pregnant cats. Releasing a pregnant cat or confining it in a foster home to have kittens only adds unnecessarily to cat overpopulation and suffering. Once trapped, many cats are extremely difficult to trap a second time. For this reason, lactating cats should also be sterilized when trapped and returned to their colonies as quickly as possible. Because cats will be released to their colony soon after surgery, incisions should be as small as possible and skin sutures should not be used.

EAR TIPPING
Feral cats may interact with a variety of caretakers, veterinarians, and animal control personnel during

their lives, so it is important that a universal method of identifying sterilized animals is adhered to. Ear tipping is the only fully reliable method and is recognized internationally (Cuffe et al. 1983). With this procedure, a hemostat is clamped across the distal centimeter of the pinna, and the tip is removed by cutting straight across with scissors (Figure 23.5a). Using scissors results in less hemorrhage than use of a surgical blade. If the ear is tipped before surgery, the hemostat may be left in place until the cat is returned to its trap. Tipping is preferred over notching, because notches may be confused with irregular pinnae caused by fight wounds, frostbite, and ear mites, whereas the tipped ear creates an unmistakable characteristic silhouette (Figure 23.5b). Tattoos and microchips may be used to identify individual cats, but this must be done in addition to ear tipping, because neither method can be read without handling the cat. If tattoos are used, it is important to sterilize the equipment between each cat to avoid the inadvertent transmission of blood-borne infectious diseases. This can be problematic in large-scale operations that are processing many cats at a time. Several types of tags and buttons designed for use in the ears of mice and rabbits have been used in cats, but these are associated with a high rate of loss and infection. Some caretakers and veterinarians have objected to ear tipping as an unnecessary and disfiguring practice. Ear tipping is performed painlessly under anesthesia and is much less invasive than the accompanying sterilization procedure. It allows the identification of sterilized cats in the field so that they do not face the trauma of unnecessary transport and surgery again. It is the standard of practice accepted by animal welfare organizations and feral cat advocacy groups in the best interest of the cats. The presence of a tipped ear does not appear to affect the adoptability of cats in the future.

VACCINATION

The AAFP recommends providing core vaccines (rabies, panleukopenia, herpesvirus, and calicivirus) to all cats (2000 Report). Non-core vaccines, such as FeLV, are recommended only for cats at risk of exposure. Since feral cats are exposed to a variety of other cats with unknown FeLV or FIV status, they would be considered at risk. However, these guidelines were developed for pet cats, not feral cats, so decisions about which

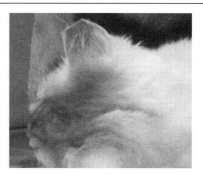

A

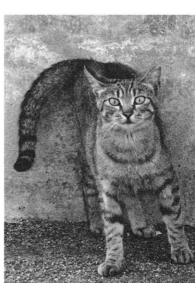

B

Figure 23.5. The internationally recognized identification mark of a sterilized feral cat is "ear tipping," in which the distal centimeter of an ear tip is removed while the cat is under anesthesia for sterilization (a). Cutting the tip straight across leaves a characteristic silhouette recognizable without having to handle the cat (b). Photos by Julie Levy (a) and John Newton (b).

vaccines to use and which cats to vaccinate should be made based on perceived cost-benefit ratios and program resources. Rabies occurs in wildlife throughout the continental United States, and feral cats may form an interface between wildlife reservoirs and humans. For this reason, rabies vaccines should be administered to all cats undergoing TNR.

Not only does this provide increased safety for the cats and their caretakers, but it also makes TNR programs more acceptable to public health officials. A rabies product with three years duration of immunity should be used, even if it is the cat's first vaccine. Many cats are difficult to retrap for booster vaccines, but a single rabies vaccine has been shown to protect cats against virulent challenge for more than three years (Soulebot et al. 1981). Some programs admit only cats three months of age and older so that the rabies vaccine is recognized by local authorities as valid. The canary pox-vectored rabies vaccine is approved for kittens as young as 8 weeks of age, but is currently labeled only for one year duration of immunity. Kittens should be vaccinated against panleukopenia, herpesvirus, and calicivirus, because of their high susceptibility and the life-threatening effects of infection in young cats. Feral cats are frequently unavailable for booster vaccines, but still benefit from a single immunization. Live-virus vaccines should be used because they confer greater immunity following a single immunization than inactivated vaccines. Whereas panleukopenia, herpesvirus, and calicivirus vaccines would also ideally be administered to adult cats, mature cats are more naturally resistant than kittens to these viruses. Program resources may dictate whether all adult cats are vaccinated against these infections. The effect of a single FeLV vaccine is unknown, and most TNR programs do not include FeLV vaccines in their programs. The first vaccine against FIV was introduced in 2002. This vaccine causes false positive FIV test results in vaccinated cats, so its use has complicated FIV testing in cats from unknown backgrounds. Similar to FeLV vaccines, the benefit of a single immunization against FIV is unknown, and this vaccine is not widely used in feral cats.

PARASITE CONTROL

Feral cats are frequently returned to their original multi-cat environment, and the advantage of a single treatment for parasites at the time of sterilization is uncertain. Parasiticides can be mixed in food for ongoing treatment of parasitism, but this is usually not practical on a large scale. Kittens are most severely affected by parasites and are likely to benefit more from treatment than are adult cats. Depopulating parasites in kittens, even transiently, may

reduce the physical stress cats experience following weaning. Adult cats are more naturally resistant to parasitism and are less likely to develop severe complications such as flea anemia, diarrhea, and weight loss. Because feral cats should only be handled after they are anesthetized, treatment of parasites at the time of sterilization is limited to topical and injectable products. Imidacloprid, selamectin, and fipronil may be applied topically for flea control. Heavily infested cats can be sprayed with a cat-safe flea spray prior to surgery. Ivermectin (0.2 mg/kg SC) may decrease roundworms, hookworms, and ear mites. Selamectin can be applied topically to anesthetized cats and is effective against roundworms, hookworms, ear mites, and fleas. Selamectin should be avoided in young debilitated kittens, as neurological side effects have been reported in this group. Single-dose ear mite treatments, such as otic milbemycin and extended action ivermectin, are ideal for feral cats that cannot be treated following recovery from anesthesia.

RECOVERY

If xylazine has been used for anesthesia, recovery can be hastened by administration of yohimbine. Prior to awakening, cats should be returned to their traps to recover in a quiet warm place and monitored until fully awake. All cats should be left in their traps overnight following surgery. If fully recovered the next day, they may be released to their colony. Although feral cats presented for sterilization are homeless, their general body condition is usually adequate, and the euthanasia rate for humane reasons is quite low. Fatal complications associated with surgery occur in feral cats at approximately the same rate as reported for pet cats undergoing anesthesia and surgery. Even though complications are uncommon, procedures should be in place for the management of surgical and medical emergencies. It is also helpful for veterinarians and cat caretakers to establish in advance protocols for unexpected findings such as cryptorchidism, pyometra, illnesses, and injuries.

CONCLUSION

Populations of feral cats exist throughout the world and are a large source of cat overpopulation. Concern about their impacts on the environment and public health, as well as consideration of the welfare of the cats themselves, has led to various efforts to reduce their numbers. TNR has emerged as one viable alternative for nonlethal cat control capable of reducing cat populations over the long term.

REFERENCES

Akucewuch, L.H., Philman, K., et al. 2002. Prevalence of ectoparasites in a population of feral cats from north central Florida during the summer. *Veterinary Parasitology* 109:129–139.

AVMA. 1996. Position statement on abandoned and feral cats. *Journal of the American Veterinary Medical Association* 209:1042–1043.

Castillo, D. 2001. *Population estimates and behavioral analyses of managed cat (*Felis catus*) colonies located in Miami-Dade County, Florida, parks.* MS thesis, Department of Environmental Studies, Florida International University, Miami, FL.

Centonze, L.A., Levy, J.K. 2002. Characteristics of feral cat colonies and their caretakers. *Journal of the American Veterinary Medical Association* 220:1627–1633.

Cistola, A.M., Golder, F.J., et al. 2002. Comparison of two injectable anesthetic regimes in feral cats at a large volume spay clinic. *Proceedings of the American College of Veterinary Anesthesiologists, 27th Annual Meeting*, Orlando, FL, October 10–1.

Clifton, M. 1992. Seeking the truth about feral cats and the people who help them. *Animal People* November: 1, 7–10.

Cuffe, D.J., Eachus, J.E., et al. 1983 Ear-tipping for identification of neutered feral cats. *Veterinary Record*; 112:129.

Dire, D.J. 1992. Cat bite wounds: risk factors for infection. *Ann Emerg Med*; 21:1008.

Dorn, A.S. 1975. Ovariohysterectomy by the flank approach. *Veterinary Medicine/Small Animal Clinician*; 70:569–573.

Hensley, J.A. 1998. Potential rabies exposures in a Virginia County. *Public Health Report*; 113: 258–262.

Jenkins, S.R., Auslander, M., et al. 2002. Compendium of animal rabies prevention and control. *J Am Vet Med Association*; 221:44–8.

Johnson, K.J., Lewellen, L., et al. 1994. National Pet Alliance survey report on Santa Clara County's pet population. *Cat Fanciers' Almanac*; (Jan): 71–77.

Johnson, K., and Lewellen, L. 2002. San Diego County survey and analysis of the pet population. Available at www.fanciers.com/npa. Accessed April 16.

Krzaczynski, J. 1974. The flank approach to feline ovariohysterectomy (an alternate technique). *Veterinary Medicine/Small Animal Clinician*; 69:572–574.

Lee, I.T., Levy, J.K., Gorman, S.P., Crawford, P.C., and Slater, M.R. 2002. Prevalence of feline leukemia virus infection and serum antibodies against feline immunodeficiency virus in unowned free-roaming cats. *J Am Vet Med Association*; 220:620–622.

Levy, J.K., Gale, D.W., et al. 2003a. Long-term control of a free-roaming cat population by trap-neuter-return and adoption. *J Am Vet Med Assoc*; 222:42–46.

Levy, J.K., James, K.M., et al. 1999. Infectious diseases of feral cats in central California. *Proc 80th Annual Meeting of the Conference of Animal Disease Research Workers*, Chicago, IL.

Levy, J.K., Richards, J., et al. 2001. Feline Retrovirus Testing and Management. *Compendium of Continuing Education Practicing Veterinarian*; 23:652–657,692.

Levy, J.K., Woods, J.E., et al. 2003. Number of unowned free-roaming cats in a college community in the southern United States and characteristics of community residents who feed them. *Journal of the American Veterinary Medical Association*; 223: 202–205.

Luria, B.J., Levy J.K., et al. 2003. Prevalence of infectious diseases in feral cats in Northern Florida. *Journal of Veterinary Internal Medicine*; 17:42.

Manning, A.M., and Rowan, A.N. 1992. Companion animal demographics and sterilization status: results from a survey in four Massachusetts towns. *Anthrozoos*; 5:192–201.

Moore, D.A., Sischo, W.M., et al. 2000. Animal bite epidemiology and surveillance for rabies postexposure prophylaxis, *Journal of the American Veterinary Medical Association*; 217:190–194.

Nassar, R., Mosier, J.E., et al. 1984. Study of the feline and canine populations in the greater Las Vegas area *American Journal of Veterinary Research*, February; 45 (2):282–7.

Patrick, G.R., and O'Rourke, K.M. 1998. Dog and cat bites: Epidemiologic analyses suggest different prevention strategies. *Public Health Report*; 113:252–257.

Scott, K.C., Levy, J.K., et al. 2002. Characteristics of free-roaming cats evaluated in a trap-neuter-return program. *Journal of the American Veterinary Medical Association*; 221:1136–1138

Scott, K.C., Levy, J.K., et al. 2002. Body condition of feral cats, and the effect of neutering. *Journal Applied Animal Welfare Science*; 5:209–219.

Soulebot, J.P., Brun, A., et al. 1981. Experimental rabies in cats: immune response and persistence of immunity. *Cornell Veterinarian*; 71:311–325.

2000 Report of the American Association of Feline Practitioners and Academy of Feline Medicine Advisory Panel on Feline Vaccines. *Journal of Feline Medicine and Surgery* 2001; 3:47–72.

Veterinary Public Health Notes, 1975, January, 1–2.

Williams, L.S., Levy, J.K., et al. 2002. Use of the anesthetic combination of tiletamine, zolazepam, ketamine, and xylazine for neutering feral cats. *Journal of the American Veterinary Medical Association;* 220:1491–1495.

Wright, J.C. 1990. Reported cat bites in Dallas: Characteristics of the cats, the victims, and the attack events. *Public Health Report;* 105:420–424.

Zasloff, R.L., and Hart, L.A. 1998. Attitudes and care practices of cat caretakers in Hawaii. *Anthrozoos;* 11:242–248.

24
Euthanasia in the Animal Shelter

Leslie Sinclair

INTRODUCTION

Perhaps no other aspect of animal sheltering is as controversial, difficult, or necessary as euthanasia. No one knows how many animals are euthanized in animal shelters annually; estimates of the number of animals relinquished to, adopted from, and euthanized by U.S. animal shelters made by various organizations vary greatly, and data collection and analysis on a national basis are limited and sparse. There are an estimated four to six thousand animal shelters in the country, most of them independently operated, and collection of data from them has proved difficult if not impossible. The most significant effort to date to accumulate and track animal shelter statistics has been made by the National Council on Pet Population Study and Policy (NCPPSP; www.petpopulation.org), but even that coalition of humane organizations, breeder groups, and veterinary associations has found that accumulating definitive statistics to characterize the euthanasia of companion animals in U.S. animal shelters and animal care and control agencies is a formidable task, although certainly one worthy of continued pursuit.

Without statistical data, only estimates are available. Patronek and Rowan compiled available statistics from several sources to estimate that 4 million dogs enter U.S. animal shelters annually, 2.1 million of whom are euthanized (Patronek and Rowan, 1995). The Humane Society of the United States (HSUS) estimates that eight to ten million dogs and cats enter shelters each year, where four to five million of them are euthanized (www.hsus.org). The American Humane Association estimates that 9.6 million animals (presumably dogs and cats) are euthanized annually in U.S. animal shelters (www.americanhumane.org).

Regardless of the numbers, however, euthanasia will undeniably always be a part of the task of sheltering animals. Animals euthanized are not just homeless offspring, disowned or displaced companions, but also victims of animal cruelty: animal fighting victims bred for aggressive tendencies who cannot be safely rehabilitated; feral and hoarded animals so unsocialized that they cannot live comfortably as companions to humans; animals who are accidentally, intentionally, or negligently injured or debilitated so severely that treatment is prohibitively costly and/or unlikely to relieve their suffering; and legions of animals discarded by the research, racing, and pet store industries and failed get rich quick schemes. Animal sheltering agencies will no doubt always be called upon to provide services for these as well as for elderly, sick, and injured animals, for whom euthanasia is often the kindest option available. Euthanasia is, and will undoubtedly always be, an inextricable part of compassionate care for animals. Even as the sheltering community makes progress in finding ways to rehome and rehabilitate more animals and to prevent relinquishment, it must continue to discuss, debate, and research the methods by which it will intentionally end the lives of a subgroup of the animals it shelters.

The debate about whether euthanasia is the appropriate approach for dealing with unowned and unwanted but otherwise healthy or rehabilitatable populations of companion animals has raged long and loud, particularly during the last decade. Animal shelters that take in limited numbers of animals, keeping each animal for as long as is necessary to find a suitable new home are referred to as limited admission, limited access, or no-kill shelters and have become more numerous and more vocal in their criticism of those shelters that accept all animals (open access or open admission shelters) but are unable to rehome all of them and, therefore, euthanize animals to make room for more. The result has been a fruitful, although often rancorous, debate about whether limited admission shelters turn their backs on animals and people in need, and whether open admission shelters do enough to find adoptive homes for animals. Both sides have benefited greatly from the conflict (and the animals most of all), as the animal sheltering community progresses toward a new model in which many types of shelters offering complementary (though not identical) services work together to provide the most possible options for each community's animals.

With a few exceptions, veterinarians have been conspicuously absent from this debate, as they have traditionally been from the field of animal sheltering altogether. The public's perception that the veterinary community is the primary source of expertise and experience regarding euthanasia disregards the millions of animals euthanized each year by nonveterinarians, in their capacity as animal shelter workers.

Who should perform euthanasia? Although veterinarians in general private practice perform euthanasia on a regular, often daily, basis, the population of animals they euthanize is for the most part far different from the population for whom euthanasia has been deemed necessary at the nearest animal shelter. Most patients euthanized in a veterinary hospital are elderly, debilitated, and/or severely sick or injured, and are accompanied by an owner familiar with their condition and their behavior. Most animal shelters routinely euthanize young puppies and kittens, dogs and cats who are feral, fractious, unsocialized, and/or aggressive (but otherwise physically healthy), severely debilitated or injured animals, wildlife, small mammals, reptiles, fish, and exotic pets. In most cases, little is known about the temperament or previous life experiences of animals being euthanized in shelters, and those persons performing such euthanasia must exercise more intuition and caution than is required for private practice euthanasia.

Private practitioners most often euthanize their patients by intravenous injection of a sodium pentobarbital formulation and have unrestricted access to drugs they may need to sedate, tranquilize, or anesthetize the patient prior to euthanasia. Rarely do private practitioners use or even consider using other routes of administration of sodium pentobarbital

(such as intraperitoneal injection) or other methods of euthanasia (such as carbon monoxide inhalation). Few veterinarians have received formal training regarding euthanasia; most veterinary curriculums include only discussion of the pharmacologic effects of sodium pentobarbital and counseling for grieving owners of animals being euthanized. Specific euthanasia techniques and methods, as well as adjunctive techniques such as pre-euthanasia chemical and physical restraint, are rarely taught in a formal veterinary curriculum.

Many experienced and properly trained shelter workers are knowledgeable about the circumstances that led to the decision to euthanize the animal, experienced at physically handling sheltered animals, and have chosen to make a career of providing for the needs of unowned and unwanted animals, even if those needs include euthanasia. To become adept at euthanasia, a shelter worker needs appropriate training and experience, proper equipment, access to drugs that enhance the safety and quality of euthanasia (including those controlled substances discussed later in this chapter), and moral and psychological support for performing an emotionally difficult task that is rarely appreciated by the general public.

A significant degree of confusion surrounds the issue of training and certification of persons who perform euthanasia. Much of the confusion stems from the fact that each state regulates training and certification, as well as access, or lack thereof, to controlled substances used for pre-euthanasia purposes, on an individual and extremely varied basis. Some states require a person who performs euthanasia—commonly referred to as a euthanasia technician, or "ET"—to receive training of specified length and content. Others require only that euthanasia technicians receive instruction from a licensed veterinarian. Still others require no training whatsoever of persons who perform euthanasia. Many states allow animal shelters direct access to sodium pentobarbital; that is, after meeting certain requirements, they may obtain and use sodium pentobarbital for euthanasia purposes without oversight by a veterinarian. Other states permit only indirect access: A veterinarian must agree to obtain, and oversee the use of, sodium pentobarbital used by the shelter. This situation is fraught with difficulty for both parties. Since few animal shelters have a veterinarian on staff, oversight is usually an act of volunteerism, and the veterinarian must trust that record-keeping and use requirements are adhered to in her absence. Likewise, the shelter must secure the trust and cooperation of a local licensed veterinarian, a task that is not always possible.

Procuring those controlled drugs other than sodium pentobarbital that are useful to the euthanasia process, such as ketamine and tiletamine-zolazepam, is even more difficult. Few shelters that do not employ a veterinarian as a member of their staff have access to these crucial drugs. Because of these difficulties, many shelters resort to the use of the carbon monoxide chamber to perform mass euthanasia.

American Humane, the Humane Society of the United States, and the National Animal Control Association all offer euthanasia training courses, the curriculums of which are usually tailored to conform to the euthanasia certification standards of those states in which they are presented (in those states that have such standards). Some states provide their own programs for training of euthanasia technicians, often offered through veterinary technician training programs. These courses are taught by both veterinarians and nonveterinarians. In California, for example, persons who are not veterinarians or registered veterinary technicians who wish to teach euthanasia must be certified as euthanasia instructors by the State Humane Association of California and the California Animal Control Directors' Association.

In those states that do not have formal training programs for euthanasia technicians, veterinarians are often asked to provide such training to prospective euthanasia technicians on an individual basis. Before accepting this responsibility, a veterinarian should be certain that he or she is knowledgeable about all of the aspects of euthanasia discussed in this chapter, and is able and willing to convey them to those who are being trained, as well as able to provide ongoing supervision and support for those persons.

When attempting to determine what the requirements are for performing euthanasia of shelter animals and for obtaining sodium pentobarbital and other controlled drugs used as pre-euthanasia agents, look no further than the boundaries of the state in which euthanasia is intended to be performed. State boards of pharmacy, departments of health, and state humane and animal control associations are usually the best sources of information regarding these issues.

PERSONAL RESPONSES TO EUTHANASIA

Euthanasia technicians must possess not only technical proficiency but also emotional stamina. End-ing any animal's life is emotionally difficult; ending the life of an animal who could be a loving companion if only a home were available is even more so. Those who are able to euthanize animals in a compassionate and technically capable manner on an ongoing basis are members of a rare breed. The task of euthanasia must be entrusted to persons who can maintain the ability to evaluate every animal on an individual basis, and provide the best possible death for each one. Euthanasia should never be performed by those who are callous or indifferent to the distress that animals may feel in a euthanasia situation, even if those persons appear outwardly to be more capable of handling the psychological effects of performing euthanasia. The best possible euthanasia experience for each animal should be the goal of those performing the task. Persons who are unable to provide such euthanasia should receive further training and be required to adhere to standards of compassion and humaneness established by the agency, or be dismissed from the task altogether.

The emotional responses of animal shelter workers to euthanasia and the "shelter culture" that allows workers (both those who actually perform the task in the shelter, and those who do not) to cope with the emotional effects of euthanasia have been studied (White and Shawhan, 1996; Arluke, 1991). Animal sheltering is a stressful occupation, and adding euthanasia to the list of duties of a shelter worker compounds the distress the occupation creates in those who choose to pursue it. The many sources of distress involved with euthanasia include, but are not limited to, making decisions about which animals must be euthanized (often based on factors that have nothing to do with the animals themselves, such as whether there are enough cages available); performing the act itself; confrontations with a public that does not understand the need for and the process of euthanasia; and providing final care (disposal) for the body after euthanasia.

Euthanasia technicians often experience feelings of anger, frustration, defeat, irritability, guilt, sadness, and remorse. These feelings can compound, or be compounded by, other stressful aspects of the euthanasia technician's life, such as relationships with spouses, children, and family members, and various life events such as divorce, moving, and illness of a family member.

Negative coping mechanisms employed by some euthanasia technicians to relieve euthanasia related stress include excessive alcohol consumption, illicit drug use, smoking, withdrawal, and denial. Chronic, severe, or even suicidal depression is possible. There have been cases of employee suicides and attempted suicides resulting from misuse of sodium pentobarbital euthanasia solution acquired from the shelter. Withdrawal from the profession entirely—burnout—is commonplace.

Positive coping mechanisms can help personnel who perform euthanasia to deal with their stress, and include regular physical exercise, engaging in hobbies, sports, or other activities unrelated to animal sheltering, adopting companion animals from the shelter who might otherwise have been euthanized and providing them with a caring home, and talking openly to those coworkers, friends, and family members who are able to understand the complex issues and emotions that surround euthanasia.

Not all of these outlets are available to all euthanasia technicians, and some shelter workers do not avail themselves of any positive coping mechanisms. Many report that finding someone appropriate to talk to about euthanasia and the stress it causes is difficult. Many euthanasia technicians have reported strained relationships with friends and family who cannot understand their role in euthanasia.

Counseling of persons who perform euthanasia can be helpful, but it must be carried out by professional counselors who are familiar with the stressors inherent to performing euthanasia, as well as the demands of a shelter career. Those who supervise shelter staff who perform euthanasia should receive training in recognizing signs of emotional distress and burnout in their staff, and be prepared to offer resources for coping with such.

There are several steps that shelter administrators can take to diminish the distress to which euthanasia technicians are subjected. Euthanasia responsibilities should be rotated as much as human resources will allow, to minimize the amount of time any one person spends performing the task. Euthanasia technicians should be given flexibility to work as a team with coworkers they like and trust, allowing them to work well together. Administrators and euthanasia technicians should maintain flexibility regarding euthanasia of individual animals, allowing technicians themselves to determine whether they do or do not wish to be involved in the euthanasia of animals to whom they have become particularly attached. Administrators should realize that technical proficiency greatly diminishes euthanasia-related stress and provide

training opportunities on a regular basis so that euthanasia technicians can acquire new information and hone existing skills and knowledge. Administrators should listen carefully to concerns expressed by euthanasia technicians and other staff with regard to euthanasia. Euthanasia technicians should return this courtesy with the understanding that supervisors and administrators may be able to see a bigger picture that encompasses the shelter's mission and resources. Administrators should enforce in an objective and consistent manner all internal policies and procedures designed to minimize stress.

The sheltering community appears to be divided on the issue of whether to offer owner requested and owner present euthanasia services, but many agencies do offer these services, and staff who perform them must be given resources that help them to deal not only with the technical difficulty of euthanizing an animal as an owner looks on, but also the emotional burden of providing assistance and support to a grieving pet owner. An excellent reference that specifically addresses this has been published (Lagoni, Butler, and Hetts, 1994), and there are many, many other resources available, including scientific literature, support groups, and telephone counseling services. The agency should also verify with their state's licensing board for veterinary medicine that owner-present euthanasia can legally be performed by euthanasia technicians and is not considered the practice of veterinary medicine, which may be the case if fees are collected to perform the euthanasia at the owner's request, regardless of whether the animal has been relinquished to the sheltering agency.

CRITERIA FOR SELECTION OF EUTHANASIA CANDIDATES

Deciding which animals are to be euthanized is the worst of the worst: the most difficult part of a difficult task. Surprisingly, many animal sheltering agencies have no formal or even informal criteria for making decisions about which animals should be euthanized, a situation laden with hazards. Some agencies have only unwritten criteria that are passed along orally from one generation of employees to another (Reilly, 1994). Lack of euthanasia criteria creates an undue legal and emotional burden on the person or persons charged with making decisions about which animals should be euthanized. It allows for inconsistency and personal bias to become factors in decisions that determine whether animals live or die. It makes it difficult for an agency to convince anyone concerned that euthanasia decisions are not arbitrary or subjective.

The criterion that determines whether an animal is to be euthanized is not simply whether he is adoptable because that term is organic and indefinable: Whether an animal is adoptable depends on factors both inherent and external to that animal. An animal's species, breed or breed-type, sex, neuter status, age, health status, physical disabilities, specific health needs, temperament, behavior and behavioral issues, background, and history all play a part in determining whether he is likely to be adopted. The sheltering agency's financial, medical, and physical (cage space) resources determine whether an animal can be held or even presented for adoption. Consideration of the characteristics of the community in which the shelter resides is crucial: the number of adoptive homes, their financial resources, their views about shelter adoption as a means of acquiring a new companion animal, and their propensity to adopt a mature animal as opposed to a juvenile. Some of these factors are unalterable, such as the animal's age. Other factors change on a daily, sometimes hourly basis: whether cage space is available, for example. Still others can be intentionally changed; for example; a public information campaign can be used to tout the benefits of adopting adult animals, thereby increasing the adoptability of the shelter's mature animal population.

Keeping in mind that the adoptability of any particular animal is an inconstant, a shelter's staff must nonetheless create criteria that will assist them in making the difficult decisions about which animals are to be euthanized. How these criteria are developed and implemented varies from one organization to the next, but it is essential that those persons who are experienced in determining which animals are to be euthanized, as well as those persons whose job it is to perform euthanasia (if these are not the same), be a part of the process of developing criteria. Once criteria are developed for an agency, it is crucial that they be accepted, implemented, and adhered to by all members (administrators, employees, volunteer workers) of the organization, for the sake of uniformity and consistency. Those who apply the criteria must be committed, supportive, and consistent in their application. All of those involved must be imbued with a sense of the value of the euthanasia criteria to the animals, the general public, the shelter as a whole, and the individuals who are associated with the sheltering agency.

Once euthanasia selection criteria are developed and implemented, they must also be reassessed on a regular basis. Because there are so many possible circumstances that might apply to any individual animal, no euthanasia criteria can be inflexible, and occasionally exceptions must be made to the rule. If it becomes apparent, however, that exceptions have become the rule, the criteria must be re-evaluated to determine why they are not functional.

METHODS OF EUTHANASIA

Just as statistics that define the population of animals that is sheltered, rehomed, and euthanized each year in the United States are difficult to obtain due to the autonomy of this nation's four to six thousand animal sheltering agencies, information about methods of euthanasia used on those populations is lacking. The injection of sodium pentobarbital appears to be the most popular and widely used method, and is mandated by law in some states. On a regular basis, isolated incidences of the use of gunshot, decapitation, freezing, electrocution, drowning, blunt trauma to the head, and injection of paralytic agents as methods of attempted euthanasia by animal care and control agencies come to light, often in rural or economically disadvantaged communities.

Like all other aspects of medicine, our knowledge of and favored methods for performing euthanasia change and grow with time. Methods that once seemed appropriate and humane are no longer deemed so, as newer methods, techniques, opinions, information, and drugs become available. The methods used by a particular animal sheltering agency vary depending on that agency's resources (physical, financial, and educational), the characteristics of the population of animals being euthanized, the skills, experiences, sensibilities, and ethics of the persons performing euthanasia, the community's involvement (or lack thereof), and any legal mandates regarding euthanasia methods that pertain to that particular state or locality.

AVMA Panel on Euthanasia

Various local, regional, and national animal protection groups have espoused different euthanasia protocols and methods of euthanasia. One widely used and accepted resource for determining what is and is not an appropriate euthanasia method is the *Report of the AVMA Panel on Euthanasia*. The report, first published in 1963 and updated in 1972, 1978, 1986, 1993, and 2000 (Table 24.1), is a review of current scientific literature regarding methods for euthanizing animals in a variety of circumstances, including

Table 24.1. Chronology of Reports of the AVMA Panel on Euthanasia

Year	JAVMA Volume and Page	Author
1963	142:162–170	AVMA Council on Research
1972	160:761–772	Smith, C.R., Booth, N.H., Fox, M.W., et al.
1978	173: 59–72	McDonald, L.E., Booth, N.H., Lumb, W.V., et al.
1986	188:252–268	Smith, A.W., Houpt, K.A., Kitchell, R.L., et al.
1993	202:229–249	Andrews, E.J., Bennet, B.T., Clark, J.D., et al.
*2000	218:669–696	Beaver, B.V., Reed, W., Leary, S., et al.

Source: Journal of the American Veterinary Medical Association
**The report is found in JAVMA 2001.*

euthanasia of animals in research facilities and animal care and control facilities, euthanasia of injured or diseased wildlife, and removal of animals (both domestic and wild) causing damage to property or threatening human safety. The report has both significant merits and faults. Its greatest value is that it is a published scientific reference presented by a credible and substantially powerful professional organization. The report is easy to access (even available as a full-text document online at www.avma.org) and well referenced. The report's faults are that it is perhaps afforded too much authority, particularly as regards euthanasia of animals by animal sheltering agencies. Although the recommendations in the report are "intended to serve as guidelines for veterinarians who must then use professional judgment in applying them to the various settings where animals are to be euthanatized", the recommendations are widely interpreted and used by several different populations of nonveterinarians in the absence of any veterinary oversight. A handful of state legislatures have even gone so far as to incorporate the recommendations of the panel report into state law, allowing little opportunity for any interpretation by any party in application to a specific agency or individual animal. While these well-intended laws were meant to ensure that animals receive the most acceptable form of euthanasia, it does allow the opposite to occur in some cases. Appropriate to its stated purpose, the report defines as acceptable many forms of euthanasia that are not appropriate for the euthanasia of companion animals in an animal shelter facility. For example, the panel mentions thoracic compression, decapitation, and cervical dislocation as conditionally acceptable methods of euthanasia for birds. These methods should be avoided because more humane methods are available. and many veterinarians have ex-

pressed concern that these methods, are in fact, inhumane (Bennett, 2001; Ludders, 2001) Those who fail to recognize the broad scope of the report— that is, a scope not limited to animal shelter euthanasia—may misinterpret these recommendations and incorrectly apply them for use in the shelter setting.

A final constraint of the report is the limited input interested parties, including the sheltering community, have to each update. Members of the panel, whose numbers have ranged from seven to 17, are appointed by the AVMA's executive board of directors, chosen from persons nominated by interested parties including animal protection organizations. The AVMA's Council on Research composes the panel to arrive at "the smallest number of people with the greatest amount of expertise on humane death" (Wollrab, 1998). Because the issues and situations examined by the report vary tremendously, the animal sheltering community and its concerns and interests (and those of any of the other concerned communities) are narrowly represented. The panel solicits comments from any interested parties but, because members of the panel are appointed, not elected by those whose concerns they are meant to represent, and because the actual proceedings of the panel are not made public, there is no mechanism to ensure that the concerns of the animal sheltering community (or of any other community that deals with the issues examined by the report) are successfully represented in the report.

Despite its limitations, the report is and will continue to be an important tool for those who must perform euthanasia or determine how it will be performed. Dr. Bonnie Beaver, chair of the panel convened in 1999 that produced the 2000 Report (published in 2001), describes the report as a work in progress: "There is no single point of time at which it is complete" (Anonymous, 2000).

One task the panel report performs well is that of presenting and classifying the myriad possible methods of killing and of euthanizing animals. It classifies euthanasia agents by three basic mechanisms: 1) hypoxia, direct or indirect; 2) direct depression of neurons necessary for life function; and 3) physical disruption of brain activity and destruction of neurons necessary for life; and evaluates them based on a list of twelve criteria that may be appropriately used by any individual who is attempting to evaluate the usefulness and appropriateness of a particular method of euthanasia for a specific purpose:

1. Ability to induce loss of consciousness and death without causing pain, distress, anxiety, or apprehension
2. Time required to induce loss of consciousness
3. Reliability
4. Safety of personnel
5. Irreversibility
6. Compatibility with requirement and purpose
7. Emotional effect on observers or operators
8. Compatibility with subsequent evaluation, examination, or use of tissue
9. Drug availability and human abuse potential
10. Compatibility with species, age, and health status
11. Ability to maintain equipment in proper working order
12. Safety for predators/scavengers should the carcass be consumed

In conclusion, the report presents in tabular form what it considers to be acceptable and conditionally acceptable methods of euthanasia, describing for each method the species to which it should be applied, but not characterizing the populations of animals within that species for which the method is appropriate. The specific recommendations of the panel report are beyond the scope of this discussion. Any person associated with the euthanasia of animals in an animal sheltering facility should obtain and become familiar with those recommendations.

Carbon Monoxide

Inhalation of carbon monoxide is still used in many locales, but is illegal for use in California, Florida, and Georgia, and its use becomes more controversial with each passing year. It is considered an acceptable method of euthanasia for dogs and cats by the AVMA, and a conditionally acceptable method by

the Humane Society of the United States. The National Animal Control Association (NACA) does not specifically approve or condone the use of carbon monoxide (it "recommends only those methods of euthanasia recommended in the current AVMA Report on Euthanasia"). American Humane (AH) has recently approved a new position statement on euthanasia that promotes euthanasia by injection of sodium pentobarbital as the only acceptable method for euthanasia of dogs and cats in animal shelters. AH explains that "we do not believe that placing a friendly and sociable dog or cat into a carbon monoxide chamber, pushing a button, and walking away rises to the strict meaning of good death because the dog or cat deserves to be held and comforted according to the needs of the individual animal." The organization assures its member agencies that it is not abandoning them for using carbon monoxide, but instead will encourage them to upgrade to euthanasia by injection and will offer information, training, and advice to help them do so. Membership in American Humane is voluntary for animal sheltering agencies and individuals; members are not required to ascribe to AH's policies.

Carbon monoxide is a colorless odorless gas that combines with hemoglobin to form carboxyhemoglobin, which interferes with the ability of the red blood cell to uptake oxygen. This leads to hypoxemia and death. Concerns about the use of carbon monoxide are multiple. It is a method that allows the person employing it to detach themselves from the animal being euthanized. This is touted as an advantage by advocates of the method, who believe this relieves somewhat the emotional distress that may be a personal response to performing euthanasia. Others see this as the method's drawback; animals are not closely monitored, nor are socialized animals provided with comforting words and physical reassurance at the time of their death. The AVMA panel report states that "carbon monoxide induces loss of consciousness without pain and with minimal discernible discomfort", yet the only study referenced by the panel report that monitored physiologic reactions to carbon monoxide inhalation identified a 20 to 25 second span of abnormal cortical function (as detected by electroencephalographic recording) prior to the loss of consciousness, occurring at the same time as the dogs in the study became agitated and vocalized just prior to loss of consciousness (Chalifoux and Dallaire, 1983). The panel report counters this concern by referencing an 1895 study that reported humans rendered unconscious by inhalation of carbon monoxide did not feel distress during this period of agitation, yet the report also states that common symptoms of early carbon monoxide toxicosis are headache, dizziness, and weakness followed by decreased visual acuity, tinnitus, nausea, progressive depression, confusion, and collapse, which may be accompanied by convulsions and muscular spasms. The report goes on to caution that carbon monoxide is extremely hazardous for personnel because it is highly toxic and difficult to detect, and because chronic low-level exposure is hazardous as well. At least one animal shelter worker has died and another (a veterinarian) has been hospitalized as a result of the use of carbon monoxide as a euthanasia method in recent years (Poole, 2000; Pawlaczyk, 1997).

Other concerns regarding carbon monoxide use are that too many animals are often placed in the euthanasia chamber together (this author has witnessed 43 dogs and cats forced into a chamber designed to hold seven animals); chambers are not properly cleaned between uses; neonatal and pediatric animals and other animals with compromised respiratory function—those whose tolerance of carbon monoxide is likely to be greater due to decreased intake of the gas—are often inappropriately subjected to this method.

Despite these concerns, many agencies continue to use this method, citing the difficulty and expense of making the change to euthanasia by injection of sodium pentobarbital. Data collected by HSUS indicate that euthanasia by injection of sodium pentobarbital is actually less expensive than by use of the carbon monoxide chamber (Rhoades, 2002). Those agencies should continue to be encouraged to adopt a more progressive method of euthanasia, and in the meantime should subscribe to standards of operation promulgated by the AVMA, AH, and the HSUS that are meant to ensure that the method is administered in the most humane fashion possible and that shelter workers are given the greatest protection possible from the potentially deadly effects of the gas. Despite the still prevalent use of carbon monoxide as a method of euthanasia by U.S. animal sheltering agencies, most euthanasia of sheltered animals is performed by injection of sodium pentobarbital. Whenever carbon monoxide is used, the precautions outlined by the AVMA panel are the minimum standards that should be employed (Table 24.2). Veterinarians working in shelters utilizing carbon monoxide should accept responsibility for ensuring the

Table 24.2. AVMA Panel Recommendations for Use of Carbon Monoxide for Euthanasia

1. Commercially compressed CO must be used.
2. Personnel must be thoroughly instructed in its use and understand its hazards and limitations.
3. The CO chamber must be of the highest quality construction and should allow for separation of individual animals.
4. The CO source and chamber must be located in a well-ventilated environment, preferably out of doors.
5. The chamber must be well lit and have view ports that allow personnel direct observation of the animals.
6. The CO flow rate should be adequate to achieve a uniform CO concentration of at least 6 percent after animals are placed in the chamber.
7. If the chamber is inside a room, CO monitors must be in place to warn personnel of hazardous concentrations.

Source: AVMA, 2000 Panel on Euthanasia, p. 679; see Table 1.

animals are humanely euthanized just as if they were utilizing sodium pentobarbital.

Euthanasia by Injection of Sodium Pentobarbital

SODIUM PENTOBARBITAL

By far, the most widely employed method for administering euthanasia to sheltered dogs and cats (and most other species) is injection of sodium pentobarbital, also known as pentobarbital sodium and pentobarbitone. When administered intravenously, sodium pentobarbital depresses the central nervous system and causes an animal to advance through all five stages of anesthesia (Table 24.3) in swift succession, resulting in rapid unconsciousness, anesthesia, and death.

Unadulterated sodium pentobarbital is a class II controlled substance. Several preparations containing sodium pentobarbital and the anticonvulsant drug phenytoin, which is cardiotoxic, are also available (see Table 26.4). The purpose of adding phenytoin is twofold: It enhances cardiac arrest and diminishes the potential for human abuse of sodium pentobarbital. Therefore, this combination of sodium pentobarbital and phenytoin is a class III controlled substance

Table 24.3. Five Stages of Anesthesia/Euthanasia

I.   Sedation: the animal becomes calm and sleepy
II.   Involuntary excitement
III. Light anesthesia
IV.   Deep anesthesia
V.   Medullary paralysis (brain death), followed by apnea (respiratory arrest) followed by cardiac arrest

and is more readily available to veterinarians and particularly to animal shelters for euthanasia.

A third combination, sodium pentobarbital plus lidocaine, was marketed briefly during the 1980s and is currently being evaluated for approval by the FDA. Lidocaine, like phenytoin, has an effect on the function of the heart and is cardiotoxic at high doses. The addition of lidocaine to sodium pentobarbital has two additional purposes: It decreases the discomfort that occurs when sodium pentobarbital is accidentally injected perivascularly, and it diminishes the abuse potential of the formulation, making it a class III controlled substance. Sodium pentobarbital-lidocaine combinations have also been shown to reduce the occurrence of the agonal gasp that is exhibited by many dogs and cats during euthanasia with sodium pentobarbital alone (Evans, Broadstone, Stapleton, et al., 1993).

Most formulations of sodium pentobarbital contain 390 mg of sodium pentobarbital (6 grains) per milliliter of solution. The manufacturer's suggested dosage for both intravenous and intraperitoneal administration should be consulted; most formulations are administered at a dose of 1 ml/10 lb of body weight for intravenous administration. A dose of 3 ml/10 lb of body weight for cats has been suggested (Grier and Schaffer, 1990) and then revised to 2 ml/10 lb of body weight in a later publication by the same authors (Grier, Colvin, and Schaffer, 1996). Some formulations have different concentrations of active ingredient, another reason for consulting manufacturers' guidelines.

ROUTES OF ADMINISTRATION
Determining the best route of administration of sodium pentobarbital is crucial to providing the best possible quality of euthanasia. The route chosen depends on many factors, including the behavioral nature of the animal, the degree of injury or illness affecting the animal, the skill and comfort of the person administering euthanasia as well as of those who are assisting, and the formulation of sodium pentobarbital that is being used. Sodium pentobarbital euthanasia formulations work best when injected intravenously. Once in the vein, sodium pentobarbital is quickly transported to the heart and then to the brain, the primary site of action. Information regarding the intraperitoneal administration of unadulter-

Table 24.4. Sodium Pentobarbital Formulations*

Class II Drug	Manufacturer	Conc. (mg/ml)
Sleepaway®	Fort Dodge Animal Health (Overland Park, KS)	260
Euthanasia®	Anthony Products Co. (Arcadia, CA)	390
Euthanasia Solution	Veterinary Laboratories (Lenexa, KS)	324
Fatal-Plus® Solution	Vortech Pharmaceuticals Ltd. (Dearborn, MI)	390

Class III Drug	Manufacturer	Conc. (mg/ml)
Beuthanasia®-D Special	Schering Plough Animal Health Corp. (Union, NJ)	390 (sodium pentobarbital) + 50 (phenytoin)
Euthasol®	Delmarva Laboratories Inc (Midlothian, VA)	390 (sodium pentobarbital) + 50 (phenytoin)

*Many sodium pentobarbital formulations have been made available by various manufacturers. This list includes the most commonly used formulations but may not be comprehensive.

ated (class II) sodium pentobarbital solution to cats has been published (Grier and Schaffer, 1990; Grier, Colvin, and Schaffer, 1996). The AVMA report acknowledges that intraperitoneal injection of a non-irritating euthanasia agent is acceptable when intravenous administration is impractical or impossible. The method is widely used in U.S. animal shelters for euthanasia of cats, kittens, and puppies. It is particularly favored by the animal shelter community as a method for providing a humane death for feral, fearful, or fractious cats, especially absent the availability of other drugs that might provide chemical restraint or sedation, because intraperitoneal administration can often be accomplished with minimal restraint of those animals.

Although no published report of the use of intraperitoneal administration for dogs has been made, anecdotal evidence suggests that they tend to struggle to right themselves as they experience the involuntary excitement stage of anesthesia (stage II). Most cats, kittens, and puppies, however, advance smoothly through all five stages of anesthesia within 15 to 30 minutes after intraperitoneal administration, especially when they are placed in a warm, dark, quiet area during induction. Concern has been expressed that when sodium pentobarbital-phenytoin combinations are administered by the intraperitoneal method, phenytoin may exert its effect on the heart before the sodium pentobarbital component has caused unconsciousness (Fakkema, 1999). The AVMA report states that the pharmacologic properties and recommended use of sodium pentobarbital-phenytoin combinations are interchangeable with those of pure barbituric acid derivatives, but it does not directly address the question of administering such a combination by the intraperitoneal route. Until more information is available regarding the absorption rates of these two drugs from the peritoneal cavity, it is prudent to use only unadulterated sodium pentobarbital (class II) for intraperitoneal injection.

Performing accurate intracardiac injection on a conscious animal is technically difficult, unpredictable, and likely to be painful. However, this method has been widely used in animal sheltering agencies for many years. Injecting directly into one of the chambers of the heart is exceedingly difficult if not impossible in most cases, especially in animals weighing less than ten pounds, although rapid absorption of sodium pentobarbital from the myocardium or from the thoracic cavity in many

instances no doubt masks misdirected injection. The AVMA panel report has since its 1978 version condemned intracardiac injection of sodium pentobarbital in conscious animals (and discouraged them in previous reports), yet this method continues to be used by many agencies, whether due to lack of training in or commitment to more appropriate methods and/or lack of access to pre-euthanasia drugs to anesthetize the animal prior to intracardiac injection. Intracardiac injection of sodium pentobarbital can only be considered acceptable when performed on a heavily sedated, anesthetized, or comatose animal.

A technique for intrahepatic administration of sodium pentobarbital in cats has been published (Grier and Schaffer, 1990) and later revised by the same authors (Grier, Colvin, and Schaffer, 1996). The use of this technique is controversial in the animal sheltering community due to concerns about discomfort induced by injection into the liver, and anecdotally appears to be less widely used now than it was a decade ago.

Because of the acidic nature of sodium pentobarbital, injection into subcutaneous tissues or muscle is painful. Slow absorption from those sites also results in slow and unpredictable advancement through the five stages of anesthesia. For these reasons, sodium pentobarbital should never be injected subcutaneously or intramuscularly. Likewise, injection into the lungs, thoracic cavity, kidneys, spleen, and spinal fluid are inappropriate methods of administration.

The cessation of life as the result of the injection of sodium pentobarbital does not necessarily constitute a humane death. When considering which route of administration of sodium pentobarbital is most appropriate, it must be kept in mind that it is possible to provide poor death—not euthanasia—for an animal by performing the injection in a manner that causes pain during administration, or that induces slow absorption of the drug, leading to prolonged involuntary excitement. The method of restraint used to position the animal for injection, the environment and circumstances surrounding the act of injection, and the route of administration all contribute to the humaneness, or lack thereof, of the procedure.

THE EUTHANASIA ENVIRONMENT AND OTHER
CONCERNS ASSOCIATED WITH SODIUM
PENTOBARBITAL INJECTION
The characteristics of the environment in which an animal's death is induced play a significant role in

the quality of that death. The physical facilities of U.S. animal shelters range from grandiose to squalid, as do the euthanasia areas within those shelters. Ideally, a room is designated specifically for the task of euthanasia. It should not be overly large, but should be spacious enough to comfortably contain two euthanasia technicians and a large dog with room to maneuver, and be well lit and well ventilated. There should be a storage area where euthanasia supplies can be stocked and readily available, as well as secured in a manner in accordance with DEA and any state requirements. There should be two counter-height surfaces made of an easily cleaned material, one for completing paperwork and one on which cats and small- to medium-sized dogs and other animals are restrained for injection. The euthanasia room should be located in an area of the shelter that sees little activity and is somewhat soundproofed from the shelter's daily activities and noise, but with easy access to holding cages and kennels and a storage area for bodies—usually a walk-in freezer, but sometimes a truck used to take bodies directly to a crematorium, landfill, or rendering facility. The room should be easy to clean and free of distractions such as ringing telephones and piped-in music. A method for signaling that euthanasia is taking place should be instituted; a locked door to the room, or a sign placed on the outside of the door usually suffices. Lighting that can be dimmed and soothing décor (such as walls painted in blues and greens) can create a peaceful atmosphere that calms both animals and people involved in the euthanasia process.

At minimum, equipment and supplies in the room should include an assortment of needles and syringes; a pair of quiet, well-maintained electric hair clippers; euthanasia and pre-euthanasia drugs and log books to document their use; a calculator and drug dosage charts; pens and blank paper; euthanasia manuals and training materials to which technicians can refer if necessary; pen lights and stethoscopes to be used in the verification of death (pen lights for examining pupillary response, stethoscope to verify cessation of a heartbeat); tourniquets (many types are available); restraint equipment including muzzles, leashes, thick gloves, thick towels, a net, a control pole, pole syringes, and a squeeze cage; diluted alcohol for wetting fur to expose veins; body bags for preparing animals for final disposition; cleaning supplies; a first aid kit; and a medical waste ("sharps") disposal container.

The euthanasia process begins long before sodium pentobarbital is injected. The manner in which the animal is transported to the euthanasia room and handled on arrival sets the tone for the quality of euthanasia that will be provided. Animals should be handled gently but reassuringly. Euthanasia technicians should take steps to determine whether a particular animal is comfortable with close handling, or with less restraint and interaction. Animals who appear to be fearful, unsocialized, or fractious should be assessed and provided with pre-euthanasia sedation, tranquilization, or anesthesia as needed. If physical restraint tools such as a pole syringe, net, or squeeze cage are used, they should be used in a calm, quiet manner, with only the necessary amount of pressure applied. As animals get excited in stressful situations, euthanasia technicians must not react in kind, but must remain calm and work in a slow and deliberate manner.

Little is known about the psychological responses of animals to euthanasia and to the death of other animals. Rats are known to show a fright reaction to blood or muscle from their own and closely related species (Stevens and Saplikoski, 1973; Stevens and Gerzog-Thomas, 1977; Hornbuckle and Beall, 1974). Some animals seem to exhibit a response to the presence or the sight of a dead animal (both those with whom they are and are not acquainted), while others seem oblivious. It is reasonable to assume that many animals experience some level of distress when exposed to the sight, smell, or presence of an animal who has already been euthanized. Ideally, an animal waiting to be euthanized (or otherwise housed in an animal shelter) should not view the euthanasia of another animal. Realistically, the physical constraints of some animal shelters make this separation of animals a difficult task; animals to whom sodium pentobarbital has been administered may need to be observed for a period of time (often while other animals are being euthanized) before death can be confirmed. Efforts to separate animals by arrangement of rooms, cages, kennels, and barriers such as doors and curtains should be made. Blood, urine, feces, and other bodily residue should be cleaned thoroughly from the surface on which euthanasia is performed with a deodorizing solution after one animal has been euthanized and before another is introduced to the same surface.

Mother animals and their neonates are an exception. When selected for euthanasia, mother animals should be euthanized prior to their offspring so that they will not be distressed at being separated from their litter, or by seeing the neonates dead. The neonates should be euthanized immediately following the mother. If they are euthanized by intraperitoneal injection of sodium pentobarbital, a procedure that will cause them to become anesthetized and then euthanized, they can be placed together with their mother's still-warm body and their other littermates for comfort.

Because sodium pentobarbital and several of the drugs used as pre-euthanasia adjuncts are substances with potential for inducing psychological and or physical addiction when administered to humans, they are controlled by the DEA pursuant to the Controlled Substances Act of 1970 and, in most states, an additional state agency, such as the department of health or board of pharmacy. Whether the drugs are available to animal sheltering agencies through direct or indirect (through a veterinarian) means, strict record keeping and security are necessary in order to maintain the privilege of access to these controlled substances. Complete details of requirements are available in Title 21 Code of Federal Regulations (CFR) Part 1300. The complete text of Part 1300 of the CFR, as well as other useful information, can be accessed from the Web site of the DEA Diversion Control Program, http://www.deadiversion.usdoj.gov.

RESTRAINT—CHEMICAL AND PHYSICAL

The quality of euthanasia an animal receives does not depend solely on the method (sodium pentobarbital injection versus carbon monoxide inhalation, for example) that is utilized. Far more important in most cases are the circumstances surrounding the euthanasia procedure, and perhaps most important of all is the method of restraint by which the animal is handled in the moments immediately prior to administration of euthanasia. Using an appropriate, effective, and humane method of restraint, whether chemical, physical, or a combination of the two, can mean the difference between a distressful and unsafe end to the animal's life, and an end that is both peaceful for the animal and safe for the person administering euthanasia.

Regardless of the method of euthanasia chosen, the animal must be restrained to some degree. The proper use of pre-euthanasia drugs and equipment is often erroneously omitted from euthanasia protocols and practices. Some agencies are not knowledgeable about or familiar with the use of specialized equipment and adjunctive drugs, some are unconvinced of the need, and too many do not have access to the drugs and equipment that improve the ease, quality, and safety of euthanasia.

Pre-euthanasia Drugs and Their Actions

A number of drugs are commonly used to provide analgesia, anesthesia, sedation, tranquilization, and/or immobilization of animals who are frightened, painful, fractious, aggressive, and/or unsocialized to human handling. Because some of these drugs can potentially be abused by humans, their availability may be restricted or prohibited for use by animal shelter workers. The most widely used drugs are acepromazine, ketamine, tiletamine-zolazepam, and xylazine.

In order to use these drugs appropriately and effectively, euthanasia technicians must understand their effects, and how those effects may vary depending upon the dose, the time and route of administration, the extent of absorption, and the individual characteristics of the animal to whom they are administered. They must also understand how to combine and administer these drugs, and how to evaluate the animal to determine what effect they have produced.

Key to understanding the actions of commonly used pre-euthanasia drugs is understanding the difference between sedation, tranquilization, analgesia, and anesthesia, and knowing which actions the drug or drug combination being used, at the dose being used, is expected to produce (Table 24.5). Understanding the five stages of anesthesia, and the clinical signs of each, is also important (Table 24.3).

COMMONLY USED DRUGS, DOSES,
AND COMBINATIONS

The inexpensive phenothiazine tranquilizer acepromazine is commonly used as a pre-euthanasia drug, either alone for its tranquilizing effect only or in combination with other pre-euthanasia drugs to enhance their effects. In particular, studies have demonstrated that premedication with acepromazine significantly enhances the quality of death induced by inhalation of carbon monoxide in dogs (Dallaire and Chalifoux, 1985). Although it is a legend drug (federal law restricts use of it to "by or on the order of a licensed veterinarian"), it is not a controlled

Table 24.5. Definitions of Actions of Pre-euthanasia Drugs

Anesthesia	Loss of feeling or sensation, especially the loss of pain sensation induced to permit the performance of a potentially painful procedure
Analgesia	Absence of sensibility to pain, particularly the relief of pain without loss of consciousness
Sedation	A state in which an animal is calm and less responsive to stimulation, usually accompanied by drowsiness or sleep
Tranquilization	A state in which an animal is calm and less responsive to stimulation usually without sleepiness (although tranquilization may allow a tired animal to sleep voluntarily)

substance, and most animal shelters obtain and use it without veterinary oversight. Acepromazine is approved for use in dogs, cats, and horses, but is used in many species for which FDA approval has not been sought or granted. It can be administered intramuscularly, subcutaneously, or orally, and therefore offers the euthanasia technician flexibility in choosing a route of administration. The tranquilizing effect of acepromazine alone will calm fractious and frightened animals, but does not protect the euthanasia technician from an aggressive animal. Occasionally an animal may develop the contradictory symptoms of aggressiveness and generalized CNS stimulation after receiving acepromazine (Plumb, 1999), and the drug may potentiate seizures in an epileptic animal. The hypotensive effects of acepromazine may make subsequent venipuncture difficult in some animals, particularly those who are already cardiovascularly compromised. Used alone as a pre-euthanasia agent, acepromazine is typically administered to cats at a dose of 0.25 to 0.50 mg/lb and to dogs at 0.5 to 1.0 mg/lb SC or IM, ten to fifteen minutes prior to restraint for intravenous or intraperitoneal injection of sodium pentobarbital. Acepromazine is also commonly mixed with ketamine to create a pre-euthanasia combination with useful properties.

The alpha-2-adrenergic agonist xylazine has similar attributes for use as a pre-euthanasia drug: It is inexpensive, a legend drug but not a controlled substance, and can be administered subcutaneously or intramuscularly. It is classified as a sedative/analgesic with muscle relaxant properties. Its effects on the cardiovascular system include an initial increase in blood pressure, followed by a longer period of lowered blood pressure (Plumb, 1999), which may make subsequent venipuncture difficult. The most significant drawback of using xylazine is that it frequently causes vomition in cats and dogs, decreasing the quality of the euthanasia procedure, but this effect can be diminished by fasting the animal for a few hours before-

hand and/or by using xylazine in combination with other drugs such as acepromazine, which has antiemetic properties, or ketamine. Xylazine is manufactured and widely distributed in two strengths, 20 mg/ml and 100 mg/ml, and those who use it must be familiar with this difference in order to dose the drug properly. Xylazine is approved for use in dogs, cats, horses, deer, and elk. Used alone as a pre-euthanasia agent, xylazine is typically administered at a dose of 1.0 mg/lb SC or IM, ten to fifteen minutes prior to restraint for intravenous or intraperitoneal administration of sodium pentobarbital. Xylazine is also commonly mixed with ketamine to create a pre-euthanasia combination with useful properties.

Ketamine is a rapidly acting general anesthetic with analgesic activity. Ketamine has been approved for use in sub-human primates and cats. Used alone, it does not induce deep anesthesia, causes increased muscle tone, and may induce seizures, therefore it is best used in combination with other drugs. As of August 12, 1999, ketamine is a controlled substance (CIII). It is a popular drug of illicit use, and has been associated with numerous scams and burglaries, affecting both private veterinary practices and animal shelters nationwide. This increased control has made it more difficult for many sheltering agencies to acquire ketamine; nonetheless, it remains a very useful and inexpensive drug for pre-euthanasia injection.

Two common uses of ketamine for pre-euthanasia purposes are in combination with acepromazine (2 ml of acepromazine added to one 10 ml bottle of ketamine, administered to cats at a dose of 0.05 to 0.10 ml/lb body weight IM) and in combination with xylazine (2 ml of 100 mg/ml concentration xylazine added to one 10 ml bottle of ketamine, administered to cats, dogs, raccoons, opossums, and skunks at a dose of 0.06 ml/lb body weight IM).

The combination of tiletamine (an anesthetic chemically related to ketamine) and zolazepam (a minor tranquilizer related to diazepam) is rapidly becoming more popular for pre-euthanasia use. Properly dosed and administered, the combination provides good anesthesia combined with muscle relaxation as well as analgesia. The greatest advantage of tiletamine-zolazepam is its small-volume dose; as little as 0.1 ml of the combination per 10 lbs body weight produces light anesthesia in most dogs and cats. Concern has been expressed that tiletamine-zolazepam is too costly for routine use by animal shelters, and it is true that the per-volume cost is significantly higher than that of the other commonly used pre-euthanasia drugs, but the low-volume dose (0.1 to 0.4 ml per 10 lb body weight) of tiletamine-zolazepam makes the cost comparable to other drug combinations (Table 24.6). The small dose also increases the ease and comfort of administration to the animal and thereby the degree of safety of the euthanasia technician. The excellent quality of anesthesia induced by the combination greatly enhances the quality of euthanasia that is provided, all factors that should be considered when making a financial decision regarding the feasibility of using tiletamine-zolazepam as a pre-euthanasia agent. Tiletamine-zolazepam is a controlled substance (CIII), approved for use in cats and dogs. It is administered intramuscularly, and may sting.

Sodium pentobarbital is sometimes used as a pre-euthanasia drug, as is the case when it is administered orally with the intention of producing sedation or light anesthesia, or when it is administered intraperitoneally (IP) and then followed with an intravenous or intracardiac injection once the animal is anesthetized. Oral administration of other combinations of the drugs discussed above have been explored (Ramsay and Wetzel, 1998; Wetzel and Ramsay, 1998; Grove and Ramsay, 2000), with good results in some cases. Other drugs that are not widely used (for myriad reasons) but may eventually prove suitable for pre-euthanasia purposes include medetomidine, butorphanol, and buprenorphine.

Physical Restraint during Administration of Euthanasia

No other aspect of euthanasia influences the quality of death an animal experiences as does the method of physical restraint used before and during the procedure. The goal of restraint is multifold: To reduce the animal's fear as much as possible (or at least avoid inducing fear), to control the animal for administration of euthanasia, to control the animal's physical response to the euthanasia method, and to protect the persons administering euthanasia from injury. The methods discussed here pertain primarily to methods used to restrain dogs and cats for intravenous, intraperitoneal, intramuscular, and subcutaneous injections as they are related to the use of pre-euthanasia drugs or drug combinations and euthanasia by injection of sodium pentobarbital, but they can also be used to restrain and prepare

Table 24.6. Cost Comparison of Ketamine-xylazine Combination versus Tiletamine-zolazepam Combination

Cost per ml of Ketamine and xylazine	Cost per ml of Tiletamine-zolazepam	Example for a 10 lb cat
Ketamine (10 ml vial) = $8.93 = $0.89 per ml	Tiletamine-zolazepam (5 ml vial) = $24.83 = $4.97 per ml	Ketamine-xylazine dose = 0.6 ml = 0.6 × $0.81 ml = $0.49
Xylazine (50 ml vial of 100 mg/ml) = $19.95 = $0.40 per ml		Tiletamine-zolazepam dose = 0.1 ml = 0.1 × $4.97 = $0.50
Ketamine-xylazine combination = 10 ml ketamine + 2 ml xylazine = $8.93 + $0.80 = $9.73/12 ml = $0.81 per ml		

Although Tiletamine-zolazepam appears to be more expensive on a volume-per-volume basis, its low dose makes it a comparably priced choice for pre-euthanasia administration.

Prices were obtained from a nationwide veterinary pharmaceutical distributor in December 2002.

animals for carbon monoxide inhalation by those agencies that use that method.

As any experienced animal care professional knows, animal restraint is as much an art as it is a skill. Some people are naturally adept at humanely and calmly restraining animals, most others can learn how to do it, and a few people will never become accomplished at animal restraint because they do not possess the intuition and compassion necessary to the task.

Evaluating the temperament of the animal to be euthanized is the first step in the process. Ideally, whatever information is known about the animal's temperament, whether gleaned from his previous owner or from those who have cared for him during his stay in the shelter, should be made available to the person(s) performing his euthanasia. Observing the animal's response to an approach to his cage or kennel, to removing him from the cage or kennel, and to normal handling should give the euthanasia technician some idea of his temperament, and his need for and tolerance of restraint efforts. When in doubt, the wisest approach is to administer a pre-euthanasia drug or drug combination that renders the animal sedated, tranquilized, or anesthetized prior to euthanasia.

Two people should work together to sedate, tranquilize, anesthetize, and/or euthanize an animal. In determining what method of restraint might work best for a particular animal, the animal's size, temperament, degree of socialization, and physical condition must be considered. Other variables are the skill and experience of the person administering euthanasia and the person assisting him or her, the equipment and drugs that are available, the environment in which euthanasia will take place, and the method by which euthanasia will be administered.

Many dogs who are socialized to human handling can be easily restrained for cephalic venipuncture and direct intravenous administration of sodium pentobarbital. Those who are somewhat fearful or fractious can often be controlled with a muzzle, perhaps aided by the administration of a dose of acepromazine. A dog who cannot be restrained by this method can be sedated, tranquilized, or anesthetized with a subcutaneous or intramuscular injection of a pre-euthanasia drug or drug combination prior to intravenous injection of sodium pentobarbital. Necessary restraint for this procedure may consist only of a leash and/or a muzzle and physical restraint, or

may require restraint of the dog with a control pole or squeeze mechanism. The noose of a control pole should be applied gently but firmly to the dog's neck and used by one technician to hold his head in a corner of the room while the other technician administers an intramuscular injection into one of the dog's thighs. Smaller dogs can be "squeezed" in the corner of a room or kennel; a rubber-coated rack—such as those designed to fit in the bottom of a stainless steel kennel cage to prevent the animal from becoming soiled—works well for this purpose, and is used to gently but firmly restrain the dog against a wall or other solid surface while an intramuscular injection is administered into the muscles of a rear leg through the grate-like openings of the rack. After the injection, the dog can be released or loosely tethered in a confined area and carefully observed until the pre-euthanasia agent has taken effect. A pole syringe can also be used to administer a pre-euthanasia agent, but it is usually necessary for the dog to be confined in such a way that he does not struggle against the needle when it is placed, the result of which can be a broken or bent needle, failed drug delivery, and significant discomfort to the animal. Alternately, an aggressive dog can be given sodium pentobarbital orally, either by placing the powdered drug in capsules and hiding them in balls of canned dog food, or by mixing sodium pentobarbital, in powder or liquid form (Ramsay and Wetzel, 1998), with canned dog food and feeding the mixture to the dog. This procedure should be performed only in a safely enclosed area, and the dog should be carefully monitored until he becomes deeply sedated or anesthetized, usually within 30 to 45 minutes of ingestion of an appropriate dose.

Once a dog is sedated or anesthetized, sodium pentobarbital can be injected into the cephalic vein or lateral saphenous vein. In a deeply anesthetized dog of medium to large size, the sublingual vein can also be easily accessed and used for injection. Administration of an intracardiac injection of sodium pentobarbital to a deeply tranquilized or anesthetized dog is considered acceptable; however, intravenous injection is usually easier to perform than accurate intracardiac injection.

Small puppies who are too wiggly or too small for cephalic venipuncture can be sedated, tranquilized, or anesthetized prior to venipuncture, or be given euthanasia solution by intraperitoneal injection (see the discussion of intraperitoneal administration to cats, later in this chapter). Intraperitoneal injection of sodium pentobarbital is a method not usually applied to adult dogs, because of the large amount of solution to be administered, and because adult dogs are purported to struggle significantly to right themselves as they move slowly through the early stages of anesthesia/euthanasia. However, the method may be applicable to adult dogs in some circumstances.

More cats are euthanized in U.S. animal shelters than any other animal, yet progressive knowledge about how to humanely end the lives of cats has advanced slowly. This author has frequently visited animal shelters where cats are inhumanely killed (drowned, or administered sodium pentobarbital by intrathoracic injection while fully conscious) because personnel are unaware of appropriate and humane methods for cat euthanasia. A large number of cats who are presented for euthanasia are feral or fractious, and even well socialized cats rarely tolerate the close restraint that is necessary to perform venipuncture. The safety hazard an agitated cat presents to the euthanasia technician is significant, but that hazard can be overcome with proper restraint techniques.

A few cats—usually large, well-socialized males—will allow cephalic venipuncture for direct administration of sodium pentobarbital; still others will allow themselves to be restrained for venipuncture of the medial saphenous vein, in which case the person providing restraint holds the cat gently but firmly by the scruff of the neck with one hand, lays her in lateral recumbency, and stretches her somewhat while holding the upper rear leg in the other hand, using the small finger to hold off the medial saphenous vein of the lower rear leg. The person performing euthanasia extends the lower rear leg with one hand and performs the injection with the other.

Conscious cats and kittens (and puppies) can also be administered sodium pentobarbital by intraperitoneal injection (Grief and Schaffer, 1990; Grier, Colvin, and Schaffer, 1996; Rhoades, 2002), either by injecting on the ventral midline caudal to the umbilicus, or on the right lateral side of the abdomen (the left lateral aspect of the abdomen is avoided to prevent injection into the stomach, where uptake may be delayed or even thwarted by the digestive process). Most puppies and kittens and many adult cats will tolerate this method of administration well. To perform the injection, an adult cat or puppy is usually placed on a counter-height surface facing away from the euthanasia technician, who lifts her cranial end by gently scruffing her or placing one hand under the chest to lift her front feet off the surface so that the belly is exposed and the injection can be made. Young kittens and tiny puppies are usually comfortable being gently held in the air by their scruff, and turned so that their belly faces the technician for injection. After intraperitoneal injection of sodium pentobarbital, the animal is placed in a warm, quiet, secure, darkened area (such as a plastic cat carrier, a stainless steel cage with a cover draped over the door, or a transfer cage with a cover draped over the entire cage) while the sodium pentobarbital takes effect and the animal advances through the five stages of anesthesia/euthanasia, a process that may take from five to twenty minutes or more. Kittens and puppies can be placed with the body of their mother (euthanized immediately prior) and/or their similarly injected littermates immediately after injection, so that they experience the warmth and familiar smell of their litter as they become sedated and then anesthetized. The animal is checked every five to ten minutes to ascertain that the drug is having the desired effect, and to verify death once it occurs. The recommended dose of sodium pentobarbital for intraperitoneal injection is two (Grier, Colvin, and Schaffer, 1996) or three (Rhoades, 2002) ml/lb body weight of a 6-grain (390 mg/ml) formulation. As previously stated, concern has been expressed that when sodium pentobarbital-phenytoin combinations are administered by the intraperitoneal method, phenytoin may exert its effect on the heart before the sodium pentobarbital component has caused unconsciousness (Fakkema, 1999). Until more information is available regarding the absorption rates of these two drugs from the peritoneal cavity, it is prudent to use only unadulterated sodium pentobarbital (class II) for intraperitoneal injection.

A cat who is too fractious or unsocialized to be handled should receive a pre-euthanasia drug or drug combination prior to sodium pentobarbital injection. The key to performing such an injection with minimal stress is the means by which the cat is confined when the process begins; the cat is not removed from the confinement until she is deeply tranquilized or anesthetized. Gloves offer little control and increase the chance of injury to the euthanasia technician, while doing nothing to minimize the cat's apprehension. Control poles and cat tongs have enormous potential for injury and abuse, and their use is not consistent with a humane death for cats.

Ideally, the cat is in a plastic carrier or metal transfer cage or trap when the euthanasia process begins; if he is in a larger enclosure, a trap or carrier can be placed in that enclosure and covered with any dark covering, whereupon a frightened cat will usually move into the darkened area. The container can be set on end so that the cat is cornered in the bottom of it and an intramuscular injection of a pre-euthanasia agent or combination of agents can be performed, with or without a pole syringe, through the mesh-like openings of the container. Alternately, the cat can be transferred into a small cage with a squeeze mechanism, and be gently squeezed into a position that allows an intramuscular injection to be performed. A squeeze mechanism can consist of a cage made expressly for this purpose, or any protective barrier (such as a piece of plywood or plexiglass, or a thick blanket) that can be used to maneuver the cat to one end of the cage without allowing her access to the euthanasia technician. A third method that can be used on cats who cannot be maneuvered into a small enclosure is netting: A fishing-style net is placed over the cat; once the cat (within the net) steps over the rim of the net, the rim is lifted so that the cat is sealed in a loop of the net, at which point he can be gently manipulated into position for intramuscular injection (Humane Society of the United States, undated).

All of these methods allow the cat to be deeply tranquilized or anesthetized, whereupon he can be safely handled for intraperitoneal or intravenous injection. The behavior of fractious and feral cats can quickly escalate, and euthanasia technicians must be careful that their own actions do not mirror those of the cat. Maintaining a calm and persistent demeanor when handling an agitated cat allows the technician to provide euthanasia in the most humane manner possible. For both humane and human safety reasons, agencies that deal with feral and free-roaming cats must commit the necessary resources of time, money, training, and equipment to this particular increasingly common aspect of shelter euthanasia.

EUTHANASIA OF SPECIES OTHER THAN CATS AND DOGS

The task of providing a humane death for species other than cats and dogs is a formidable one. Shelter staff are less accustomed to handling these animals, to dealing with their natural behaviors, and to

protecting themselves from them. Anatomical variation also complicates the task. Euthanasia methods are presented here by species.

Guinea pigs are usually calm animals who can be euthanized by intraperitoneal administration of sodium pentobarbital; as with puppies, cats, and kittens, they should be handled on a counter-height surface and placed in a warm, dark, quiet area while they advance through the five stages of anesthesia/euthanasia. Some hamsters, gerbils, rats, mice, and other small rodents can be held cupped in a hand or by their scruff for an intraperitoneal injection, but some will be quite unsocialized to handling and others will be too fearful of a stranger to allow it. These small animals can be maneuvered or gently "squeezed" with objects such as a plastic margarine dish or lid, a small piece of hardware cloth, or any mesh-like object that can be used to move them into a position that allows access to the abdomen. Because these animals can easily be dropped or quickly escape over the edge of a raised surface, it is a good practice to work with them inside an open-top box or cage placed on a counter-height or lower surface. One milliliter of sodium pentobarbital is an adequate dose for these tiny animals. Careful verification of death should be performed. If death cannot be confirmed, the animal should be set aside in a secure place until rigor mortis has occurred.

Ferrets can be euthanized with an intraperitoneal injection of sodium pentobarbital; restraint is the same as that for a cat or kitten. Ferrets who are not comfortable being handled can be given a pre-euthanasia drug or drug combination appropriate for cats, administered by the same techniques.

Rabbits are notoriously resistant to the drugs commonly used for sedation, tranquilization, and anesthesia. In general, the same pre-euthanasia drugs and drug combinations used for dogs and cats can be used for rabbits, but doses should be doubled. The same is true for sodium pentobarbital, which may be easily given intraperitoneally to rabbits who tolerate handling. Rabbits have large veins in their ears; once they are deeply tranquilized or anesthetized, it is often possible to inject sodium pentobarbital into these veins.

Raccoons, squirrels, and opossums can be tranquilized or anesthetized in the same manner as feral cats: By maneuvering them within a small cage or squeeze mechanism, a pre-euthanasia drug or drug combination (any of those appropriate for cats) can be injected intramuscularly. Death is induced by intraperitoneal injection of sodium pentobarbital once the animal becomes anesthetized. Appropriate care should always be taken to avoid being scratched or bitten when euthanizing wild animals considered to be local rabies vector species.

Skunks are euthanized in the same manner as are raccoons, squirrels, and opossums, but care must obviously be taken by the euthanasia technician to avoid being sprayed. Covering the cage in which the skunk is confined with a dark cloth, working in a quiet area, and proceeding in a calm, quiet, and deliberate manner greatly diminishes the possibility of being sprayed. Once the skunk is maneuvered into position for injection, a pole syringe will keep the technician somewhat out of the line of fire, should there be one.

The "fad pet" popularity of iguanas, other lizards, and snakes over the past few years has left many shelters with unwanted reptiles who must be euthanized. Non-native, venomous lizards and snakes should be handled by a herpetologist who specializes in their care. Contact the nearest large zoo for referral to someone who can help you with these species. Local authorities should be contacted for information about the legalities of handling native snakes and lizards.

Methods for euthanasia of reptiles have been described (Mader, 1996; Burns and McMahan, 1995). Contrary to popular belief, freezing is not considered an acceptable, humane means of euthanizing reptiles. Mader recommends pre-euthanasia anesthesia induced by intramuscular injection of tiletamine-zolazepam (25 mg/kg) or ketamine (100 mg/kg), which should require 15 to 20 minutes to take effect, whereupon sodium pentobarbital is administered by the intravenous, intracardiac, or intracoelemic (intrapleuroperitoneal) route. The location for intracardiac injection of snakes depends on the particular species; a snake's heart is generally located 1/3 of the distance from the head to the tail, and can usually be located by palpation. A lizard's heart can also be palpated, or euthanasia solution can be injected into the ventral tail vein. Intrapleuroperitoneal injection is performed by inserting the needle lateral to the ventral midline in the caudal one-third of the body for snakes and lateral to the ventral midline in the abdominal region of lizards (Burns and McMahon, 1995).

Because of their very slow metabolism, reptiles may seem dead when they are not. Reptile bodies should be secured in a room-temperature enclosure for 24 to 48 hours for observation to verify euthanasia. When euthanasia of a snake or lizard is performed at the owner's request, the owner should be advised to pick up the body at a later date, rather than taking it home with them immediately.

Although Vietnamese potbellied pigs, fad pets of the 1980s, are no longer so fashionable, many are still kept as pets, and pet domestic pigs may also be relinquished to animal shelters. Decreased popularity means that adoptive homes may be easier to find (since fewer pigs are homeless), but euthanasia is occasionally still necessary. A 1:1 mixture of ketamine and acepromazine given at a dose of 1 ml per 10 lbs IM will provide deep sedation/light anesthesia and allow intravenous administration of sodium pentobarbital. The intramuscular injection should be given into the muscles of the thigh. Most pigs scream loudly when handled, no matter how gently; the best way to perform this injection is to maneuver the pig into a corner using a large barrier, such as a piece of plywood or a sorting panel (a plastic barrier designed expressly for the purpose of maneuvering pigs about, commercially available). The euthanasia technician should reach over the barrier and inject into the rear leg muscles while the person holding the barrier distracts the pig's attention. Using a 1-1/2 inch needle will ensure injection is made into muscle rather than overlying fat. Once the pig is sedated/anesthetized, sodium pentobarbital is injected into the cephalic vein, which is obscure but found in the same location as that of a dog.

Birds can be considered in three classes: tiny birds (parakeets, canaries, cockatiels, lovebirds, finches, and so on), mid-sized birds (parrots, cockatoos, macaws, pigeons, small chickens), and large birds (ducks, geese, guineas, peacocks, larger chickens). The more "exotic" mid-sized birds (parrots, cockatoos, macaws) are rarely candidates for euthanasia, and should be referred to a veterinarian who works with those species. The other birds listed here are occasionally euthanized in shelters. Consult with someone who is experienced in handling these types of birds for information about restraint.

All birds have a brachial (wing) vein located on the medial side of the wing near the cubital joint that can be used for intravenous injection of sodium pentobarbital. Severely injured or frightened birds can be anesthetized first with an intramuscular injection of a mixture of ketamine and xylazine, at a dose of 0.05 ml of each per lb for large birds, 0.1 ml of each per lb for small and mid-sized birds. The bird is placed in a cardboard box in a quiet place until anesthetized, and then given sodium pentobarbital into the brachial vein.

Only one drug is approved by the Food and Drug Administration for euthanasia of fish—the anesthetic MS-222, also known as Finquel or tricaine methanesulfonate (Argent Chemical Laboratories, Inc., Redmond, WA). Immerse the fish in a container of 350 ppm MS-222 (350 mg MS-222 per liter of water) for 10 minutes. MS-222 immersion is also an appropriate euthanasia method for amphibian species.

Equine euthanasia is an often inelegant and always potentially dangerous procedure. Even when properly tranquilized prior to sodium pentobarbital injection, a horse can fall suddenly or violently, or rear up, potentially striking his handlers. Horses should be euthanized by two experienced horse handlers, at least one of whom is experienced with equine euthanasia. A pre-euthanasia tranquilizer (xylazine, detomidine, and/or acepromazine) is recommended in all cases. A large volume of sodium pentobarbital must be injected (typically 60–120 milliliters or more); placement of a jugular catheter facilitates injection and enhances the safety of the person performing the injection. An important practical consideration is that arrangements for the final disposal of the body must be made prior to euthanasia, and the horse should be euthanized in a location that allows for removal of the body.

Sheep, goats, and cattle must sometimes be euthanized in a shelter environment. Sheep, goats, and calves who are tractable can be manually restrained and euthanized by intravenous injection of sodium pentobarbital into the cephalic or jugular vein. These species are extremely susceptible to the effects of xylazine, and can be tranquilized prior to euthanasia with an intramuscular injection of a volume as small as 0.05 ml of a 100 mg/ml formulation per 100 lb body weight (0.05 mg/lb). As with horses, disposal considerations must be made before euthanasia of larger members of these species.

VERIFICATION OF DEATH

There is no single method for verifying death immediately after it occurs; a combination of observations is necessary. The corneal and pupillary reflexes as well as the femoral pulse should be absent. There should be no signs or auscultable sounds of respiration. The heartbeat should neither be palpable nor auscultable. Mucous membranes should be pale or cyanotic; the color of the gums, conjunctiva, penis, and vulva may be examined. Rigor mortis, when it occurs, is the most reliable sign; it usually develops within a few hours after death. Rigor mortis may fail to develop in juvenile animals or in animals who are elderly or severely debilitated. Hypothermia at the time of death may slow the onset of rigor mortis, and hyperthermia may speed its appearance and disappearance. When doubt exists as to whether death has occurred, the animal's body should be set aside in a safe place and should be periodically reexamined until death has been absolutely verified. A needle attached to a syringe may be inserted into the heart of an unconscious and presumed deceased animal (and blood aspirated to verify penetration of the heart) to make certain there is no movement indicating a heartbeat is still present. Failure to carefully and accurately verify death of an animal is an unacceptable error. Regardless of the effectiveness of the method of euthanasia used, errors in administration, as well as individual physiological peculiarities of the animals to whom euthanasia is administered, will occur, on occasion resulting in the failure of usual euthanasia procedures to cause the death of the animal.

PERSONAL SAFETY DURING EUTHANASIA

Like many aspects of shelter work, the task of euthanasia is laden with opportunities for injury. Possible injuries include bite and scratch wounds; exposure to zoonotic diseases such as rabies, scabies, ringworm, and leptospirosis; back injuries that result from lifting or restraining large animals; traumatic injuries that result from wrestling to restrain a large dog; punctures or lacerations from needles; mucous membrane exposure to sodium pentobarbital and other drug substances; inhalation of carbon monoxide; and slipping, tripping, and falling, particularly on debris that results from the euthanasia process such as urine, feces, and saliva. The emotional hazards of performing euthanasia have already been discussed.

Many of the hazards associated with euthanasia can be avoided with good work practices, such as proper lifting techniques, keeping work areas clean, well lit and uncluttered, and working together as a team to perform a physically challenging task. Appropriate animal restraint equipment in good working condition, as well as chemical restraint options, are tools essential to euthanasia safety, as is proper instruction in how to use those tools humanely and effectively. Good hygiene practices prevent the bulk of zoonotic disease transmissions. Pre-exposure rabies vaccination is essential for any person expected to perform euthanasia of animals of unknown origin and health history (the population of almost all shelters).

BODY DISPOSAL

Euthanasia does not end when death has been verified; the body of the animal must be disposed in some fashion. Most U.S. animal shelters dispose of animal carcasses in one of three ways: cremation, landfill burial, and rendering. None of these methods is easy or aesthetic; all three have significant drawbacks. Each agency must determine for itself which method is most appropriate for the animals it shelters. A fourth method for disposing of a large mass of bodies—composting—has been described (Glanville and Trampel, 1997). Concerns that the rendered remains of shelter animals might find their way back into commercial pet foods in the form of bone meal or fat have been widely circulated, often in a sensational manner. The FDA's Center for Veterinary Medicine found no evidence of cat or dog remains in the commercially available dog foods it recently sampled; the CVM developed technology for detecting dog and cat DNA in the protein of dog food as a part of this study (FDACVM, 2002), and that technology could potentially be used to alleviate concerns about the final destination of products that are the result of rendering the bodies of animals euthanized by animal shelters.

CONCLUSION

Euthanasia of animals in an animal shelter environment is a vastly different task from euthanasia of owned animals in a private veterinary practice, as different as is euthanasia of animals in a research environment. All of these populations deserve the best quality of death that we can offer them, but the methods for achieving that humane death differ markedly. The greatest incongruity of shelter euthanasia is that research—of the methods, equipment, and drugs that might better serve this popula-

tion of animals and the people who euthanize them—is so desperately needed, yet any form of clinical research performed on sheltered animals undermines the public's trust in the mission of that particular shelter (and of every other shelter, no matter the universal autonomy of U.S. animal shelters), even if such research will benefit animals who will require euthanasia at some time in the future. This accounts for the painfully slow progress of the art and science of euthanasia. We have only one opportunity to end the life of each animal we euthanize; to sacrifice that opportunity to provide a better death for another animal is a difficult choice.

Veterinarians are uniquely poised to bridge the gap between formal knowledge of pharmacology and anesthesiology, and the wealth of knowledge about how to best end an animal's life that this nation's animal sheltering professionals possess. It is hoped that the increased activity and visibility of the subcommunity of veterinarians whose focus is animal shelter practice, manifested recently by the creation of a formal organization, the Association of Shelter Veterinarians, will bring those two populations closer together, for the greater good of the animals they both seek to shelter.

REFERENCES

Anonymous. 2000. Dissents over review process for euthanasia report; board revisits issue. *Journal of the American Veterinary Medical Association* 217(5): 636–637.

Arluke, A. 1991. Coping with euthanasia: A case study of shelter culture. *Journal of the American Veterinary Medical Association* 198: 1176–1180.

Bennett, R. A. 2001. Association disagrees with euthanasia method for avian species. *Journal of the American Veterinary Medical Association* 218:1262.

Chalifoux, A., and A. Dallaire. 1983. Physiologic and behavioral evaluation of CO euthanasia of adult dogs. *American Journal of Veterinary Research* 44: 2412–2417.

Dallaire, A., and A. Chalifoux. 1985. Premedication of dogs with acepromazine or pentazocine before euthanasia with carbon monoxide. *Canadian Journal of Comparative Medicine* 49: 171–178.

Evans, A. Thomas, Broadstone, R., et al. 1993. Comparison of pentobarbital alone and pentobarbital in combination with lidocaine for euthanasia of dogs. *Journal of the American Veterinary Medical Association* 203: 664–666.

Fakkema, D. 1999. *Operational Guide for Animal Care and Control Agencies (Euthanasia)*. American

Humane Association, Englewood, CO, p. 7.

Food and Drug Administration/Center for Veterinary Medicine. 2002. *Report on the risk from pentobarbital in dog food*. February 28.

Glanville, T. D., and Trampel, D. W. 1997. Composting alternative for animal carcass disposal. *Journal of the American Veterinary Medical Association* 210: 1116–1120.

Grier, R. L., and. Schaffer, C. B. 1990. Evaluation of intraperitoneal and intrahepatic administration of a euthanasia agent in animal shelter cats. *Journal of the American Veterinary Medical Association* 197: 1611–1615.

Grier, R. L., Colvin, T. L., et al. 1996. *Euthanasia Guide (for animal shelters)*. Ames, IA: Moss Creek Publications.

Grove, D. M., and Ramsay, E. C. 2000. Sedative and physiologic effects or orally administered (2-adrenoceptor agonists and ketamine in cats. *Journal of the American Veterinary Medical Association* 216: 1929 Ames, IA.1932.

Hornbuckle, P. A., and Beall, T. 1974. Escape reactions to the blood of selected mammals by rats. *Behavioral Biology* 12: 573–576.

Humane Society of the United States. Undated. How to use a net, in *How to do Almost Anything in the Shelter*.

Lagoni, L., Butler, C., et al. 1994. *The Human-Animal Bond and Grief*. Philadelphia, PA: W.B. Saunders Co.

Ludders, J. W. 2001. Another reader opposing thoracic compression for avian euthanasia *Journal of the American Veterinary Medical Association* 218:1721.

Patronek, G. J., and Rowan, A. N. 1995. Determining dog and cat numbers and population dynamics. *Anthrozoös* 8: 199–205.

Pawlaczyk, G. 1997. Gas sickens pound director. *Belleville (OH) News-Democrat* Saturday, July 12.

Plumb, D. C. 1999. *Veterinary Drug Handbook*, 3rd edition. Ames, IA: Iowa State University Press.

Poole, J. 2000. Man succumbs to fumes while putting dogs to sleep. *The Times & Free Press (Detroit)*, Wednesday, March 29.

Ramsay, E. C., and Wetzel, R. W. 1998. Comparison of five regimens for oral administration of medication to induce sedation in dogs prior to euthanasia. *Journal of the American Veterinary Medical Association* 213: 240–242.

Reilly, A. 1994. Making the hard decisions. *Shoptalk* 2nd quarter.

Rhoades, R. H. 2002. *The Humane Society of the United States Euthanasia Training Manual*. Washington, DC: Humane Society Press.

Stevens, D. A., and Gerzog-Thomas, D. A. 1977. Fright reactions in rats to conspecific tissue. *Physiological Behavior* 18: 47–51.

Stevens, D. A., and Saplikoski, N. J. 1973. Rats' reactions to conspecific muscle and blood: Evidence for an alarm substance. *Behavioral Biology* 8:75–82.

Wetzel, R. W., and Ramsay, E. C. 1998. Comparison of four regimens for intraoral administration of medication to induce sedation in cats prior to euthanasia. *Journal of the American Veterinary Medical Association* 213: 243–245.

White, D. J., and Shawhan, R. 1996. Emotional responses of animal shelter workers to euthanasia. *Journal of the American Veterinary Medical Association* 208: 846–849

Wollrab, T. 1998. Euthanasia panel report (Report of the AVMA's April 3–4, 1998 board meeting). *Journal of the American Veterinary Medical Association* 212(11): 1670.

25

Disaster Medicine for Animal Shelter Veterinarians

Mark Lloyd

INTRODUCTION

Disaster veterinary medicine is a growing discipline within both public health and veterinary medicine. Unfortunately it has grown by necessity responding to environmental disasters and growing societal threats. The American Society for the Prevention of Cruelty to Animals (ASPCA), United States National Disaster Medical System (NDMS) and other animal welfare organizations have rallied to provide guidance and funding for disaster medical preparation and response. The Veterinary Medical Assistance Teams (VMAT), supported by the American Veterinary Medical Foundation (AVMF), are just one example of the growing area of disaster veterinary medicine. Taking advantage of resources such as these will facilitate creation of your own veterinary disaster management plan.

An appropriate response is no accident. It requires critical thinking and physical preparation. This chapter is intended to be a starting place for shelter veterinarians. The diverse nature of potential disasters requires diverse planning. Geographic parameters dictate the most likely type of disaster for individual shelter locations. However, the severity of many disasters is the direct result of an unusual occurrence for that geographic area which might be common in another area. For example, four inches of snow in Montana may barely cause one to lift an eyebrow, but in Florida it may have devastating effects.

It is the reader's responsibility to verify all information herein. Lists, dosages, product information and recommendations are subject to the shelter veterinarians' confirmation. Ensure the accuracy of all information prior to use. The shelter veterinarian should use this and other references as a starting place to build their own disaster plan, collect references and create emergency preparation lists.

Unfortunately, demographics and transportation services may also exacerbate a disaster. A focus on elderly or special needs residents in a concentrated area may hinder evacuation. Likewise, escape routes may be overwhelmed for metropolitan areas, coastal areas, or peninsular locations that limit egress. Escape and alternative evacuation routes should be identified and discussed with the staff. A road map clearly marked with the potential escape routes should be included in the disaster plan and discussed. A third-party contact in a distant (safer) location should be used to verify all staff have been accounted for. The disasters most difficult to prepare for are those of malintent. Agri-terrorism is now considered one of the most likely and most effective forms of terrorist activity.

DESIGNING A PLAN

Disaster plans for other entities may be valuable templates from which individual plans can be created and customized. In addition to using another

411

animal shelter's disaster plan, municipal, state and institutional plans are frequently excellent references. A written document plan is the first step to sound preparation. Each plan must be tailored to the location and resources.

Back up provisions may have to be set up well in advance. Trying to purchase an electric generator after a hurricane has been named may be futile or expensive. Plan early.

Don't hesitate to seek assistance. Pride has no place in an emergency situation. Disaster teams like Veterinary Medical Assistance Teams (VMAT) and federal disaster responders were established to assist you. Don't wait until all reserves are empty before asking for assistance from other SPCAs or humane organizations. Ask for help early. That's what they are there for.

ANIMAL CONTAINMENT

Human shelters typically do not allow animals to accompany owners. Potentially traumatic interactions between animals and humans preclude mingling of pets and people. Because of this exclusion, some animal owners may release their pets when they must evacuate. Escaped animals may also be displaced and disoriented by the destruction. They too end up with the animal influx to a shelter in a disaster. It is not recommended that human shelters voluntarily board privately owned animals during a potential disaster.

All animals should receive redundant identification to insure rapid reunion with their owners. Identification collars can be removed, cage cards can be damaged or lost and even transponder ID chip readers can have dead batteries. At least two forms of identification are prudent in a disaster situation. Polaroid[R] or digital photography of each new arrival is ideal and allows assessment by potential owners without entering the animal holding area. Neither requires sending out for photo developing, although a computer is required for printing with digital cameras. The location where the animal was rescued is equally critical information to the signalment. As with all shelter acquisitions, accurate and complete records are critical to reuniting owners and pets.

The animal cages or kennels must be secured with failsafe enclosure locks. Structural challenge to the building can facilitate animal escape if enclosures are not secure. Building collapse is a primary cause of animal mortality in a disaster. Redistribution of animals as space allows can decrease the likelihood of trauma from falling debris. Locations close to interior walls, door frames and wall intersections offer the most protection for both animals and personnel.

New animals that arrive at the shelter should be examined closely, triaged and quarantined as the shelter veterinarian directs. Rabies quarantine or suspect animals must remain in quarantine. They do not yet belong to the shelter. If they must be euthanized, the brain must be submitted for histopathology, and any individual bitten should initiate rabies prophylaxis.

Any animals that must be euthanized or die present a significant disposal challenge in a disaster situation. Electric freezers may be out of service, waste disposal services can be unable to transport refuse, and burial may be impractical. Heavy body bags may contain a carcass for a short time, but standard trash bags lack the integrity required. Consider removal of all carcasses that are stored at the shelter prior to a potential disaster. If frozen carcasses are in a defunct freezer or refrigerator, leave them undisturbed until a better location is determined. The insulation will delay the defrosting and decomposition.

SPECIES

Most shelters are designed as domestic canine and feline husbandry and holding facilities. Disasters may concentrate wildlife on high ground or they may be driven to a protected location. Small mammals, birds and reptiles may be brought to the shelter under unusual conditions. Indiscriminate euthanasia should be avoided if possible. Most states legally protect all indigenous wildlife. Many birds are also protected by the Migratory Bird Act. Special facilities may be required if wildlife is held on site. Rabies vector species cannot legally be translocated in some states to limit the spread of disease. These may include foxes, skunks, raccoons, bats and woodchucks.

Local wildlife officials should be contacted prior to a disaster to make appropriate arrangements. If wildlife species are maintained at a shelter they should be held in quarantine for the duration of their stay. Only a paid, experienced and vaccinated staff member should be allowed to work with captive wildlife.

Birds may be severely affected in a disaster and present a challenge with the limited resources of many shelter veterinarians. Birds have a high metabolic rate and require frequent meals and ad lib water. Birds should be housed in a quiet location. Covering the cage may calm birds. Short transport can be accomplished by placing small birds into a cloth bag. Always check for loose strings that could strangulate the legs. Turn the cloth bag inside out to eliminate risk of the stitching catching bird nails or toes. Handled with care, the forgiving walls of an opaque bag minimizes visual excitation and safely transports many small birds. Wild birds should never be removed from the cage except for medical examinations or treatments. Wrapping birds in a cloth will prevent them from hurting themselves while resisting restraint. Don't wrap too tightly. Birds lack a diaphragm and depend on thoracic excursion to respire. After the wings are examined, they may be folded against the body and the entire bird can be lightly rolled up like a bird burrito to force feed them or perform other procedures. This controls both the talons and the beak if done correctly and increases safety for both the bird and the shelter veterinarian.

Most reptile species, other than venomous snakes, can be safely and efficiently kept in a cloth bag for several days. Most reptiles rest calmly in an opaque soft enclosure. They may be soaked every day or two for rehydration while still inside the bag. Place them in a shallow container of 75–85°F water for 15 minutes. Keep at least half of the bag out of the water to allow easy elevation of the head above the water inside the bag to breathe. Wet bags can become too heavy to lift above the water to breathe without help for small specimens. Soaking 10–15 minutes should be adequate. Rubber or plastic containers with sealable perforated tops also make excellent small reptile or amphibian enclosures and may be stacked. Tight fitting lids on containers are essential for reptiles kept for extended periods. Reptiles should be kept at an ambient temperature of 75–85°F. Feeding should be unnecessary for a week or two at least. If an individual specimen appears grossly or morbidly emaciated, rehydrate first; then a small amount of meat baby food may be administered via gastric tube.

Small mammals may do best if provided with copious amounts of bedding or substrate and a small opaque hiding area. Minimal supplementary heat should be necessary for small mammals unless they are hypothermic, wet or neonatal. Dietary needs vary with species. Shelter veterinarians should familiarize themselves with the most likely species in their area.

REMOTE DRUG DELIVERY SYSTEMS

Shelter veterinarians may be asked to assist in the capture of animals in a disaster situation. Not only wildlife, but domestic species as well, may become displaced and disoriented. Shelter veterinarians should not enter disaster areas, nor should any staff member or the public, without directly notifying the emergency management personnel *first*. A human rescue attempt creates unnecessary risk for emergency personnel trying to save a veterinarian who went out to save a pet. If an attempt is feasible, emergency personnel must be aware, approve of the plan and accompany as needed. Wildlife displacement into urban areas brings humans and animals into close quarters. Most animals wish only to escape, but behavior can be erratic and animals may exhibit a strong fight-or-flight reaction. Carefully and patiently "hazing" the animal toward a perceived exit can be very effective to move animals away from a high-risk area. Push boards (half sheets of plywood with handles on the back) are very effective and safer for personnel than an unprotected approach.

Wildlife or domestics in locations that pose a human hazard may require intervention. Domestic species frequently revert to wild behavior such as fight-or-flight reactions. Following a traumatic event, a thoroughbred may act more like a zebra. Even domestic animals can be dangerous or difficult to manage in a disaster situation without proper restraint. Nets, noose poles, capture sticks or rabies poles may be used if manual capture can be accomplished safely. Manual capture may place personnel or public at unacceptable risk of injury. If the animal must be relocated, remote anesthetic delivery by pole syringe or dart may be the safest choice. The shelter veterinarian must be involved in any use of projectile anesthetic darts. The shelter veterinarian must prescribe the drug, dose and method of delivery.

If the veterinarian is less skilled with the pole syringe, blowpipe or dart rifle, another staff member may be the shooter, but they must work under the direct supervision of the veterinarian. Whether the veterinarian either administers the drug or supervises, he or she bears the responsibility for a safe procedure. It is critical to consider human safety first and foremost. No drug should be used without first making sure that critical emergency information is on site in case of accidental human exposure to the drug. Injecting a human with a large animal dose of anesthetic can be lethal. Dart pistols and rifles should be handled with the same respect accorded any firearm. The user as well as the audience should be muzzle aware at all times, loaded or not.

The perimeter of the scene must be free of onlookers and staff, and evaluated for safety. The shelter veterinarian should receive instruction in the use of projectile darts. Several training programs are available throughout the country, including some by the author. Training is highly recommended for the shelter veterinarian prior to the purchase of any darting equipment.

Two pieces of information should be immediately available to the shelter veterinarian considering use of a remote drug delivery system. First, the shelter veterinarian should have a reference for the pre-calculated doses of the veterinarian's drug(s) of choice for all species likely to be encountered in a disaster, and potentially requiring immobilization. See Table 25.1. The combination of tiletamine and zolazepam (Telazol) is a frequent choice. The lyophilized form is very stable, stores well and allows multiple dilutions and variable potency. Other drugs can be freeze dried by pharmaceutical companies according to the preference of the shelter veterinarian. Opiates and alpha-2 agonists are common choices for hoof stock remote immobilization.

Second, the shelter veterinarian should have accidental human drug exposure information on site prior to the use of any projectile drug delivery device. This should include every drug that may be used. The information should include trade name, chemical and/or generic description, emergency treatment for human exposure, contact information

for the manufacturer and antidote/reversal agent if available. The author recommends that the information on both the dose and the emergency procedures be printed on laminated cards for durability and kept with the immobilization equipment. See Table 25.2.

INFECTIOUS DISEASE

Infectious disease is always a concern in any transient animal facility such as a shelter. This concern is compounded by the potential contamination of water and food supplies. Disaster conditions may enhance disease transmission. Vectors may multiply rapidly to carry transmissible diseases. Flooding may act as a mechanical vector to spread disease into and throughout a shelter. Moist conditions may promote fungal and bacterial growth in the environment. Wet conditions may also compromise disease defenses. Wet conditions cause maceration of skin and nails. Nails and hooves are more susceptible to fungal and bacterial invasion.

Diseases of particular concern for wet conditions include arthropod vector diseases such as malaria, West Nile virus, equine encephalitis, and other arboviruses. Water contamination by flooding may contain giardia, coccidia, *E.coli*, and vermiform ova.

TRAUMATIC INJURIES

Traumatic injuries may occur from falling objects or from structural damage. Climbing or walking across wreckage and sharp objects can cause lacerations.

Table 25.1. Sample Emergency Dose Chart for Dart Immobilization of Wild or Dangerous Animals

Telazol: For darting, reconstitute to 500 mg/ml by adding one ml sterile water

Animal	Dosage (mg/kg)	Dose (mg)	Volume (ml)
Dog small	3–6	50	0.1
Dog medium	3–6	100	0.2
Dog large	3–6	200	0.4
Dog giant	3–6	400	0.8
Domestic cat	4–7	50	0.1
Skunk	4–7	50	0.1
Opossum	4–7	50	0.1
Raccoon	4–7	100	0.2
White tail deer	1–4	500–100	1–2 (1–2 entire vials)
Black bear	2–4	1000–1500	2–3 (2–3 vials)
Moose	2–4	1000–2000	2–4 (2–4 vials)

Note: No claim is made for dosages or product information accuracy, for example only.

Table 25.2. Sample Human Exposure Emergency Information Card

Front	

Telazol: Tiletamine hydrochloride and zolazepam hydrochloride	

Concentration	500 mg / vial, variable reconstitution dilution
Pharmacological description	Injectable dissociative anesthetic tiletamine and nonphenothiazine tranquilizer zolazepam. Nonnarcotic, Nonbarbiturate.
Action	CNS and respiratory depression, tachycardia, muscle fasciculations, emesis, salivation
Specific antagonist	None
Manufacturer	A.H. Robins (312) 299-2206

Back	

Emergency Human Medical Treatment for Accidental Exposure	

1. Place patient in a recumbent position, lying down if unconscious. Loosen belt and collar.
2. Wash exposure site with copious water.
3. Observe for abnormal behavior, vomiting, somnolence, drowsiness, and hallucinations.
4. Call for emergency medical assistance if symptoms occur or drug has been injected.
5. Administer CPR and prevent aspiration.
6. Transport to hospital.

Do not leave the patient alone for at least one hour after exposure to ensure no delayed reaction occurs.

Note: No claim is made for specificity or medical information accuracy, *example only*.
Consult appropriate medical professional before recommending any medical treatment.

Hypothermia may be caused by the combination of exhaustion and excessive heat loss from adverse environmental conditions. The most common causes of large animal deaths in disasters are traumatic injuries. According to Hurricane Action Guidelines for Country Property, most fatalities are victims of structural collapse, electrocution from downed wires or auto collision due to fence compromise (see Appendix 25.1). If the pasture is free of hazards and enclosed with a sound fence, it is the safest place for large animals in most severe weather with the exception of blizzard. Entanglement in fence wire or other debris is also a common cause of trauma to the extremities. Horses often have trauma to the rump from flying debris because of their tendency to face downwind.

Small animals and many large animals experience severe effects from exposure. The most common manifestations are renal failure from dehydration and hypothermia. The initial examination and treatments should be based on the assessment of hydration and core body temperature. Absence of external traumatic injuries may be a poor indicator of physical condition.

Minimize flying debris inside the shelter and around the perimeter by removing potential projectiles from the area. Loose objects on the wall or on shelving should be stored. Unanchored landscape or cleaning tools, buckets, planters and other items in the general vicinity can pose a safety hazard if not stored.

WATER

Many types of disasters can precipitate water contamination. Flooding is the most obvious source of contaminated wells and water systems. Contamination may also occur with any hazardous material spillage, carcass runoff and salination.

Sufficient water should be stored for 14 days consumption by all animals and staff. A conservative estimate of at least 50 ml/kg/day per animal can be used for estimation of water requirements. This is in addition to any alternate water requirements. Water for personal hygiene, cleaning, dishes, flushing toilets and cooking are in addition to the metabolic needs of animals and staff. Water for some alternative uses may utilize nonpotable water.

Sealed plastic drums are readily available and can be used to hold large volumes of both potable and nonpotable water. Chemical disinfectants such as sodium hypochlorite 5.25 percent (laundry bleach) may be used to preserve water for consumption. For small volumes to consume immediately, 2 drops per quart for 30 minutes can be used to disinfect drinking water. For water storage containers, one teaspoon per gallon can be used. Organic compounds inactivate chlorine. It is essential that water to be disinfected is free of organic debris. Other disinfectants include iodine. Plastic containers may adsorb the iodine in long-term storage. The plastic may become stained and make it difficult to tell that the water has clarified and may no longer be protected by the iodine for safe storage. Iodine may be best used for immediate consumption but the flavor is distasteful to many people. Thyroid disease may be incompatible with consumption of iodine. It may be used as a secondary choice.

Water can also be purified using appropriate micro-filtration. Several manufacturers have inexpensive hand pump models (under $100) available from camping/backpacking stores. When considering purchase of a water filter, examine the claims and terminology. Two key factors should be considered: the effectiveness and the estimated gallon life. A micro-filter may be ceramic or made of paper reinforced with plastic. The term "water filter" indicates adequate filter materials to remove particulate matter and pathogens over about 10 microns in diameter. This excludes giardia and most vermiform ova from the filtered water. A "water purifier" indicates removal of bacteria and may also remove viruses. Filters must be labeled with the efficacy information. Examine them carefully. Water purifiers may "remove" viruses and bacteria with disinfectants such as iodine. Removal of elemental and pollutant contaminants is available with some purifiers (heavy metals, minerals, odiferous sulfur compounds). Activated charcoal or other chelators are used to remove many contaminants and may drastically improve palatability.

The approximate gallon life is available from most manufacturers as well. It is a measure of how much water the filter can "clean" before becoming clogged or otherwise expired. The manufacturers' estimate is a convention under a standard set of conditions that allows model comparison. The exact life span in total gallons filtered will depend on a number of factors. The most effective filters also are the most easily clogged by sediment because of the microscopic pore size. Salts and mineral deposits such as calcium carbonate can obstruct the filter but their concentration in water varies. A prefilter or sedimentation tank can greatly extend filter life. Calcium deposits can be removed with a mild acid such as vinegar pumped through the filter, then rinsed with water to remove the vinegar. Evaluate the filter to match your needs.

Emergency water sources may be available in a disaster. If water quality concerns arise, use the most contaminated for the least critical requirements. Save the cleanest water source for human consumption. Potential sources include toilet tanks and roof runoff. Toilet tanks on the back of the unit may hold a small volume of emergency water. Prepare for loss of water pressure by saving water in troughs, aluminum boats/canoes and trashcans. If large containers such as these are filled prior to a wind emergency (hurricane, tornado), the water will stabilize the containers in the wind and provide emergency water after the primary event. Empty soda bottles and rinsed milk containers may be filled with water and placed in the freezer. The frozen water containers will act as emergency clean water sources. They also provide a supply of sealed ice containers that keep the well-insulated freezer cold, long after it may be nonfunctional. Always leave freezers and refrigerators closed if power is interrupted to insulate the contents. Ice may remain frozen for several days in a closed freezer.

FOOD

Assume that food availability will be interrupted for two weeks. Even in a disaster of short duration, the domino effect on public services can be extended. Food storage should be in waterproof containers and elevated from the floor. Vermin proof storage is essential to decrease the risk of contamination. If canned food is used, a manual can opener should be available if the electric can opener is nonfunctional.

Refrigeration will be lost if electric power has been interrupted. Nonrefrigerated food is highly preferable. If foods require refrigeration, frozen water containers can be employed as a refrigerant. Dry extruded or pelletized food is voluminous, but the least expensive form of reliable nutrition. Canned food is more durable and will tolerate total immersion in water. However, cans are heavy and create more refuse.

NATURAL DISASTERS

Tornadoes

Tornadoes are one of the most devastating local disasters. Strong winds from any cause may create similar damage. Very few causes other than tornadoes create wind speeds over 150 mph. The localized and episodic nature of a tornado requires planning and preparation well in advance of the event, in lieu of any specific warning of imminent danger. In areas prone to tornados, specific shelter reinforcement may mitigate the damage from high winds. Tornado strapping for the building, strong shutters for the windows and an emergency sub-floor escape room for staff, are shown to limit structural damage and save lives.

In the event of a direct tornado impact, a small emergency shelter below ground level may be the cheapest, most effective protection available. A space just large enough for all staff to hide for a few minutes during the short tornado passage over the building is all that is required. However, the construction of a sub-floor emergency shelter may require integration into the original construction plan. It is difficult and expensive to design an above ground tornado shelter as safe as one below ground level. Shelter veterinarians should be involved in shelter design.

The shelter veterinarian should also be familiar with the tornado classification scale. Unfortunately the scale has only limited predictive value. Tornadoes give little warning, although documented weather systems provide conducive conditions for tornado formation. However, tornadoes occasionally come as clusters in a geographic area. A severe tornado in the vicinity should alert a shelter veterinarian to prepare for the potential of another near them. The local emergency management agency (EMA) should be consulted for specific advice on tornado preparation for that area. See Table 25.3.

Hurricanes

Hurricanes combine the force of the wind with torrential rain and flooding. Although the wind speeds seldom rival those of a severe tornado, the sustained structural challenge may last for hours or days. Structures such as animal shelters and caging are frequently rated for wind speed tolerance. Keep in mind that a 100 mph wind is not the same as a 100 mph tree limb. As with a tornado, potential flying debris should be removed from the general vicinity of the shelter. Shelter structural modifications should be utilized in

Table 25.3. Fujita-Pearson Tornado Scale

Scale	Wind speed (mph)	Expected damage
F0	40–72	Light
F1	73–112	Moderate
F2	113–157	Considerable
F3	158–206	Severe
F4	207–260	Devastating
F5	261–318	Catastrophic

locations prone to tropical storms. The local EMA should be consulted concerning structural modifications appropriate for the area. Near coastal areas, saltwater storm surges can salinate an otherwise safe water source as well. Storing water for a rainy day may sound strange, but it is prudent for a hurricane.

Hurricanes, as well as other causes of flooding can cause electrical malfunction and pose a shock risk. Electrical panels (breakers or fuse boxes) should be turned to the off position as soon as flooding is expected. Adequate supplemental lighting must be available.

Unlike tornadoes, advance warning and storm monitoring of hurricanes is extensive. However without a reliable form of communication, updates and information are unavailable. The shelter veterinarian should ensure a battery-operated radio with a backup set of batteries is on the premises. Weather alert radios are inexpensive but limit types of information available. Automobile radios are reliable as a last resort for weather information. Mobile phones may be nonfunctional and should not be relied upon as the emergency backup. Inexpensive short-range walkie-talkie type radios may enhance communication among staff in larger facilities or if individuals must venture outside alone. However, they are incapable of providing outside contact in most situations.

Shelter veterinarians should be aware of the category and relative severity of hurricanes to help evaluate the preparation and determine whether evacuation may be prudent. Evacuation should occur at least 72 hours prior to hurricane landfall. If any staff remain they must contact the local EMA to advise them how many personnel are there and the immediate plan for the animal shelter in the storm. EMA instructions should be followed completely. See Table 25.4.

Table 25.4. Saffir-Simpson Hurricane Scale

Category	Wind speed (mph)	Tidal surge (ft)	Expected damage
1	74 – 95	4 – 5	Minimal
2	96 – 110	6 – 8	Moderate
3	111 – 130	9 – 12	Extensive
4	131 – 155	13 – 18	Extreme
5	>155	>18	Catastrophic

Earthquakes

Earthquakes are relatively frequent in active tectonic locations. The shelter veterinarian should be aware of the earthquake potential for that area. Most earthquakes in North America occur in Alaska. However, tectonic activity and earthquakes can occur in almost any location. Strict construction requirements usually support earthquake safe structures. Many shelters are older buildings that may have been built prior to new regulations. A walk through assessment by an EMA representative and written evaluation can be used for seeking funding for improvements to comply with newer construction requirements.

Tsunami created by deep-sea earthquakes can affect coastal community shelters. Seward, Alaska received the 1963 All American City award only to be destroyed by a tsunami in 1964. The city was rebuilt and won the 1965 award, too. Check with your local EMA for the tsunami warning system in your area. Shelter veterinarians should have a good comprehension of the relative strength of earthquakes according to a standard Richter scale. It is a logarithmic scale; each number represents a 10-fold intensity increase over the last. See Table 25.5.

MANMADE DISASTERS

Fire

Fire is the most common disaster and almost always caused by humans. A comprehensive fire prevention program should be in place for every shelter. Maintaining an area free of combustible materials around the shelter can decrease wildfire risk. The shelter veterinarian should be involved in a complete fire inspection by the local Fire Department and be included in planning shelter fire drills.

Hazardous Materials

Hazardous material spills, including oil spills, are serious business. Haz-mats should be left to

experts (Fig. 25.1). If you suspect a hazardous material accident has occurred, use the following as guidelines.

- Protect yourself—If you get hurt, you immediately become a victim instead of a responder.
- Move upwind and upgrade from the location.
- Call for assistance. Use any means available.
- Report: exact location, number of casualties, signs and symptoms, and weather conditions.
- Isolate the area. Set perimeter limits to exclude all individuals.
- Avoid becoming contaminated yourself.
- Do not touch the container. Look for other containers.
- Gather any victims upwind.
- Avoid or preserve any evidence.
- Assist EMA upon arrival in cold zone: decontamination, first aid.

Chemical-Biological Disasters

Shelters are unlikely targets for intentional chemical and biological dispersal. However, they may be close to a potential target. The El Paso Animal Control kennel is only a few hundred yards from the busiest international bridge in the US, the Bridge of the Americas. Shelters may also receive animals that have been contaminated or exposed, and brought to the shelter following a chemical or bio-

Table 25.5. Richter Earthquake Scale

Scale	Relative severity
4	Minor tremors
5	Moderate intensity
6	Strong earthquake
7	Severe damage in urban areas
8	Devastating in urban areas

logical agent release. In either case, the response should be similar to a haz-mat accident.

- Protect yourself. Use personal protective equipment before you think you need it.
- Contact the local EMA. Report: exact location, number of casualties and signs/symptoms.
- Establish a generous "hot zone" in which everything is considered contaminated, consider it a reverse sterile field.
- Triage and quarantine all animals and personnel within the hot zone.
- Establish a "warm zone" in which decontamination can occur to move patients out.
- Allow only properly equipped emergency personnel to enter hot or warm zones.
- Allow only uncontaminated or decontaminated animals, personnel or items to enter the cold zone.

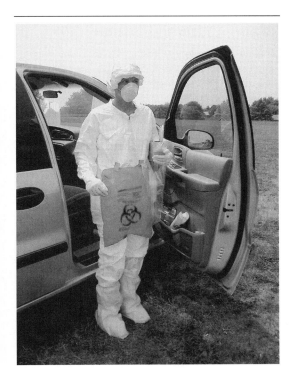

Figure 25.1. VMAT teams are available within hours to support the shelter veterinarian in distress, and they are trained in biosecurity, haz-mat, and natural disaster response. Photo courtesy of Mark Lloyd, DVM.

Chemical weapons are unfamiliar to most veterinarians. A shelter veterinarian should be familiar with a few of the most common types. There is a great deal of concern about the use of certain zoonotic disease agents as biological weapons, and shelter veterinarians would be well advised to familiarize themselves with the appropriate measures to take and contacts to make whenever such an incident is suspected, but it is beyond the scope of this textbook to discuss in detail. The ASPCA Animal Poison Control Center (APCC) is an excellent resource to contact whenever the use of chemicals or biological agents is suspected (888 426-4435 or www.appc.aspca.org; there is a fee.). Another useful source of information is the Center for Disease Control (www.cdc.gov). The AVMA also has extensive information available for veterinarians regarding the zoonotic diseases most likely to be of concern: plague, anthrax, tularemia, and Q fever. They also issue biosecurity alerts (www.avma.org). It is particularly important that shelter veterinarians be familiar with these diseases because of their contact with strays and other animals with unknown medical histories.

Examination of an animal in question may enable the shelter veterinarian to treat in lieu of confirmation of the diagnosis. If any question exists of possible chemical or biological contamination, examine animals only using personal protective equipment. See Table 25.6. Caps, masks, gowns, and other protective garments should be worn whenever dealing with animals that may be suspect for any zoonotic disease.

Petroleum product spills occur relatively frequently. Because of the familiarity of these compounds it is easy to forget they are hazardous chemicals and they should be handled as such. Whether the petroleum contamination is the disaster itself or the consequence of a larger catastrophic event, due care should be exercised in personal contact with the product. Often contaminated animals are handled extensively by well meaning individuals who have come to the rescue.

Do not touch contaminated animals or objects without protective equipment. Do not allow any staff member or volunteer under your supervision to touch anything contaminated with petroleum products. Every drop of water that runs off an oiled duck's back is hazardous waste. Before handling or attempting to decontaminate oiled animals, contact appropriate authorities.

Table 25.6. Common Chemical Agents Signs and Symptoms

Agent	Odor	Symptoms/Signs	Therapeutics
Nerve agents	Fruity	Miosis, salivation, vomiting, diarrhea, urination, twitching	Atropine 2-PAM
Vesicants (blister agents)	Garlic, geraniums, new cut hay	Immediate or delayed reaction, swelling and fluid filled vesicles, coughing, choking	British-Anti-Lewisite, external decontamination
Cyanide	Bitter almonds	Bright red mucus membranes and skin, gasping for breath, nausea	Sodium nitrite, sodium thiosulfate, decontamination

Respiratory mycoses with opportunistic fungi such as Aspergillus are common sequelae to a toxic insult. Delayed mortality can be high in apparently recovered animals. Immediate treatment with an antifungal may be most effective.

Decontamination of animals should be left to professionals specially trained in hazardous material disposal. Tri State Bird Rescue and Research is one organization dedicated to treating animals and training responders to handle petroleum product spills (www.tristatebird.org). If a veterinarian wishes to be involved in treating oiled animals, specific training should be obtained.

VOLUNTEERS

Many shelters are understaffed and may depend heavily on volunteers. Use of volunteers is discouraged in a disaster situation. If volunteers must be used, they must follow strict guidelines for their own safety. A strong volunteer coordinator is essential to maintain order in a disaster situation. The shelter veterinarian may have too many other responsibilities to directly coordinate volunteers effectively. Each volunteer should comply with the following:

- Agree to work assignments solely under the discretion of the volunteer coordinator.
- If uncomfortable with an assignment, agree to notify coordinator immediately.
- Agree not to leave the area without notifying the volunteer coordinator.
- Agree not to enter the shelter without notifying the volunteer coordinator.
- If unable to fulfill a scheduling obligation, agree to make every reasonable effort to contact the volunteer coordinator to allow time for a replacement to be found.
- Agree to sign in upon arrival and sign out if leaving the immediate area.

- Understand not to be compensated for time or expenses incurred while volunteering.
- Provide critical emergency information:
  - Emergency contact and relationship (name, address, phone)
  - Blood type
  - Drug allergies, other allergies
  - Medical conditions

CONCLUSION

A shelter veterinarian should seek and request assistance early and involve local responders in the planning stage. They should be made aware of your final disaster plan. Communicate with them immediately prior to a disaster and inform them of the shelter location, situation and immediate plans. Emergency planning agencies exist at every level of government. Many humane organizations have assistance readily available. Take advantage of their work.

Make your own plan from the resources available. If local responders are overwhelmed, other emergency groups are available as well. The Veterinary Medical Assistance Teams (VMAT) sponsored by the AVMF and deployed by the NDMS, are available at all times to respond to veterinary emergency situations throughout the US and its territories. Make a formal request for support *before* you think you need it. Remember, there will be a lag time in the response. Emergency responders are usually glad you have the situation under control by the time they arrive. Again, don't be afraid to ask for help early. Be prepared. Appropriate Disaster Response is No Accident.

Tables 25.7 and 25.8 are intended as template lists of suggested equipment that a shelter veterinarian may require in a disaster situation. Modify lists to suit individual needs.

See Appendix 25.1 for a list of references and suggested reading.

Table 25.7. Shelter Veterinarian Personal Jump Kit

Personal Protective Equipment (PPE)
PPE is essential to personal safety. A basic set of PPE should be included in individual Jump Kits

Item	Description	Comments
Highly Recommended		
Particle masks	Particle filter masks (sx) adequate Charcoal masks remove odors and some noxious chemicals	Soil quickly both inside and out, more than one may be useful
Eye protection	Light goggles preferred Glasses with side protection may suffice	May be required even with prescription lenses, may be more critical for contacts
Eye wash	Sterile saline or lens solution, Use with or without contact lenses	Cup attachment enhances rinsing performance
"Rubber" gloves	Individual preference: Latex, PVC, Powder free, hypoallergenic	Several pair may be useful Sterile gloves not typically required
Surveyor's flagging tape	Any bright color, A partial roll is adequate (10 ft)	Easy distance identification of locations, equipment or individuals in lighted locations
Safety lights	Cylume-type cool light sticks and/or battery operated safety lights	For identifying personnel, equipment or location in limited light conditions
Ear plugs	Working, traveling or sleeping in high noise areas is common	Helpful even for snoring cohorts when in close quarters
Fire	Two clear large butane lighters	Water proof matches are a second choice
Whistle	Loud simple whistle allows location in distress, high noise areas or in poor visibility	Yelling only leads to rapid laryngitis
Personal knife and / or multitool	Pocket folding knife, one or more	May include other components (can opener, screw drivers, etc.)
Sunscreen	SPF 15 or greater	User dependent but prudent for most individuals to carry
Waterless disinfectant	For hands, work surfaces	Access to soap and water may be intermittent on work site
Personal first aid kit	Commercially available or individually prepared	Personal first aid supplies and medications 14+ days, examine contents of commercial types
Flashlight(s)	Both hand held types and headlamps are useful, water resistant/proof, lightweight	Identical batteries in all electronics allow interchange, plus one spare set
Water resistant/proof watch	Durable, light weight, with fast drying band	Essential to medical procedures and rendezvous
Optional PPE		
Tyvek coverall suit	1-2 sizes larger facilitates wearing over uniform	Useful even without bio-chem contamination concerns
Disposable bonnet	Useful in contaminated or dirty conditions	Washable hat may be second choice
Disposable boot covers	Useful in contaminated environment	May be used to keep shoes clean of simple debris / mud
Candles	Inexpensive tea candles avoid waste and dripping	Long periods w/o electricity will drain flashlight batteries quickly

(*continues*)

Table 25.7. (*continued*)

Personal insect repellent	D.E.E.T. most effective, eucalyptus-based also proven effective	Pump spray or creams preferred. Sonic repellents ineffective.
Mosquito head net	Arthropod population blooms may be sequel to flooding	Small volume, disaster dependant
Emergency mini-strobe light	Personnel or Location beacon in poor light conditions	Inexpensive small models available (especially around Halloween)
Plastic bags	Several 30 gallon trash, and heavy gallon resealable, quart resealable	1001 uses: trash, poncho, wet cot or seat cover, visual barrier, equipment cover, clothing protection, warmth, etc.
Hard hat	Seldom required, but may enhance safety in disaster areas of structural compromise	Personal hard hat may be more comfortable or convenient. Require large packing space. Attachable headlamps available.
Duct tape	Regarded by many to be an essential	1001 uses

Personal Needs

Highly recommended

Sunglasses	Light and UV protection type	
Extra eyes	Extra contacts or eye glasses	Second pair prudent
Toilet paper	Small personal amount prudent to be able to cover your needs	Don't leave home without it. Keep in waterproof container.
Personal prescription medications	Two week supply in waterproof containers	May be refilled in emergency situation by emergency medical staff *IF* available
Over-the-counter Medications	Especially analgesics, antacid, antidiarrheals, antihistamine, etc.	May be redundant with first aid kit.

Optional Personal Needs

Regional topographic and road maps	Lat-long maps may be useful if a GPS is avail. Directional sign are often the first structures lost.	Even if shelter is not flooded, escape routes may be. Alternate routes should be discussed.
Compass	Light, simple, inexpensive	Useful even in urban locations
Small portable radio *with earphones*	Real-time weather / news may be valuable but unavailable	Interchangeable batteries with other electronics (flashlights, and so on)
Hygiene products	14 day + supply, towelettes, toothpaste, deodorant, talcum, personal hygiene	Stressful situations may precipitate diarrhea, menstruation, viral out-breaks etc.
Suture material	Swaged needle, NON-absorbable, braided suture most versatile	Multiple uses: wound closure, pack or clothing repair, floss, etc.
Hemostat / forceps	Non-sterile, multiple uses	Delicate manipulations
Scissors	Personal and professional uses	Several sizes may be useful
Mirror	Personal Hygiene, Emerg. signal	Unbreakable preferred over glass
Small cooler	Drugs, drinks, food, hot or cold	Soft compressible pack best
Water sterilization chemicals	Iodine tablets, sodium hypochlorite (chlorine bleach)	Prudent to use if any question of contamination exists
Water filtration / purification	Inexpensive lightweight models available which remove protozoa, bacteria, viruses, and many contaminants	Water (including tap) may be contaminated in disaster. Boiling much more difficult and does not remove most contaminants.
Personal water container	Every individual should maintain a personal water cache (1–2 liters)	Hydrate early and often

Table 25.7. (continued)

Travel-size laundry detergent	Occasional hand washing of clothes may be required even in urban areas	Laundry facilities may not be readily available.
Personal soap	Sm. liquid soap in reseal bag facilitates dry packing	Accommodation dependent
Camera and extra film	Dry bag may be prudent to keep camera in for safety	Photos of pets, facility, damage. Water resistance consideration.
Small collapsible cooler	Pharmaceuticals, personal drinks	Soft side coolers fold for storage
Small pack	Hip pack, backpack (2500-3500 cubic inch), carry bag, etc.	Paperwork, PPE, other key items may be more easily transported.
Foam pad	Thin, waterproof, ultra light, small, greatly increases comfort	Mission dependent, cot or seat cushion pad. Large pack volume.
Useful		
Cash	Small bills. Hard currency may be unavailable. Banks closed.	Computer connections for "plastic $" may be lost.
Moist towelettes	Bathing facilities availability variable.	Personal reusable wash cloth and hand towel second choice.
Snacks (human, nonperishable)	Restaurants and grocery may be closed for extended times	Some to share (?)
Identification including affiliation	Must be provided upon request at any disaster scene	Wearing I.D. as necklace en route and on site assists security
Uniforms / work clothes / boots	14 + day supply	Multiple changes optimal.
Seasonally appropriate personal clothing	Synthetics dry most rapidly. Two changes per day optimal in hot or dirty conditions	You never have too much clean underwear or dry socks. In resealable waterproof plastic bags.
Raingear	Lightweight compressible	Prudent in any environ. or season
Hat with brim	Rain or sun protection	Season / user dependent
Warm layers of clothing	Layers allow comfort control	Season / disaster dependent
Shoes	Second pair to allow boots/feet to dry out	Light weight, quick drying

Table 25.8. Task-Oriented Checklists

Animal handling and restraint equipment

Ropes	Collars	Tranquilizer dart equipment	Burlap bags, towels
Halters	Gloves	Muzzles and/or	and blankets
Lead rope	Push boards	construction materials	Portable fence
Leashes	Dog control stick/ rabies pole	Crates/animal carriers	Portable dog runs

Equipment for escue operations

Fire extinguisher	Tie-down straps	Wire cutters	Leather punch
Flares	Bungie cords	Bolt cutters	Crowbar
Sling	Tarpaulin	Shovels	Car jack/pneumatic jack
First aid (personal)	Rope	Hammer	Channel lock pliers
Axe	Gloves	Nails	Lock grip pliers
Sledgehammer	Knife	Saw	Hand winch "come-along"

Appendix 25.1:
Resources for Disaster Planning
(Including Acquisition Information)

MANUALS AND BOOKS

1. Auerbach, P. S., and Geehr, E. C., eds. 1989. *Management of Wilderness and Environmental Emergencies* 2nd ed. St. Louis, MO: C.V. Mosby.
2. AVMA. 1991. *AVMA Emergency Preparedness and Response Guide*. 1931 N. Meacham Rd., Suite 100, Schaumburg, IL 60173-4360. (847) 925-8070, Fax (847) 925-1329.
3. Chan, S.D., Baker, W.K. Jr., and Guerrero, D.L., eds. 1999. *Resources for Crisis Management in Zoos and Other Animal Care Facilities*. American Association of Zoo Keepers. 635 W. Gage Blvd. Topeka, KS 66606-2066. www.aazk.org.
4. Rhode Island Disaster Animal Response Team. 1994.*RIDART Manual*. 120 Haswill Street, Providence, RI 02886. (401) 738-2513.
5. U.S. Department of Transportation, Research and Special Programs Administration, Office of HazMat Initiatives and Training (DMH-50). 2000. *2000 Emergency Guidebook*. Washington, DC 20590-0001. (202) 366-4900, fax (202) 366-7342. http:\\hazmat.dot.gov.

BROCHURES AND PAMPHLETS

1. California Veterinary Medical Association, *Disaster Planning for Horses*. 5231 Madison Avenue, Sacramento, CA 95841. (916) 344-4985.
2. California Veterinary Medical Association, *Disaster Planning for Dogs, Cats and Other Pets*. 5231 Madison Avenue, Sacramento, CA 95841. (916) 344-4985.
3. Sarasota County Emergency Management, *You and Your Pets Preparing for Hurricanes*. 1660 Ringling Blvd., Sarasota, FL 34236. (941) 951-5283. Fax (941) 366-7383.
4. Sarasota County Emergency Management and A.H.O.O.F. The Sunshine State Horse Council, *Hurricane Action Guide for Country Property*. 1660 Ringling Blvd., Sarasota, FL 34236. (941) 951-5283. Fax (941) 366-7383.
5. Schroeder, R. J., ed. 1987. Veterinary services in disasters and emergencies in *Journal of the American Veterinary Medical Association*, 190(6):701–799.
6. Humane Society of the U.S., Southeast Regional Office, 1624 Metropolitan Circle, Suite B, Tallahas-

see, FL 32308. (904) 386-3435. (Some materials also available online at www.unr.net/~Lbevan/adpac.)
   Guidelines for Developing an Animal Disaster Plan for Your County
   Disaster Planning for Animal Shelters
   Disaster Planning in Shelter Design
   Guidelines for Evacuation or Euthanasia of Shelter Animals in Disasters
   Guidelines for Pet Friendly Public Evacuation Shelters
   Guidelines for Developing a Community Animal Disaster Plan for People with Special Needs
   Animal Health Alert
   The Humane Society of the U.S. Offers Disaster Planning Tips for Pets, Livestock and Wildlife
   Disaster Relief Incoming Form
   HSUS Emergency Disaster Care Card
   HSUS / Red Cross, Pets in Disasters: Get Prepared
   HSUS Brochure, Disaster Relief: Every Victim Counts
   HSUS Booklet, Disaster Relief: Designing a Disaster Plan for Your Community
   June 1994 HSUS Close-up Report: Surviving Disasters
   November 1994 Shelter Sense Issue on Hurricane Andrew
   Spring 1996 HSUS – Southern Regional Office Report on Hurricane Opal
   A Suggested Checklist for Items and Supplies Needed in a Disaster Involving Animals and the Community

SELECTED ONLINE REFERENCES FOR DISASTER AND EMERGENCY INFORMATION AND INTERNET LINKS

1. American Society for the Prevention of Cruelty to Animals: www.aspca.org/site/emergency
2. Bioterrorism Learning Center: http://bioterrorism.digiscript.com/
3. American Veterinary Medical Association (AVMA): www.AVMA.org
4. Center for Disease Control: www.cdc.gov
5. Veterinary Medical Assistance Team 1 (VMAT1): www.VMAT1.org
6. American Humane www.americanhumane.org

Section 5:
Animal Cruelty

INTRODUCTION

The AVMA has several policy statements regarding its position on various animal welfare issues. Its policy on reporting animal abuse states "The AVMA recognizes that veterinarians may observe cases of animal abuse or neglect as defined by federal and state laws, or local ordinances. When these situations cannot be resolved through education, the AVMA considers it the responsibility of the veterinarian to report such cases to appropriate authorities. Disclosures may be necessary to protect the health and welfare of animals and people. Veterinarians should be aware that accurate record keeping and documentation of these cases are invaluable" (AVMA 2002 Membership Directory and Resource Manual). Most texts on veterinary ethics also support the position that veterinarians are morally bound to report suspicions of animal abuse to the appropriate authorities. The AVMA's Model Veterinary Practice Act (AVMA 2002) and the American Association of Veterinary State Board's Practice Act Model (www.aavsb.org) both recommend that cruelty to animals be considered grounds for disciplinary action against a veterinary licensee. Many state practice acts have actually done so, and some states mandate reporting animal fighting or animal abuse to the appropriate authorities.

Despite these positions and increased awareness about the link between animal abuse and human violence, the growing strength of the human animal bond and the elevation of penalties for animal abuse from misdemeanors to felonies in many states, veterinarians remain uncertain about their role in reporting animal abuse. The concerns exist for a number of reasons; lack of recognized, published standards defining animal neglect versus abuse, concerns about confidentiality clauses in veterinary practice acts regarding medical records and the civil liability attached to reporting, concerns about personal safety or retaliation when dealing with poten-

tially violent clients, loss of personal income, concern about time lost testifying in court, and so on. A key point that is frequently misunderstood by veterinarians is that reporting is justified if a reasonable "suspicion" of abuse exists based upon the results of the physical examination. The veterinarian need not be certain that abuse has occurred in order to make a report. The report simply launches the investigation that will uncover the facts necessary to determine whether or not criminal abuse has indeed occurred.

The veterinarian who works for a shelter is usually confronted with animal abuse in a much more direct fashion—animals are typically presented for an assessment of their condition where abuse is already suspected and a confirmation is sought based on the physical evidence in the form of the victim, whether deceased or alive. This section in the textbook attempts to bring together information that both private practitioners and shelter veterinarians will find useful when dealing with animal abuse. Patronek provides an overview of the laws governing abuse as well as a description of the common types of abuse and methods of dealing with them in chapter 26. Reisman describes the examination of the live patient, record keeping and documentation of the evidence in a manner consistent with the successful prosecution of a cruelty case in Chapter 27. Leonard provides the veterinarian with a new perspective on performing forensic necropsies by including information about crime scene investigation in chapter 28. In chapters 29 and 30, Cheever and Dinnage rely heavily on their own experiences investigating equine abuse and animal fighting to provide background information on these activities, guidelines on how to recognize the characteristic injuries associated with them and management recommendations.

The reader is referred to the 1997 American Humane Association publication, "Recognizing and

Reporting Animal Abuse, A Veterinarian's Guide"
for a much more comprehensive discussion of the
link between animal abuse and human violence and
other issues related to recognizing and reporting
animal cruelty. Other references for more information are included at the end of chapter 27.

REFERENCES

AVMA, 2002. Membership Directory and Resource
    Manual. Schaumburg, IL AVMA.
AAVSB, www.aavsb.org.

26
Animal Cruelty, Abuse, and Neglect

Gary J. Patronek

INTRODUCTION

This chapter will discuss three scenarios that every veterinarian working in a shelter must be familiar with in some depth—abuse arising from husbandry-related neglect, the special case of neglect due to animal hoarding, and allegations of abuse arising from the challenges of delivering routine care, handling and restraint in the shelter environment. One other area, deliberate or intentional cruelty will be discussed only briefly.

Complexity of Shelter Practice

Animal shelters operate near the extremes or margins of human-animal interaction. Because of their role as both a safety net and avenue of last resort for animals, they encounter the best as well as the worst of human behavior. For veterinarians, animal shelters bring challenges that differ qualitatively and quantitatively from those encountered in private practice. Shelter culture is vastly different from private practice, and this adds an unexpected level of emotional intensity to the medical care of animals and interaction with the public (Balcom and Arluke, 2001). The simple fact that healthy animals must sometimes be euthanized adds enormous stress and creates an environment where caregivers often must construct complex psychological coping mechanisms to get through their day. Employees, volunteers, board members, and myriad community groups involved with shelters often have very strong feelings about the efforts spent on care, rehabilitation, and adoption of animals perceived to have been abandoned, abused and rescued, particularly when euthanasia is a possibility (Arluke, 1991). Shelter veterinarians will inevitably need to deal with the medical aspects of various forms of abuse, ranging from deliberate cruelty to unintentional neglect. On a technical level, abused animals presented to a shelter may include a surprising variety of domestic, wild, and exotic species, with diverse temperaments, husbandry needs and inclination to cooperate for medical care. The care that is given will be delivered in what has been termed a very public "fishbowl" where the decisions and actions of the veterinarian may be subject to close scrutiny coupled with sometimes unrealistically high expectations. Shelters with government funding are likely to operate with an even greater degree of formal or ad-hoc public oversight than private shelters.

Regulatory Issues

From a regulatory perspective, shelter veterinarians are likely to work in an environment that may put them square in the middle of a complex web of municipal, state, federal, and potentially even international laws and treaties. Ironically, despite this complexity, the general practice of sheltering lacks universally agreed upon standards of practice and an overarching regulatory body. The primary federal law that affects some companion animals in at least a limited capacity, is the Animal Welfare Act (AWA). The AWA regulates the care of warm-blooded animals used in exhibition to the public (zoos, circuses), scientific research (universities, industry), transported commercially, or bred commercially for resale (www.aphis.usda.gov). The AWA requires that covered species must be provided with adequate care and treatment in the areas of housing, sanitation, nutrition, water, veterinary care, and protection from extreme weather and temperatures. In 2002, an amendment to the Farm Bill codified in law prior U.S. Department of Agriculture (USDA) regulatory policy to exclude rats, mice, and birds from protection. The AWA does NOT regulate animal care by private pet owners, local kennels, hobby breeders, retail pet stores, or shelters. However, the current trend for some shelters to import large numbers of animals from other states or other countries for adoption has some industry and breeder groups claiming that they are in effect acting as dealers, and should be regulated under the AWA (Strand, 2002). To date, this has not occurred.

To help prevent trade in lost or stolen pets, the AWA provides for licensing of 'Class B dealers', that is, individuals who sell former pets to research facilities. When these former pets are obtained from shelters, the practice has been termed 'pound seizure'. To date, 14 states have passed legislation prohibiting pound seizure (Table 26.1). In the states where animal shelters are either required to comply (five states) or are not specifically prohibited from complying (31 remaining states) with requests from research facilities for unclaimed animals, then private shelters who provide animals for research are regulated as dealers and have certain reporting and holding requirements for animals. If you believe that you are dealing with a situation covered under the AWA and have questions, it is best to contact a regional USDA veterinarian for advice (www.aphis.usda.gov).

The regulatory environment is more complex at the state level. Twenty states have some kind of state law regulating animal shelters, thirteen states require animal shelters be registered or licensed, fourteen states authorize the inspection of animal shelters, four states require the establishment of an advisory board, and three states also require shelter personnel to complete some training (Table 26.1). At least seven states require some form of training for animal control officers and two provide for regulation of foster care groups (Pullen, 2002). Two states have statutes that mandate reporting of shelter intake and exit statistics to the state. Colorado has one of the most comprehensive statutes defining shelters and various other forms of pet rescue groups (Colorado Pet Animal Care and Facilities Act, 1999). California recently instituted a far

Table 26.1. Distribution of State Laws Affecting Shelter Operations in the United States

States with laws regulating animal shelters[a]	CT, FL, GA, IL, IA, KS, LA, ME, MD, MI, MO, NH, NJ, NY, NC, RI, SC, TX, VT, VA
States requiring licensing of animal shelters	GA, IL, IA, KS, ME, MD, MI, MO, NH, NJ, NC, RI, VT
States in which animal shelters are inspected	CT, FL, GA, IL, KS, MD, MI, MO, NH, NY, RI, SC, TX, VA
States requiring an advisory board for shelters	LA, ME, MO, TX
Training required for shelter personnel	LA, TX, VA
Training required for animal control officers	CA, FL, ME, MI, NJ, NM, VA
States with some regulation of fostering organizations	VA, CO
States in which shelter statistics must be reported	VA, MI
States with consumer protection laws applicable to pets	AR, AZ, CA, CT, DE, FL, ME, MN, NH, NJ, NV, NY, PA, SC, VT, VA
States in which pound seizure is prohibited	CT, DE, HA, ME, MD, MA, NH, NJ, NY, PA, RI, SC, VT, WV
States in which pound seizure is required for government-run shelters	IA, MN, OK, SD, UT
States in which customary farming practices are exempted from cruelty statutes	AZ, CO, CT, ID, IL, IN, IA, KS, MD, MI, MO, MT, NE, NV, NJ, NC, OR, PA, SC, SD, TN, UT, WA, WV, WY

[a]Some state statutes (for example, PA) may indirectly regulate shelters if they cover any facility that kennels dogs

reaching statute that regulates many aspects of animal shelter operation, including the provision of veterinary care, but so far laws of this scope are the exception rather than the rule (Balcom, 2000). Some states or municipalities may have regulatory language for licensing of kennels and retail pet stores that may also include shelters because they "kennel" dogs, even though shelters are not specifically named.

Seventeen states have remedies for consumers who purchase certain species of pets from a commercial establishment (Table 26.1). Sixteen are state laws and one is by regulation (MA). All seventeen states cover dogs but three (CA, DE, PA) do not cover cats. One (NH) includes ferrets. In all seventeen states, a consumer can exchange the dog or cat for another dog or cat, or get a refund (HSUS Government Affairs Section, Email Communication 2002). It is believed that these laws have not yet been applied to shelters or similar non-profit rescue groups. However, it would be worthwhile for shelter veterinarians to be aware of the statutes in their states, since it is not unreasonable that as the line between shelter and rescue and pet stores becomes more blurred, these statutes could be extended to cover shelters or remote, off-site adoptions of shelter animals located at pet stores. At minimum, shelters should consider how they measure up to these standards.

HUSBANDRY-RELATED NEGLECT

Shelters receive animals from several different sources (animals turned in by owners, strays brought in by animal control or the public, and animals rescued by humane agents or police), and inevitably some will be victims of various degrees of cruelty. In addition to just receiving animals, some shelters proactively investigate situations where animals may be suffering because of deliberate, intentional cruelty or neglect. As a result of their investigations, shelters may remove animals from at-risk situations and take them into custody for protection, rehabilitation or medical care. Taking an animal into protective custody against the owner's wishes may involve a variety of administrative, civil or criminal procedures that will be unique in each state. Therefore, the specifics of the process, and the agency with the statutory authority to seize a neglected animal, may vary considerably. In cases where animals are removed as the first step in a criminal proceeding, the animals seized have a special status—they are evidence that a crime has been committed, and as such, it is essential that veterinarians take great care to document their condition in ways that will stand up in court. These precautions have been covered in several references (Stroud, 1998; Munro, 1998b) and in chapters 27 and 28 in this text.

Which Animals Are Protected

Although the majority of animals handled by local shelters are domestic pets that will be covered by state anti-cruelty laws and/or local ordinances, exceptions are becoming increasingly frequent as the public becomes more enamored of exotic pets, wildlife, and even endangered species that may be excluded by cruelty statutes or subject to regulation under other laws. Any of these can, and do, end up in shelters, and the regulatory authority surrounding their ownership and care can become complex. A thorough discussion of the web of local, state, national, and even international laws and treaties that may regulate or otherwise affect care and ownership of exotic species is beyond the scope of this chapter, and the reader is referred to several excellent web sites (www.le.fws.gov, www.ipl.unm.edu, www.endangered.fws.gov). Only the most salient points are summarized below.

Language in individual state animal cruelty statutes will determine whether a specific animal is protected under state law (www.megalaw.com). In some states, ownership per se is required in order for the duty of care provisions to apply. This definition can be quite broad, and there may be language stating that anyone who cares for, possesses, controls, or otherwise has or assumes custody of an animal is considered legally responsible for its care. Therefore, it is possible for someone feeding stray animals (for example, feral cats), or caring for the animals of a friend, to have the same duty of care as if they were the owner. Not all species of animals will be protected, or protected to the same degree, in every state. The seemingly simple task of even defining an "animal" is not always straightforward. Some state statutes simply say "animal", while others go to great lengths to specify which animals are included or excluded. For example, the Delaware statute defines animals as "excluding fish, crustaceans, and mollusks", the Kentucky statute refers to "every warm-blooded creature except a human being", the Indiana statute specifies "vertebrates", the South Dakota statute specifies "mammals, birds, reptiles, amphibians, and fish", the Georgia statute specifies that animal "shall not include any fish nor shall such term include any pest that might be exterminated or removed from a business, residence, or other structure" whereas the New Jersey statute defines animal as the "whole brute creation". Louisiana and South Carolina specifically exclude poultry. Other factors that may determine whether an animal is protected include ownership and/or domestication status, and in some cases the intent of the perpetrator (for example, if the act was committed willfully or maliciously).

The definition of which wild animals are covered under the state anti-cruelty statute is inconsistent from state to state. For example, the New Hampshire statute covers a "wild animal in captivity", whereas Oklahoma covers any "mammal, bird, fish, reptile, or invertebrate including wild and domesticated species". In Texas, an animal includes a "wild living creature previously captured"; in Iowa, the statute includes non-human vertebrates but excludes game unless it is controlled or confined by a person; and in Tennessee, an animal includes a "captured wild creature". These distinctions are often critical. On March 19, 2002, a jury in McLennan County, Texas, found a former Baylor University baseball pitcher innocent of misdemeanor cruelty for shooting, beating, and then decapitating a cat, because the court found that the statute, which defined animals as "domesticated or captured creatures" did not apply to feral cats (Animal People, 2002).

The protection of wildlife will also be determined by whether or not they are a federally protected or endangered or threatened species. For example, the federal Migratory Bird Treaty Act covers all migratory birds except for pigeons, house sparrows, and starlings (Bean and Rowland, 1997). It is illegal to possess or trade in any of the above migratory birds (dead or alive), their eggs, nests, or feathers without a permit for rehabilitation, education, or scientific research. Exceptions would include regulated hunting (for example, waterfowl) or special permits to remove nuisance birds. In the event a veterinarian was asked to provide care to an injured bird, a grace period would apply to allow for emergency medical care, with the understanding that the bird would be transferred to a licensed rehabilitator as soon as practical after stabilization (O'Rourke, 2002). The permit process is regulated by the U.S. Fish and Wildlife Service (USFWS) (www.permits.fws.gov) and permits can be obtained through 7 regional bird permit offices (www.permits.fws.gov).

The US Fish and Wildlife Service works with states and other governments to prevent illegal take or trafficking in protected species, to protect wildlife from environmental hazards and safeguarding critical habitat for endangered species, and works to solve wildlife crimes, among other things. This is accomplished through a central and seven regional law enforcement offices (www.le.fws.gov). Under the U.S. system of government, federal law regulates interstate and international commerce and trade in animals, but other than the licensing provisions previously mentioned in the AWA, generally does not regulate ownership per se, which is left up to the states. Under federal law, importation and interstate sale of endangered or threatened species is prohibited, except for the offspring of animals present in the US prior to the 1973 law (www.endangered.fws.gov). This "offspring" provision, as well as the failure of federal law to regulate ownership per se, leaves a large loophole that has fostered a thriving traffic in exotic pets, both on the Internet and via animal auctions and dealers.

Each state has the authority to regulate the use of its native wildlife and to prohibit possession of certain species of wildlife. Typically, these prohibitions are included due to concerns about public safety or the potential impact on native wildlife if released. Occasionally, these statutes can affect animals considered pets. For example, private ownership of the domestic ferret remains illegal in California and Hawaii because those states continue to define these animals as wildlife. In many states, it is illegal to translocate or re-release certain species after capture, especially rabies vectors, locally or across state lines.

The offices of the state veterinarian (responsible for animal disease control and outbreak investigation, particularly in farmed species), the state public health veterinarian if one exists (responsible for public health concerns and zoonoses), and the department of fish and wildlife (both game and non-game wildlife) are also very useful contacts to establish for information concerning regulation of wildlife species. The on-line directory of state and local officials is an easy way to locate these individuals (www.fda.gov).

Actions Prohibited by Cruelty Statutes

Anti-cruelty statutes in every state have established certain duties and responsibilities for owners towards animals in their care, and also prohibit certain acts. All statutes have at least broad language prohibiting deliberate acts of cruelty and inflicting unnecessary physical pain and suffering. There will also be some language specifying that covered animals be provided adequate food, shelter, and necessary veterinary care to relieve suffering, or conversely, prohibiting depriving an animal of food, water, or shelter. What exactly constitutes "necessary pain and suffering" is left to interpretation. This is exactly the type of situation where veterinarians should be considered the experts. In addition to ambiguity within states, laws across different states are not consistent in their language or scope. Some statutes try to specifically define terms such as "cruel", "neglect", "abandonment", and "proper shelter". Regardless of the level of detail in the language, there is always room for some interpretation, which is where the professional judgment of a veterinarian is critical.

Actions Exempted by Cruelty Statutes

Thirty states specifically exempt all or some normal or customary agricultural practices (Wolfson, 1999). Twenty-five of these states prohibit the application of cruelty laws to all customary farming practices (Table 26.1) (Wolfson, 1999). However, deliberate cruelty or extreme neglect can still be prosecuted, as long as it does not fall under the customary practice exemption. There is at least one recorded case of a successful felony prosecution of workers on a large scale industrial hog operation, but the offenses involved deliberate mistreatment that was not part of normal husbandry procedures (www.peta-online.org). Other practices commonly exempted from state anti-cruelty statutes include biomedical research, hunting and trapping, and pest control. New Jersey is currently the only state that exempts dog training:

> The training or engaging of a dog to accomplish a task or participate in an activity or exhibition designed to develop the physical or mental characteristics of that dog. These activities shall be carried out in accordance with the practices, guidelines or rules established by an organization founded for the purpose of promoting and enhancing working dog activities or exhibitions; in a manner which does not adversely affect the health or safety of the dog; and may include avalanche warning, guide work, obedience work, carting, dispatching, freight racing, packing, sled dog racing, sledding, tracking, and weight pull demonstrations (New Jersey Permanent Statutes).

Evaluating Husbandry Standards

The first line of reference should always be any applicable state or local statute or code, although as previously mentioned, these are often vague. Another point of reference is the AWA. AWA guidelines provide specific details for the care of hamsters, guinea pigs, and rabbits, in addition to dogs and cats. It is essential to recognize that the standards promulgated in the Act do not specifically apply to privately owned pets, and that it would be a mistake to infer that they do. They could, however, be used to bolster a veterinarian's opinion of proper care, particularly in non-regulated institutional settings such as shelters or sanctuaries, since the AWA standards are understood to represent minimum, not optimal, care (www.aphis.usda.gov/ac/cfr/9cfr3.html#3.1, www.aphis.usda.gov/oa/pubs/awact.html).

Livestock provide a special challenge, since anything that can be considered "customary practice" in a farming situation is often exempted. Animal science textbooks and agricultural extension services, as well as any veterinary library, are a good source of information about customary practices. For livestock, there are well-accepted body condition scales for horses (Henneke, 1995; www.ihahs.org, equinenet.org) and cows (Wildmann et al., 1982) that could assist in documenting failure to provide proper nutrition.

For native wildlife, the two main national bodies governing wildlife rehabilitation, the National Wildlife Rehabilitators Association and the International Wildlife Rehabilitation Council (IWRC), publish joint husbandry standards (www.iwrc-online.org) intended for anyone engaged in rehabilitation of wildlife. Some state statutes have incorporated these standards by reference, and they will be incorporated in an upcoming revision of the federal Migratory Bird Treaty Act (MBTA), making the bird portions binding on all federally licensed rehabilitators. A key point here is that proper standards are based on the animals' needs, regardless of numbers and types of wildlife cared for, budget size, number of paid or volunteer staff, and size and location of activity.

Surprisingly, universally accepted husbandry standards may be the most lacking for the most commonly kept domestic animals—pet dogs and cats. In one study, dogs were the animal most commonly reported being neglected (Donley, Patronek, and Luke, 1999). This is probably because of the greater visibility of dogs compared to cats, and the belief that outdoor cats can fend for themselves. A determination of whether or not the caretaker's duty of care has been breached and criminal negligence exists will be heavily influenced by a subjective assessment of the animal's physical state and living conditions. In order to establish the presence of neglect, a good rule of thumb is to consider three factors: the number of problems present, the duration of the problems, and the severity of the problems. It is this last factor that poses the greatest challenge for quantification. At the most basic level, it is the veterinarian's training and professional opinion about proper care and housing that will guide the evaluation. However, making such distinctions has been shown to be an area of great discomfort for veterinarians. Surveys of veterinarians have indicated that published guidelines would greatly increase their confidence in where to draw the line between an explainable lapse in normal care vs. neglect (Donley, Patronek, and Luke, 1999; Sharpe, 1999)

In order to more objectively gauge severity of husbandry-related neglect for dogs, a simple system, the Tufts Animal Condition and Care (TACC) scales, has been developed to allow for easy scoring of the degree of neglect in 4 different areas: body condition, weather safety (exposure to temperature extremes), environmental health, and physical care. (See Appendix 26.1.) The scales were developed with the assistance of the Fort Wayne Department of Animal Care and Control in Fort Wayne, Indiana and the Law Enforcement Division of the Massachusetts Society for the Prevention of Cruelty to Animals. The TACC scales originally appeared in the first manual on animal abuse issues for veterinarians (Patronek, 1998). Since then, hundreds of copies of laminated TACC scales have been ordered by animal shelters and control agencies for field use throughout the US. A modified version has been implemented for all cruelty cases brought into the ASPCA hospital in New York City (Reisman,

2001). They have been published by the animal welfare committee of the Canadian Veterinary Medical Association (Crook, 2000), as well as in *Animal Sheltering Magazine* (Humane Society of the United States, 1998).

Body Condition

The most obvious indicator of probable neglect for any species of animal is body condition. The responsibility of an owner or caretaker to ensure that an animal receives proper nutrition is specified either implicitly or explicitly in state anti-cruelty statutes that impose a duty to provide necessary food, or prohibiting starving an animal, depriving it of necessary sustenance, or failing to feed an animal properly. A 9 point scale has been developed to assess body condition in dogs and has been shown to be reproducible and to be highly correlated with radiographic measurements of body fat, with each point representing a 5 percent increase in body fat (Laflamme, 1993). Five points of this scale, representing ideal to emaciated body conditions, combined with elements of another scale (Armstrong and Lund, 1996), have been adapted in TACC (Appendix 26.1). Scoring should be based on both palpation and visual evaluation, particularly for long-haired dogs. A thorough veterinary examination is important for determining whether poor body condition can be explained by reasons other than failure to provide proper nutrition. In the absence of such an exculpatory explanation, the TACC score provides a means of quantifying the extent of the neglect in this domain.

Weather Safety

Most state cruelty statutes impose a duty of care for providing proper shelter for a companion animal. (Note that normal or customary agricultural practice is the standard that will likely apply for livestock species kept as pets.) Regardless of the specific wording, the main point of imposing a duty for proper shelter is to ensure that an animal can maintain normal body temperature, or thermal homeostasis. Thermal homeostasis occurs when there is a balance between heat load and heat dissipation. Heat load is the sum of environmental and metabolic heat (Krum and Osborne, 1997), and heatstroke occurs when heat load exceeds heat dissipation. Clinical signs of heat stroke develop when a dog's body temperature exceeds the species-specific critical threshold (109°F). Physiologically, heat stroke is a multi-systemic disorder precipitated by generalized cellular necrosis. Disorders of acid-base balance and primary renal failure are common sequelae, and even with aggressive immediate treatment, heat stroke is often fatal. The typical case history of naturally occurring heatstroke in dogs often involves forced confinement to a hot environment, such as a parked car, exercise, or tethering in the sun (Krum and Osborne, 1977; Drobatz and Macintire, 1996; Magazanik, Shapiro, and Shibolet, 1980). In these high risk situations, a dog's body temperatures can exceed lethal levels in a matter of minutes. However, there have also been reports of pets suffering severe heat stroke in circumstances that appear to be low risk, including walking with their owner on a hot day (Bardsley and Saunders, 1987), exposure to direct sun through the window of a car while riding with their owner (Caird and Mann, 1987), or even a heavy coated dog walking with its owner on an apparently cool evening (Pengelly, 1987). In a review of 42 canine cases, exercise was a factor in 45 percent, 28 percent involved confinement in a closed environment, and 19 percent were just exposed to a warm environment (Drobatz and Macintire, 1996).

Dogs cool themselves primarily through panting, which increases heat loss from the respiratory epithelium in the lungs and nasal turbinates. Therefore, dogs with a brachycephalic conformation have lower heat tolerance than dogs that are phenotypically moderate. In general, dogs are much more sensitive to heat stresses than cold stresses, and have a much lower temperature comfort range than humans. There are size-related differences in heat and cold tolerance as well. Large dogs have more difficulty radiating heat than small dogs, whereas smaller dogs have more problems conserving heat (Phillips, Coppinger, and Schimel, 1981). Large breed dogs with a tendency toward brachycephalic conformation, such as the St. Bernard, may be at very high risk. In conjunction with exercise or high ambient temperature, a heavy hair coat, coupled with large size or obesity, can contribute to a rapid increase in body heat. Exposure to direct sun and inability to reach shade will greatly increase risk, even at temperatures a person might consider comfortable. Experimentally, lack of water in conjunction with high external temperatures has been shown to exacerbate the situation by expediting

dehydration, circulatory collapse, and shock (Assia, Epstein, Magazanik, and Sohar, 1989).

Hypothermia occurs when an animal is unable to conserve heat. In general, dogs are better able to withstand cold stresses than heat stresses. The first line of defense is a normal hair coat. Therefore, if the animal is exposed to sleet or rain in cold temperatures and becomes wet, it can compromise the substantial natural protective ability of a dry coat.

When phrasing such as "proper shelter" must be interpreted in the absence of explicit statutory standards, the provisions in the AWA are a useful baseline reference for evaluating temperature safety since dogs and cats used in research are physiologically no different from pets. The AWA specifies that housing facilities must be sufficiently heated and cooled when necessary to protect them from temperature or humidity extremes and to provide for their health and well-being (www.aphis.usda.gov). The ambient temperature in the sheltered part of the facility must not fall below 50° F for dogs and cats not acclimated to lower temperatures, for those breeds that cannot tolerate lower temperatures without stress and discomfort (such as short-haired breeds), and for sick, aged, young, or infirm dogs or cats, except as approved by the attending veterinarian. Dry bedding, solid resting boards, or other methods of conserving body heat must be provided when temperatures are below 50°F. The ambient temperature must not fall below 45°F nor rise above 85°F for more than 4 consecutive hours when dogs or cats are present. The relative humidity must be maintained at a level that ensures their health and well-being. Outdoor shelters must protect them from the direct rays of the sun, contain a roof, four sides, and a floor, and provide the dogs and cats with adequate protection and shelter from the cold and heat and the direct effect of wind, rain, or snow and provide a wind break and rain break at the entrance. Outside housing areas must contain clean, dry, bedding material if the ambient temperature is below 50° F and additional clean, dry bedding is required when the temperature is 35° F. A lower limit of 50° F is specified for short-haired dogs, for dogs not acclimated to lower temperatures, and for young or aged dogs.

For dogs in particular, it is also important that any evaluation of risk account for the greater heat sensitivity and cold tolerance among breeds with heavy hair coats, compared with short-haired breeds. There is precedent for establishing differential safe temperatures based on dog hair coat and phenotype. For example, the guidelines published by the International Air Transport Association (IATA) for air transport of dogs and other species indicate that the minimum and maximum temperatures for journeys of > 30 minutes duration are 50–75°F for brachycepahlic dogs, 40–80° F for long-haired dogs, and 50–90° F for short-haired dogs (International Air Transport Association, 2002). Temperature safety indices have been developed as tools to determine when it is safe to ship livestock, and these are another published tool that can be used as part of a comprehensive evaluation of care (Grandin, 1995).

The weather safety TACC scale (Appendix 26.1) takes into account the standards promulgated by the AWA as well as various transport regulations to evaluate risk. It also considers a dog's size, age, phenotype, the availability of water, and exposure to direct sunlight when evaluating the effect of temperature. In order to use this scale, the best estimate of the temperature that the dog is exposed to in whatever shelter is available, should be used. For example, the fact that a dog is indoors may be irrelevant if the environment does not allow the animal to maintain thermal homeostasis (for example in an unventilated garage or shed). Conversely, a dog that has access to a well constructed dog house with sufficient hair coat and thick bedding may be able to maintain thermal homeostasis even though it lives outdoors during winter months. It is critical to remember that a dog may be susceptible to heat stroke under conditions that might not be uncomfortable, much less life threatening, for humans. Therefore, it is advisable to err on the side of caution when evaluating the risk of heat exposure for dogs. Small mistakes with heat may cause a dog its life, whereas dogs subjected to cold temperatures may be uncomfortable, especially if they are not acclimated to cold, but the experience is much less likely to prove rapidly fatal.

ENVIRONMENTAL HEALTH

An owner's duty to provide an environment that is sanitary, dry, and safe may be explicitly stated in cruelty statutes, or be implicit in the general duty to provide proper shelter. For example, the cruelty statute in Maine specifies a duty to provide humanely clean conditions, in Maryland it specifically includes a duty to provide proper air and

space, and in Minnesota and Ohio it imposes a duty for providing proper air. Massachusetts requires a sanitary environment. The Michigan statute prohibits overcrowding and specifically defines sanitary conditions as "free from health hazards including excessive animal waste or other conditions that endanger an animal's health". However, all of this wording still leaves much to interpretation, and that is where expert veterinary opinion is essential.

In any cruelty case, it is critical to link prohibited actions or required duties of care in state statutes with the actual conditions observed. Information in the AWA about proper housing and environmental conditions can be a useful checklist and roadmap for a veterinarian evaluating a situation (www.aphis.usda.gov). Factors to consider include:

- Are building surfaces in contact with animals in outdoor housing facilities impervious to moisture?
- Are any non-acceptable structures (for example, metal barrels, cars, refrigerators or freezers) used as shelter structures?
- Are the floors of outdoor housing facilities of suitable material (for example, compacted earth, absorbent bedding, sand, gravel, or grass) and are they replaced if there are any prevalent odors, diseases, insects, pests, or vermin?
- Are surfaces of outdoor housing facilities that cannot be readily cleaned and sanitized replaced when worn or soiled?
- Are structures accessible to each animal in each outdoor facility, and are they large enough to allow each animal in the shelter structure to sit, stand, and lie in a normal manner, and to turn about freely?
- Are floors constructed in a manner that protects the dogs' and cats' feet and legs from injury, and that, if of mesh or slatted construction, do not allow the dogs' and cats' feet to pass through any openings in the floor?

The TACC environmental health scale (Appendix 26.1) provides a rapid method of summarizing these various characteristics. It is a useful supplement to, but not a replacement for, a detailed written narrative accompanied by high quality photographs.

PHYSICAL CARE

When dealing with allegations of inadequate physical care, the courts may not realize that the development of purebred dogs has resulted in some coat types that make it impossible for the dog to adequately self-groom. Therefore, periodic grooming and nail trimming by humans is required in order to maintain health and well-being. Since cruelty laws do not generally impose a specific duty to groom a dog, it is important to explain in some detail how deficiencies in grooming or other physical care cause unnecessary pain or suffering, as opposed to a purely cosmetic situation. It is also important to establish the commonsense nature of these concerns, as opposed to requiring specialty knowledge, as much as possible. For example, a heavily matted dog is under extreme discomfort because of the tension on its skin, interference with normal mobility, and inability to relieve any discomfort or irritation by scratching. Irritation from embedded foreign material, external fecal impaction, and urine scald will be extremely painful. A heavily matted coat will make external parasite control impossible. It is not uncommon for fecal impaction in the perineal hair to lead to maggot infection of the flesh in the perineal region. In the natural state, a dog's nails are kept short through the course of normal movement. However, many domestic pets, particularly those that are confined for extended periods and receive little exercise, require periodic nail trimming. When extreme, overgrown nails can penetrate the footpad, causing pain, lameness, and possibly infection. They also force the feet into an unnatural position, causing gait alterations and discomfort. The TACC scale for evaluating the condition of the dog's coat and nails is shown in Appendix 26.1.

INTERPRETATION AND CAVEATS OF TACC

The method of deriving and interpreting the TACC score is shown in Appendix 26.1. The TACC score is intended to be a simple screening device for developing an index of suspicion that intentional or unintentional neglect may be present. It is important to consider the following caveats. The TACC score is not intended to replace definitive assessment of any animal's situation by a veterinarian or trained law enforcement agent. A low (normal) TACC score does not preclude a diagnosis of neglect or abuse upon more careful examination of the animal and its living situation. For example, an indoor pet in good body condition with sanitary living conditions could still be at risk of many forms of mental and physical abuse. Similarly, a high TACC score indicates a strong suspicion of either acute or chronic neglect,

although it is not necessarily pathognomonic for neglect, particularly if only one scale is used. However, if an animal receives a high TACC score on multiple scales, the probability of neglect is very likely. When multiple scales are used to obtain a TACC score, a dog whose care or condition is sub-optimal in multiple areas is at greater risk of neglect than a dog with the same degree of neglect in only one area. For example, a malnourished dog will be less tolerant of environmental stress than a well-nourished dog of normal body weight, as will a dog whose thermoregulation is impaired by a dirty, heavily matted coat.

UTILITY OF TACC

The TACC system is ideal for initial screening of a dog that may be in danger and for prioritizing reports of neglect for definitive assessment. It has also proven particularly useful when it is necessary to systematically evaluate large numbers of animals rescued in hoarding situations. Because it is based on objective standards, it hopefully will remove much of the subjectivity that has made evaluating cases of animal abuse so challenging.

Psychological Well-Being

One emerging area of concern that most current cruelty statutes do not adequately address is psychological well-being. Although some progress has been made concerning providing exercise for dogs used in research, there is much less legal precedent for addressing quality of life for domestic pets. Some municipalities (www.hsus.org) have prohibited or limited tethering of dogs because of recognition that the frustration produced through chronic chaining poses a threat to human safety. The AWA also prohibits tethering as a primary means of confinement (www.aphis.usda.gov). New Jersey recently incorporated language into a statute regulating pet stores, kennels, and shelters that requires regulated agencies to provide a disease control program that addresses physical and psychological well being (www.hsus2.org). Regulated agencies are required to reduce the negative impact of excess noise, smells, visual stimuli, and perceived threats. The science behind evaluation of stress and distress as a result of confinement, lack of socialization, and the links to behavioral abnormalities is just beginning to be appreciated, and there are now calls for much more attention to this area. However, in most states, once minimum standards of cleanliness, nutrition, and veterinary care are met, there are few avenues available to help a companion animal perpetually confined to a chain, cage, or crate, and deprived of exercise and socialization. Even in child protection, where the issue of psychological well-being is specifically mentioned in state laws, it does not appear that prosecution purely on grounds of psychological distress has been successful (Lockwood 2002). Fortunately, in many cases where psychological distress is present due to neglect, other more actionable violations of the law are also present.

ABUSE FROM ANIMAL HOARDING

There is probably not a shelter in the country that has not had to deal with the problem of animal hoarding. Shelters are often the primary point of intervention for these cases. In these situations, dozens—and sometimes hundreds—of animals are accumulated (sometimes under the pretext of being a legitimate shelter or rescue group), until the individual or agency becomes unable to provide even minimal standards of care. They differ from the run-of-the-mill neglect case because of the number and variety of animals, the severity of their health problems and lack of socialization, the determination of the hoarder to resist all attempts to help, and the tendency for municipal authorities to dismiss the cases as anomalies rather than something part of a larger pattern of abuse.

Most cases are identified because of a complaint by a neighbor, service worker, landlord, or sometimes a family member. When the hoarder claims to be operating a shelter or rescue operation, members of the public or volunteers may make a report. In a typical case, a person is discovered living in squalid conditions with dozens to hundreds of animals, both dead and alive. Animals are frequently ill and malnourished to the point of starvation. Floors may buckle from being soaked with urine and feces, and the air may be difficult to breathe without respiratory protection. By any measure, these cases violate the most basic requirements for sanitary, safe shelter, breathable air, potable water, adequate food, and necessary veterinary care. Cats and dogs are the most commonly hoarded species, but domestic wildlife, dangerous exotic wildlife, and farm animals have been discovered, even in urban situations.

Who Are Animal Hoarders?

Dealing with the animal component of a hoarding case, no matter how extreme, may still be the easy part. The human component is likely to be much more difficult. Hoarding cases are different from other types of abuse because of the lack of intent to cause harm and often a claim of intending to help or rescue the animals. Yet despite these claims of good intentions, hoarders are by definition oblivious to extreme animal suffering that is obvious to the casual observer. The denial seems to serve as a vehicle for continuing to accommodate their own needs to acquire animals. Hoarding is a problem that transcends multiple pet ownership as well as legitimate animal sheltering or rescue, and should not be confused with either. There is mounting evidence that, in at least some of these cases, a mental health component may be present. Unfortunately, until recently, there has been little awareness of the sentinel role animal neglect can play for a range of human health problems. An interdisciplinary research team, the Hoarding of Animals Research Consortium (HARC), was established in Massachusetts in 1997 to study this issue and to increase awareness among mental health and social service professionals and municipal officials. Their definition of animal hoarding was incorporated in a revision of the Illinois cruelty statute in August, 2001 (Illinois Public Act 92-0454). This was the first time animal hoarding was defined in any state law. According to HARC, an animal hoarder is someone who (www.tufts.edu and Patronek, 1999):

- Accumulated a large number of animals that overwhelmed their ability to provide even minimal standards of nutrition, sanitation, and veterinary care
- Failed to acknowledge the deteriorating condition of the animals (including disease, starvation, and even death) and the household environment (severe overcrowding, very unsanitary conditions)
- Failed to recognize the negative effect of the collection on their own health and well-being and on that of other household members.

Although the stereotypical profile of a hoarder is an older, single female living alone and known as the neighborhood "cat lady", in reality this behavior seems to cross all demographic and socioeconomic boundaries. This behavior has been discovered among doctors, nurses, public officials, college professors, and veterinarians, as well as among a broad spectrum of socioeconomically disadvantaged individuals (Patronek and the Hoarding of Animals Research Consortium, 2001). It is unknown if people involved in legitimate sheltering or rescuing efforts are at greater risk than others for becoming hoarders. However, given the fact that this behavior has been documented in a variety of people associated with animal care and rescue, and the tendency of hoarders to gravitate to enablers or enabling situations, every veterinarian should aware of certain warning signs (Table 26.2). Although much remains to be learned about animal hoarding, veterinarians are in an ideal position to communicate the complexity of hoarding situations to the media, public health authorities, and the justice system.

Removal or Rescue of Animals

Ideally, veterinary involvement should occur at the earliest possible stages when a rescue is being contemplated. If possible, it is helpful to include the veterinarian on the investigative team to view the conditions on site. Proper planning is the key to making what will always be a challenging process go as smoothly as possible. You need to be ready for anything and everything—expect the unexpected. Preparation for a large scale rescue is not unlike disaster planning in its complexity and scope. Issues that need to be considered include the following:

SPECIES AND JURISDICTION

Although hoarders tend to concentrate on one species, for example, dogs or cats, it is not uncommon for a menagerie to be discovered. In one recent case, a total of 259 animals, including many exotic and endangered species, were removed from a townhouse by a humane society in Canada (Steinbachs, 2002). The collection was so diverse that expert zoologists were called in just to aid with identification of the species. Proper identification of species is important for providing proper husbandry as well as to determine the legal status of the animal. It is wise to check ahead of time to verify which other parties, if any, need to be notified or involved. The Fish and Wildlife Department in each state or the state veterinarian are probably the best sources of information about which animals are specifically permitted or exempted at the state level. The US Fish and Wildlife Service has seven regional offices that handle law enforcement issues as well as the permitting process for federally regulated species (www.le.fws.gov).

SPECIFIC HUSBANDRY NEEDS

Be sure to familiarize yourself with the normal husbandry of each species present or suspected to be present prior to intervention. Some species may be inherently difficult to handle because of their tem-

Table 26.2. Warning Signs for Animal Hoarding Among Veterinary Clients

Constantly changing parade of pets with few repeat visits
Visits mainly for problems due to trauma or infectious diseases indicating a lack of preventive health care
Rarely see the same animal for diseases of old age like cancer or heart disease
May travel great distances to the practice, come at odd hours, and use multiple vets so as not to tip them off about the number of animals
May seek heroic and futile care for animals they have recently found
Perfuming or bathing animals prior to a visit to conceal odor[a]
Bringing in a relatively presentable animal in an attempt to get medication for more seriously ill animals at home and trying to persuade the vet to provide medication or refills without seeing the animals[a]
Being unwilling or unable to say how many animals they have[a]
Claiming to have just found or rescued an animal in obviously deplorable condition (strong odor of urine, overgrown nails and muscle atrophy), which may be more indicative of chronic confinement in filthy conditions than of wandering the streets[a]
Having an interest in rescuing even more animals, including checking the office bulletin board and questioning staff or other clients in the waiting room[a]

Sources: Patronek, G.J., and Irwin, A. Animal Hoarding—A Hidden Problem. *Keystone Veterinarian-Journal of the Pennsylvania Veterinary Medical Association.* September/October, 2001, p. 22.

[a] Denotes contributions by Irwin (2001).

perament or size. If exotic species, farm animals or birds are to be removed, the standard shelter housing conditions may not be suitable, and special arrangements will need to be made. Depending on the numbers and husbandry needs, can you adequately house the animals at the shelter or will alternative housing be required? Is temporary MASH-type housing an option using portable or collapsible cages or fencing? Would it be preferable to house the animals on-site to provide care? If so, can the site be adequately secured to protect the health and security of the animals and safety of staff? Special accommodations may need to be made if nursing mothers, sexually intact males, females in heat, neonatal animals, or geriatric animals are present. If exotic animals are present, it may mean obtaining special diets and bedding ahead of time. Will the services of a zoo or specialty sanctuary be required? If large animals are unable to rise or need to be removed from confined spaces, will special rescue equipment (hoists, sliding supports, winches) be needed?

CONTAGIOUS AND ZOONOTIC DISEASES

Particularly if species other than those you are completely familiar with are present, it is worth reviewing what types of zoonoses could be present and the diagnostic tools necessary to rule out infection or contagion. For example, in March 1996 in San Mateo County, California 230 goats were seized by a shelter. Subsequently, at least 10 people became ill and were serologically confirmed to have Q fever, which was also documented in the herd (Deresinski 1996). If zoonotic diseases are believed to be present or can be anticipated, what special precautions may be necessary to protect the safety of staff and other animals? Will you need special equipment, protective clothing, new training or staff education to minimize risk of transmission?

Diseases that are contagious to other animals should probably be expected to be present until proven otherwise. What implications will this have for isolation and housing at the shelter or for veterinary treatment? Will you have the required medications in stock in sufficient quantity? Particularly if agricultural species are kept, are there any notifiable or reportable diseases of concern to the agricultural industry in the state that you should be looking out for? The risk of a problem is enhanced when diverse species of unknown origin are mixed and kept under questionable circumstances. It is probably worth

contacting both the state veterinarian and the state public health veterinarian if you anticipate such a situation. If certain contagious diseases are present, the office of the state veterinarian may be able to add some regulatory leverage to your efforts by imposing and enforcing a quarantine of the premises.

CONFINEMENT STATUS

Consider whether the animals are free roaming, tied, or confined in some manner. If free roaming, how will the environmental conditions help or hamper removal? Are certain animals or types of animals confined to specific areas for some reason? Is there an order that must be preserved? Will animals need to be trapped, removed from tight or inaccessible spaces such as walls or ceilings, or lured to a confined area? What kind and how much special equipment will be necessary to accomplish this? This could include traps, baits, squeeze cages, protective gloves or clothing, catch poles, nets, and tranquilizing devices. Will controlled substances be needed for capture? Is there any danger to neighbors or the community if there is an escape? Do you need secondary barriers brought in to prevent escape during capture? Have you allocated sufficient time and staff for a patient and humane capture process? If trapping will be required, is there a plan for access during the extended rescue?

SOCIALIZATION AND TEMPERAMENT

In hoarding situations, you can expect to encounter everything from calm socialized pets to exotic species that cannot be handled without sedation. Your plan must protect the animals from each other as well as protect staff from the animals. What are the implications for the skill level of personnel needed to safely remove the animals, the expected time frame for rescue, transport, veterinary examination, treatment, and housing? If intact males are present, this may pose additional constraints on how quickly and safely the animals can be moved. Consider whether conditions require special capture equipment or personnel with training in capture of difficult or dangerous species, customized transportation and housing, and the availability of veterinary specialists for those species.

COORDINATION WITH OTHER AGENCIES

One of the factors that inhibit optimal resolution of hoarding cases is that shelters tend to tackle these problems alone. A better approach is to identify and coordinate with all relevant agencies and individuals. The list will vary with each situation and each community, but the following should be considered: Health Department, State Veterinarian, State Public Health Veterinarian, State Wildlife Agency, Department of Aging or Adult Protective Services, Child Protection, Mental Health, Sanitation, Zoning, Code Enforcement, and Hazardous Waste management. All of this will be much simpler if the shelter veterinarian has existing professional relationships with some of these agencies. A good place to start would be to introduce yourself to the local health department or public health veterinarian.

EXAMINATION OF ANIMALS

Despite the fact that you may be dealing with a "herd" of animals, it is still important to carefully examine each animal and document its condition in a medical record. Particularly when large numbers of animals and/or multiple veterinarians are involved, triage may be more easily accomplished using an easily scored instrument like the TACC scales. The veterinary examination needs to be done in a careful, systematic manner and documented extensively. These records may end up as evidence in a criminal prosecution or a civil administrative proceeding. A thorough physical examination should be supported by accurately labeled photographs containing unambiguous identification of the animals pictured, and documented in clearly written medical records suitable for presentation in court. A minimum database would include estimated age, an accurate body weight and body condition score, a fecal examination, and a thorough oral examination to establish condition of the teeth. Be sure to review any species-specific features that should be examined and noted.

It is important that the examination be done prior to any treatment that would alleviate or mitigate the conditions present, providing the delay is not contraindicated on humane grounds. Since in the majority of these cases, animals will have been living in the conditions for many months or years, a careful methodical exam should not be contraindicated. Since socialization and temperament may become a factor in the eventual placement of the animals, these characteristics should be noted. If dead animals are present, the bodies should undergo a forensic necropsy to establish cause and approximate time of death. Note any unusual placement, ordering, or attempts to conceal bodies that suggest awareness of the deaths. The evidence collection procedures should be coordinated with law enforcement agencies and prosecuting attorneys to ensure that all relevant evidence is collected and documented in a way that will stand up in court.

THE MEDIA

One additional complication of dealing with hoarding cases is that they are often very newsworthy and become high profile in the media. This will bring a level of public scrutiny to the cases that veterinarians may not expect. Therefore, it is important that they develop good skills in communicating the details of the situation and condition of the animals when the press calls. With media attention, there will likely be a public response to adopt or foster the rescued animals. There may also be great public interest in their health and progress. If euthanasia is likely to be necessary, it is important to remember that the interested public will ultimately become part of that dialogue. A recent article describing how the media have typically reported these cases may be useful to better understand how a well-written medical record can better reflect the extent and duration of neglect and contribution of the hoarder to the situation (Arluke and the Hoarding of Animals Research Consortium, in press).

EUTHANASIA

It is important to have a plan in place regarding euthanasia if it becomes necessary. When an animal is seized under a warrant, then it is technically part of the evidence in the case and cannot be euthanized except in extreme medical circumstances. It is important to consult with the prosecuting attorney ahead of time to develop mutually agreed upon guidelines when euthanasia is necessary to relieve suffering. In some cases, when an animal is in extremis and natural death is imminent, you may have no choice. It is absolutely essential to completely document why this was necessary. However, a more typical presentation is that the animals may not be in extremis, but severely debilitated or very ill. In these cases, saving some lives may be technically possible but not feasible from a practical standpoint because of the severity of their condition. Sheer numbers may sometimes preclude treatment for less serious ailments. All of these scenarios should be discussed ahead of time, and a clear plan of approach documented. In order to protect yourself, it may be advisable to obtain a supporting opinion from a second veterinarian before any animal is euthanized.

All too frequently, euthanasia may be necessary primarily because the shelter is already overwhelmed with adoptable pets, and not because the rescued animals are beyond rehabilitation. In those situations, the ethical dilemma is that making room for a large number of unhealthy, poorly socialized animals would not be justifiable if it meant euthanizing pets that may be more adoptable. This is a very slippery slope, and one that should be considered carefully before a rescue is attempted. It may cause conflict among the shelter staff and volunteers, criticism from the public and adverse attention from the media. It can be difficult to explain why animals that were rescued and that are medically treatable need to be euthanized because there is not sufficient room. Alternative plans should be considered as much as possible ahead of time to see if foster homes, rescue groups, or some form of temporary housing could be arranged that would allow rehabilitatable animals to be saved. If mass euthanasia is necessary, the veterinarian will ultimately be called on to justify it.

Euthanasia in these situations poses logistical challenges that must be addressed as well. At minimum, it should be performed in a manner consistent with the AVMA panel guidelines and all applicable state laws. Where will it be done? If it is done on site, is there a place where it can be done in a quiet, private manner so that animals are not stressed and not in view of each other or onlookers? Have you reviewed techniques for birds, reptiles, or exotic species? Are sufficient drugs available, and if controlled substances are needed, are you prepared for adequate record keeping? How will carcass transport and disposal be handled?

EXAMINATION OF THE ENVIRONMENT

Most of the time, this part of the investigation will be handled by humane officers, animal control, or other police agency. However, since the environment of the animals is intimately linked to their health status and the adequacy of their care, it is advantageous if the shelter veterinarian can personally view and document conditions at the site. Veterinarians are the best trained individuals to comment on sanitation;

water and air quality; adequacy of protection from the elements consistent with the laws governing various species; safety; and general husbandry. Particularly since starvation is such a prominent feature of many hoarding cases, it is essential to carefully document the quantity, quality, and availability of all food on the premises for each species kept. If possible, examine receipts or other evidence of purchase of food. Anything removed from the premises needs to be properly stored, labeled, and secured as it may be needed as evidence.

Humans at Risk

In order to build the most effective case, it is important to take a broad approach to the situation and pay attention to the human and public health aspects that are likely to be present. The public health and elders neglect issues are important aspects of animal hoarding that go largely unrecognized and that may provide avenues for intervention. Careful documentation of the human living circumstances can go a long way to eventually helping the animal victims.

For most hoarders, living spaces are often compromised to the extent that they no longer serve the function for which they were intended. Appliances and basic utilities (heat, plumbing, and electricity) frequently are inoperative. Household functioning is often so impaired that both food preparation and maintaining basic sanitation are impossible. Rodent and insect infestations as well as odors can create a neighborhood nuisance. The clutter can pose a fire hazard, especially if utilities are not working and fireplaces or kerosene heaters are used for heat. Access to electrical outlets, heating ducts, and exits to the building are often absent in hoarding situations and violate municipal codes. Municipal plumbing, electrical, sanitation, and public nuisance codes are often quite specific and can be an avenue for access and intervention.

Despite the high degree of impairment in household functioning, few hoarders seem to meet criteria for mental incompetence or immediate danger to the community, so options for intervention along those lines are limited. The criteria for an administrative search warrant to check for code compliance are typically less stringent than a criminal warrant, so familiarizing yourself with local regulations for human housing can be very helpful when trying to improve conditions for animals. What is not yet widely appreciated is that in many animal hoarding situations other family members, for example, minor children, dependent elderly or disabled adults, are present and are also victims of this behavior (Hoarding of Animals Research Consortium, 2002). The conditions may well meet criteria for adult self-neglect, child neglect and/or elder abuse. In one state (Illinois), veterinarians are among the mandated reporters of elder abuse, and have a legal duty to report these situations (IL Elder abuse and neglect act).

Due to the substantial accumulation of feces and urine in hoarding households, environmental ammonia levels may be dangerously high. Workplace health references list from 35 to 50 ppm as the maximum average occupational exposure during an 8 hour workday (www.cdc.gov). Levels above 25 ppm begin to irritate the nasal passages. The US Occupational Safety and Health Administration (OSHA) lists 50ppm as the maximum workplace exposure (www.osha-slc.gov) and further defines a concentration of 300 ppm as a concentration 'immediately dangerous to life or health' (www.cdc.gov). There is ample evidence in the animal science literature on the detrimental effects of elevated atmospheric ammonia on appetite and weight gain in farm animals. Pigs exposed continuously to 103–145 ppm reduced their consumption of feed and had weight loss. In many hoarding situations, it is difficult for a non-acclimated person to breathe without respiratory protection. This suggests there is good reason to believe ammonia levels may be very high. In one case, an ammonia level of 152 ppm was recorded after the home had been ventilated by the fire department (Lembke, 2001). Measuring environmental ammonia is not technically difficult and could be a valuable tool for supporting the need for veterinary intervention. It can be done with the cooperation of an industrial hygienist or anyone dealing with hazardous materials management. There is also a small self-contained measuring device can be purchased for under $500 (Giangarlo Scientific Co. Incorporated).

ROOTS OF THE BEHAVIOR

Despite the oversimplification that often occurs in media reports and the provocative evidence for a mental health component to hoarding, it is important to note that animal hoarding is not yet recognized as indicative of any specific psychological disorder. It is not yet understood how, or why, the behavior develops. Preliminary work has suggested that animals may have been the only stable feature in some hoarders' chaotic childhoods. Perhaps the most prominent psychological feature of these individuals is that pets (and other possessions) become central to the hoarder's core identity. They develop a strong need for control, and even the thought of losing an animal can produce an intense grief-like reaction.

In a recent monograph, HARC outlined possible psychological models for animal hoarding (Hoarding of Animals Research Consortium, 2000). One argument is that a focal delusional disorder could be present, since claims that animals are healthy and well cared for in the face of clear evidence to the contrary are consistent with a belief system that is out of touch with reality. Similarities have been noted between hoarders and substance abusers, others with impulse control problems, or compulsive gamblers. An attachment disorder could also be present, such that relationships with animals are preferred because they are safer and less threatening than relationships with people. Perhaps the most parsimonious explanation is obsessive compulsive disorder (OCD). Hoarding of inanimate objects is seen in a variety of psychological disorders, but is most commonly seen in OCD. 2–3 percent of the human population suffers from OCD, and 15–30 percent of those have hoarding as a primary symptom (Frost and Steketee, 1998). It is unknown what proportion of these individuals hoard animals. In the face of numerous competing hypotheses, at this point, it seems that hoarding is best understood as a behavior that represents the final common pathway of a variety of disorders.

Resolution of Cases

Penalties in the event of a guilty finding can range from a nominal fine to forfeiture of the animals and jail time. Some states mandate psychological counseling of offenders, whereas other states make it an option for the court. It is unknown how effective this is, or to what degree there is even compliance with court orders for counseling. Some state statutes provide for recovery of cost of boarding and medical care for animals in cruelty cases. Occasionally there may be prohibitions on future pet ownership or limitations imposed on the number of animals, along with provision for periodic monitoring of the situation by authorities. However, when prohibitions are enacted, it is usually in a local jurisdiction and can easily be circumvented by moving to a nearby community. Supervised probation has been recommended over court probation as a better way to ensure compliance.

It is unknown what types of strategies are most effective in preventing recurrence of hoarding. What does seem fair to say is that with a penalty-based intervention strategy, rapid recidivism is the rule rather than exception. Prohibitions against future pet ownership are effective only to the extent that monitoring is practical. Even when monitoring is practical, hoarders can escape enforcement by moving (often only across town or county lines) to a new jurisdiction. Some communities attempt to either prevent or remedy hoarding situations by passing ordinances that limit the number of pets a person can own. It seems unlikely that these measures are effective, and they are wildly unpopular, difficult to enforce, and likely to be opposed by a broad coalition of dog and cat fanciers, breeders, rescue groups, and animal protection organizations. Restricting ownership or caretaking based solely on numbers is a harsh and probably ineffective remedy that needlessly penalizes responsible pet owners and rescue groups.

Licensing requirements and comprehensive standards for the operation of animal shelters or pet rescue organizations are another tool for prevention. The Colorado statute is a model (Colorado Pet Animal Care and Facilities Act). By stipulating housing, sanitation requirements, veterinary care, and providing for regular inspection of licensed facilities, the worst situations may be avoided. Such criteria could also help the media and the public as well as the courts distinguish between legitimate sheltering efforts and hoarding.

ABUSE FROM ROUTINE HANDLING

As advocates for the better treatment of non-human animals, shelters have the added responsibility of maintaining the highest possible internal standards for care. For veterinarians, often this must be accomplished with more limited resources than they would have in private practice. There will be additional hurdles because the animals may not be easy to handle for treatment, either because of aggression, fear, or lack of socialization and training. Therefore, delivering even routine care can be quite challenging. A shelter veterinarian will prac-

tice in a much more public environment than in private practice and may also be surrounded by people who either are, or believe themselves to be, very knowledgeable about animal care, husbandry, and training. Staff members, volunteers, board members, shelter clients, municipal officials, rescue groups, and the media may all at one time or another have reason or opportunity to observe you in action, to take an interest in a particular individual or type of animal. Regardless of their actual level of expertise, it is guaranteed that they will have strong opinions that need to be respected. Therefore, it is essential to practice in a manner that seeks to prevent any misinterpretation of your decisions or actions.

Although any area of animal care and handling can be sensitive, particularly fertile ground exists surrounding euthanasia, which has the potential for great controversy and misunderstanding. Even when the most pressing medical or humane indications exist, there may be people who disagree with a completely appropriate decision to euthanize an animal. In many ways, euthanasia is the standard by which all other aspects of shelter operations are judged. Improper euthanasia can become a lightning rod for attention to real or perceived deficiencies in other areas of shelter operation. Despite great improvements in the professionalism of shelters and the growth of shelter veterinary practice as a legitimate arm of veterinary medicine, the fact remains that shelters as a group have no accrediting or regulating body that ensures compliance to specific performance standards. Although relatively few cases of grossly substandard practices have been documented involving shelters, every shelter veterinarian should be aware of these situations in order to guard against them effectively. These include staff found to be inadequately verifying death prior to disposal (for example, animals with beating hearts found in the freezer), use of intracardiac injection in conscious animals, and euthanizing animals in the presence of other animals. Other problems that have been documented in media reports about shelters include housing cats together regardless of age, temperament, health, or gender; lack of isolation/vaccination protocols, deviation from accepted standards of preventive health care, cleaning practices such as hosing down cages with cats still inside which soaked the cats and produced great stress, use of catch poles around the neck to control, restrain or move cats, picking dogs up by the neck skin to move them, and generally non-compassionate handling of animals with use of excessive force. When such situations are brought to public attention, the public reaction is likely to be severe, and the institutional and professional consequences for the veterinarian substantial.

Resources for Veterinarians

Euthanasia

Improper euthanasia may be the most controversial charge to be levied against a shelter or a shelter veterinarian, and is also the most preventable. The AVMA Panel Report on Euthanasia (www.avma.org) is a universally accepted guideline for minimum standards for humane euthanasia. In some states, it is even incorporated by reference into state statutes and therefore has the force of law. There is really no excuse for deviating from these minimum standards. However, the AVMA Panel document was not developed with animal shelters or animal control facilities in mind, and various animal protection groups have outlined deficiencies in this document that shelter veterinarians should be aware of if they are seeking to meet the most rigorous standards for humane euthanasia. The reader is referred to chapter 24 in this text for a fuller discussion of euthanasia.

Dog Handling and Training

Dog training is generally not dealt with in most state cruelty statutes. New Jersey is one exception, where, as already discussed, the statute specifically exempts most training practices (New Jersey Permanent Statutes). Until recently, dog training practices were not considered of major concern in the field of animal abuse prevention. However, in the late 1990's, a national panel of prominent dog trainers, behaviorists, animal protection representatives, and others knowledgeable about dog training issues convened under the joint auspices of the American Humane Association and the Delta Society to examine issues related to appropriate dog training methods. One of the events that sparked this initiative was a case where a dog trainer was prosecuted for cruelty to animals because a dog was blinded after being lifted off the ground and spun around by his choke collar ("helicoptering"). At the trial, he was acquitted of the charges, in part because common dog training books available at popular chain bookstores listed this as a legitimate training practice. The lack of any published literature or widely accepted standards to the contrary did not help. Thus, a broad working group was convened in an attempt to reach some consensus about appropriate training methods. The two organizations eventually produced separate summary reports with a somewhat different focus (American Humane Association, 1998–2001, www.deltasociety.org). Nevertheless, despite minor differences in wording, both documents did agree on many points. The actions listed in Table 26.3 were deemed as inhumane or cruel due to their potential to cause lasting harm or severe distress. In addition, the AHA report rated equipment as either recommended, conditionally recommended, or not recommended. Two pieces of commonly used equipment that received the not recommended rating were the choke collar (unlimited slip) and the shock collar. The shock collar has been outlawed in Switzerland, and the RSPCA in England has had the collars banned in police dog training schools. The use of

Table 26.3. Possible Actions During Dog Training Considered Inhumane or Cruel

Hanging or choking a dog with a collar or leash
Choking a dog with hands or arms or depriving of oxygen from near drowning
Helicoptering (lifting a dog off the ground with a leash and/or collar and swinging in a circle)
Using devices or hands to pinch or squeeze sensitive parts of the body, such as ears or genitals
Biting or throwing a dog against a solid object
Rubbing a dog's face in urine or stool; intentional prolonged social isolation
Hitting a dog to the point of inflicting pain

Source: American Humane Association's Guide to Humane Dog Training; Englewood, CO: American Humane Association, 1998–2001 and Delta Society. "Professional standards for dog trainers." http://www.deltasociety.org/standards/standards.htm

various training devices as well as the balance of aversive vs. reward based techniques is an area of ethics that will continue to evolve in dog training as well as in veterinary medicine.

RESTRAINT FOR CARE

Much less guidance is available concerning proper handling and restraint in the delivery of medical care. Although the focus of the Delta and AHA recommendations was dog training, it seems reasonable that the prohibited actions clearly could apply and be used as a guide to any situation involving restraint or handling of a dog. There have been several recent high profile cases that received wide attention in the media where shelter veterinarians, if for no other reason than guilt by association and/or their position regardless of their level of authority, were accused of, or held responsible for, cruel or improper treatment of animals. Shelters and shelter veterinarians are by no means unique in this risk. In 1999, a veterinarian in private practice was prosecuted and found guilty of cruelty to animals due to his handling and discipline of companion animals during routine medical procedures in his hospital (Nolen, 1999). (It should be noted that this veterinarian was subsequently acquitted of all charges after another judge reviewed the lower court proceedings on appeal [Brakeman, 2000]).

In recognition of the importance of this discussion, the emerging controversy, and lack of guidance in this area, the AVMA recently came out with a preliminary policy statement, along with a pledge to continue examining this issue. The policy approved by the executive board November 2001, states:

> Humane and safe physical restraint is the use of manual or mechanical means to limit some or all of an animal's normal voluntary movement for the purposes of examination, collection of samples, drug administration, therapy, or manipulation. The method used should provide the least restraint required to allow the specific procedure(s) to be performed properly, and should protect both the animal and personnel from harm. In some situations, chemical restraint may be the preferred method. Whenever possible, restraint should be planned, formulated, and communicated prior to its application.

Why Is This Happening Now?

A quarter century of dialogue about the human-animal bond and the concurrent growth of companion animal medicine as the mainstay of veterinary practice are evidence of societal concern. This history provides some clues about why scrutiny of veterinary care is increasing. As a profession we have heard that pets are family members for so long that we tend to accept that premise without even considering its implications. Perhaps the most visible implication is the phenomenal growth of veterinary specialties and specialty practices delivering high end care that rivals what is available for human family members. Although not widespread at this time, there have been veterinary practices that place video cameras in hospital treatment and ward areas, similar to the nanny-cams for child caregivers, to reassure anxious owners about their pet's well being. Overall, scrutiny of animal caregivers in the US is increasing (Brakeman, 2000). Public concern for animal well being is also reflected by the increase in the size, number and budgets of animal-related charities. The recent establishment of Maddie's Fund, with an endowment of over $200 million dollars targeted at eliminating the euthanasia of unwanted animals, has brought the public dialogue to protect companion animals to a new level (www.maddiesfund.org). Public outrage over mistreatment of animals, although not a new phenomenon, can be rapidly disseminated via the Internet and result in massive media attention. This concern has been instrumental in increasing the number of states with felony-level penalties for some forms of animal cruelty from about 15 in the mid-1990's to 35 in 2002. By the time this text reaches print, the number will undoubtedly be higher. This concern has culminated in several very public, scathing critiques of practices in prominent shelters in New York (Office of the Comptroller 2002) and Indiana (Harris and Theobold 2001).

Concern for the mistreatment of other vulnerable family members (children, battered women, and dependent elderly) has also exponentially increased. The status of companion animals has even symbolically changed with the replacement of the word "owner" with "guardian" in municipal statutes in Boulder, Colorado; West Hollywood and Berkeley, California; Amherst, Massachusetts; Menomonee Falls, Wisconsin; and in a state statute in Rhode Island (In Defense of Animals 2002).

Within the past decade, animal rights law classes have been added to the curriculum at eighteen law schools (Hoffman and Wolfson, 2002), and well respected legal scholars are weighing in to support the notion that at least some animals are more than property. On a more pragmatic level, it has been noted that many pet owners and animal caregivers share the commonsense view that animals experience positive, as well as negative, emotional states (McMillan, 1996). The increasing attention given to provision of adequate pain control in animals in clinical situations is a final piece of evidence of how important the subjective experiences of animals are to society and the veterinary profession (Holton, Scott, et al., 1998).

As a result of this evolving attitude, it is essential that the manner in which veterinarians care for and handle animals be in keeping with current sensibilities about appropriate treatment. State anti-cruelty laws generally provide little help, as their wording is frequently quite broad and often does not address specific situations or acts related to restraint and discipline. At best, the use of force is a muddy area. Based on the prevailing social ethic, a number of actions were proposed as inappropriate when handling or restraining companion animals (Table 26.4) (Patronek and Lacroix, 2001). Conditions that have been identified as facilitating the improper use of force in other situations (Table 26.5) clearly have the potential to be present in shelters.

There may be times when the use of force is unavoidable in order to protect the safety of animals, staff or the public. However, the force used should be limited to the extent needed, and force should never be used as a form of punishment. They are consistent with other proposed standards on the use of force during clinical procedures in which the use of force has been described as permissible if caregivers using force are in full control of their emotions, only the minimum amount force needed to achieve compliance is used, and force is used with an understanding of the animal's nature, with empathy for the animal's feelings, with the goal of animal care, and as if the owner were observing or the patient were an infant (McMillan, 1996).

There are many resources available to assist with the humane restraint of animals and mitigate the need for force. Companies such as Animal Care and Equipment Services (ACES) (www.animal-care.com) make a wide variety of nets, bite-proof gloves with extraordinary flexibility, squeeze and transfer cages, and a variety of remote delivery systems for tranquilizers to protect the safety of both animals and shelter staff and minimize stress when handling scared, aggressive, or fractious animals. Shelters should make use of the broad array of tranquilizing and sedative drugs that are available that offer various combinations of cost effectiveness, safety, and reversibility.

Several steps that shelters as well as veterinary practices can take to minimize liability and optimize the treatment of animals have been identified (Patronek and Lacroix, 2001). The first is to provide professional and lay staff with written guidelines for proper handling, restraint, and discipline of animals. A model shelter policy should include definitions from the state statute on cruelty to animals, as well as any additional features that are needed to clarify any vague language used in the state statute. A whistle blowing or employee reporting policy should be implemented, and state to whom the report should be made, and specify that no punitive

Table 26.4. Inappropriate Actions During Handling or Restraint of Companion Animals in Veterinary Practice

Use of force that exceeds that necessary for self-defense or the protection of others.
Use of force as punishment.
Punishment delivered in anger and with the intent to cause pain.
Striking animal on the head or other sensitive or injured body parts.
Choking an animal.
Shaking an animal violently.
Striking an animal with an object.

Source: Patronek, G.J., and C. Lacroix. Developing an ethic for veterinarians and other animal caregivers on abuse, discipline, and restraint. *J Am Vet Med Assoc* 218:1–4; 2001.

Table 26.5. Workplace Conditions that Contribute to Inappropriate Use of Force

Inadequate training in working with animals and defusing tension
Lack of skills that reduce the necessity for use of force
Overcrowding, which increases tension and likelihood of violence
High turnover of staff with loss of expertise
Weak systems of accountability and inspection

Source: Patronek, G.J., and C. Lacroix. Developing an ethic for veterinarians and other animal care-givers on abuse, discipline, and restraint. *J Am Vet Med Assoc* 218:1–4; 2001.

action will be taken for a report made in good faith. In addition to establishing internal policies, shelters should also include in employment contracts a provision that states that mistreating an animal is grounds for immediate termination. Such a provision would sensitize employees to the gravity of the offense and discourage them from acting inappropriately. More and more veterinary employers are including such provisions in their employment agreements as they become aware of how devastating the negative publicity surrounding allegations of animal abuse by veterinarians, technicians, or lay staff members can be to their practices.

DELIBERATE CRUELTY TO ANIMALS

Deliberate cruelty to animals occurs all too frequently in our society, ranging from overly harsh training methods, to exploitation via dog fighting, intensive commercial breeding and excessive labor, to impulsive acts of violence, instilling mental anguish or willful deprivation of companionship and socialization, to almost every imaginable form of sadistic physical torture. A variety of reasons have been proposed to explain deliberate cruelty by adults and children (Table 26.6).

Over the past decade, there have been increasing calls for veterinarians to recognize and report this type of abuse (Arkow, 1996; Rollin, 1994; Ascione, Thompson, and Black, 1997; Reisman and Adams, 1996). Much of this concern has arisen because of increased recognition of the interconnectedness of all forms of violence in the family and the sentinel value of animal maltreatment (Arkow, 1994; Kellert and Felthous, 1985). It has been suggested that veterinarians could make a contribution to increasing the protection of animals, similar to how physicians and other health care workers revolutionized the protection of children when they became mandated reporters of suspected child abuse following the publication of Kempe's landmark paper in 1962 (Kempe et al., 1962). Mainstream veterinary medicine has cautiously endorsed this role, with the AVMA issuing a supportive position statement (AVMA, 1997; Stultz, 1995). The Canadian Veterinary Medical Association has gone a step further and made animal abuse one of its top three priorities for the period

Table 26.6. Reasons for Deliberate Cruelty or Killing of Animals by Children and Adults

By Adults	By Children
To threaten, intimidate, or control a person	Curiosity or exploration
To satisfy a prejudice against a species	Peer pressure
To retaliate against the animal	Relieve boredom or depression
Nonspecific sadism	To protect the animal from worse abuse in the family
To control an animal	Fear of the animal
To shock people for amusement	Forced abuse by a more powerful person
To enhance their own aggression	Reenacting their own experience of being abused
To enhance their aggression via an animal	Regaining a sense of power after abuse
Sexual gratification	

Source: Dr. Randall Lockwood and Dr. Frank Ascione, numerous personal communications, published papers, and conference presentations

1999–2001 (Crook, 2000). However, despite these calls for action, private practitioners remain wary of greater involvement. Some of this stems from concerns about repercussions and some from lack of training or published reports. Unfortunately, the pathognomonic criteria listed by Kempe for child abuse have not yet been identified for veterinary medicine. It has been noted that "veterinary forensic medicine is not yet a bona fide discipline within the veterinary curriculum, and this lack of status, coupled with the paucity of data, hampers the ability of the veterinarian to contribute his or her skills and knowledge" (Cooper and Cooper 1998). Several recent papers have begun to lay an excellent foundation for this discussion (Stroud, 1998; Munro, 1998a; Miller and Zawistowski, 1998; Cooper, 1998; Stroud, 2001; Forbes, 1998; Leonard, 2001; Munro, 1998b; Munro and Thrushfield, 2001a; Munro and Thrushfield, 2001c; Munro and Thrushfield, 2001d). Papers detailing guidelines for being an expert witness have been published, and should be part of the library of any shelter veterinarian (Hannah, 1998; Lockwood, 2001; Harris, 1998). A new website at Tufts is being developed to link this disparate material together (www.tufts.edu).

One of the most unusual forms of deliberate cruelty to animals is Munchausen syndrome by proxy. This syndrome is well described in people, usually involving a parent and child. The parent, usually the mother, falsifies or induces an illness or injury in her child in order to gain attention and sympathy. According to Munro (Munro and Thrushfield, 2001b), the preferred terminology is factitious illness by proxy, but this has gained little acceptance because the previous terminology is ingrained. A distinctive feature of this syndrome is the excessive repetition of the behavior, sometimes involving hundreds of visits to physicians and hospitals. This syndrome has only rarely been documented among veterinary clients, but this may be because of lack of awareness of the syndrome among veterinarians. Some suggested mechanisms could include, and certainly are not limited to, adding blood to a urine specimen to create hematuria, application of irritants to the skin, induction of neurological, gastrointestinal, or biochemical disorders by administration of chemicals, drugs, or toxins. According to Munro (Munro and Thrushfield, 2001), the index of suspicion for this behavior should be raised when clinical signs and history do not follow any known or previously described pattern, the signs improve when the patient is separated from the client, and there is excessive attention-seeking behavior by the client.

CONCLUSION

Although shelter veterinarians may actually see more abused animals than private practitioners, they are less likely to be hobbled by some of these constraints since the abuse is likely to be more obvious and the perpetrator, if one can be identified, unlikely to be a client. As the penalties for certain forms of deliberate animal abuse increase throughout the US, this will mean that the standards for proof will increase proportionately. Shelter veterinarians will play a critical role in performing a complete and thorough forensic examination and will have to become expert in the collection and documentation of evidence suitable for presentation in a court of law. Currently, the field of veterinary forensic investigation is in its infancy. There are no training programs in veterinary forensics, and the professional literature is almost nonexistent. Veterinary pathologists, who will play a critical role in this evolving field, have been slow to take up the call. Shelter veterinarians are in an ideal position to move this field forward. Hopefully, as others contribute to this knowledge base, sufficient material will accumulate to engage a broad spectrum of veterinarians in forensic investigation.

REFERENCES

American Humane Association's Guide to Humane Dog Training; 1998–2001 American Humane Association, Englewood, CO.

American Veterinary Medical Association. 2000 Report of the AVMA panel on euthanasia. http://www.avma.org/resources/euthanasia.pdf.

American Veterinary Medical Association. 1997 Animal welfare positions. www.avma.org.

Animal Care and Equipment Services, Inc. http://www.animal-care.com/.

Arkow, P. 1994. Child abuse, animal abuse, and the veterinarian. *J Am Vet Med Assoc* 204:1004–1007.

Arluke, A., and the Hoarding of Animals Research Consortium. In press. Animal hoarding in the media. *Society and Animals*.

Arluke, A. 1991. Coping with euthanasia: A case study in shelter culture. *J Am Vet Med Assoc* 198:1176–1180.

Armstrong, P.J., and Lund, E.M. 1996. Changes in body composition and energy balance with aging. *Vet Clin Nutr* 3:83–87.

Ascione, F.R., Thompson, T.M., Black, T. 1997 Childhood cruelty to animals: Assessing cruelty dimensions and motivations. *Anthrozoos* 10: 170–177

Assia, E., Epstein, Y., Magazanik, A., and Sohar, E. 1989. Plasma cortisol levels in experimental heatstroke in dogs. *Int J Biometeorol* 33:85–88.

AVMA. 1997. Positions on animal welfare. *AVMA Membership Directory and Resource Manual.* Schaumburg, IL: The American Veterinary Medical Association, 58.

Balcom, S., and Arluke, A. 2001. Animal adoptions as negotiated order: A comparison of open versus traditional approaches. *Anthrozoos* 14:135–150.

Balcom, S. 2000. Legislating shelter animal welfare: A review of SB 1785 in California. *Society and Animals* 8:139–150.

Bardsley, M.E., and Saunders, S.M. 1987. Heat stroke in a dog. *Vet Rec,* August 8:135.

Bean, M.J., and Rowland, M.J. 1997. The evolution of national wildlife law. Westport, CT: Praeger Publishers.

Brakeman, L. 2000. A new ethic. As societal views change toward animal welfare, DVM's are being targeted, second-guessed on medical decisions. *DVM Newsmagazine* March, 1, 9, 10, 16.

Brakeman, L. 2000. Three-year nightmare ends in acquittal for NJ DVM. *DVM Newsmagazine,* June, 35–6.

Caird, J.J. and Mann, N. 1987. Fatal heat stroke in a dog. *Vet Rec* July 18, 72.

Center for Animals and Public Policy, Animal hoarding research. http://www.tufts.edu/vet/cfa/hoarding/index.html

Center for Wildlife Law, University of New Mexico. State Wildlife Law Handbook. http://ipl.unm.edu/cwl/statbook/intro.html

Colorado Pet Animal Care and Facilities Act § 35-80-109, C.R.S. (1999 Supp.).

Cooper, J.E., and Cooper, M.E. 1998. Future trends in veterinary forensic medicine. *Sem Avian Exotic Pet Med* 7:210–217.

Cooper, J.E. 1998. What is veterinary forensic medicine? Its relevance to the modern exotic animal practice. *Sem Avian Exotic Pet Med* 7:161–165.

Crook, A. 2000. The CVMA animal abuse position— How we got here. *Can Vet J* 41:631–635.

Delta Society. Professional standards for dog trainers. http://www.deltasociety.org/standards/standards.htm.

Deresinski, S. 1996. Q fever—San Mateo County (USA) 9/20/96 PROMED-AHEAD Archive 19960920.1609 http://www.fas.org/promed/.

Donley, L., Patronek, G.J., and Luke, C. 1999. Animal abuse in Massachusetts: A summary of case reports at the MSPCA and attitudes of Massachusetts veterinarians concerning their role in recognizing and reporting abuse. *J Applied Animal Welfare Science* 2:59–73.

Drobatz, K.J., and Macintire, D.K. 1996. Heat-induced illness in dogs: 42 cases (1976–1993). *J Am Vet Med Assoc* 209:1894–1899.

Equine Rescue Net. 1998. Henneke scoring report. http://www.equinenet.org/ernet/henneke.html

Forbes, N.A. 1998. Clinical examination of the avian forensic case. *Sem Avian Exotic Pet Med* 7(4):193–2000.

Frost, R.O., Steketee, G.S. 1998. Hoarding: Clinical aspects and treatment strategies. In M.A. Jenike, L. Baer, W.E. Minichiello, eds. *Obsessive-compulsive disorders—practical management.* New York: Mosby, 533–554.

Giangarlo Scientific Co Incorporated. 1995. Sensidyne Gastech. http://www.giangarloscientific.com/sensidyne/images/gasbro.pdf.

Grandin, T. 1995. Humane transport good business as well as welfare practice. *DVM* December 2f–3f.

Hangin' Judge Roy Bean. 2002. "Justice" prevails in Texas for feral cats *Animal People,* 20, May.

Hannah, J. 1998. The veterinarian as an expert witness. In *Recognizing & Reporting Animal Abuse: A veterinarian's guide.* Englewood, CO: American Humane Association, 60–62.

Harris, B. and Theobald, B. 2001. Destined to Die. *Indianapolis Star* (series). October 14–16. http://www.indystar.com/library/special/destinedtodie/.

Harris, J.H. 1998. The role of the practicing veterinarian as an expert witness. *Sem Avian Exotic Pet Med* 7:176–181.

Henneke, D.R. 1995. A condition scoring system for horses. *Equine Pract* 7:14–16.

Hoarding of Animals Research Consortium. 2000. People who hoard animals. *Psychiatric Times.* April 17:25–29.

Hoarding of Animals Research Consortium. 2002. Health implications of animal hoarding. *Health & Social Work,* Volume 26, 125–136, May.

Hoffman, J.E., and Wolfson, D.J., eds. 2002. The legal status of nonhuman animals. *Animal Law* 8:46.

Holton, L.L., Scott, E.M., Nolan, A.M., et al. 1998. Comparison of three methods used for assessment of pain in dogs. *J Am Vet Med Assoc* 212:61–66.

HSUS Government Affairs Section, 2002. Email Communication, June 20.

Humane Society of the United States. 2000. In New Jersey, Stress Management is Now Required. *Animal Sheltering Online* Jul.–Aug. http://www.hsus2.org/sheltering/magazine/currentissue/jul_aug00/frontlines_newjersey.html.

Humane Society of the United States. 1998. Concepts that have worked for others. *Animal Sheltering Magazine,* July/August, 21–23.

Humane Society of the United States. The Facts About Chaining or Tethering Dogs, http://www.hsus.org/ace/11865.

Illionois Elder abuse and neglect act, Chapter 320 ILCS Sec 2 f-5.

Illinois Public Act 92-0454: An act concerning cruelty to animals. 510 ILCS 70/2.10.

In Defense of Animals, 2002. Amherst, MA, becomes Sixth City to Recognize Concept of Animal Guardianship. News release, May 15, http://www.idausa.org/newsarchives.html.

Indiana Hooved Animal Humane Society. The Henneke Body Scoring System. http://www.ihahs.org/henneke.html.

International Air Transport Association. 2002. (IATA) *Live Animal Regulations. Appendix C.* 29th Edition, October 1.

Irwin, A. 2001. Animal Hoarding—A Hidden Problem. *Keystone Veterinarian-Journal of the Pennsylvania Veterinary Medical Association.* September/October, 22.

Kellert, S.R., Felthous, A.R. 1985. Childhood cruelty toward animals among criminals and noncriminals. *Human Relations* 38:1113–1129.

Kempe, C.H., Silverman, F.N., Steele, B.F., Droegemuller, W., Silver, H.K., 1962. The battered child syndrome. *J Am Med Assoc* 181:17–24.

Krum, S.H., and Osborne, C. 1977. Heatstroke in the dog: A polysytemic disorder. *J Am Vet Med Assoc* 170:531–535.

Laflamme, D.P. 1993. Body condition scoring and weight maintenance. *Proceedings of the North American Veterinary Conference*, 290–291.

Lembke, L. 2001. Stautzenberger State College, Personal Communication, February 23.

Leonard, E.A. 2001. An approach to forensic necropsy *Proceedings of the Tufts Animal EXPO,* 834–837.

Lewis, B. 2002. Fort Wayne Department of Animal Care and Control. Email communication, July 3.

Lockwood, R. 2001. Veterinary forensics: testifying in court. *Proceedings of the Tufts Animal EXPO*, 825–826, 838–840.

Lockwood, R. 2002. Humane Society of the United States, Email communication, June 25.

Maddies Fund, The Pet Rescue Foundation. http://www.maddiesfund.org/.

Magazanik, A., Shapiro, Y., and S. Shibolet. 1980. Dynamic changes in acid base balance during heatstroke in dogs. *Pfluger Arch* 388:129–135.

McMillan, F.D. 1996. Compassionate animal care in veterinary practice. Part II. Expectations and goal setting. *Vet Technician* 17:259–265.

MegaLaw.com Lawyers window to the web. http://www.megalaw.com/.

Miller, E.A. 2000 Edition Minimum Standards for Wildlife Rehabilitation, 3rd Edition. National Wildlife Rehabilitators Association, St Cloud, Minnesota, 77 pages. http://www.iwrc-online.org/standards.html.

Miller, L., and Zawistowski, S. 1998. A call for veterinary forensics: The preparation and interpretation of physical evidence for cruelty investigations and prosecution. In *Recognizing & Reporting Animal Abuse: A veterinarian's guide.* Englewood, CO: American Humane Association, 63–67.

Munro, H.C. 1998a. The battered pet syndrome. In *Recognizing & Reporting Animal Abuse: A veterinarian's guide.* Englewood, CO: American Humane Association, 76–81.

Munro, H.C. 1998b. Forensic necropsy. *Seminars in avian and exotic pet medicine.* 7(4):201–209.

Munro, H.M.C., and Thrushfield, M.V. 2001a. Battered pets: Features that raise suspicion of non-accidental injury. *J Sm An Pract* 42:218–226.

Munro, H.M.C., and Thrushfield, M.V. 2001b. Battered pets: Munchausen syndrome by proxy. *J Sm An Pract* 42:385–389.

Munro, H.M.C., Thrushfield, M.V. 2001c. Battered pets: Non-accidental physical injuries found in dogs and cats. *J Sm An Pract* 42:269–290.

Munro, H.M.C., and Thrushfield, M.V. 2001d. Battered pets: sexual abuse. *J Sm An Pract* 42:333–337.

National Institute for Occupational Safety and Health Documentation for immediately dangerous to life or health concentrations (IDLH's). Introduction. http://www.cdc.gov/niosh/idlh/idlhintr.html.

National Institute for Occupational Safety and Health. Ammonia. http://www.cdc.gov/niosh/pel88/7664-41.html.

National Institute for Occupational Safety and Health. Documentation for immediately dangerous to life or health concentrations (IDLHs). http://www.cdc.gov/niosh/idlh/intridl4.html.

New Jersey Permanent Statutes. Title 4 Agriculture and domestic animals 4:22–16 Permitted Activities.

Nolen, R.S. 1999. New Jersey veterinarian convicted of animal cruelty. *J Am Vet Med Assoc.* 7:918.

O'Rourke, K. 2002. A little bird told me, you'd better listen to the law. *J Am Vet Med Assoc* 220:436–438.

Occupational Safety and Health Administration. 2002. Chemical Sampling Information: Ammonia http://www.osha-slc.gov/dts/chemicalsampling/data/CH_218300.html.

Office of Regulatory Affairs. Director of State and Local Officials 2002 Edition. http://www.fda.gov/ora/fed_state/directorytable.htm.

Office of the Comptroller, City of New York. 2002. Audit report on the shelter conditions and adoption efforts of the Center for Animal Care and Control

June 6, http://comptroller.nyc.gov/bureaus/audit/PDF_FILES/ME01_109A.pdf.

Patronek, G.J., and Lacroix, C. 2001. Developing an ethic for veterinarians and other animal caregivers on abuse, discipline, and restraint. *J Am Vet Med Assoc* 218:1–4.

Patronek, G.J., and the Hoarding of Animals Research Consortium. 2001. Understanding hoarders. *Municipal Lawyer* May/June. 6–9,19.

Patronek, G.J. 1999. Hoarding of animals: an under recognized public health problem in a difficult to study population. *Public Health Reports* 114:82–87.

Patronek, G.J. 1998. Issues and guidelines for veterinarians in recognizing, reporting, and assessing animal neglect and abuse. In *Recognizing and reporting animal abuse—A veterinarian's guide*. Denver, CO: American Humane Association, 25–39.

Pengelly, J. 1987. Heat stroke in a dog. *Vet Rec* August 8:135–136.

People for the Ethical Treatment of Animals. Pig farmers plead guilty in landmark cruelty case. http://www.peta-online.org/news/500/500belguilt.html.

Phillips, C.J., Coppinger, R.C., et al. 1981. Hyperthermia in running sled dogs. *J Appl Physiol.* 51:135–142.

Pullen, K. 2002. Humane Society of the United States (HSUS), Email communication, June 21.

Rauch, A. Veterinary forensics research. http://www.tufts.edu/vet/forensics.

Reisman, R., Adams, C.A. 1996. Part of what veterinarians do is treat animal victims of violence. Should they also report abusers? *Latham Letter* XVII: 1, 8–11.

Reisman, R. 2001. Evaluation of cruelty cases. *Proceedings of the second annual Tufts Animal EXPO*, 841–846.

Rollin, B. 1994. An ethicist's commentary on whether veterinarians should report cruelty. *Can Vet J* 35:408–409.

Sharpe, M. 1999. A survey of veterinarians and a proposal for intervention. In *Child abuse, domestic violence, and animal abuse*. Frank R. Ascione and Phil Arkow, eds. West Lafayette, IN: Purdue University Press, 250–256.

Steinbachs, J. 2002. Zookeeper is again home alone. *Ottawa Sun*, Saturday, June 15.

Strand, P.L. 2002. Pet overpopulation crisis is artificially sustained by animal rights activists. *National Animal Interest Alliance (NAIA) News* 11:1,14.

Stroud, R.K. 2001. Wildlife forensics techniques at the USFWS laboratory *Proceedings of the Tufts Animal EXPO* 847–851.

Stroud, R.K. 1998. Wildlife forensics and the veterinary practitioner. *Seminars in avian and exotic pet medicine* 7(4): 182–192.

Stultz, T.B. 1995. Veterinarians say abuse clause "step in the right direction" for AVMA. *DVM* 26:1, 12.

United States Department of Agriculture. Animal Care Regional Map and Addresses. http://www.aphis.usda.gov/ac/acorg.html.

United States Department of Agriculture. The Animal Welfare Act. http://www.aphis.usda.gov/oa/pubs/awact.html.

United States Department of Agriculture. Animal Care Publications and Policy http://www.aphis.usda.gov/ac/publications.html#awa.

United States Department of Agriculture. Title 9—Animals and animal products, Chapter 1—Animal and plant health inspection service, Department of agriculture, Part 3—Standards. http://www.aphis.usda.gov/ac/cfr/9cfr3.html#3.1.

United States Department of Agriculture. Title 9—Animals and animal products, Chapter 1—Animal and plant health inspection service, Department of agriculture, Part 3—Outdoor housing facilities. http://www.aphis.usda.gov/ac/cfr/9cfr3.html#3.4.

U.S. Fish & Wildlife Service. Office of Law Enforcement. http://www.le.fws.gov/.

U.S. Fish & Wildlife Service. Endangered Species Related Laws, Regulations, Policies & Notices. http://endangered.fws.gov/policies/index.html.

U.S. Fish & Wildlife Service. Migratory Bird and Eagle Permits. http://permits.fws.gov/mbpermits/regulations/regulations.html.

U.S Fish & Wildlife Service. Regional Bird Permit Offices. http://permits.fws.gov/mbpermits/addresses.html.

U.S. Fish and Wildlife Service. Office of Law Enforcement Regions. http://www.le.fws.gov/le_chart.htm.

Wildmann, E.E., Jones, G.M., Wagner, P.E., Bowman, R.L., Trout, H.F., and Lesch, T.N. 1982. A dairy cow body condition scoring system and its relationship to selected production variables in high producing Holstein dairy cattle. *J Dairy Sci* 65:495–501.

Wolfson, D.J.1999. Beyond the law. Agribusiness and the systemic abuse of animals raised for food or food production. Farm Sanctuary, Inc. 26.

Note: All Internet sites were accessed July 1, 2002.

Appendix 26.1:
Tufts Animal Care and Condition (TACC)

Tufts Animal Care and Condition (TACC) scales for assessing body condition, weather and environmental safety, and physical care in dogs

I. Body condition scale (Palpation essential for long-haired dogs; each dog's condition should be interpreted in light of the typical appearance of the breed)

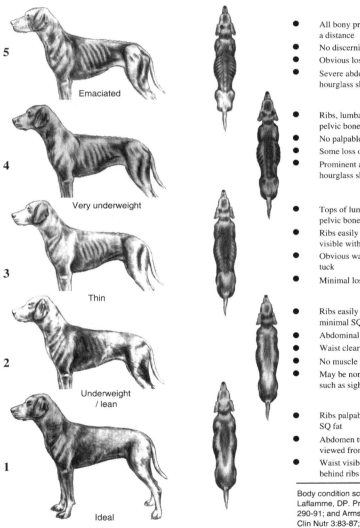

5 Emaciated
- All bony prominences evident from a distance
- No discernible body fat
- Obvious loss of muscle mass
- Severe abdominal tuck and extreme hourglass shape

4 Very underweight
- Ribs, lumbar vertebrae, and pelvic bones easily visible
- No palpable body fat
- Some loss of muscle mass
- Prominent abdominal tuck and hourglass shape to torso

3 Thin
- Tops of lumbar vertebrae visible, pelvic bones becoming prominent.
- Ribs easily palpated and may be visible with no palpable fat
- Obvious waist and abdominal tuck
- Minimal loss of muscle mass

2 Underweight / lean
- Ribs easily palpable with minimal SQ fat
- Abdominal tuck evident
- Waist clearly visible from above
- No muscle loss
- May be normal for lean breeds such as sighthounds

1 Ideal
- Ribs palpable without excess SQ fat
- Abdomen tucked slightly when viewed from the side
- Waist visible from above, just behind ribs

Body condition scale adapted from Laflamme, DP. Proc. N.A. Vet Conf 1993, 290-91; and Armstrong, PJ., Lund, EM. Vet Clin Nutr 3:83-87; 1996. Artwork by Erik Petersen.

II . Weather safety scale
(read score off diagonal bars.
by dog size)

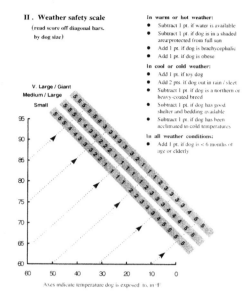

In warm or hot weather:
- Subtract 1 pt. if water is available
- Subtract 1 pt. if dog is in a shaded area protected from full sun
- Add 1 pt. if dog is brachycephalic
- Add 1 pt. if dog is obese

In cool or cold weather:
- Add 1 pt. if toy dog
- Add 2 pts. if dog out in rain / sleet
- Subtract 1 pt. if dog is a northern or heavy-coated breed
- Subtract 1 pt. if dog has good shelter and bedding available
- Subtract 1 pt. if dog has been acclimated to cold temperatures

In all weather conditions:
- Add 1 pt. if dog is < 6 months of age or elderly

V. Large / Giant
Medium / Large
Small

Axes indicate temperature dog is exposed to, in °F

To determine score, draw a line up from the current temperature and parallel to the dotted lines, and read score on bars. Common sense must be used to take into account the duration of exposure to any given temperature when assessing risk; even brief periods of high heat can be very dangerous, whereas a similar duration of exposure to cold temperatures would not be life-threatening.

Interpretation of the TACC score from scales I - IV:

The Tufts Animal Condition and Care (TACC) score is assessed from the number of points read off either the **Body Condition, Weather Safety, Environmental Health,** or **Physical Care** Scale. When multiple scales are evaluated, the highest score on any scale should be used to determine the risk of neglect. Multiple high scores are indicative of greater neglect, risk, or inhumane treatment than a single high score.

Score	Body condition, physical care, environ. health scales	Weather safety scale
≥5	Severe neglect and inhumane treatment. An urgent situation that justifies an assertive response to protect the animal.	Potentially life-threatening risk present. Immediate intervention to decrease threat to the animal required (provide water, shelter).
4	Clear evidence of serious neglect and / or inhumane treatment (unless there is a medical explanation for the animal's condition). Prompt improvement required.	Dangerous situation developing. Prompt intervention required to decrease risk (e.g. provide water, shade, shelter, or bring indoors). Warn owner of risk and shelter requirements.
3	Indicators of neglect present. Timely assessment; correction of problems and/or monitoring of situation may be required.	Indicators of a potentially unsafe situation, depending on breed, time outdoors. Inform owner of risk and proper shelter requirements.
2	A lapse in care or discomfort may be present. Evaluate, and discuss concerns with owner. Recommend changes in animal husbandry practices, if needed.	Risk unlikely, but evaluate the situation, and if warranted, discuss your concerns and requirements for proper shelter with the owner.
≤1	No evidence of neglect based on scale (s) used	No evidence of risk

Disclaimer: The TACC score is intended to be a simple screening device for determining when neglect may be present, for prioritizing the investigation of reported animal cruelty cases, and as a system for investigative agencies to use to summarize their case experience. The TACC score is not intended to replace definitive assessment of any animal by a veterinarian or law enforcement agent. A low TACC score does not preclude a diagnosis of abuse, neglect, or a dog requiring veterinary care upon more careful examination of an animal and its living situation.

III. Environmental health scale

5   **Filthy** - many days to weeks of accumulation of feces and / or urine. Overwhelming odor, air may be difficult to breathe. Large amount of trash, garbage, or debris present; inhibits comfortable rest, normal postures, or movement and / or poses a danger to the animal. Very difficult or impossible for animal to escape contact with feces, urine, mud, or standing water. Food and / or drinking water contaminated.

4   **Very unsanitary** - many days of accumulation of feces and / or urine. Difficult for animal to avoid contact with waste matter. Moderate amount of trash, garbage, or clutter present that may inhibit comfortable rest and / or movement of the animal. Potential injury from sharp edges or glass. Significant odor, breathing unpleasant. Pools of water, mud difficult to avoid.

3   **Unsanitary** - several days accumulation of feces and urine in animal's environment. Animal is able to avoid contact with waste matter. Moderate odor present. Trash, garbage, and other debris cluttering animal's environment but does not prohibit comfortable rest or normal posture. Clutter may interfere with normal movement or allow dog to become entangled, but no sharp edges or broken glass that could injure dog. Dog able to avoid mud or water if present.

2   **Marginal** - As in #1, except may be somewhat less sanitary. No more than 1-2 day's accumulation of feces and urine in animal's environment. Slight clutter may be present.

1   **Acceptable** - Environment is dry and free of accumulated feces. No contamination of food or water. No debris or garbage present to clutter environment and inhibit comfortable rest, normal posture, and range of movement or pose a danger to or entangle the animal.

"Environment" refers to the kennel, pen, yard, cage, barn, room, tie-out or other enclosure or area where the animal is confined or spends the majority of its time. All of the listed conditions do not need to be present in order to include a dog in a specific category. The user should determine which category best describes a

IV. Physical care scale

5   **Terrible** - extremely matted haircoat, prevents normal motion, interferes with vision, perineal areas irritated from soiling with trapped urine and feces. Hair coat essentially a single mat. Dog cannot be groomed without complete clipdown. Foreign material trapped in matted hair. Nails extremely overgrown into circles, may be penetrating pads, causing abnormal position of feet and make normal walking very difficult or uncomfortable. Collar or chain, if present, may be imbedded in dog's neck.

4   **Poor** - substantial matting in haircoat, large chunks of hair matted together that cannot be separated with a comb or brush. Occasional foreign material embedded in mats. Much of the hair will need to be clipped to remove mats. Long nails force feet into abnormal position and interfere with normal gait. Perineal soiling or irritation likely. Collar or chain, if present, may be extremely tight, abrading skin.

3   **Borderline** - numerous mats present in hair, but dog can still be groomed without a total clip down. No significant perineal soiling or irritation from waste caught in matted hair. Nails are overdue for a trim and long enough to cause dog to alter gait when it walks. Collar or chain, if present, may be snug and rubbing off neck hair.

2   **Lapsed** - haircoat may be somewhat dirty or have a few mats present that are easily removed. Remainder of coat can easily be brushed or combed. Nails in need of a trim. Collar or chain, if present, fits comfortably.

1   **Adequate** - dog clean, hair of normal length for the breed, and hair can easily be brushed or combed. Nails do not touch the floor, or barely contact the floor. Collar or chain, if present, fits comfortably.

All of the listed conditions do not need to be present in order to include a dog in a specific category. User should determine which category best describes a particular dog's condition. This scale is not meant for assessment of medical conditions, e.g., broken limb, that clearly indicate a need for veterinary attention.

27

Medical Evaluation and Documentation of Abuse in the Live Animal

Robert W. Reisman

INTRODUCTION

A veterinary forensic evaluation of an animal victim is one part of the veterinarian's role in assisting in an investigation of alleged animal cruelty, abuse, and/or neglect. A veterinarian is one member of a team of professionals involved in cases of cruelty, abuse, and neglect. Many aspects of a successful veterinary evaluation of an animal victim of abuse are procedural. If a person is responsible for an animal's pain and suffering, medical problems become intertwined with problems of society and law. This chapter will cover both the medical and procedural aspect of the veterinarian's role in animal abuse cases.

THE PROCESS — AN OVERVIEW

The Complaint

The simple picture is that a person (e.g., a neighbor, a passerby, a veterinarian) makes a complaint to law enforcement that they suspect an animal has been mistreated. A law enforcement officer listening to the complaint and knowing the laws of the state that pertain to animal mistreatment decides whether to investigate the complaint. A veterinarian participates by evaluating the animal's health. If the complaint is found to be legitimate, the case is presented to the district attorney's office.

There must be a team of professionals to manage these cases, and the reality is it is often not clear who these individuals are; they vary from town to town and state to state. It may be difficult just to identify the person(s) in law enforcement who have

the responsibility of handling animal cruelty complaints. And, the individuals in law enforcement and others in the criminal justice system who have been designated to act on complaints of animal abuse may not be familiar with the specific laws that pertain to animal care and treatment. Additionally, the veterinary role in animal abuse cases is, in this country, to a large extent undefined.

Child abuse case management may serve as a model. A significant governmental (federal and state) effort is being made to reduce child abuse. The National Center on Child Abuse and Neglect (NCCAN), created by the Child Abuse Prevention and Treatment Act of 1974, is the federal agency responsible for coordinating the effort to reduce child abuse and neglect. No similar effort has been made to reduce the occurrence of animal abuse. NCCAN developed *The User Manual Series: A Coordinated Response to Child Abuse and Neglect: A Basic Manual*—Twenty-one manuals designed to provide guidance to professionals involved in the child protection system and to enhance community collaboration and the quality of service provided to children and families (1992). This manual is a good introduction to establishing a multidisciplinary team to manage abuse cases. These manuals are available in PDF format at http://www.calib.com/nccanch/pubs.

The Investigation

A law enforcement investigation of a complaint may support a finding of animal mistreatment, and a request may be made for a veterinary evaluation

453

of the alleged animal victim of abuse. There are many difficult, unresolved issues as to the veterinary involvement in animal cruelty cases. Which veterinarian in a specific community will be asked? What are that person's qualifications? Who pays the costs for the forensic veterinary evaluation and the animal's medical care? What is the state law with regard to medical record confidentiality and abuse case reporting? There are generally answers to these questions when there is a human victim of abuse or neglect. It is not so straightforward with animal victims. These are important questions because the investigation can falter at any step along the way.

The veterinarian evaluating the alleged victim of abuse will be asked to write a statement of their findings. The medical findings and evidence the law enforcement officer has gathered during her or his investigation is presented to the district attorney's office. The veterinarian is generally not aware of all aspects of the investigation, and should not feel that the case depends solely on their findings. It does not.

The Prosecution

The district attorney's office evaluates the evidence presented within the context of the state's laws that pertain to animal mistreatment and decides whether to pursue a criminal prosecution. Arrest and prosecution result when evidence documents that a crime has been committed. Veterinary medical evidence is one part of a body of evidence. A veterinary statement of findings must be produced in a timely fashion (approximately one week to 10 days after the animal presents if not sooner), so that the legal case can proceed. A more complete statement of findings (i.e., a final veterinary statement) may need to be written later when all medical issues associated with the abuse or neglect issues of the case are resolved. If more than one statement is written, the statements must not contradict each other. The first or preliminary statement should not overreach. It is not unusual for an animal cruelty investigator to request an immediate veterinary statement. It is appropriate for the veterinarian to delay writing a first statement until the medical aspects of the case are clear. Starvation or extreme malnutrition is a common finding in an animal abuse case. Generally, it is known within the first week whether an emaciated animal has a serious underlying medical condition, or whether (in the absence of findings of underlying medical pathology) the conclusion is that the emaci-

ation is due to lack of proper nutrition. In starvation cases, a preliminary statement should communicate that the emaciated condition is solely a result of inadequate nutrition. A final statement should document the weight increase that results from feeding a balanced diet. Arrests are made both before and after the district attorney's evaluation of evidence. The timing of the arrest depends on the specific circumstances of the crime. An arrest and criminal prosecution may or may not result in a trial. The majority of prosecuted cases of animal abuse do not go to trial. Most of these crimes have misdemeanor penalties, and plea agreements are often made. In cases that do go to trial, the trial does not typically occur for many months (frequently 12 or more months) from the time when the criminal case is initiated.

Neglect, Abuse, and Cruelty—Legal Terms

Laws are society's statements of acceptable human behavior and for our purposes humane care and treatment of animals. Although we may live in the same country, the laws that define unacceptable care or treatment of animals vary from state to state (Anti-Cruelty Statutes by State; Rutgers University; Federal Animal Welfare Act). Neglect, abuse, and cruelty are legal terms for which there is not a uniform set of definitions. Whether a case is prosecuted is not determined by veterinarians, but by law enforcement individuals and district attorneys.

Veterinarians should be familiar with the laws that are applicable to animal neglect and abuse prosecutions in their home state. Every affidavit that you sign attesting to your findings in a criminal complaint of animal abuse has at the beginning, the law under which the complaint is being filed. If you ever have the opportunity to testify in a criminal trial, you will find that the defense attorney will choose unexpected topics to question you about, for example, the legal text at the beginning of the affidavit that bears your signature.

MEDICAL EVALUATION OF LIVE ANIMAL VICTIMS OF CRUELTY, ABUSE AND NEGLECT

How Animal Victims of Abuse Present to the Veterinarian

Veterinarians are presented with animals in the exam room that have been abused or neglected or, they may be asked to evaluate animals presented by law enforcement that are alleged to be the victims of abuse or neglect (see Figure 27.1).

Animals that present in the exam room are suspected to have been the victims of abuse or neglect, either because of

1. Information gathered during history taking. Note: History taking includes statements made in person or on the telephone to staff and statements made to staff or other clients in the reception area.
2. Physical examination findings
3. Disparities between the medical history and exam findings

Goals

The following are the veterinarian's goals in examining the animal suspected of being the victim of abuse or neglect:

1. Accurate identification of the animal victim
2. Documentation of the animal's medical condition upon initial presentation
3. Documentation of the animal's medical condition during treatment and recovery
4. Statement of medical findings
5. Preparation of the animal for adoption to a new home

Abuse and neglect have a serious negative impact on the victim's health. The medical findings are consequently an integral part of the legal proceeding. By using an organized approach to the medical evaluation and using clearly defined medical terms to describe findings, the examining doctor should be able to write a statement that, if appropriate, supports the legal case against the perpetrator. Additionally a well-documented case will give the doctor the necessary confidence to respond to questions about the medical findings in a court of law. Although there are currently few established standards, ideas are provided in this chapter that will be useful in medical evaluations of abuse cases.

At the time of law enforcement seizure, the owner may surrender an animal to the shelter. Many animals are therefore not returned to their owners. These animals need to be prepared for eventual adoption to new homes. In addition to medical care specific to the consequences of neglect and abuse, at the ASPCA, all animals are vaccinated, microchipped, and dewormed. In addition, there is ongoing evaluation of their behavior, and they are neutered before being rehomed.

Veterinary Forensics

Veterinarians are experts at diagnosis and treatment of animal disease. Differences between a standard medical evaluation and abuse case evaluation exist because the latter requires answers to non-medical questions. Forensic medicine is the wedding between medicine and law. A forensic evaluation provides medical answers to legal questions. For example, questions of time are frequently asked: How long did it take for this animal to develop this emaciated body condition? How long has the collar been embedded in this animal's neck? Questions also may be asked about animal pain and distress. Veterinary forensics is the application of veterinary medical knowledge to the legal determination of whether an animal's pain and distress has been caused by a person's cruel, abusive, or neglectful behavior.

Medical Record-Keeping

The medical record and all additional case documentation, such as radiographs and photographs, are legal documents. This is true of all medical records, but in this situation of the medical documentation of an abuse case, medical records are by nature of the case part of a legal proceeding. As with any medical case, a medical record should be prepared before any work is done with the animal.

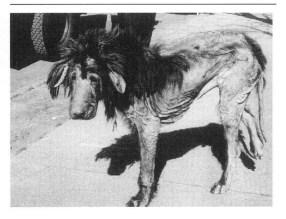

Figure 27.1. A severe case of neglect. This dog was seized by Humane Law Enforcement agents and brought to the hospital for care. Photo credit: Mark MacDonald.

If multiple animals are involved in the case, each animal should have a separate medical record.

In addition to being legal documents, all medical records, including laboratory reports, radiographs, and so on, are part of the evidence and must be maintained as such. The chain of custody of the evidence must be maintained so that the whereabouts of the evidence are known at all times. This concept is more fully explored in chapter 28 on forensics and by Miller and Zawistowski (1998).

It is not unusual for a particular abuse case to involve more than one animal. Because these animals that present as a group must 1) be medically managed as individuals, and 2) will eventually go their separate ways, they must be individually identified with their own unique identification number. This means they cannot be animals A, B, C, and so on with the same identification number.

When the medical aspects of the abuse case are resolved, the original medical record should be photocopied. The original record should be stored securely for use in future legal proceedings, and the photocopy should travel with the animal to a better life. All abuse case documentation should be stored separately from other medical records. This includes the medical record, laboratory reports, radiographs, photographs, and so forth. Medical records can be misplaced. This is an unacceptable response to a subpoena in a criminal case.

DOCUMENTATION OF MEDICAL FINDINGS

At the ASPCA, we have used both computer spreadsheet and word processing programs to create medical record forms for use in medical management of abuse cases. The forms include: Intake evaluation (SOAP), body condition scoring, weight change, condition of skin, condition of haircoat and nails, a preliminary veterinary statement, a final veterinary statement, the euthanasia certification, and medical record certification. Photographs are taken of the animal at the time of presentation, during treatment (if changes are appropriate to document), and when the animal has been returned to good health.

MEDICAL HISTORY

In situations where abuse victims present in the exam room, the veterinarian may be speaking with the abuser or someone who knows the abuser. Forty years ago, physicians found themselves in a situation similar to the one veterinarians face today.

"Physicians have great difficulty both in believing that parents could have attacked their children and undertaking the essential questioning of parents on this subject. Many physicians find it hard to believe that such an attack could have occurred and they attempt to obliterate such suspicions from their minds, even in the face of obvious circumstantial evidence." (Kempe et al., 1962)

"Furthermore, the physician's training and personality usually makes it quite difficult for him to assume the role of policeman or district attorney and start questioning patients as if he were investigating a crime. The humanitarian-minded physician finds it most difficult to proceed when he is met with protestations of innocence from the aggressive parent, especially when the battered child was brought to him voluntarily." (Kempe et al., 1962)

In a recent case at the ASPCA, a woman with a young child presented with a Cocker Spaniel that was a victim of neglect. The animal had a terribly objectionable odor that could be smelled in the hospital the next day. The haircoat was severely matted, especially around the ears. The ear mats were soiled with blood and feces. Sarcophagid fly larvae were feeding on ulcerated and necrotic tissue at the base of the right ear. The woman's story at presentation is that she had left the animal with someone for a period of months and had returned to find the animal in a severe state of neglect. She expressed outrage at the animal's condition. In addition to the hair and skin problems, the dog had an oral tumor, severe dental disease, and a chronic cystitis. Our humane law enforcement department was notified of the case. After an investigation into the whereabouts of another individual proved fruitless, the woman was re-interviewed and this time confessed that she had been solely responsible for the dog's welfare. The dog was legally seized, a criminal summons was served and child welfare was notified of the case. Animal abuse is often the first clue that human violence, including spousal, child, or elder abuse, may be occurring in the household. This is commonly referred to as the "link" between animal abuse and human violence. It is beyond the scope of this textbook to discuss the link, but there are several excellent references and articles available that veterinarians should be familiar with, especially as the American Veterinary Medical Association (AVMA) encourages veterinarians to report animal abuse, and more and more states contemplate mandating reporting of animal abuse and child abuse. (AVMA position statements on reporting animal abuse, Petrovski 1997/1998; Reisman, Summer 1996; American Humane Association, 1998. See also the link references)

"A marked discrepancy between clinical findings and historical data as supplied by the parents is a major diagnostic feature of the battered child syndrome." (Kempe et al., 1962)

In *Recognizing and Reporting Animal Abuse: A Veterinarian's Guide*, Dr. Helen Munro (in The Battered Pet Syndrome) lists the following reasons a veterinarian might suspect physical abuse:

1. The account of the accident does not fit with the injury observed.
2. The owner refuses to comment on how the injury came about.
3. The owner shows a lack of concern for the animal's injuries.
4. There is a delay in seeking veterinary treatment.

In another case at the ASPCA, a veterinarian was presented with a young adult, indoor-only cat with a broken leg. The veterinarian was uncomfortable with the client's lack of interest in the circumstances that resulted in the injury. The staff psychologist was asked to speak with the client, a twenty-something, Caucasian woman who had recently relocated from the Midwest to New York City. The woman revealed that she had turned to prostitution to support herself. A man in her apartment injured the cat. As a result of the veterinarian's observations and actions, the woman reestablished her relationship with her mother (who helped pay for the cat's medical bills), and moved back home. Two lives were saved.

Questions about behaviors that put an animal at risk in the presence of an abusive individual may provide information about the circumstances of the animal's condition. It is recommended that veterinarians incorporate questions about these behaviors into their routine history taking and not just in instances of suspected abuse. Routinely asking these questions will make it easier to ask the ques-

tions in the difficult circumstance of suspected abuse. By routinely asking these questions, responses also may be easier to interpret, and in cases where there is no abuse the veterinarian may learn about problems of which they otherwise would have been unaware. Behaviors that may put an animal at risk include the following:

1. The need for constant supervision
2. Urination and defecation in the house
3. Chronic illnesses that may result in diarrhea, and/or vomiting, or result in a significant financial burden
4. Resistant or destructive behavior
5. Aggressive behavior
6. Excessive noise

Note that these same behaviors put children, the elderly, and disabled persons at risk. "Problems stem from the limitations of the parents or other caregivers in meeting these demands" (Loar, 1999).

Legal counsel at the ASPCA (Melissa Rubin JD, Humane Law Enforcement ASPCA, personal communication) recommends that the veterinarians not alert a suspected abuser to the suspicions of abuse or accuse a person of any criminal wrongdoing. In addition to questions about animal behavior, the veterinarian should try to ascertain the person's relationship with the animal—are they the animal's primary companion? How long have they been with the animal? Are there other animals at home?

A careful review of an animal's medical record is essential to determine if there is a history of repeated abuse. Medical records of other animals in the family should also be reviewed to determine if there is evidence of abuse present in different animals.

If a humane law agent or investigator requests a veterinary evaluation of a live animal, a medical history should be taken as you would any medical history. Veterinarians are experts at medical history taking. Use this expertise. There are two parts to the history given by a humane investigator: 1) the investigator's observations, and 2) the information that was provided by the person(s) the investigator interviewed. The veterinarian should try to differentiate between the information provided by the investigator as a result of direct observation and information obtained from witnesses.

Humane investigators or agents do not have the same understanding of the clinical signs of disease as veterinarians. They may be more concerned about neglect of an obvious medical problem and may not realize the account of the accident does not fit the injury observed. It is the veterinarian's responsibility to accurately evaluate the animal and draw his or her own conclusions. Remember that law enforcement functions to determine if a crime has been committed and if an arrest should be made. That is their job. Significant resources are expended if a criminal prosecution is initiated. There will be instances when the medical determination will support a finding of abuse and/or neglect. There will be instances when the medical determination will not support a finding of abuse and/or neglect. Law enforcement and the prosecuting attorney are relying on veterinarians to give an accurate assessment of the animal's medical condition.

Physical Findings

ANIMAL IDENTIFICATION
The animal victim should be identified by species, breed type, color, sex, and estimated age. A separate animal identification form may be helpful. It is not unusual for the client (in the case of an exam room presentation), a receptionist, or the investigator to inaccurately identify the animal. The veterinarian must take responsibility for complete and accurate victim identification. If it is not known, an estimate of the animal's age should be made. A year down the road when the case goes to trial, you do not want to look at a medical record and wonder about the animal's age. A defense

attorney questions a witness with the goal to call into question the witness's integrity and knowledge. Animal misidentification or incomplete identification is grist for the criminal defense lawyer's mill. A photograph of the animal with an identification card (listing a date and case number) in the picture should be made.

Age determination is frequently an estimate. In young animals, the tooth eruption process allows a reasonably accurate estimate of age (see Tables 27.1 and 27.2.) This is the type of information that should be used for forensic determinations. When a veterinarian is questioned as to why an animal is estimated to be a certain age, this kind of reference is invaluable.

PHYSICAL EXAM
An intake form for abuse cases is similar to other physical exam forms. There is a checklist for all body systems and detailed findings of the checked abnormal systems are recorded in the space found below the checklist. The differences from a standard physical exam form are specific for its use for neglect and abuse cases. There is space to record behavior, pain, and body condition score. Injuries must be carefully documented. We use separate forms for skin problems and problems with the haircoat and nails (see section titled "Body Conditions" in this chapter). Musculoskeletal abnormalities and/or neuromuscular abnormalities, which can result from physical abuse, should be carefully documented. Radiographs should be a standard part of abuse case evaluation.

Table 27.1. Canine Dental Formula and Eruption Schedule

Canine dental formula
Deciduous teeth 2 × (I 3/3, C 1/1, P 3/3) = 28
Permanent teeth 2 × (I 3/3, C 1/1, P 4/4, M 2/3) = 42

Tooth	Deciduous Teeth	Permanent Teeth
	Age in weeks	Age in weeks
Incisors (I)	3 – 6	12 – 20
Canine (C)	3 – 5	12 – 24
Premolars (P)	4 – 12	16 – 24
Molars (M)	Not applicable	16 – 28

Table 27.1. Age estimate based on tooth patterns. Composite of information from five veterinary dental texts (Bojrab and Tholen, 1990; Emily and Penman, 1990; Harvey, 1985; Kertesz, 1993; Mulligan et al., 1998).

BEHAVIOR

Although the association between behavior, abuse, and neglect may not provide strong evidence of neglect or abuse, the animal's behavior at presentation and afterwards should be documented. Pain and distress may cause some abnormal behaviors.

PAIN AND DISTRESS

Because cruelty, abuse, and/or neglect of animals cause animals pain and distress, there must be an attempt to describe this aspect of an animal victim's condition. A variety of terms can be used to describe the negative consequences of neglect, abuse, and cruelty on an animal's welfare. As much as possible, the use of these terms should be as consistent as the use of terms to describe body condition, bite wounds, burns, and so on. The Institute of Laboratory Animal Research of the National Research Council (NRC) has chosen the terms *pain* and *distress* to describe the negative effects of research procedures on animals. An animal's state varies across a continuum from comfort through discomfort to distress and pain (NRC, 1992). As a result, an accurate description of an animal's pain or distress is complicated.

Definition of Pain and Distress

The following are the definitions of pain and distress, as defined by the NRC (1992, 2000).

Comfort is a state of equilibrium in which an animal is in good health, accustomed to its environment, and engages in normal activities (such as feeding, drinking, grooming, social interaction, sleeping-waking cycles, and reproduction).

Stress negatively affects an animal's comfort and may result in discomfort, distress, or pain. Injury, disease, starvation, and surgery cause physiologic stress. These, in turn, may result in the stressors of pain and dehydration. Fear, anxiety, boredom, loneliness, and separation cause psychological stress. Environmental stressors can result from restraint, noise, odors, habitat, people, other species, chemicals, and pheromones.

Discomfort describes a minimal change in an animal's comfort as a result of stress from environmental changes or alterations in its physical, or psychological state. Physiologic or behavioral changes that indicate a state of stress may or may not be observable.

Distress describes a state in which an animal cannot escape from or adapt to external or internal stressors that result in negative effects on its well-being (NRC 2000). This aversive state may result in an animal showing maladaptive behaviors or illness. It can be evident as abnormal feeding, absence or reduced postprandial grooming, inappropriate social interaction with other animals of the same species or human handlers (e.g., aggression, passivity, or withdrawal), and reproductive problems. Distress may result in pathologic conditions such as gastric and intestinal lesions, hypertension, and immunosuppression. Maladaptive responses that briefly reduce an animal's distress can become permanent parts of the animal's behavior and threaten its well-being. Generally, any behavior that relieves the intensity of distress is likely to become habitual, regardless of its long-term effects on an animal's

Table 27.2. Feline Dental Formula and Eruption Echedule

Feline dental formula
Deciduous teeth 2 × (I 3/3, C 1/1, P 3/2) = 26
Permanent teeth 2 × (I 3/3, C1/1, P 3/2 M 1/1) = 26

Tooth	Deciduous Teeth	Permanent Teeth
	Age in weeks	Age in weeks
Incisors (I)	2 – 4	11 – 16
Canine (C)	3 – 4	12 – 20
Premolars (P)	3 – 6	16 – 24
Molars (M)	Not applicable	16 – 24

Table 27.2. Age estimate based on tooth patterns. Composite of information from five veterinary dental texts (Bojrab and Tholen, 1990; Emily and Penman 1990; Harvey, 1985; Kertesz, 1993; Mulligan et al., 1998).

well being. Examples of such behaviors are coprophagy, hair pulling, self-biting, and repetitive stereotyped movements.

Pain Physiology

Pain is a complex experience that results from mechanical, chemical, or thermal stimuli that damage tissue or, have the potential to damage tissue (NRC, 1996; Lamont et al., 2000). *Physiologic* or *nociceptive pain* occurs when a nociceptive or noxious stimulus (i.e., painful or injurious stimulus) threatens tissue health. The neurons responsible for pain sensation are called nociceptors. Because they only respond to injurious stimuli, they are considered high-threshold sensory neurons. Low-threshold sensory neurons respond to noninjurious stimuli such as the stimulation derived from brushing up against a solid object or the stimulation of air movement. Nociceptors are located in skin, peritoneum, pleura, periosteum, subchondral bone, joint capsules, blood vessels, muscles, tendons, fascia, and viscera. Their distribution varies with anatomic location and species. Physiologic pain is a defense mechanism that warns of potential injury and initiates reflexes to avoid injury. It is transient and distinctive from pain that occurs from tissue injury. Physiologic pain ends when the nociceptive stimulus ends. If pain continues after the nociceptive stimulus ends, there must be tissue injury.

Tissue pathology results in *pathologic or clinical pain*. Ongoing discomfort and post-injury hypersensitivity to external stimuli, including harmless stimuli such as gentle palpation, are features of pathologic pain. *Acute pathologic pain exists* subsequent to recent injury. With the development of acute pain, the injured area and surrounding tissues become hypersensitive to all stimuli. As a result, external stimuli are avoided, which facilitates undisturbed healing. Acute pain serves a useful biologic function. Pain caused by a stimulus that is normally not noxious (e.g., gentle palpation) is termed *allodynia*. Spontaneous pain that may be dull or intense is called *causalgia*.

Chronic pain is pain that persists for many months. There may or may not be an ongoing noxious stimulus, such as inflammation, present. Chronic pain offers no useful biologic or protective function. The nervous system itself becomes the focus of the pathology. Chronic pain implies more than just duration—it is debilitating and has a significant negative impact on a patient's well-being. Chronic pain is often characterized by poor response to analgesic therapy.

Pain Assessment

Pain assessment is essential to the medical evaluation and treatment of neglected or abused animals. In people, the "gold standard" for pain assessment is verbal communication between doctor and patient. As animals are unable to communicate what they have experienced, it is left to the veterinarian to assess and describe the animal's pain and distress. This assessment will aid treatment and support the prosecution of the abusive individual.

Animals feel and anticipate pain similar to people (Matthews 2000). Unless the contrary is established, investigators should consider that the procedures that cause pain or distress in people cause pain or distress in animals (NRC, 2000). There are behavioral and physiologic characteristics associated with pain and distress. Some behavioral manifestations of pain or distress are vocalization, depression, abnormal appearance or posture, and immobility (NRC, 1992). Pain assessment is complicated because animal species differ in how they manifest pain and distress. Pain scales for specific species have been evaluated (Cambridge et al., 2000; Firth et al., 1999; Holton et al., 1998; Conzemius et al., 1997). Treatment of pain can be considered successful if the animal resumes engaging in relatively normal activities, such as eating, sleeping, ambulating, grooming, and interactions with other member of its species or its caregivers (American College of Veterinary Anesthesiologists, 1998). Response to analgesics can be useful in pain assessment. Indeed, successful treatment of pain requires an assessment of the animal's response to analgesic administration (Nolen, 2001).

Pain scales are used for assessing pain in animals and people (Flaherty 1998). Human patients score their own pain on the various scales, but assessment in animals requires an observer (Cambridge et al., 2000; Conzemius et al., 1997). One method used is a **simple descriptive scale** where observers apply values to multiple described behaviors, the sum of which provides the final pain score. Another method of assessing pain uses a **visual analogue scale**. In this method, there is a 100 mm line with 0 mm representing no pain and 100 mm representing maximal pain. The observer places a mark on the line that represents the severity of pain the patient is experiencing. Any scoring system requires that the observer is experienced and trained in interpreting the signs of pain.

A pain assessment scale used by the University of Florida Institutional Animal Care and Use Committee (IACUC) is based on work from the Colorado State Veterinary School (French 2000). This is a simple descriptive scale that is used to recommend analgesic therapy based on pain score. A pain scale for the following scenarios is presented: Dogs following stifle surgery, large animals following stifle surgery, rodents with arthritis, rabbits following femur surgery, and birds following humerus surgery.

0 – 3 total score or <1 score in a category:
No intervention
4 – 9 total score or >1 score in a category:
Administer buprenorphine—two doses (0.05 mg/kg), at 12-hour intervals for 24 hours, and re-evaluate pain score.
10 – 11: Administer buprenorphine—one dose (0.05 mg/kg, subcutaneously) and re-evaluate pain score in one hour. If pain is not controlled, administer flunixin meglumine (1.1 mg/kg subcutaneously) and re-evaluate in one hour. If pain is still not controlled, then euthanize the animal. If pain is controlled after either of the above treatments, re-evaluate at six and 12 hours and administer second dose of buprenorphine at eight hours. Re-evaluate the animal's pain score at 12 hours after second dose. If pain is controlled, continue with two or more doses over 24 hours. Discontinue at 24 hours after first dose and re-evaluate pain score.

The parameters used during pain score observations are outlined here:

1. **Activity:** Overall activity level will generally decrease with pain. Some animals may show restlessness (pacing in cage) or agitation, or be nonweight bearing.
2. **Appearance:** Animal may be hunched, have a rough hair coat, have discharge around eyes and nose (i.e., porphyrin staining in rats may indicate stress from pain), or be recumbent.
3. **Temperament:** Animal may become more aggressive (biting, scratching); it may shy away from being handled or it may become apathetic.

4. **Vocalizations:** An animal in pain may make auditory noises (teeth grinding) while undisturbed in cage or when being handled. Some animals that would normally vocalize may not when pain is present such as birds.
5. **Feeding behavior:** Water and food intake is often decreased when an animal is in pain. A reduction in body weight, hydration, urine, or feces may be measured.
6. **Physiological changes:** Respiration rate and pattern, blood pressure, pulse, heart rate, skin color, and body temperature can all change considerably from normal when an animal is in pain.
7. **Appearance of surgery site:** Erythema, swelling (joint effusion), or swelling of tissue around incision and discharge may indicate pain in an animal; animal may show excessive licking and/or chewing at incision site or an affected limb if it is painful.

BODY CONDITION SCORING

All states have laws that require animals to be provided with food, water, and shelter. As a result, starvation cases are the most straightforward abuse cases to prosecute. The hallmark of starvation is weight loss manifested as poor body condition—a reduction in body fat and/or muscle mass. Body condition scoring is a subjective, immediate, determination of the consequences of weight loss. There are many ways to verbally describe an underweight animal. For consistency, the scoring system used at the ASPCA is based on the Tufts Animal Condition and Care Scoring (TACC) system (Patronek, 1997; see chapter 26 appendices). The Tufts system is similar to the simple descriptive scale used for pain assessment in that the different scores for body condition, physical condition, and environment score are totaled to help determine if the animal is a victim of neglect. This is helpful to investigators evaluating animals in their environment. In the animal hospital, we use the body condition scale and physical condition scale separately as part of the overall medical evaluation. The benefit of using the scales in this way is that we are able to use clearly defined terms to describe an animal's body condition and physical condition (i.e., skin, haircoat, and nails). The body condition score and term are written on the intake form. A separate form of the body condition definitions is included in every medical record.

The TACC body condition scale is a five-point scale. Ideal body condition has a score of one. An emaciated body condition has a score of five (see Figure 27.2). At the ASPCA, we rely more on the definitions of the terms than the pictures.

All animals have a weight chart placed in their medical record. Confirmation of the accuracy of body condition scores is demonstrated by weight gain following hospitalization. Weights are taken weekly. In the final veterinary statement, significant weight gains are emphasized. We calculate the percentage of admitting weight that the animal gains during hospitalization. Between four to six weeks post-hospitalization, we have a good idea of the animal's ideal mature body weight. If the standard work-up does not demonstrate any significant underlying disease process, and treatment is basically supportive, a weight gain of 30 percent or more is proof of starvation-neglect. We have had animals whose weight has increased 90 percent from their presenting weight to a normal weight.

CONDITION OF SKIN

We use separate forms, one for cats and one for dogs, to document all skin abnormalities. An outline of a dog or cat is used to diagram the skin lesions. (Note: Haircoat and toenail abnormalities are separately documented on a physical condition form). The types of problems we use the skin form for are embedded collars, wounds, and external parasites. The number and type of wounds, estimates of the number of external parasites, identification of the external parasites, and the type of collar should be documented. It may be necessary to send the parasites to a diagnostic laboratory for identification. We frequently test for tick-

borne diseases. Because the animal's skin is visible to the animal's caretaker, unattended abnormalities are strongly supportive of neglect and/or abuse.

The extent of skin pathology can only be determined if the haircoat is shaved. Skin wounds change over time. The extent of injury may not be apparent upon initial presentation. This is especially true of burns. Documentation by description, diagrams, and photographs must continue until the extent of the injury is known. The length of time that a wound has existed can be estimated, based on the principle that it takes approximately one week for a granulation bed to form. Granulation tissue grows at a rate of about 1 mm per day and 1 cm per month (i.e., the rate of growth slows as the lesion ages) (McDonough, 2002).

In the case of an embedded collar, the length of the embedded part of the collar and the circumference of the neck where the collar is embedded (which is greater than the collar length) should be recorded. Photographs of the collar with blood and tissue attached are particularly helpful in documenting the severity of the problem. Embedded collars generally occur in young animals. The problem develops because the animals grow and the collar doesn't accommodate the change in the animal's neck size (See Figure 27.3). In cases where a very heavy chain is attached to the collar, the length and weight of the chain also should be recorded. The wounds from an embedded collar are generally on the ventral surface of the neck, because the animal pulls against its restraint. A recent case of a neck wound was initially misidentified as a wound from an embedded collar. The wound extended around the left side of the neck of a five-year-old dog. The law enforcement officer who seized the dog was informed that the wound was consistent with an incised wound. The person responsible for the dog's care confessed to using a box cutter on the dog's neck.

Good quality, close-up photographs should be used for documenting skin abnormalities. Photographs should be taken before and after wounds are shaved and cleaned and during the treatment and healing process. All photographs should be properly illuminated, with a date and case identification number included in the picture.

The following bite wound classification is recommended (Griffin, 2001):

- Class 1-Partial-thickness laceration (without penetration of the dermis)

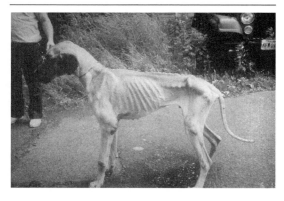

Figure 27.2. Tufts Animal Care and Control (TACC) body condition score of 5-Emaciation. Photo credit: Mark MacDonald.

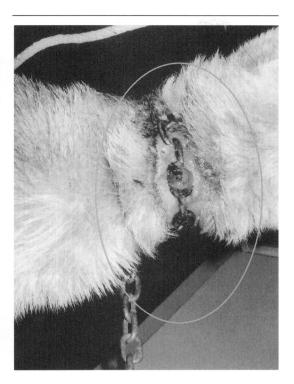

Figure 27.3. A chain embedded in the neck. Photo credit: Mark MacDonald.

- Class 2-Full-thickness laceration (with penetration of the dermis)
- Class 3-Full-thickness puncture wound
- Class 4-Full-thickness puncture or laceration with avulsion of underlying tissues and dead space

Burns should also be classified. This may require a skin biopsy. Burn histopathology will benefit both treatment and the legal case. There are two burn classifications methods used. The older classification system refers to first, second, and third degree burns (Di Maio and Dana, 1998). A newer classification uses the terms, superficial, partial superficial, partial deep, and deep (Saxon and Kirby, 1992). An estimate should be made of the body surface area involved in the burn lesion.

Condition of the Haircoat and Nails

The ASPCA uses a modification of the TACC physical condition scale. (See chapter 26 for a description of use of this score, and the chapter 26 appendices.) The difference is that embedded collar injuries are included on the skin form. We use separate forms, one for cats and one for dogs, to document all haircoat and nail abnormalities. An outline of the animal is used to diagram the abnormalities. This is an excellent scoring system, because it gives you the language you need to describe an animal whose haircoat and nails have been neglected. There are frequently assumptions that can be made based on your findings that will support neglect. One is that animals with matted coats that limit limb movement, or medium- or large-sized dogs with overgrown nails have not had the opportunity for any reasonable amount of physical exercise. Physical exercise contributes to an animal's well-being and state of comfort.

LABORATORY TESTING
A standard work-up for a cruelty, abuse, and/or neglect case includes, in addition to a physical exam, a complete blood count (CBC), chemistry panel, urinalysis, fecal, occult heartworm for a dog, retrovirus screen for a cat, and survey radiographs.

We routinely find that starved animals are anemic, and have low blood albumin and/or low blood protein values. We also find a very high percentage of neglected or abused animals with intestinal parasitism.

RADIOLOGY
All neglect and abuse cases have at least a chest radiograph to look for rib fractures. Lameness should be evaluated by physical exam and radiographs. If one fracture is found anywhere, then all bones are radiographed. The hallmark of physical abuse is multiple fractures at different stages of healing (Kempe et al., 1962; Munro, 1997). Begin with a chest radiograph to look for rib fractures and proceed from there.

We frequently submit radiographs through our commercial lab for review by a radiologist. In these cases, we are careful not to write anything in the medical record that might differ from the radiologist's report. Conflicting interpretations will hurt the legal case.

TOXICOLOGY
Toxicology is another important area of forensic medicine. Miller and Zawistowski (1998) provide a list of samples recommended for submission by the ASPCA National Animal Poison Control Center (NAPCC) in their chapter on veterinary forensics in the American Humane Guide *Recognizing and Reporting Animal Abuse: A Veterinarian's Guide*.

Veterinary Statement

The veterinary statement has an audience of humane law agents, district attorneys, defense attorneys, judges, psychologists, and social workers. It must be written in detail, but in a way that non-medically trained persons can understand. The statement should be typed and if possible printed on letterhead stationery. The typed statement should be dated, identified by case number, and signed. This is a statement of medical evidence that supports a prosecution of animal neglect or abuse. You do not state normal findings (e.g., The chemistry panel was normal; The fecal exam was negative for parasites.), unless it is to emphasize the significance of an abnormal finding (e.g., There is no explanation for the poor body condition other than starvation).

It may be necessary to write more than one statement for a case. A preliminary statement is written because law enforcement needs a veterinary statement to make an arrest and/or submit the case to the district attorney's office. This must be written within days of the case being presented to the veterinarian. I always recommend that clinical laboratory work results be available before the statement is written. A final veterinary statement is written when all medical issues are resolved. It is in this statement that complete weight gains to ideal body condition are included to support neglect cases.

THE USE OF THE BODY CONDITION DEFINITION IN A VETERINARY STATEMENT

The following statement is an example of the language that should be used when incorporating the TACC body condition score in a veterinary statement.

The dog's prominent abnormality at presentation was an emaciated body condition, Tufts Body Condition Score number 5. An ideal body condition has a score of 1. The scale is from 1–5 with 5 being the worst score—see attached form.

The definition for emaciation is

1. *Visual prominence of skeletal structures (ribs, vertebral spines, pelvic bones, spine of scapula, and femur) from a distance*
2. *Obvious loss of muscle mass*
3. *No discernible body fat*
4. *Severe abdominal tuck and extreme hourglass shape*

Skeletal structures are prominent because of the loss of fat and muscle. Fat is stored energy, and muscle is not. Muscle is a structural tissue. When weight loss proceeds to the point of muscle tissue being used as an energy source, an extreme, abnormal state of metabolism exists.

THE ASSOCIATED STATEMENT OF WEIGHT GAIN

An example of a veterinary statement that provides dramatic evidence of the animal's weight gain is furnished here.

At presentation (7/14/01), the dog's weight was 23 lb. As of the writing of this statement (8/2/01), the dog's weight has increased to 38.2 lb. This is a 15-pound weight gain in 19 days. This is a 66 percent increase in weight in less than three weeks.

THE ASSOCIATED STATEMENT OF TREATMENT

There has been no treatment other than feeding a balanced diet and a vitamin supplement.

THE ASSOCIATED STATEMENT OF ANEMIA

Statements that provide documentation and an explanation of the significance of a notable abnormality should be conscise, but thorough and understandable, such as the example that follows.

A complete blood count performed at admission showed that the dog was anemic (i.e., too few red blood cells). On 7/14/01, the dog's packed cell volume (a measure of red blood cell number) was 27 percent. Normal packed cell volume is 36 - 60 percent. As of the writing of this statement, the dog's packed cell volume has increased to 40 percent. The anemia is secondary to starvation. The increase of the packed cell volume to 40 percent has resulted solely from feeding a balanced diet. (There was a negative fecal exam in this case and this was included in the statement.)

Photography

As mentioned previously, photographs are essential to the proper documentation of animal victims of abuse at the time of presentation and during treatment and healing. Digital photography is beginning to be used by law enforcement (Kershaw 2002).

Digital photography provides tremendous advantages over Polaroid® or 35 mm photography. The number of pictures that can be taken is unlimited. The pictures, because they are in a digital format, can be easily organized and stored on a computer. Copies of the images can be transferred by CD, or via e-mail. The question of alteration of digital images is still under discussion. See chapter 28 for more information on this subject. In Wake Forest County, North Carolina, they have set up a system for securely handling images that is intended to address the issue of image alteration (Eaton 2002). The memory card for the digital camera is dropped in a safe. The one individual who has access to this secure storage immediately burns a CD. The CD is put in a time-dated, sealed envelope, which is put in secure storage. This becomes the reference CD for all copies of the images.

Medical Record Certification

All medical records that are submitted as evidence in a court case must be certified as accurate records of the medical management of the case. A hospital owner or director, or office manager can certify the records. This is the text for our certification form (also found in Appendix 27.7):

I, Dr. Robert Reisman, the Medical Coordinator of Abuse Cases, at the Henry Bergh Memorial Animal Hospital of the American Society for the Prevention of Cruelty to Animals, 424 East 92nd Street, New York, New York, 10128, certify that the attached document is a true and accurate copy of the medical record of:

ANIMAL IDENTIFICATION

Humane Law Enforcement case I.D. _____
Bergh Memorial Animal Hospital patient I.D. _____

CONCLUSION

Attention to detail, organized and thorough documentation of abuse victims' medical status, and building working relationships with other team members who manage animal abuse cases, will result in successful prosecutions of those responsible for the cruel treatment of animals. Because the same individuals frequently are responsible for animal and child abuse, domestic violence, elder abuse, and abuse of disabled individuals, many lives will be saved in the process by successful prosecution of animal abuse cases (Ascione 1999, Lockwood 1998, Reisman 1996).

The appendixes for this chapter contain forms that the reader can adopt for use in their own shelters and hospitals when documenting abuse in both living and deceased animals.

REFERENCES

American College of Veterinary Anesthesiologists. 1998. American College of Veterinary Anesthesiologists' position paper on the treatment of pain in animals. *JAVMA* 213 (5): 628 – 630.

Cambridge, Anthony J., Karen M. Tobias, Ruth C. Newberry, Dipak K. Sarkar. 2000. Subjective and objective measurements of postoperative pain in cats. *JAVMA* 217 (5): 685– 690.

Conzemius, Michael G., Chris M. Hill, Jill L. Sammarco, and Sandra Z. Perkowski. 1997. Correlation between subjective and objective measures used to determine severity of postoperative pain in dogs. *JAVMA* 210 (11): 1619 – 1620.

Di Maio, Vincent J. M., and Suzanna E. Dana. 1998. *Forensic Pathology*. Austin, Texas: Landes Bioscience, pp. 161 – 173.

Eaton, Nancy. 2002. *Digital Detectives in Wake County, N.C.* Available at http://www.apple.com/hotnews/articles/2002/09/forensics/

Firth, Ava, M. Haldane, and L. Sarah. 1999. Development of a scale to evaluate postoperative pain in dogs. *JAVMA* 214 (5): 651 – 659.

Flaherty, Derek. 1998. Comparison of three methods used for assessment of pain in dogs. *JAVMA* 212 (1): 61 – 66.

French, Elisa, Sue VandeWoude, Julia Granowski, and Don Maul. 2000. Assessment of Pain in Laboratory Animals, abstract P50. *Contemporary Topics* 39: 85. Ft. Collins, CO: Laboratory Animal Resources, Colorado State University. Available at website: http://nersp.nerdc.ufl.edu/~iacuc/painassessment.htm

Griffin, Greg M., and David E. September/October 2001. Dog-bite wounds: Bacteriology and treatment outcome in 37 cases. *Journal of the American Animal Hospital Association* 37: 453–460.

Holton, Louise L., Ethyl M. Scott, et al. 1998. Comparison of three methods used for assessment of pain in dogs. *JAVMA* 212(1): 61–66.

Institute of Animal Research, National Research Council (NRC). 1992. *Recognition and Alleviation of Pain and Distress in Laboratory Animals*. Washington, DC: Institute for Laboratory Animal Research, NRC, National Academy Press. Available at http://www.nap.edu/catalog/1542.html

Institute for Laboratory Animal Research, National Research Council (NRC). 1996. *Guide for the Care and Use of Laboratory Animals.* Washington, DC: Institute for Laboratory Animal Research, NRC, National Academy Press. Available at http://www.nap.edu/catalog/5140.html

Institute for Laboratory Animal Research, National Research Council (NRC). 2000. *Definition of Pain and Distress and Reporting Requirements for Laboratory Animals: Proceedings of the Workshop.* Washington, DC: Institute for Laboratory Animal Research, NRC, National Academy Press. Available at http://www.nap.edu/books/0309072913/html/

Kempe, C. H., F. N. Silverman, B. F. Steele, W. Droegemuller, and H. K. Silver. 1962. The battered child syndrome. *Journal of the American Medical Association (JAMA)* 181: 17 – 24.

Kershaw, Sarah. 2002. Digital Photos Give the Police an Edge in Abuse Cases. *The New York Times*, September 3, 2002.

Lamont, Leigh A., William J. Tranquilli and Kurt A. Grimm. 2000. Management of pain. *Veterinary Clinics of North America: Small Animal Practice* 30 (4): 703 – 728.

Loar, Lynn. 1999. I'll only help you if you have two legs. In Frank Ascione and Phil Arkow (eds.), *Child Abuse, Domestic Violence, and Animal Abuse, Linking the Circles of Compassion for Prevention and Intervention.*West Lafayette, IN: Purdue University Press.

Mathews, Karol A. 2000. Physiology of Pain, Pain Assessment and General Approach to Management. *Veterinary Clinics of North America: Small Animal Practice* 30 (4): 729 – 756.

McDonough, Sean. 2002. Pathology Chairperson–New York State College of Veterinary Medicine. Personal communication.

Miller, Lila, and Stephen Zawistowski. 1998. A call for veterinary forensics. *Recognizing and Reporting Animal Abuse: A Veterinarian's Guide.* Englewood, NJ: American Humane Association.

Munro, Helen. 1997. The battered pet: Signs and symptoms. *Recognizing and Reporting Animal Abuse: A Veterinarian's Guide.* American Humane Association.

National Center on Child Abuse and Neglect (NCCAN). 1992. *The User Manual Series: A Coordinated Response to Child Abuse and Neglect: A Basic Manual.* McLean, VA: U.S. Department of Health and Human Services Administration for Children and Families Administration on Children, Youth and Families. Available at http://www.calib.com/nccanch/pubs

Nolen, R. Scott. 2001. The problem with pain. *JAVMA* 219 (3): 288 – 289.

Patronek, Gary. 1997. Issues and guidelines for veterinarians in recognizing, reporting, and assessing animal neglect and abuse. *Recognizing and Reporting Animal Abuse: A Veterinarian's Guide.* Englewood, NJ: American Humane Association.

Rubin, M. 1999. Humane Law Enforcement ASPCA personal communication.

Saxon, William D., and Rebecca Kirby. 1992. Treatment of acute burn injury and smoke inhalation. *Current Veterinary Therapy XI.* Philadelphia, PA: W.B. Saunders Company, pp. 145 – 154.

LAW REFERENCES

Anti-Cruelty Statutes by State, Rutgers University. Available at http://www.animal-law.org/statutes/index.html

Federal Animal Welfare Act. Available at http://www.nal.usda.gov/awic/legislat/awa.htm

New York State Law. Available at http://assembly.state.ny.us/leg/?cl=4&a=58

DENTAL REFERENCES

Bojrab, M. Joseph, and Mark Tholen. 1990. *Small Animal Oral Medicine and Surgery.* Philadelphia, PA: Lea & Febiger.

Emily, Peter, and Susanna Penman. 1990. *Small Animal Dentistry.* Oxford: Pergamon Press.

Harvey, Colin E. 1985. *Veterinary Dentistry.* Philadelphia, PA: WB Saunders.

Kertesz, Peter. 1993. *A Colour Atlas of Veterinary Dentistry & Oral Surgery.* London: Wolfe Publishing.

Mulligan, Thomas W., Mary Suzanne Aller, and Charles A. Williams. 1998. Atlas *Canine & Feline Dental Radiography.* Trenton, NJ: Veterinary Learning Systems.

LINK REFERENCES

American Humane Association. 1997. *Recognizing and Reporting Animal Abuse: A Veterinarian's Guide.* Englewood, CO: American Humane Association.

Ascione, Frank R., and Phil Arkow. 1999. *Child Abuse, Domestic Violence and Animal Abuse, Linking the Circles of Compassion for Prevention and Intervention.* West Lafayette, IN: Purdue University Press.

Lockwood, Randall, and Frank Ascione. 1998. *Cruelty to Animals and Interpersonal Violence: Readings in Research and Application.* West Lafayette, IN: Purdue University Press.

Petrovski, Leslie. December 1997/January 1998. The silent link. *American Animal Hospital Association (AAHA) Trends*, pp. 7 – 11.

Reisman, Robert. Summer 1996. Part of what veterinarians do is treat animal victims of violence. Should they also report abusers? *ASPCA Animal Watch*, pp. 19 – 21.

Appendix 27.1:
History/Cover Sheet

Label	Name of hospital
	address
	telephone number
	Doctor _____

Necropsy of Humane Law Case

History

Time of necropsy	:	AM PM	/ /
Time dog last seen alive	:	AM PM	/ /
Time animal found dead	:	AM PM	/ /

Describe circumstances of death below

Preliminary conclusion   *Physical Findings on following pages*

Histopathology pending?	Y	N
Toxicology pending?	Y	N

7/24/2003

Appendix 27.2:
Gross Examination Worksheet—Necropsy

PROSECTOR: Date: Time: _____ a.m.   p.m.

GENERAL CONDITION: (Nutritional condition, physical condition)

Neonates: examine for malformations (cleft palate, deformed limbs etc)
Weight: _____ #

BODY CONDITION
Ideal (1) Underweight/Lean (2) Thin(3) Underweight (4) Emaciated (5)

SKIN: (haircoat, skin, pinna, feet, subcutaneous fat and subcutaneous bruising)
Attach separate sheet for wound/injury and distribution   Yes   No

MUSCULOSKELETAL SYSTEM: (Bones, joints, and muscles)
Radiographs: Yes (see separate form)   No

BODY CAVITIES: (Fat stores, abnormal fluids)
Neonates: assess hydration (tissue moistness)

HEMOLYMPHATIC: (Spleen, lymph nodes, thymus)

RESPIRATORY SYSTEM: (Nasal cavity, larynx, trachea, lungs, and regional lymph nodes)
Neonates: Did breathing occur (i.e., do the lungs float in formalin)?   Yes   No

CARDIOVASCULAR SYSTEM: (Heart, pericardium, and great vessels)

DIGESTIVE SYSTEM: (Mouth, teeth, esophagus, stomach, intestines, liver, pancreas, mesenteric lymph nodes).
Diarrhea _____
Intestinal parasites _____
Feces submitted for ova and parasites?   Yes
Neonates: is milk present in stomach?   Yes   No

URINARY SYSTEM: (Kidneys, ureters, urinary bladder, and urethra)

REPRODUCTIVE SYSTEM: (Testis/ovary, uterus, vagina, penis, prepuce, prostate, mammary glands, placenta)

ENDOCRINE SYSTEM: (Adrenals, thyroid, parathyroids, pituitary)

NERVOUS SYSTEM: (Brain, spinal cord, and peripheral nerves)

SENSORY ORGANS (Eyes, ears)

LABORATORY STUDIES: (List bacterial and viral cultures submitted and results, if available)

Attach sample submission checklist

After Munson - http://www.vetmed.ucdavis.edu/whc/Necropsy/AppIIe.html

Appendix 27.3:
External Wounds—Cats and Dogs

Label	Name of hospital
	address
	telephone number

Necropsy of Humane Law Case External Wounds/Lesions

1) Show location, size, and distribution of skin wounds or lesions (Describe on diagram or in Comments section)

2) External parasites Yes No (Describe in comments section or next to diagram. Include estimate of numbers)

COMMENTS

Label	Name of hospital
	address
	telephone number

Necropsy of Humane Law Case External Wounds/Lesions

1) Show location, size, and distribution of skin wounds or lesions (Describe on diagram or in Comments section)

2) External parasites Yes No (Describe in comments section or next to diagram. Include estimate of numbers)

COMMENTS   **separate page for description of hair ;**

Appendix 27.4:
Fixed Tissue Checklist for Histology—Necropsy

Preserve the following tissues in 10 % buffered formalin at a ratio of 1 part tissue to 10 parts formalin. Tissues should be no thicker than 1 cm.

INCLUDE SECTIONS OF ALL LESIONS AND SAMPLES OF ALL TISSUES ON THE TISSUE LIST.

__**Salivary gland**

__**Oral/pharyngeal mucosa and tonsil** - plus any areas with erosions, ulcerations or other lesions.

__**Tongue** – cross- section near tip including both mucosal surfaces.

__**Lung** - sections from several lobes including a major bronchus

__**Trachea**

__**Thyroid/parathyroids**

__**Lymph nodes** - cervical, mediastinal, bronchial, mesenteric and lumbar. Cut transversely.

__**Thymus**

__**Heart** - Sections from both sides including valves

__**Liver** - sections from 3 different areas including gall bladder

__**Spleen** - Cross sections including capsule.

__**GI Tract** - 3 cm long sections of:
    Esophagus
    Stomach - multiple sections from all regions of the lining
    Intestines - multiple sections from different areas

__**Omentum** - ~3 cm square

__**Pancreas** - sections from two areas

__**Adrenal** - entire gland with transverse incision.

__**Kidney** -cortex and medulla from each kidney

__**Urinary bladder, ureters, urethra** - cross section of bladder and 2 cm sections of ureter and urethra.

__**Reproductive tract** - Entire uterus and ovaries with longitudinal cuts into lumens of uterine horns. Both testes (transversely cut) with epididymis. Entire prostate, transversely cut.

__**Eye**

__**Brain** - cut longitudinally along midline.

__**Spinal cord** (if neurologic disease) - sections from cervical, thoracic and lumbar cord.

__**Diaphragm and Skeletal muscle** - cross section of thigh muscles

__**Opened rib or longitudinally sectioned femur** - marrow must be exposed for proper fixation

__**Skin** - full thickness of abdominal skin, lip and ear pinna.

__**Neonates: umbilical stump** - include surrounding tissues

After Dr. L. Munson - http://www.vetmed.ucdavis.edu/whc/Necropsy/AppIIb.html

Appendix 27.5:
Preliminary Statement—Necropsy

Label	**Name of hospital** --- address telephone number

Preliminary Veterinarian Statement - NECROPSY

On   /   /   I evaluated a _____ (*age, breed, species*)

I found the _____ (*species*) to be (*general appearance, temperament etc.*), _____

List specific findings below

Attach external wound form   **Y NA**   Radiology   **Y NA**   Histopathology   **Y NA**

Body condition at presentation: Ideal **(1)** Underweight/Lean **(2)** Thin **(3)** Very Underweight **(4)** Emaciated **(5)**

Description of body condition on next page

Pending   Histopathology   **Y N**   Radiographs   **Y N**   Toxicology   **Y N**

Preliminary Conclusion

The above statement is an accurate summary of my findings

		/ /
Stamp of veterinarian	Signature of veterinarian	Date

Appendix 27.6:
Final Statement—Necropsy

Label	**Name of hospital** address telephone number

Final Veterinarian Statement - NECROPSY

On / / I performed a post-mortem evaluation on a _____ (*age, breed, species*)

I found the _____ (*species*) to be (*general appearance*), _____

List specific findings below

Attach External wound form **Y NA** *Internal wound form* **Y NA** *Histopathology results* **Y NA**

Attach Radiology interpretation **Y NA** *Radiology consult* **Y NA** *Toxicology results* **Y NA**

Body condition at presentation: Ideal (1) Underweight/Lean (2) Thin (3) Ve

Description of body condition on next page **Weight at Presentation** _____ #

Conclusion

The above statement is an accurate summary of my findings

/ /

Stamp of veterinarian   Signature of veterinarian   Date

Appendix 27.7:
Certification of Medical Record

I, *Name and address of hospital*, certify that the attached document is a true and accurate copy of the medical record of;

ANIMAL IDENTIFICATION

Humane Law Enforcement   AO200_____

<<Name of Hospital>>   _____

Animal Placement   A01_____

I also certify that this record was made in the regular course of business of this Hospital. That, it is the regular business of this Hospital to make and keep such a record, and that the record was made upon the dates set forth or within a reasonable time of the condition, act, transaction, occurrence, or event.

Signature: _____

Date: _____

Appendix 27.8:
Live Animal Forms

INTAKE—SOAP

Label	Name of hospital
	-----------------------------
	address
	telephone number
	Doctor _____

Medical Evaluation of Humane Law Enforcement Seizure

Medical History

Exam	T	P	R	

Behavior   - Assess strength, activity and interaction with people and animals

Sensorium	N Abn	Integ.	N Abn	Ears	N Abn	Heart	N Abn	MuscSkel	N Abn
Pain	Yes No	**L. nodes**	N Abn	**Nose**	N Abn	**Lungs**	N Abn	**Neurol.**	N Abn
Hydration	N Abn	**Eyes**	N Abn	**Mouth**	N Abn NE	**Abdomen**	N Abn	**Urogen.**	N Abn

Body Condition: Ideal **(1)**   Underweight/Lean **(2)**   Thin **(3)**   Very Underweight **(4)**   Emaciated **(5)**

Record abnormal findings below

Attach skin/haircoat forms if appropriate ☐   *Physical Findings continued on second page* ☐

Assessment

Plan

CBC/Chem ☐	UA ☐	Fecal ☐	Dog - DAG ☐	Cat - FeLV/FIV ☐	Microchip ☐
Rabies / /	**DHPP** / /		**B. bronchisep.** / /	**FVRCP** / /	

Label	Name of hospital address telephone number Doctor _____

Medical Evaluation of Humane Law Enforcement Seizure

Continuation of physical findings

Assessment and Plan - see first page

WEIGHT CHANGE

Label	Name of hospital
	address telephone number

Weight Change	
Weight (#)	

Date   /   /   _____

Date   /   /   _____

Date   /   /   _____

Date   /   /   _____

Date   /   /   _____

Date   /   /   _____

Date   /   /   _____

Date   /   /   _____

Date   /   /   _____

CONDITION OF SKIN—CAT

Label	**Name of hospital** address telephone number

Condition of skin

1) Show location, size, and distribution of skin wounds or lesions (Describe on diagram or in Comments section)

2) External parasites Yes No (Describe in comments section or next to diagram. Include estimate of numbers)

COMMENTS   **separate page for description of hair and nails**

CONDITION OF SKIN—DOG

Label	Name of hospital
	address
	telephone number

Condition of skin

1) Show location, size, and distribution of skin wounds or lesions (Describe on diagram or in Comments section)

2) External parasites Yes No (Describe in comments section or next to diagram. Include estimate of numbers)

COMMENTS   **separate page for description of hair and nails**

CONDITION OF HAIRCOAT AND NAILS—CAT

Label	Name of hospital address telephone number

Condition of haircoat, and nails

Physical care scale (see definitions next page)

1) Adequate   **2) Lapsed**   **3) Borderline**   **4) Poor**   **5) Terrible**

After Dr. G. Patronek, Tufts Care and Condition Scoring Scales, American Humane Association, 1998.

COMMENTS

CONDITION OF HAIRCOAT AND NAILS—DOG

Label	Name of hospital
	address
	telephone number

Condition haircoat and nails

Physical care scale (see definitions next page)

1) Adequate   **2) Lapsed**   **3) Borderline**   **4) Poor**   **5) Terrible**

After Dr. G. Patronek, Tufts Care and Condition Scoring Scales, American Humane Association, 1998.

COMMENTS

DEFINITION FOR USE WITH PHYSICAL CARE SCALE FOR HAIRCOAT AND NAILS

Label	
	--

Physical care scale - Haircoat and Nails
After Dr. G. Patronek, Tufts Care and Condition Scoring Scales, American Humane Association, 1998.

☐ 5 Terrible

Haircoat a single mat that prevents normal movement and interferes with vision. Soiling of hind end and legs with trapped urine and feces.
A complete clipdown required.
Nails extremely overgrown into circles and may be penetrating pads causing pain and infection. Nails interfering with normal gait.

☐ 4 Poor

Substantial matting of haircoat. Large sections of hair matteed together. Occasional foreign material embedded in mats. Much of the hair will need to be clipped. Fecal and urine soiling of hind end and legs.
Long nails that interfere with normal gait.

☐ 3 Borderline

Numerous mats, but animal can still be groomed without a total clip down.
No significant fecal or urine soiling. Nails are overgrown which may alter gait.

☐ 2 Lapsed

Haircoat may be somewhat dirty or have a few mats present that are easily removed. Remainder of coat can be easily brushed or combed.
Nails need a trim.

☐ 1 Adequate

Dog clean. Hair can be easily brushed or combed. Nails okay.

RADIOLOGY

Label	Name of hospital
	address
	telephone number

Radiograph Label	*Radiograph Consult? Yes No* *Please Attach*

Radiographic View	Interpretation	

PRELIMINARY VETERINARY STATEMENT

Appendix 27A.8 Preliminary veterinary statement

Label	**Name of hospital** address telephone number
Preliminary Veterinary Statement	

Brief summary of animal's condition at presentation. Include description of animal.

List specific findings below

Body condition at presentation: Ideal **(1)** Underweight/Lean **(2)** Thin **(3)** Very Underweight **(4)** Emaciated **(5)**

Weight at presentation _____ #

Veterinary statement attached

Other attachments

Body condition definitions

Skin and or haircoat form   Y   NA

Radiology   Y   NA

Histopathology   Y   NA

Other

Pending   **Blood tests**   ☐ **Urinalysis**   ☐**Fecal**   ☐**Radiographs**   ☐

The above statement including all attachments is an accurate summary of my)

/   /

Stamp of veterinarian   Signature of veterinariar   Date

FINAL VETERINARY STATEMENT

Label	Name of hospital address telephone number
Final Veterinary Statement	

Brief summary of animal's condition at presentation. Include description of animal.

List specific findings below

Body condition at presentation: Ideal **(1)** Underweight/Lean **(2)** Thin **(3)** Very Underweight **(4)** Emaciated **(5)**

Weight at presentation _____ #

Veterinary statement attached

Other attachments

Body condition definitions

Skin and or haircoat form   Y   NA

Radiology   Y   NA

Histopathology   Y   NA

Other

The above statement is an accurate summary of my findings

/   /

Stamp of veterinarian   Signature of veterinarian   Date

28
Veterinary Forensics

Edward A. Leonard

INTRODUCTION

Forensics pertains to the law. From time to time practitioners may perform examinations on the instruction or order of a legal authority. It is beyond the scope of this text to outline a complete necropsy or all the lesions associated with a nonaccidental traumatic incident or other forms of animal abuse. Whenever possible, veterinary or other specialists (veterinary pathologists, radiologists, medical examiners, and so on) should be called in to perform the necropsy or to assist in the finding's interpretation. This chapter highlights the common points relating to veterinary postmortem examinations from a legal aspect.

The point of the forensic necropsy goes beyond determining just the cause of death. It tries to recreate events close to the death, and to reveal any part that trauma, poison, disease, or neglect may have played. This reconstruction must remain within a legal and sometimes medical-criminal frame.

Do your examination with an open mind. Base your opinions on your own findings, trying not to approach the situation with preconceived views.

> *"When you have eliminated the impossible, whatever remains, however improbable, must be the truth."*
> — Arthur Conan Doyle
> (Sherlock Holmes)

SAFETY

Safety is the first concern in all cases. Always act with an awareness of three types of hazards: biological, chemical, and physical. If something killed an animal, our aim is to prevent it from killing again.

Make use of a three-layer border to isolate and secure a scene in the field. The outer border is a region much larger than the actual site itself. This is the safe area for bystanders, media, and nonessential personnel. The middle zone is a control buffer and work area. The inner zone is the core—the site surrounding the event itself. When the scene is stable, close off any areas that may yield evidence: driveways, surrounding yards, pathways, and so on. Use barricade tape or ropes to prevent unauthorized people from entering the area and potentially contaminating it or themselves.

Eating, drinking, or smoking is never appropriate at a site. For involved cases, a break area should be available somewhere outside the restricted areas. It could be a vehicle, picnic table, room, tent, and so on. It can be a gathering place for noninvolved personnel; a place for investigators to take breaks, eat, drink, or smoke; a communication center; a place for press conferences; and so on.

Part of the work area (away from the public area) may need to be a cleansing area, for the disinfection of gear and the removal of dangerous matter. Levels of protective clothing vary from a coverall-type garment with no respirator to the highest-level fully encapsulated suit with a self-contained breathing apparatus. Use rubber boots, coveralls, protective gowns, aprons, facemasks, eye/face protection, and cut-proof gloves under rubber gloves as needed. Too much protection is better than not enough. Shoe covers, outer footwear, and ordinary footwear dedicated for wear at contaminated scenes and necropsies are best. Put these with other items that staff can disinfect.

Pens, notes, sketches, and cameras can become sources of contamination when examining areas and bodies. Try to have someone else take notes and photos and make sketches. Tell them what to record. At least use a disposable pen, and dispose of it in a safe manner along with the gloves and other equipment before leaving the scene. Wearing protective gear is almost pointless when a contaminated pen, pencil, or marker ends up in our pocket or its cap is between our teeth. Wipe the outside of all equipment with an appropriate disinfectant before leaving the area.

Bodies covered with a tarp, or in a bag, need airing. Handle with care, and wait until the fumes have dissipated. Experience will tell when something smells familiar or "wrong." Blackleg, Salmonellosis, Ascariasis, septic mastitis, urea poisoning, myiasis, mange, onion poisoning, motor oil toxicity, and many other conditions each have a characteristic odor. With unrecognized odors, continue the examination as if dealing with a toxic substance.

Assume the animal has a contagious disease and proceed accordingly. For example, if anthrax is a problem in the area, get blood smears from the peripheral areas (in ungulates) or from areas of swelling (in carnivores) before opening a carcass. When the smears are dry, label one end of the slide with the date, species, animal ID, and location. Transport the slides to a laboratory or stain them in the field. If anthrax bacteria are present on blood smears, do not open the carcass. (Opening a carcass with anthrax will cause the bacteria to form spores and disperse the spores throughout the environment.)

FIELD BASICS

Veterinarians are typically more accustomed to working in hospitals or laboratories than in the field gathering information from a possible crime scene. The following basic guidelines provide information about crime scene investigation from a veterinary standpoint.

Identification

The proper tagging, labeling, and marking of the "evidence" enable us later to easily identify those items. Marking and labeling begins our control and custody of the items of evidence. A chain of custody is a witnessed, written record of all of the individuals who maintained unbroken control over the items of evidence. It establishes the proof that the items of evidence collected at the crime scene is the same

evidence presented in a court of law. Who, what, when, where, and the case number or identifier belongs on each evidence tag. Seal all evidence containers at the scene.

The Search

The search should be careful and methodical. Be aware of people's expectation of privacy and legal standing. A search warrant or proper consent to search may be necessary. Work with law enforcement investigators to ensure compliance on this part of the investigation. After talking to the people first on the scene and learning from them of any changes made to the scene since their arrival, then enter the scene using care not to disturb or destroy any evidence. Ideally, only one investigator should initially approach a body. To avoid destroying evidence, a pathway may be marked off using barricade tape, ropes, string, or flags, and used as the sole entrance and exit to the scene until the search is over. Find out if anyone has moved or altered anything prior to arrival. If so, find out who moved it and why. Carefully observe the walls and floor or ground. Look up as well—every scene is three-dimensional. Look for stains, marks, and so on. Photograph them using a scale. Shining a flashlight or reflecting sunlight with a hand mirror across the floor or ground highlights details (also known as side lighting).

Initially do not move or alter the body's position. Make a thorough visual examination of the body and the area immediately around it. Look between the legs without moving them. Look for struggle signs. Examine the scene for the presence or absence of body fluids. If any is present, note the amount, size, shape, and direction of flow patterns. Is the pattern consistent with gravity? Photograph fluid spots using a scale or ruler.

Sketching

Make a sketch of the scene. It may be rough and freehand, or on graph paper with so many squares representing so many square feet or inches. Include the location of doors, windows, furniture, the body, and anything else significant. A sketch can cover a large area and leave out clutter that appears in photographs. Measure the size of the area, and the width and height of doors, windows, furniture or other items. Locate the body and any items of evidence within the scene. Include notes on the location, date, time, case number, preparer, weather, lighting, scale (or scale disclaimer), compass orientation, evidence, measurements, and so on.

Photographs

Keep a photo log. Use rulers, index cards, and a felt pen to identify items. Photos of the scene should show the approach to the area, signs, lights, and all identifying objects in relation to the actual scene. Photograph the scene in a clockwise overlapping pattern before altering the body's position or any other evidence within the scene. Photograph the scene from at least two opposite corners. Leave nothing photographically hidden behind other objects. Photograph the body and the immediate vicinity around the body. Take pictures from directly above the body and other evidence as well as from ground and eye level.

Photograph a ruler with items where relative size is important or on items that need to have one-to-one comparison photographs. Photograph the object first as is, then with the ruler and identification. Always identify similar bodies and important objects with cards displaying the location, date, time, and case and identification numbers.

Take pictures of every room and building you have access to, even if the relationship of them to the scene is not readily apparent. When photographing the exterior, take surreptitious photos of the spectators and vehicles. A perpetrator may return to observe the actions of investigative personnel. Photos may also help identify reluctant witnesses. Film is cheaper than lost cases.

Federal Rules of Evidence, Article X (Contents of Writings, Recordings, and Photographs), Rule 1001 permits photographs stored digitally in a computer. A digital photograph stored in a computer is an original, and any exact copy of the digital photograph is admissible evidence. However, always check state's rules of evidence for specifics on digital photographs. Keep images in an unalterable, archival form. Include all information regarding their creation. Control custody of all image records at all times.

The principal requirements to admit a photograph (digital- or film-based) into evidence are relevance and authentication. Unless both parties stipulate admission of the photograph, the party attempting to admit the photograph into evidence must be ready to offer testimony that the photograph is an accurate representation of the scene. This usually means someone must testify that the photograph accurately portrays the scene as viewed by that witness.

The videotaping of the scene should never replace still photography. Common errors committed when videotaping a scene include poor focus, lighting, and panning and zoom techniques. Once the video camera begins recording, it should not stop until the taping is complete. The camera operator should describe each room and view of the scene. However, everyone else should be silent during the taping. The key to good videotaping is slow camera movement.

Examination of the Body

After photographing everything, begin a detailed examination of the body. Take careful notes of the external appearance of the body. Look for blood pooling and decomposition. Describe the location and appearance of injuries, wounds, missing body parts, and so forth. Describe just what is there, and draw no conclusions yet. If some common item may be missing, note it. For example, are there signs of a missing collar or strap? Record postmortem changes (rigor mortis). The pooling of the blood within the body fixes with time, and may show someone or something moved the body after death. Note the presence or absence of blood, saliva, vomit, urine, and their direction and flow. What are the odors emanating from the carcass and surroundings? Are there foreign materials on the body (e.g., powders, leaves, grass, soil)? Collect any easily lost evidence from the body. Record maggot activity. When moving the body, check the underside for injuries and evidence. Obtain an air temperature. Then, record the temperature of the body, the surface it is lying on, and the area between the two. If a maggot mass is present, take the temperature of the mass.

Virtually any biological evidence found at a crime scene can have DNA to be tested. Given the sensitive nature of DNA evidence, contact laboratory personnel or evidence collection technicians whenever collection questions arise. DNA contamination easily happens when someone sneezes or coughs over evidence, or touches his or her own body before touching an area that may contain the DNA for testing. Keep the evidence dry and at room temperature. Secure the evidence in paper bags or envelopes, then seal, label, and transport it properly. DNA evidence placed in plastic bags may experience damage from moisture. Direct sunlight and warmer conditions also may be harmful.

Burial Sites

Estimate the probable dimensions (length, width, and depth) as closely as possible. Examine the ground surface for any evidence before slow and careful excavation. In some cases, especially those of large graves, heavy equipment (e.g., a backhoe) may help initially to remove the topsoil, with a monitor watching carefully for evidence or remains exposed by the machinery. Then, probe the removed soil carefully with pick and shovel and finally, with trowel and brush.

Burying usually protects bodies from animals, insects, or changes in surface temperature. The rate of decomposition relies solely on the activity of microorganisms and soil structure. In mass or deep graves, often there is little oxygen to promote the growth of organisms and decomposition, and the bodies may stay well preserved. In single or shallow graves, the process of decomposition is more rapid.

Unburied bodies experience the destructive effects of insect, climate, and animal activity. The potential for animals to destroy or scatter body parts increases with time. Small bones and loosened teeth may "sink" below a soil surface worked by insects. Rain and wind mixes earth and decayed plant matter to cover bones. Gravity helps scatter remains located on a slope.

Expand the Search

Search the immediate area, and work outward in circles through the remainder of the building or scene. The scope or intensity of the search depends on the particular situation and the conditions present. It is difficult to conduct a detailed examination of a scene without adequate lighting. Inadequate lighting may result in the overlooking or destruction of evidence. When indoors, note the type of heating or air conditioning available and the thermostat setting. Check the contents of wastebaskets and trashcans. Note the presence of items that do not "belong" there. Search hidden places around large appliances, and behind, on top of, and under furniture (use a hand mirror), on the roof, and so on.

Reports

A generic animal diagram form makes it easier to record observations. As always, detailed information includes dates and times, names and addresses, individual identification (species, breed, age, sex, color, tag number, marks, weight, and so on), and history (if available).

Extras

A kneeling pad saves knees. Magnifying devices aid vision. Always carry spare batteries and replacement bulbs.

NECROPSY ESSENTIALS

A standard necropsy has a basic format common to all species. However, each varies with different species anatomy, the particular case history, and the discoveries made. A generic necropsy findings check-off form makes it easier to record observations. The best time for a necropsy is as soon as possible after death. Even with refrigeration, lesions steadily become more and more difficult to assess. Do not freeze the carcass or specimens.

Records

Begin with information from the evidence tags, bands, tattoos, and the officer in charge. Scan the carcass for microchips. Add information from observations (e.g., species, breed, gender, estimated age, markings, and so on) and at each step in the necropsy process. Accurately describe all abnormalities and collect samples where possible. Remember, interpretation should not appear in the description of lesions.

Weight and Temperature

Weigh the body on a scale and record its temperature. (Later compare this temperature to field notes on body temperature, the surface it was laying on, the area between the two, and the air temperature at the site, for consistency.) Organ weight data are optional. Collect it when appropriate.

Radiographs

X-ray the entire body if possible. Note newly broken or dislocated bones, healing and healed fractures, as well as foreign objects. Is there any potential pattern of abuse? Dental development (calcification and eruption of teeth) can give accurate age information in pre-adults. The appearance of ossification centers and epiphyseal unions may be comparable with available age standards.

Images

Photograph the body and significant findings throughout the process and keep a photo log. Use rulers, index cards, and a felt pen to identify the items.

Measurements

Log the length (tip of nose to base of tail), height (at shoulder), and girth as appropriate for the species.

Assessment

Record the animal's nutritional condition (using a scale such as the *Nestlé Purina Body Condition System* or *Tufts Animal Care and Condition Scales*) if possible, as well as state of rigidity and extent of postmortem decomposition. Rigor mortis usually begins with the jaw and spreads from the extremities to the trunk. Loss of rigor is a result of the putrefaction process. The onset and duration, or absence, of rigor depends on the environment, the animal's physical condition at death, and the handling of the body after death.

Surfaces

Comb the body for tattoos, scars, abnormalities, discharges, discolorations, nodules, masses, and anomalies. Hold paper under the area you are combing. Shave, count, measure, and photograph all wounds and lesions. (Bruising and bleeding in the tissues near the wounds indicate that they occurred before the animal died.) Look for and preserve any external parasites.

Openings

Note the condition and changes of the eyes, ears, nose, mouth, anus, and urinary and genital tracts.

Samples

Collect representative specimens if indicated. Collect external foreign substances such as dirt, blood, insects, and so on. The femur, rib, sternum, and vertebra are sites for collection of bone marrow. Take blood samples from the chambers of the heart or major vessels and urine samples from the bladder or kidneys. Some laboratory values remain stable after death. Save gastrointestinal contents for identification and for analysis of toxic substances. Use saline to rinse the tissues during the necropsy. (Rinsing with tap water will cause artifacts.) If needed, collect eye specimens carefully without puncturing the globe to document disease or trauma. Take the microbiologic samples as soon as possible during the necropsy. Use sterile instruments to cut away contaminated surfaces. Collect specimens with additional sterile instruments or culture swabs. Take samples from any abnormal areas. Autolysis can cause many artifacts in tissues that can look like a disease process. However, it is always best to take a sample from an area that looks abnormal rather than assume that the change was autolysis. Histopathology will be able to distinguish between true lesions and postmortem changes.

The Necropsy

Use sharp, clean and, if possible, sterile instruments. Begin to skin the body, looking for signs of trauma, wounds, and lesions. With the body on its back, make a ventral midline incision from the tip of the jaw to just below the anus. Spread the skin from the abdomen, thorax, and neck region, exposing underlying tissues and lymph nodes. Note the amount and color of the subcutaneous adipose tissue. Cut the muscles between the scapula and thorax and the soft tissues surrounding the hip joint to allow the pelvic and thoracic limbs to lay flat and maintain the body in a steady position.

Carefully remove the muscles ventral to the trachea to examine the thyroid and parathyroid glands. Locate and examine the salivary glands and regional lymph nodes.

Completely expose the abdominal viscera with a ventral midline incision through the abdominal wall from the sternum to the pubis. From the thoracic end of this incision, cut laterally along the posterior margin of the ribs. From the pubic end of the incision, cut laterally just anterior to the pubis.

Methodically examine all viscera in situ and observe for correct anatomic size and position. Record any abnormal characteristics of the fluids present. Locate and examine both adrenal glands. Demonstrate wound paths with rods and photograph them.

Verify negative thoracic pressure by carefully observing and listening for air rushing into a small stab incision made through the nonmuscle portion of the diaphragm. Using bone cutters, remove the ventral third of the rib cage.

Examine the thoracic viscera in situ and observe for correct anatomic size and position. Record any abnormal characteristics of the fluids present. Demonstrate wound paths with rods and photograph them.

Dissect through the soft tissue between the tongue and mandible, across the soft palate and through the hyoid apparatus to free the tongue and larynx. Then, remove a "block" of thoracic viscera, including the tongue, larynx, trachea, esophagus, heart, aorta, and lungs. Tying off the distal esophagus helps prevent spillage of gastric contents. Examine the oral cavity, teeth, pharynx, and tonsils.

Incise the pericardial sac. Check for abnormal fluid accumulation. Reflect the pericardium over the base of the heart. Examine the base of the heart, the great vessels, and atria. Then, examine the cardiac surface and coronary arteries. Carefully dissect the heart following the path of normal blood flow and examine all inner surfaces. Next, section the thymus.

Examine and open the trachea from the larynx to the level of the primary bronchi. Palpate all lung lobes. Dissect the lung lobes by opening all major bronchi. Next, open and examine the esophagus.

Locate the foramina on either side of the ventral pelvis. Using bone cutters cut the pubis caudally and cranially into one foramen. Repeat this cutting on the opposite side. By blunt and sharp dissection, remove the freed section of bone to expose the pelvic canal.

Incise the skin and subcutaneous tissues around the external genitalia. Then, free both kidneys from their attachment sites. Dissect the ureters and excise at the urinary bladder. On both kidneys, incise and reflect the renal capsule and examine the ureters and renal vasculature.

Section the kidneys to the renal pelvis, cutting one kidney longitudinally and the other kidney transversely for identification. Then, extend the renal pelvic incisions into each ureter. Next, serially section the kidneys and ureter.

Remove the remaining urinary and genital organs. Record any signs of reproductive system surgery. Next, examine the urinary bladder, urethra, and prostate gland (if applicable). Open the bladder and urethra along their ventral aspects and re-examine the urethra and urinary bladder, then examine the male or female genitalia.

Next, examine the anus and rectum. Incise the skin and subcutaneous tissues around the anus and remove the abdominal viscera as a "block". Examine the remaining lymph nodes and the abdominal aorta.

Next, examine the pancreas. Apply pressure to the gallbladder, while observing for bile expulsion at the major duodenal papilla. Open and examine the gallbladder. Then, open the large hepatic arteries and veins (visceral surface) and examine them. Serially section the liver, and examine and serially

section the spleen. Examine the omentum, mesentery, the root of the mesentery, and mesenteric lymph nodes. Then, open and examine the distal esophagus, stomach, and small and large intestines. Collect fecal samples. Rinse the specimens with physiologic saline, not tap water.

Open the hip, stifle, shoulder, and elbow joints to examine for abnormal fluid; and for ruptured, stretched, or frayed ligaments; eroded and ulcerated cartilage; thickened joint capsules; and other abnormalities. Document any evidence of disease or trauma.

Afterwards, examine the brain in all cases that suggest neurological disease or trauma. First, remove the head. Making a dorsal midline incision from the nose to the foramen magnum, reflect the skin ventrally. Then, transect and examine the ear canals, and remove the temporal muscles from the cranium. To remove the brain, make bilateral cuts in the cranium. One additional cut into the cranium just behind the orbits connects the two previous cuts. Pry the top off the skull and examine the internal surface. Allow the brain to fall gently into the examiner's hand and then serially section the brain. Saw across the frontal and maxillary bones in front of the orbits, and then examine the nasal cavity and sinuses.

Following the examination of the brain, examine the ventral surface of the vertebral column and record any abnormalities. Remove the skin remaining on the carcass and also examine the dorsal subcutaneous tissue and musculature for any abnormal signs.

If the case suggests spinal disease or trauma, remove the spinal cord by cutting through the cervical, thoracic, and lumbar vertebral arches at different angles. Removing the thoracic section allows the easier placement of the saw blade for the subsequent removal of the cervical and lumbar sections. Use care not to cut the spinal cord upon entering the canal.

LESIONS

After death, the temperature in the body starts to drop. Variations in live body temperature, the ambient temperature in the hours after death, and the insulation and weight of the body all factor into temperature changes. For some species, such as deer, standards for temperature change can help determine time of death. After the onset of putrefaction, the body temperature will increase again due to the metabolic activity of the bacteria and other decomposing organisms. Rigor mortis depends on the temperature and concentrations of lactic acid. High metabolic activity in the time just before death (e.g., running) leads to higher levels of lactic acid, and shorter time for the rigor mortis to develop. Higher environmental temperature also leads to a shorter reaction time. In temperate regions, the following very general rules of thumb may help in estimating death (use with caution): Warm means dead for not more than eight hours. Stiff means dead for not more than three days.

Starvation

Malnourishment over time produces an extremely thin body, lacking both fat and lean body mass. The cause may be inadequate food or a disease process, but the result is from the lack of essential nutrients. Upon examination, the organs and muscular tissue appear thinner, moist, and glossy. There is an obvious atrophy of fat, especially around the heart and kidneys. Any remaining fat appears watery, translucent, or like jelly. Anemia and edema may also be present.

Wounds from Guns

Flame, soot, unburned gunpowder, and a bullet all exit out of the barrel of a gun. Flaming gas goes only a few inches and can produce a burn. Soot goes six or so inches from most handguns and can produce a smudge. Unburned powder travels up to three feet for a handgun, and may produce powder stippling (not powder burns). Contact wounds of air guns would lack these features. Roughing the skin as the bullet pulls it inward may appear as an abraded ring around the entry wound when the skin returns outward.

If the muzzle of the gun is tight against the skin, the gas, soot, and powder pass through the broken skin. When the blast enters the confined space, it can create a star-shaped entry wound as the skin turns backwards and tears. If the muzzle is not hard against the skin, there may be a small amount of soot at the edges, but no dispersed powder stippling. Star-shaped bursting is less likely, but it can still occur.

Exit wounds may be primary or secondary missiles. Fragments of a bone struck by a bullet pass through, and damage tissue as bullets do. An examination for gunshot residue may aid in distinguishing entrance from exit wounds, for the entrance wound will have more than the exit, or the exit will have none. Of course, residue is lacking in entrance wounds from air guns.

Entrance wounds into bone may produce beveling, or coning, of the bone at the surface away from the weapon. This may permit the determination of the direction of fire. In some situations, these findings may help to establish in what sequence the bullets entered. For example, multiple gunshot wounds to the head may produce fracture lines, and a subsequent fracture line will not cross a pre-existing fracture line.

As a bullet passes through the body, energy will transfer to the tissues and disperse in radial fashion. A temporary cavity occurs with a diameter many times that of the bullet. The faster the bullet, the worse is the damage. If the bullet exits the body, it will carry some of its energy with it, sparing the tissues. If the bullet yaws (tilts) as it enters the body, more energy will disperse over a shorter area resulting in greater tissue destruction.

At close range, a shotgun causes the most destructive civilian gunshot wound. The weight of the pellets, and the energy in the gas, almost never leave the body, so their entire energy damages the tissue. At greater distances, the shotgun pellets fan out—fewer pellets hit the target.

Do not attempt to clean bullets before sending them to a laboratory. Washing them may destroy trace evidence. Air dry the bullets, wrap each in paper, and seal them in separately labeled envelopes. Never mark the bullets unless directed to do so by the local authorities. Be careful to follow their instructions as to where and how to mark the bullets. Send all the bullets recovered to the laboratory. A conclusive identification may be possible on only one bullet, even when they all appear to be in good condition.

Remember that the orientation of a bullet track is positional. The wound may have happened while the animal stood or ran, but at necropsy the soft tissues can shift position. The more difficult problem is distinguishing a distant from a contact wound when the body is decomposed or the victim survived long enough that healing of the wound began. Take care to avoid misinterpretation of the bullet wounds and when rendering opinions as to direction of fire.

Wounds from Blunt Trauma

The amount of damage delivered by a blow from a blunt object varies directly with the force used in delivering the blow and the surface area that receives the blow. Blows from a rounded pipe or a knob on a club do more damage than the side of a board by directing the larger mass of the object to a smaller area on the body.

Before death, abrasions (scrapes) are reddish from inflammation and perhaps minor bleeding. After death, abrasions are yellow, with a fibrin coating resembling parchment. An abrasion may be the only external sign of blunt force injury, which may have done serious internal damage. Patterned abrasions may tell the nature of the object causing the injury (e.g., tire tracks, pipes, even rings on a fist). Claw marks are deeper, U-shaped lesions that penetrate the outer skin layers.

Contusions (bruises) are areas of hemorrhage in soft tissue due to ruptured blood vessels from blunt trauma. If it is palpable, it is a hematoma. Like abrasions, bruises may or may not have a pattern. Remember that bruises are often hard to see. The rate of color change is tremendously variable, and cannot be used to estimate the time of an injury.

Even heavy trauma may not produce a bruise. Conversely, bruises can be much larger than the object that produced them, due to stretching and avulsion of nearby vessels. One can produce a bruise on a newly dead body. Without blood pressure, it will not be as impressive as one produced by the same force in life. Advanced decomposition and pooling of the blood can produce lesions similar to bruises.

Lacerations are splits and tears of the skin or soft tissue, due to stretching-shearing or crushing, on the body's surface or deep inside. Do not call an incised wound (cuts), produced with something sharp, a laceration. Lacerations have irregular, crushed, abraded, undermined, bruised edges and elastic connective-tissue bridges in their depths. Lesions produced by very dull knives or the edges of boards may appear similar. The wound's shape does not tell the exact shape of the instrument that produced it. An example is a Y-shaped lesion produced by a metal pipe.

Stomping or kicking may cause brutal injuries. Brain hemorrhage, fractures, a pneumothorax, and extensive visceral damage may all be present. Hit-by-a-car injuries, on the other hand, may show damage only corresponding to the height of a bumper or the width of a tire.

Wounds from Sharp Objects

Pointed and sharp objects produce stab wounds, incised wounds (cuts), and chop wounds (incised wounds plus an underlying bone fracture or groove, made by heavy instruments). We differentiate wounds by sharp instruments from lacerations by clean, sharp margins; absence of bruising at the edges; and absence of bridging deep in the tissues.

It is difficult to determine the size or shape of a knife from the wounds produced. With an incompletely inserted blade, the track will be shorter and narrower than the blade. With great force, the track will be longer than the blade. If the knife does not move straight in and out, the skin wound may be wider than the blade. The sharper the knife, the easier it is to penetrate the skin. A dull knife will cause abraded, bruised margins, and a very dull knife will cause jagged, contused margins.

If there are multiple stab wounds, it is easier to make an educated guess about how thick and how long the weapon was. Probe knife wounds gently. We can easily make them deeper and thereby learn nothing useful.

Incised Wounds

Hesitation marks are superficial cuts made before the lethal deep cut. Perpetrators tend to use their dominant hand and locate their cuts accordingly.

Most incised wounds have very shallow ends. A wrinkle wound is several discontinuous incised wounds, caused when a knife wrinkles the skin, cutting only the crests. The dimensions of an incised wound tell us nothing about the weapon that made it.

Chop Wounds

Chop wounds are placed in a separate category because they combine features of incised wounds and lacerations, or they may appear intermediate. Machete and meat cleaver wounds belong in this category.

Typically, a chop wound will produce an obvious defect in the underlying bone. Depending on how sharp the instrument is, the outer wound may appear to be an incision or laceration.

Suffocation and Drowning

Suffocation is failure of oxygen to reach the uppermost airway. With smothering (death from occlusion of the mouth and nose), the necropsy findings may be entirely negative.

In hangings, the pressure is often great enough to prevent most arterial flow to the head. Therefore, we may not see bruising. In lethal ligature and manual strangulation (not necessarily suffocation), there may be bruising on the conjunctivae. This finding is by no means specific. Sphincter incontinence may or may not happen with strangulation.

With hanging, the compression of neck structures is secondary to a noose tightened by body weight. We will usually find the noose above the larynx. Look for marks, unless the ligature is soft and the body is taken down soon after death. Authentic-looking noose marks can appear on a body if hanged two hours or less after death by some other means.

Ligature strangulation is compression of the neck structures secondary to a noose (collar) tightened by something other than body weight. The appearance of the mark can be highly variable. With a towel, there may be none at all.

With ligature or manual strangulation or hanging, lesions may sometimes include fractures of the hyoid bone of the larynx, episcleral or subconjunctival hemorrhage, petechial hemorrhage of the internal eye, crushing injury of the larynx, laryngeal edema, and lingual swelling, or edema of the lips and eyelids (Munro and Thrusfield, 2001a; Spitz, 1993). In two cases of cats that were manually strangled, the tympanic membranes were ruptured and hemorrhages were found in the middle ear in both (personal communication with Dr. Andrew Newmark). These findings in cases of strangulation were also reported by Spitz (1993). Absence of the lesions does not rule out the diagnosis.

Drowning may result in subtle signs of water inhalation. Look for froth in the airways. Peripheral displacement of air by water can over inflate the lungs. The presence of diatoms (tiny plants) in inhaled water also may help the diagnosis.

Injury due to Fire

A house fire's temperature is usually around 1200°F, and this is usually not hot enough to ash a 60-pound animal body in less than one hour. Animals caught in a burning building inhale smoke, fumes, and heat. Animals dying in fires typically have soot in the airways, and they will always have elevated carboxyhemoglobin levels (greater than 50 percent). This carbon monoxide poisoning may cause a bright pink discoloration of light-colored tissues. Arson is a time-honored means of trying to conceal a crime. A dead animal burned by a perpetrator will not have soot in the airway or high carboxyhemoglobin levels (normal is less than 10 percent).

Many arsonists assume that after an intense fire only negligible amounts of fire accelerants will remain. The amount of accelerant remaining depends on the quantity and type of compound used, the nature of material it was on, the time since the fire, as well as the severity of the fire. Normally, the fire department conducts an investigation into the cause and origin of a suspicious fire. Investigators have been able to detect trace amounts of liquid hydrocarbons in soil beneath a gutted house months after a fire.

Electrical Injuries

High-voltage alternating current (7,680 volts from the generator plant) kills by generating heat. Low-voltage alternating current (110-volt household current) kills by inducing ventricular fibrillation; or if the amperage is high, the heart simply cannot repolarize. Electrical burns are generally small, gray, charred marks with a grayish-white rim. Lightning (direct current) produces fern-shaped burns.

Insects

One of the first groups of insects that arrive on a dead vertebrate is blowflies. Usually the female lays eggs within two days after death of the vertebrate. If we know how long it takes to reach the different stages in an insect's life, the age of the insects can be an estimate of the animal's time of death. Unfortunately, this period is quite variable and depends on temperature, time of day and year, and exposure. However, insects can also be of help in establishing whether someone or something moved the body after death, by comparing the local fauna around the body and the fauna on the body. Dead bodies found in covered environments should have no blowflies.

After the initial decay, the body begins to smell and attracts different types of insects. The insects that usually arrive first are the flies, in particular the blowflies and the flesh flies. The females will lay their eggs on the body, particularly around the natural orifices such as the nose, eyes, ears, anus, penis, and vagina. If the body has exposed wounds, the eggs also will appear there.

One important biological phenomenon that occurs on cadavers is a succession of organisms that thrive on the different parts. For example, beetles that specialize on bone will have to wait until bone is available. Predatory beetles or parasites that feed on maggots will have to wait until the blowflies arrive and lay their eggs. The succession on cadavers happens in a predictable sequence and can help in estimating the time of death, even if the body has been lying around for some time.

In northern regions, dead bodies may appear in spring, after the snow melts. If the death occurred before winter, it is possible to find dead insects in and on the body. By analyzing the dead insects, and estimating when the insects probably died (by looking at meteorological records), we have a clue to when the death happened.

Sexual Assault

Sexual assault should be suspected when the history is suggestive of sexual activity or unusual injuries are found around the anus, vagina, penis, or testicles. In cases of known or suspected sexual assault, some of the findings reported by Munro and Thrusfield (2001b) include gross vaginal injuries such as trauma from knife wounds and other injuries, sudden onset hemorrhage from the vulva, multiple hemorrhages around the vulva, foreign objects retrieved from the vagina (including a candle and pieces of a broomstick), necrotic tissue around the anus or other perianal wounds consistent with stabbing, and cord ligatures or elastic bands around the base of the penis or scrotum.

NON-LESIONS

A bloody nasal discharge may be due to nasal congestion at death with the subsequent rupture of congested vessels. Advanced decomposition and pooling of the blood produces lesions similar to bruises. Gray to black discoloration of tissues may be due to postmortem decomposition of blood by bacteria.

CONCLUSION

The key to a good forensic necropsy is attention to small details in the forest of normal changes present from decay. We have to be able to see both the forest and the trees as we reconstruct the landscape of events prior to death. Our best tools are a keen eye and an open mind. Forming your opinions from real findings, free of predetermined notions, will lead you closest to the truth. The reader is strongly encouraged to use the following references cited for additional information.

REFERENCES

Adrian, William J., ed. 1996. *1996 Wildlife Forensic Field Manual,* 2d ed. Denver, CO: Association of Midwest Fish and Game Law Enforcement Officers.

Castner, James L., and Jason H. Byrd. 2000. *Forensic Insect Identification Cards.* Gainesville, FL: Feline Press.

Catts, Paul E., and Neal H. Haskell. 1990. *Entomology and Death, a Procedural Guide.* Clemson, SC: Joyce's Print Shop, Inc.

Eliopulos, Louis N. 1993. *Death Investigator's Handbook: A Field Guide to Crime Scene Processing, Forensic Evaluations, and Investigative Techniques.* Boulder, CO: Paladin Press.

King, John M., David C. Dodd, and Lois Roth. 2000. *The Necropsy Book.* Illustrated by Marion E. Newson, Betsy Uhl, and Mike Simmons. Gurnee, IL: Charles Louis Davis, D.V.M. Foundation.

Munro, H. M. C., and M. V. Thrusfield. 2001a. Battered Pets: Non-accidental physical injuries found in dogs and cats. *Journal of Small Animal Practice* 42: 279 – 290.

Munro, H. M. C., and M. V. Thrusfield. 2001b. Battered Pets: Sexual assault. *Journal of Small Animal Practice* 42: 333 – 337.

Newmark, A. 2003. Personal communication with Dr. Andrew Newmark. April.

Scene of the Crime: U.S. Government Forensic Handbook. 1992. Boulder, CO: Paladin Press.

Spitz, Werner W. 1993. *Spitz and Fisher's Medicolegal Investigation of Death, Guidelines for the Application of Pathology to Crime Investigation,* 3rd ed. Springfield, Illinois Charles A. Thompson, Chapter 11.

Strafuss, Albert C. 1988. *Necropsy: Procedures and Basic Diagnostic Methods for Practicing Veterinarians.* Springfield, IL: Charles C. Thomas.

TB MED 283, Veterinary Necropsy Protocol for Military Working Dogs and Pathology Specimen Submission Guidelines. 2001. Washington, DC: Headquarters, Department of the Army.

Title 28—Appendix, Federal Rules of Evidence, Article X, Contents of Writings, Recordings, and Photographs. Rule 1001.

Williams, David J., Anthony J. Ansford, David S. Proday, and Alex S. Forrest. 1998. *Colour Guide Forensic Pathology.* Toronto, Ontario: Churchill Livingston.

29
Recognizing and Investigating Equine Abuse

Holly Cheever

INTRODUCTION

Historically, horses have occupied a broad niche in our lives and have played a critical role in human social evolution. As draft animals, modes of transportation, battle adjuncts, entertainers, and (increasingly) beloved companion animals, they have been intricately involved with many aspects of our lives and achievements. Their place in our cultural development, agriculture, and economy has been so crucial that equines were the primary focus for veterinary practice until well into the twentieth century. Reading the author's comments in James Herriot's books as to the relative importance of livestock versus companion animal medicine during the first half of the last century underscores the horse's prominent position. Only in the latter half of the 20th century did companion animals (household pets) replace horses as the preeminent focus for veterinary research and treatment—the changing demographics of human society brought more people into cities and away from farms, with working livestock being replaced by indoor pets. In addition, the increased displacement of horse-drawn machinery by automotive technology diminished the horse's critical role in our lives.

Because of their many varied uses, ranging from beasts of burden to treasured pets, horses are placed in a paradoxical position legally. There are five legislative acts that apply specifically to horses with four on the federal level: horses are included in the Animal Welfare Act (if used for entertainment or research but not for agriculture), the Horse Protection Act, the Wild Free Roaming Horses and Burros Act, and the Humane Slaughter Act. In addition, each state covers horses under their own state anti-cruelty laws. Horses are usually classified as agricultural animals for the purposes of both state and federal anti-cruelty or regulatory laws, and are therefore accorded only a minimum standard of humane care. Increasingly, however, these animals are regarded by the public as cherished companion animals and splendid athletes who deserve a higher level of protection. Public debate often develops over alleged horse abuse cases, as the demands for humane treatment by the horse-loving public conflict with the standards mandated by statute.

The use to which a horse is put determines whether it will be accorded pet or agricultural animal status, its degree of protection, and the severity of the punishment for a convicted abuser will vary accordingly. Some states define who has "animal" status for the purposes of their animal cruelty laws, and further refine their terminology as to what constitutes a "pet" versus a "farm" animal. In New York, for example, if you douse a pet pony with gasoline and set it afire, you have committed a felony as long as the owner can prove that the pony is considered a companion. However, performing the same violent act on a "farm" horse makes you guilty only of a misdemeanor. Similarly, under the federal Animal Welfare Act, a circus owner can be prosecuted for overdriving a horse during training and performance sessions, but if the equine's performance is rendered by a racing thoroughbred on a racetrack or by a draft horse pulling a plow in an agricultural setting, the Animal Welfare Act no longer applies.

To add to the challenge involved in the successful investigation into and prosecution of equine abuse cases, many law officers and animal control agents do not feel as confident in evaluating "farm" animals (including horses) as they do working with the more familiar dog and cat cases. I have found that the law officers' willingness to investigate these cases is enhanced if they know that there is a veterinarian willing and able to assist in the evaluation of the evidence and to provide expert testimony, if needed, in case of a trial. This chapter is intended to assist the veterinarian in investigating and evaluating equine abuse cases and includes the following topics:

• The evolution of the horse as a key to understanding both physiological and behavioral needs; this understanding is crucial for the recognition of abuse and also provides the background for designing optimal husbandry protocols once the horses are brought to a shelter or foster home.
• An overview of the categories of abuse.
• Welfare concerns in specific areas such as show horse training and commercial uses of equines (e.g., mule diving, donkey basketball, carriage horse operations).
• An effective strategy for evaluating backyard horse abuse cases and typical lesions to look for in such cases.

The information included herein is intended to be a very practical and elementary guide, thus providing a framework upon which to build as experience dictates. Together with the resources listed in the references as aids for the practitioner, I hope it will encourage and assist veterinarians to become proactive in promoting the humane treatment of horses.

EQUINE EVOLUTION: UNDERSTANDING THE BASIC REQUIREMENTS FOR PHYSICAL AND PSYCHOLOGICAL HEALTH

Horses evolved as ungulates with a simple stomach and a specialized large intestine and cecum. Their large body size and metabolic requirements for speed to escape predators demanded large volumes of forage to provide sufficient energy from a low-density energy source. Their diet consisted of grasses and shrubs lacking the concentrated energy sources seen in modern feeding programs that rely heavily on concentrates. Therefore, without the advantage of the ruminants' four-chambered stomach and rumination cycles, horses required long

time periods for food prehension each day to allow them to ingest sufficient bulk for energy. Though they are now primarily a grazing species, their prehistoric ancestors were browsers. Feral horses still browse extensively when cold weather makes other food sources scarce, and domestic horses overwintered without access to hay and grass strip bark from trees and nibble on branches and fence posts. The typical natural grazing pattern consists of tearing off a few mouthfuls of grass while standing in one spot, then moving a few steps while chewing to select the next mouthfuls. Food prehension is thus a process requiring motion in the form of walking while ingesting nutrients (Houpt 2002).

Therefore, based on these needs, an ideal management program will provide constant access to grazing or at least several feeding opportunities per day of forage (hay), for optimal digestive function. It will also provide plenty of opportunity for the horse to move freely, as opposed to being confined for 24 hours daily in a stall (e.g., inadequate "turnout" is a primary concern with urban carriage horses and Premarin mares). A well-sheltered run-in shed in a large paddock provides an ideal housing situation, with compatible horses and adequate manger space to permit even the subordinate group members adequate access to food supplies. Note that a bare paddock with no food access does not satisfy the horse's need to move about during the process of food prehension: If there is nothing to eat, the horse will remain stationary during its turnout period after an initial investigation of the enclosed space (Houpt 2002).

The horse has a highly evolved lower limb with elongated third metacarpal and metatarsal bones, which have powerful muscles proximally and elongated tendons and ligaments distally. These form an efficient system of levers and drivers with which to produce a longer stride per unit of muscle exertion than a shorter-limbed animal (Getty 1975). This specialized anatomy produces great speed over relatively short distances as well as the capacity for long distance travel. Because their lower limb development is so specialized and so lacking in protective soft tissue padding, horses are particularly prone to injury in this area, and lameness is a common sequela to overuse, improper training, and poor husbandry practices. Many areas of equine use (e.g., urban carriage horses, thoroughbred racers) produce typical limb injuries, as will be discussed later.

Ideally, the less the horse is exposed to hard concussive surfaces (such as city streets or excessively hard, fast tracks) during bony growth and development, the better. Ideal housing must provide dry, clean, nonslippery footing with a yielding surface to minimize stress on the limbs and prevent hoof infections. Unless a lameness dictates the need for special therapeutic shoeing, shelter horses generally do better if left unshod, but they will still require regular farrier care, usually starting immediately upon arrival because many horses coming into the shelter environment are suffering from neglect.

As a prey species, horses have an exaggerated startle "fright or flight" reflex, which causes them to bolt when scared. If they are inadequately controlled in a busy urban or otherwise congested environment, disastrous results occur. Because their eyes are positioned on the sides rather than the front of their skulls, they can visualize a wide field around them, even when grazing, but have a blind spot close to and directly in front of them. Horses are particularly susceptible to spooking when startled by noises behind or above them (such as snow sliding off a roof or cracking branches overhead), having evolved with predators who attacked from high perches. Therefore, if horses are used in environments where startling stimuli are likely to exist, the driver or rider must pay particular attention to the horse to maintain control at all times. Urban carriage horse operations have had countless instances of motor vehicle—horse collisions, sometimes fatal for human or horse, initiated by a carriage horse's spooking into an uncontrollable gallop (Newspaper Accounts).

Horses are intensely social animals. Wild bands travel together, including a stallion, several mares, and their offspring, with individuals occupying a hierarchical position within the group. Horses enjoy playtime, particularly when young, and exhibit a competitive love of speed as part of their play behavior. They spend time in mutual grooming rituals that strengthen their bonds and provide both physical and psychological pleasure. The frequency of grooming is affected by season and by individual preferences (friendships) within the band (Houpt 2002). Therefore, although there is no legislation mandating that horses be kept with conspecifics, a humane housing situation will provide company, preferably equine, although goats will serve as an improvement over solitary housing. Katherine Houpt (personal communication) notes that chickens also serve as an acceptable substitute for a conspecific companion, but they may be dominant over the horse so the practitioner must ensure that the horse is permitted access to the food supply. Whatever the species used, particular attention must be paid to grouping compatible individuals together to prevent injury, inadequate food intake, and stress in the subordinate animals.

TYPES OF ABUSE

One of the primary factors bringing horses to a shelter is their seizure as evidence in an animal abuse investigation. Whether or not the alleged defendant (the owner) agrees to turn these animals over to the shelter to dispose of as its resources allow, or whether these animals must be held as the defendant's private property and as evidence pending a hearing and trial, they will need to be evaluated by the shelter veterinarian upon arrival. The evaluation may be needed to substantiate the charges in a cruelty case and must therefore be recorded in an accurate and precise manner for the trial. If the horse(s) are dead or must be euthanized, a thoroughly documented necropsy may be necessary for evidence; cruelty cases have been lost solely due to the failure to perform a proper necropsy and to document the findings. For the living animals, the New York State Humane Association has published a cruelty investigation manual that contains a useful veterinary evaluation form, expediting the recording of one's findings on the physical examination and also reminding the attending veterinarian of specific lesions to itemize (NYS Humane Association 1996) (See Appendix 29.1). In addition to codifying the evidence, a thorough examination will form the basis for the determination of the optimal program to rehabilitate any injured or malnourished victims by identifying their deficiencies and lesions.

As with all other species, horse abuse comes in a distressingly wide variety of forms. The American Humane Association (AHA) has published an excellent resource for veterinarians who wish to become involved in the reporting, investigation, and prosecution of equine abuse cases entitled *Recognizing & Reporting Animal Abuse: A Veterinarian's Guide* (AHA 1998). Any veterinarian working in this field would do well to obtain a copy. This guide includes a very useful reference chart entitled "Typology of Companion Animal Abuse", originally developed by Vermeulen and Odendaal, which aides the practitioner in categorizing and defining different forms of cruelty (Vermeulen and Odendaal 1993). It also reminds the practitioner what types of equine use might merit investigation and where to look for lesions.

In this classification system, abuse is divided into two broad categories with multiple subheadings, specifically physical abuse (active, passive, and commercial) and mental abuse (active maltreatment and passive neglect). Although most states do not include an evaluation of an animal's mental state in anti-cruelty legislation, it is always important for the veterinarian to evaluate and stress this parameter, especially when testifying before a judge or jury in a case in which a horse's degree of physical suffering may not be obvious. A horse kept in total isolation for years is arguably abused because, as a highly social species, the company of conspecifics is critical for the horse's well being. The Vermeulen and Odendaal categories of abuse are self-explanatory, but I would like to expand on some specific references in the order listed in their typology.

Active Maltreatment

INCORRECT METHOD OF TRAINING

Veterinarians should be aware of the inhumane training practices used to prepare some horses for show ring competition. The federal Horse Protection Act, passed in 1970 and amended in 1976, was introduced to address this form of abuse. For a full discussion of the myriad of cruel training procedures associated with specific breeds and their shows, I refer the practitioner to the American Horse Protection Association in Washington, D.C. This organization was a prime force in the passage of the Horse Protection Act and is a good source of information on typical abusive practices inflicted on some equine performers to make them more "competitive". Because many of these training methods leave no detectable lesions, the practitioner should know of their existence in the hopes of uncovering evidence that such practices have been used on the animals under investigation. The following practices are undeniably unpleasant at best and cruel at worst.

In the world of "gaited" performance horses, the exaggerated flexion action in the gaits may be produced by painful methods, including "soring" (creating painful abrasions in the forelimb pastern area during training) and the use of nails driven into the horse's frog or sole to make each step too painful to bear weight for more than an instant. Horses also wear irritating chains, wires, or wooden beads around their front pasterns in training. A hoof radiograph of the front feet and the use of the USDA/APHIS booklet "Understanding the Scar Rule" (USDA 2001) will help the veterinarian determine if an animal has been abused in this manner. Although there are guidelines from breed organizations for each show breed as to acceptable hoof length and maximum permitted weights, there are no actual legal statutes regulating the overgrowing and weighting of the hooves in competing Morgans, Saddlebreds, and Tennessee Walkers. However, the veterinarian can still attempt to prove that these practices contribute to an animal's lameness and reflect care that constitutes improper husbandry.

For the desired elevated tail carriage seen in the gaited Tennessee Walkers and American Saddlebreds, the practices of breaking and resetting the tail vertebrae as well as partially cutting the tail tendons are still popular, as is the old trick of inserting ginger in the anus to irritate the mucosa, encouraging greater lift of the tail. Horses are trussed in restrictive harnessing (tail sets or braces) that inhibit natural body postures for 23 out of 24 hours during the show season (Pagelsen 2002). It is clear from observing horses who wear this tight and restrictive apparatus that they are unable to adopt a natural and relaxed body posture. All of these techniques combine to produce an animal in the top gaited show rings (as well as in some Arabian, Morgan, and Hackney shows) that sweats profusely during competition, has flared nostrils and dilated eyes, and moves with every sinew taut. The stress in these horses' movements is self-evident, reflecting the pain to which they are subjected.

At the opposite end of the stylistic spectrum of equine performance, Western pleasure classes call for a low head and tail carriage. The lowered head may be produced either by elevating the horse's head and restricting any vertical and lateral movement in the stall for hours to fatigue the neck muscles or by attaching heavy hanging weights to the halter for the same purpose (Pagelsen 2002). The Quarter Horses and Paints performing in these classes may have tail blocks, in which rubbing alcohol is injected as a primitive nerve block to deaden the tail muscles. In the English show world, a hunter may also be "surgically" altered in this manner.

These blocks must be repeated every few months, frequently become abscessed, and can produce the undesired effect of impeding defecation because the limp tail may obstruct the anus (Pagelsen 2002).

For some horses in both the English and Western halter classes, cosmetic surgery is becoming more common. An Arabian, Morgan, or Saddlebred that lacks a sufficiently clean throatlatch contour may be surgically reshaped to improve their conformation. If an undesirable degree of white sclera is visible, producing the ring of white around the eye indicating (supposedly) an uncertain temper, the sclera may be darkened by tattooing. The eyes and ears are also targets for surgical reshaping (Pagelsen 2002). A veterinarian may be called by the prosecution to determine if a horse has been surgically altered; if it has, it is imperative to identify the perpetrator who may not be a veterinarian and can therefore be prosecuted under most state laws for practicing veterinary medicine without a license.

The preceding examples of abuse in show preparation and training are hardly exhaustive; unfortunately, many other "tricks of the trade" are employed to increase the owners' chances of winning the all-important ribbon, cup, or monetary prize and to boost their prestige. Any veterinarian involved with investigating these training methods should do everything possible to get media attention on this issue in an attempt to educate the public and thereby eliminate these cruel traditions from the show ring repertoire.

BESTIALITY

One of the categories that is most overlooked is bestiality. According to Stephanie LaFarge, Ph.D. (personal communication), it is increasingly reported, although there is no way to tell whether or not there is an actual increase in incidence. It even has dedicated websites with a distressingly large audience of subscribers; equally distressing is the fact that many of them are youths in their teens (LaFarge 2002). This practice was common enough to deserve mention as a lesion meriting investigation (under the heading of sadism) in the large animal surgery textbook used at Cornell's College of Veterinary Medicine in the 1970s (Oehme and Prier 1974). Bestiality (defined as interspecies sexual *assault*) should be distinguished from zoophilia, which is defined as interspecies sexual contact *without detectable physical or behavioral signs of abuse*. A detailed discussion of these two forms of interspecies sexual contact is beyond the scope of this chapter, but the veterinarian should be aware that, in the states where sexual contact with animals is illegal, bestiality and zoophilia are both equally and emphatically against the law and the veterinarian's role may be to determine if sexual contact has occurred. Bestiality should be suspected whenever the practitioner discovers rectal or vaginal tears without a history of breeding or birthing trauma, which may present as a case of diffuse peritonitis with sudden onset. Other animals on the premises should be thoroughly examined for these lesions if one individual is found with this presentation, because the perpetrator may well be committing these acts on multiple victims.

COMMERCIAL EXPLOITATION: MULE (HORSE) DIVING

The commercial category includes a myriad of areas in which horses may be misused or overused while serving as a form of entertainment or tourist attraction. Mule (horse) diving acts still make the rounds of some county fairs and community fundraisers or serve as a featured act at amusement parks. In this event, horses must climb a ramp and jump into a pool of water. Horses do not naturally back down and around corners to exit the ramp, as they would have to do to avoid the plunge, and are trained not to attempt it. Aside from the associated abuses of improper housing, feeding, and transportation, which are common among many of these operators, the act itself can be determined to be very frightening to an equine if the response to the prospect of the dive is flared nostrils, strained head carriage, white-rimmed eyes, and nervous defecation at the top of the diving ramp (personal observations, a). The veterinarian's role, if sought, in investigating these acts is to underscore and interpret the equine's "body English" for the layman as exemplifying heightened fear and to inform the public that this activity is entirely unnatural. Educating sponsors to eschew this kind of "entertainment" may be more effective in putting an end to this practice than attempting to prosecute operators under state anti-cruelty laws.

DONKEY BASKETBALL

Similarly, donkey basketball has survived into the twenty-first century as an entertainment venue and fundraiser, often for local schools, charities, or churches whose members are unaware of the animals' treatment. For those who have not had the opportunity to witness this event, participants mount donkeys divided into two teams, and can only pass, dribble, and shoot baskets while mounted. The welfare and treatment of the donkeys is entirely dependent on the nature of their riders. Some donkeys are therefore treated roughly in the riders' attempts to maneuver their mounts into position for the perfect shot, and both donkey and human injuries have been documented (Bangor Daily News 1996). Feed and water may be withheld if the event is to be staged on an indoor surface to minimize soiling. As with mule diving, the housing, feeding, and transportation may be substandard and should be evaluated to assess if the animals' needs are being met. Measuring the inside temperature of the "semi" vans in which these animals are carried is important because historically, donkeys have been exposed to extremes of temperatures during transport, thus providing an unacceptable environmental stress. The veterinarian's role, as with mule diving, is to evaluate the animals for signs of physical and psychological abuse, and to educate the public as to the inherently inhumane nature of forcing equines to participate in such an unnatural event.

RODEOS

Rodeos represent a controversial arena of equine use, even within the veterinary profession. Supporters defend the use of bucking horses, while opponents express anger over the injuries sustained during performance and over the use of bucking straps (flank straps) and electric shock prods employed to enhance the bucking action by the application of an unpleasant stimulus while waiting in the chute. The Professional Rodeo Cowboys Association (PRCA) has published a welfare guide for participants in its sanctioned rodeos that expressly forbids this use of the electric shock prod (PRCA 2002). However, humane law officers and lay observers have noted (and videotaped) multiple instances in which the prod is used repeatedly in the chute, despite the recommendations of the welfare guide to the contrary. Although the flank strap is covered with a padded material and does not pinch the genitals, as some activists have claimed, it still represents a noxious stimulus, evinced by the horse's continuing to buck after dumping the rider until a second rider comes alongside to release the strap. Only after the removal of the noxious stimulus does the horse cease to buck.

Lesions that might be observed in rodeo stock include traumatic injuries (leg and spinal fractures and severe bruising) and the more chronic lower limb injuries expected in animals who compete at an advanced level in events requiring quick stops and rapid turns (such as barrel racing and cutting contests). Please note that such chronic injuries from these events do not, in themselves, constitute abuse; I can attest to my own pony's intense enjoyment of barrel racing competitions. As for the controversy surrounding the bucking horses, each practitioner must come to his or her own conclusions as to whether or not the horse is enjoying the performance. For a spirited debate on the pros and cons of rodeo, I recommend the article and consequent exchange of letters between Peggy Larson, a veterinarian and ex-bronco rider (adamantly opposed), Dr. James Furman (in support), and others in the *Journal of the American Veterinary Medical Association* (Furman 2001).

CARRIAGE HORSES

Carriage horses are often featured in cities with a historic character to permit tourists to see the sights in a supposedly nostalgic setting. The health, housing, and husbandry of these animals vary enormously from city to city. In my experience over a 15-year period of inspecting carriage horse operations across the country, I have found that cities such as New York, Atlanta, and Boston have shown the worst track records for humane treatment of their carriage horses, while the city of Philadelphia has been laudably proactive in implementing humane standards of care and operation. Although carriage horses comprise a small number of the total horses encountered in abuse work, their lives are arguably the most hazardous and their sphere of operation the most inhospitable. They often represent, unfortunately, a classic model for heat stress in equines when working in urban environments with high heat and humidity in summer months.

The draft horses from farming communities and Standardbreds retired from the racetrack are seen as ideal animals for urban carriage horse operations because they are already familiar with harnessing and hitching and therefore require little additional training (personal conversations 1988–1992). Many operators in the northeast find their replacement animals primarily at auctions where those horses no longer fit enough for the Amish farming community or the Standardbred tracks are brought for sale to private owners or for slaughter. Some carriage horses, therefore, enter the tourist trade with pre-existing lesions, usually in the form of old soundness problems and "heaves" (chronic obstructive pulmonary disease [COPD]) (personal observations, b). The primary health stresses they encounter while pulling carriages through congested urban streets are (1) exacerbation of lameness from pounding the hard concussive pavement surfaces, (2) respiratory disease from their nose-to-tailpipe existence in urban traffic, and (3) heat prostration in hot and humid environments. Atlanta, Boston, and New York have all experienced fatalities from heat stress in their carriage horse populations.

It is critically important for an attendant veterinarian to recognize that the ambient air temperature announced by the U.S. Weather Bureau's official report may be radically different from the microenvironment that the horse experiences on the street. A study conducted by Cornell's Urban Horticultural Institute between 1983 and 1985 revealed that the temperature at New York City's street level could be as much as 45°F higher than the temperature recorded by the U.S. Weather Bureau, taken in Central Park (Sandler 1989). Furthermore, New York's former Transportation Commissioner, Ross Sandler, was quoted in the *New York Times* (7/9/89) as stating that asphalt temperatures could reach "well over 200 degrees" in summer months. With such high temperatures radiating up from the street surfaces, heat stress in horses standing in this microenvironment for an eight- to 10-hour work shift is not unexpected.

The effect of high temperatures on the horses' ability to keep cooled is exacerbated by the high humidity that is a common occurrence in the three cities named previously. With the surrounding air already saturated with high levels of moisture, horses cannot be cooled by the evaporation of their sweat. Draft breeds in particular have difficulty in dissipating their heat loads due to their proportionally larger increase in body mass relative to their surface area compared to lighter horses. Therefore, if asked to assist a city council in promulgating regulations for humane working environments for the city's carriage horses, it is important to specify both temperature and humidity limits. A combined reading known as the "THI" (Temperature-Humidity Index) should be used, with the temperature in degrees Fahrenheit added to the percentage humidity; 150 is a THI value that has been proposed, above which the risk for heat stress rises significantly (especially if the humidity value is greater than half of the combined sum) (Mackay-Smith and Cohen 1982).

In addition to the physical challenges that these horses face, they also must encounter the psychological stresses of sudden motions and loud noises provided by motor vehicles and large crowds. There are numerous accounts of horses spooking due to automobiles backfiring or to minor collisions with motor vehicles causing accidents when the horses panic and bolt through a series of intersections. Many humane organizations attempt to change city codes to permit carriage horses to operate only in areas and in time periods with minimal, if any, competition with traffic.

If asked to investigate the condition of any carriage horses, I recommend that the veterinarian start with the stabling and inquire into the provision of daily turnout, stall size, temperature in the barn during extreme hot and cold spells, ventilation, and the availability of water and trace mineral salt blocks at all times. After assessing the horse's living conditions, a thorough physical examination of the horses themselves should be performed, looking for the presence of COPD, chronic lameness, dental problems, inadequate farrier care, and harness sores. Check the condition and cleanliness of the harness as well and note any harsh bits (e.g., the chain or wire bits) or harness repairs done with tape and twine that may irritate the horse's skin. Request the veterinary records and evaluate the frequency of deworming and routine care such as hoof trims and dentistry. The best urban operations that I have inspected provide box stalls and daily turnout, with good quality concentrates and hay utilized in the feeding programs. Water (sometimes with electrolyte solutions available as well) and trace mineral salt should be available at all times. Some operators even permit "R & R" time for the horses, with a two- to three-month rotation out of the city onto a farm. One role in which a knowledgeable veterinarian's assistance can prove invaluable is in assisting a city council or health department in promulgating regulations for the humane operation, handling, and housing of these animals.

THOROUGHBRED AND STANDARDBRED RACING

The horse racing industry is based on an activity that horses love to perform. However, because the top purses are for two- and three-year olds for whom growth plates are still open, and because training therefore begins with intensity at a very young developmental age, many race horses trained inappropriately may experience significant limb injuries that eliminate them from competition before they have even reached their prime. Racehorses that don't earn money are at risk for abandonment and neglect. An examination of the upper lip tattoo may aid the investigator in tracing the origins of a retired racer.

Racing injuries run the gamut of lower limb breakdowns, including fractured sesamoid bones, bowed tendons, "popped" splints, swollen joints, and chronically torn ligaments with thickened sheaths and scar tissue. As a general rule, the Thoroughbreds' injuries will be mostly in the forelimbs, while the Standardbred trotters and pacers have more hind limb injuries. An examination of the metacarpal/metatarsal, pastern, knee, and hock areas may reveal the symmetrical punctate scars of pin firing. This controversial treatment, in which thermocautery is applied to an injured ligament, tendon, or joint and a blistering agent then applied, is said to heal the injury by an excessive provocation of the inflammatory response. It is excruciatingly painful once the local anesthetics have worn off, and too often is used in place of an adequate rest period for proper healing. Horses who end their racing careers with a final sanctuary at a shelter will need considerable attention paid to pain relief with the use of analgesics (particularly the nonsteroidal anti-inflammatory drugs [NSAIDS]) and nutraceuticals such as the glucosamine chondroitin preparations.

Passive Neglect or Ignorance (Backyard Horse Abuse): A "How-To" Approach for Investigating a Cruelty Complaint

The preceding overview of specific areas of equine abuse is hardly exhaustive and may be considered by some to be controversial. Additional examples of active horse abuse vary from the common to the bizarre, such as abuse performed for initiation rites or satanic rituals. However, the overwhelming majority of cases that the average practitioner will encounter are examples of neglect, abandonment, and starvation, which fall under the general heading of "backyard horse abuse." This section provides an outline for investigating and quantifying the degree of suffering experienced by horses seized in such situations.

Many judges and juries remain unconvinced that neglect can constitute cruelty, and therefore are reluctant to convict a perpetrator for violation of their state's anti-cruelty laws. It is incumbent upon the investigating veterinarian to communicate the degree of suffering experienced by the animal(s) and to make that suffering intelligible to a lay audience. As far as the horse is concerned, whether the neglect resulted from malicious intent or simple ignorance and lack of care is irrelevant—the degree of suffering is the same. Evaluating the degree of suffering is aided by the systematic "macro to micro" approach—starting with the big picture and refining the focus of the investigation—that I teach four times annually in seminars offered by the New York State Humane Association for animal control officers, law officers, and veterinarians in New York State.

A typical scenario involves the request for a veterinary opinion from an animal control or law enforcement officer who, in turn, responded to a complaint from neighbors or passersby. The gathered evidence is then turned over to the district attorney's office for prosecution. The horses and their environment must be evaluated in exacting detail to improve the chances for a successful outcome in proving that the state's animal cruelty laws have been violated. Starting with the "macro" (big picture) analysis, the first step is to examine the premises in which the animals are held. Take note of the presence or absence of pasture, and take the time of year into account. Is grass available? How long will the grass last? Is the footing dry and clean or is the pasture little more than a mud hole? Will the surfaces be slippery and hazardous in the wintertime? Is the area going to be deluged during seasonal runoff?

The availability of water is the next crucial determination, again taking seasonal variation into account. Claims that water is always available due to the presence of a small stream running through their pasture should be investigated to make certain that the water is really potable, and whether it is present in the wintertime (or frozen) and in the summertime (or dried up). One comment about winter water access: Frozen water and snow do not provide a humane and effective cold weather water source, as defendants often try to claim, and in fact are contraindicated for malnourished animals because ingesting sufficient snow and ice to satisfy water needs can produce hypothermia. Check water tubs for evidence that they are filled and cleaned regularly. Water buckets containing fecal contamination and large algae populations are not acceptable.

Next, check for feed sources and have the law enforcement officer request evidence of hay and feed purchase and delivery. Evaluate the quality of the hay and grain and their storage facilities: Are they dry and rodent-proof for the concentrates? If the hay is essentially no better than baled weeds and twigs (as I have frequently observed), the veterinarian's expertise is required to explain why a barn full of non-nutritional stems does not satisfy nutritional needs. Note also if trace mineral salt blocks are readily available to satisfy micronutrient needs.

Finally, examine the premises from the safety angle, including the shelter and fencing. One reason why neighbors may call the local law officers is because the horses continually break out and damage adjacent property. If this is the case, keep in mind that the horses may be straying because their feed intake is insufficient and they are trying to satisfy their hunger. Rickety boards with exposed nails, miscellaneous trash, and junked cars in the pasture all provide an environment that is hazardous to equine health. Obviously, fencing should be safe, secure, and well maintained, and barns or run-in sheds should provide good protection from adverse weather with no surfaces (broken boards, protruding nails) that might cause an injury. Look for signs of superficial abrasions and deeper cuts on the limbs if the construction of the barn or shed seems hazardous and ensure that the court is aware of the cause. If the horses are sheltered, assess the adequacy of their ventilation, again factoring in the effects of seasonal temperature changes. Finally, note the bedding (if any) and the amount of fecal and urinary waste upon which the horses must stand. If the manure has built up to the point that the horse has to stand with his head lowered due to the inadequate space between footing and ceiling, stress this lack of hygiene and comfort in your report.

The veterinarian's investigative focus should then be refined from concentrating on the horse's setting to evaluating the horse himself in his entirety. Starting again with the big picture, assess the horse's demeanor (Is the horse depressed? Dull? Bright and alert?), as well as the body weight and condition of the skin and coat. The use of the Henneke scale, developed originally in 1983 to quantify a horse's body condition, is a highly recommended tool that can be found on the websites of several horse protection organizations (Henneke Scale). The horse's weight is scored on a scale of 1 (emaciated) to 10

(obese), with a concise description pertaining to each numerical value. The use of this scale as evidence in a trial is an effective adjunct because it implies an objective quantitative evaluation rather than a subjective determination of an animal's physical state. An elderly horse's lack of proper condition will be characterized by the defense as uncorrectable due to the alleged inevitability of poor condition in geriatric horses. However, the truth is that with frequent dental examinations and treatment, coupled with proper deworming programs and the use of a feeding program designed for older equines (including the use of complete pelleted feeds, senior rations, and the addition of corn oil and water to soften the food), even elderly horses can appear well conditioned in most cases.

As for the skin, look for evidence of "rain scald" (pityriasis), "rain rot" (dermatophilosis), ectoparasites, and fungal infections that indicate poor husbandry practices and inadequate hygiene and shelter. Scars that may be due to unsafe construction, bullying by herd mates, or physical abuse by the owner, should be documented precisely. Poor shedding with the retention of a wooly winter coat into the summer may indicate a hormonal imbalance (Cushing's Syndrome) that requires treatment. A coat that is either filthy and caked with mud and manure, or patchy due to alopecia, cannot piloerect normally to provide the insulating layer of air that helps horses stay warm in cold weather. It is the veterinarian's job to interpret the significance of a poor coat condition so that it is clear that it derives from poor nutrition and care, thereby adding to the burden of suffering, and is not a matter of cosmetic appearance only.

At this point, the physical examination becomes increasingly focused on the "micro" details. Ear infections, ocular diseases, dental abnormalities, the pitting edema known as "bottle jaw" (sometimes due to the hypoproteinemia of endoparasitism), degenerative joint disease, thrush (*Fusobacterium necrophorum*), laminitis, and so forth should all be detailed in each animal. If a repeating pattern of neglect and insufficient veterinary care can be established (e.g.,, if every animal on the premises shows signs of rain rot or laminitis), it becomes simpler to prove that the animals are suffering consistently from sufficient neglect to violate the state's anti-cruelty laws. No detail is too small, so be as inclusive as possible in citing any lesions. Intact stallions should be clearly noted because some states' laws (e.g., the laws of New York) require special enclosures for them to ensure that they can't escape to attack or breed adjacent horses. Necropsies should be performed and recorded with the same precision.

After the pertinent details have been reported, recorded on an official investigation sheet, and photographed, hopefully there will be enough evidence to prove a failure to provide proper sustenance on the owner's part. With verification of the horses' condition as given by the prosecution's veterinarian, the animals can be seized as evincing sufficient neglect to be removed from the property for placement in a shelter or foster home. They may then be adopted out to new owners if the defendant agrees to surrender them to the shelter, or will be held there pending the hearing if the defendant refuses to relinquish them. If no shelter or foster home is available, the court may order the horses to be detained *in situ* (i.e., on the defendant's property), with oversight responsibility for their rehabilitation, care, and feeding delegated to the local shelter staff. The veterinarian then faces the considerable task of restoring these horses to health, as will be discussed in the Chapter 14 on shelter health protocols for equines.

CONCLUSION

An effective and professional affidavit or testimony from a knowledgeable veterinarian may be the deciding factor in the successful outcome of a cruelty investigation case. As discussed, the veterinarian must be thorough, including all relevant details and interpreting their signficance for the prosecuting attorney, the jury, and the judge. There is no one involved in the prosecution who knows better than the expert witness (the veterinarian) why a training method, stabling situation, or a particular activity involving horses is inhumane. The veterinarian's job is to make this information intelligible to the court, and to work with the prosecuting attorney to make as solid a case as possible to relieve the suffering of the equine victims in each case.

REFERENCES

American Humane Association (AHA). 1998. *Recognizing and reporting animal abuse: A veterinarian's guide.* Englewood, CO: American Humane Society. Also available at www.americanhumane.org.

Bangor Daily News, May 9, 1996.

Bassuk, N. and Whitlow, T. 1988. Environmental stress in street trees. *Arboricultural Journal* 12:197–200.

Furman, J. W. 2001. Rodeo cattle's many performances. *Journal of the American Veterinary Medical Association* (JAVMA) 219 (10):1394–1397.
> Larson, P. W. 2002. Letters to the editor. *JAVMA* 220 (2):166–167
> Furman, J. W. 2002 Letters to the editor. *JAVMA* 220 (2):166–167.
> Taylor, M. B. 2002. Letters to the editor. *JAVMA* 220 (5):594.
> Cobb, D. B. 2002. Letters to the editor. *JAVMA* (5): 594.
> Larson, P. W. 2002. Letters to the editor. *JAVMA* (5): 594–595.
> Walker, J. A. 2002. Letters to the editor. *JAVMA* (6): 741–742.

Larson, P. W. 2002. Letters to the editor. *JAVMA* (6): 741–742.

Getty, R. 1975. In Sisson and Grossman's *The Anatomy of Domestic Animals,* 5th edition. Philadelphia, PA: WB Saunders, 253.

Henneke Scale available at the Equine Protection Network, www.equineprotectionnetwork.com; also at Indiana Hooved Animal Humane Society, www.ihahs.org.

Houpt, K. 2002. Director, Animal Behavoir Clinic, College of Veterinary Medicine at Cornell. Personal conversation with author in June.

LaFarge, S. 2002. Senior Director of Counseling Services, American Society for the Prevention of Cruelty to Animals (ASPCA). Telephone conversation with the author in June.

Mackay-Smith, M., and Cohen, M. 1982. Exercise physiology and diseases of exertion. In R. A. Mansmann, E. S. McAllister, and P. W. Pratt (eds.), *Equine Medicine and Surgery,* 3rd edition. Santa Barbara, CA, I: 125–129.

Newspaper acounts of accidents involving horse-drawn carriages and motor vehicles can be obtained by contacting People for the Ethical Treatment of Animals (PETA) at www.peta.org and by contacting Redwings Horse Sanctuary at www.redwings.org.

New York State Humane Association. 1996. *How to Investigate Animal Cruelty in New York State: A Manual of Procedures.* Kingston, NY: New York State Humane Association, 351.

Oehme, F. W., and Prier, J. E. 1974. *Textbook of Large Animal Surgery.* Baltimore, MD: Williams and Wilkins Company, 498.

Pagelsen, K. 2002. Director of Communications, American Horse Protection Association. Telepheone conversation with author in June.

Personal conversations with carriage hourse owners and drivers in New York, conducted during inspections of the carriage horse industry by the author in conjunction with the American Society for the Prevention of Cruelty to Animals (ASPCA) 1988–1992.

Personal observations (a) by the author on multiple occasions of live acts at the Magic Forest, Lake George, NY (August 2002) and videotaped performances of the traveling Tim Rivers' Mule Diving Act (dates unknown).

Personal observations (b) from inspections performed by the author on New York's carriage horses, 1988–1992.

Professional Rodeo Cowboys Association (PRCA). 2002. *Animal Welfare: The Care and Treatment of Professional Rodeo Livestock*. Colorado Springs: CO, 7. Also available at www.prorodeo.com.

Sandler, R. 1989. *New York Times,* July 9.

Vermeulen, H. and Odendaal, J. S. J. 1993. A Proposed typology of animal abuse. *Anthrozoos* (6):248–257.

United States Department of Agriculture (USDA) Animal and Plant Health Inspection Service (APHIS). 2001. *The Horse Protection Act: Understanding the Scar Rule*. Riverdale, MD. Also available at www.aphis.usda.gov/ac.

Appendix 29.1

VETERINARIAN'S STATEMENT
ANIMAL EVALUATION FORM

Animal belonging to: _____

Animal found on the premises of_____

Located at (complete address) _____

ID# assigned to animal _____ Species_____ Breed_____ Sex_____ Weight_____

Approx. age_____ Description (color/markings)_____

_____

I, _____, am a veterinarian licensed in the State of _____.
  (please print name)

I am responding to a request by (agency)_____ to evaluate the above-identified animal.

I hereby certify that this animal exhibits the following:

☐ presumed neutered/spayed ☐ unneutered/unspayed
☐ pregnant ☐ nursing ☐ in heat
☐ evidence of previous litters (enlarged nipples/vulva)

☐ emaciation   ☐ multiple bite wounds   ☐ arthritis, other lameness
☐ dehydration   ☐ tumors, other growths   ☐ overgrown nails/hooves
☐ excessive hair loss ☐ abscesses   ☐ earmites/infection
☐ severe itching   ☐ diarrhea   ☐ eye infection
☐ mange   ☐ urine scalding   ☐ generalized debility
☐ dermatitis   ☐ dental problems   ☐ internal parasites
☐ flea dirt   ☐ respiratory infection   (Indicate type below)
☐ ticks   ☐ heartworm symptoms

Other (e.g., other afflictions, comments on weight, observations of behavior, etc.):_____

_____

_____

Check here if animal was euthanized : ☐   I hereby certify that this animal is so maimed, diseased, disabled, or infirm as to require euthanasia to be spared suffering. Euthanasia is appropriate for this animal, whose symptoms are as described above.

In a written instrument, any person who knowingly makes a false statement herein which such person does not believe to be true has committed a crime under the laws of the State of New York punishable as a Class A Misdemeanor. (PL § 210.45)

_____   _____
Signature of Veterinarian   Date

☐ Animal kept on premises
    or
☐ Relocated to _____ Date _____

Form prepared by New York State Humane Association, PO Box 3068, Kingston, NY 12402 — 8/2000

30
Animal Fighting

Julie Dinnage, Kelley Bollen, and Scott Giacoppo

INTRODUCTION

Investigation and prosecution of animal fighting cases can be difficult and lengthy. When fighting animals are seized as evidence and held for evaluation, medical care, and impounding, the animals and the staff are faced with many challenges to provide adequate and safe housing. This chapter discusses the background, care, and housing of two more common fighting animals—pit bulls and fighting cocks. Much of the information presented is based on the personal experience of the authors gathered from years of experience handling these animals for the Massachusetts Society for the Prevention of Cruelty to Animals (MSPCA).

DOG FIGHTING

History of the Breed

Knowledge of the pit bull's ancestral roots can help animal shelters house and handle these dogs in a manner that is equally safe for the animals and their handlers. In addition, insight into the history of the breed will help to more effectively provide for their physical and psychological well-being while in a shelter. We can learn a great deal about the dogs of today by studying the origins and the history of the "sport" of dog fighting.

The origins of the pit bull date back to England around the mid 1800s when bull-baiting events were popular. Bull-baiting, as it was called, pitted two or more bulldogs against a tethered bull. This all occurred in an arena for entertainment purposes. The 1800s fighting bulldogs were very different from the bulldogs of today in size and

structure and more closely resembled today's bullmastiff.

The sport of bull baiting was outlawed with the passage of the Humane Act of 1886. No longer able to participate legally in bull-baiting competitions, the owners of these highly aggressive animals attempted to find an alternative use for their dogs. There remained a high demand for barbaric bloody sporting events that would provide a venue for gambling. That demand was eventually met with a new alternative dog-fighting event in which owners pitted the bulldogs against one another as spectators wagered bets on the outcome. The new sport, however, failed to be as exciting because the bulldogs were rather large and clumsy. The fights were viewed as slow, cumbersome, and less thrilling for spectators.

As a result, bulldog owners looked for ways to change the breed altogether in order to make a better fighter and to subsequently attract spectators and gamblers back to the sport. The goal was to create a dog that maintained certain characteristics of the traditional bull-baiting bulldog with additional traits that would make the dog a more effective fighter in the pit. It was in a coal mining section of England called Staffordshire that a selective breeding practice began. The bulldog was crossed with various terrier type dogs, and the ideal new fighting dog, the Staffordshire bull terrier, was born (Fig. 30.1). The following characteristics were originally and continue to be selected for a fighting dog:

1. Strength in relation to size:
   The fighting dog needed to maintain the strength of the bulldog but be smaller and more compact.

2. Bite style:

   Typically a dog bite causes a series of puncture wounds. This would not be effective in combat. Instead, the style of bite needed to inflict maximum muscle and tissue damage. An example of a more damaging biter is the rat terrier, who characteristically bites down and vigorously shakes its prey.

3. Agility and athleticism:

   This new breed needed to be extremely agile to avoid serious injury during a fight. These dogs have a high level of athleticism and endurance.

4. Aggression toward other animals:

   Like the bulldog, it was imperative that this new breed be highly aggressive toward other animals, especially dogs, without showing even the slightest signs of aggression toward humans. This disposition would enable the dog's handler to more safely separate the dogs during a fight.

5. Ignore signs of submission:

   Dogs typically fight until one shows signs of submission such as rolling over and exposing the abdomen. Submissive postures normally indicate to another dog that the fight is over. Fighting dogs, however, are selectively bred to ignore these signs and will instead continue attacking causing serious, if not fatal injuries.

6. Give no warning that an attack is imminent:

   In normal dog behavior, adversaries display physical cues such as bearing teeth or raising hackles that warn another dog that an attack will occur. In the fighting dog, these behavioral cues were considered undesirable and again selectively removed from the breed.

7. Gameness:

   This is by far the most sought after trait of all the fighting dogs' characteristics. Gameness refers to the dog's willingness to continue fighting regardless of the pain and suffering it is enduring. *Deep game* (also referred to as *Dead game*) indicates that the dog has been bred to continue fighting until death.

With the birth of this new breed of dog, organized dog fighting successfully took the place of bull baiting, and the sport began to grow. As the Staffordshire bull terrier breed became more popular, further attempts were made to create an even better fighting dog. Since breeding was now taking place outside Staffordshire and the dogs were bred prima-

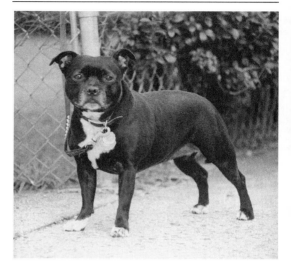

Figure 30.1. Staffordshire Bull Terrier. Photo credit Marion Lane.

rily for the pit, the term pit bull terrier was used to describe these newer breeds.

All of these aggressive and athletic traits can still be found in the professionally bred fighting dogs of today. It is important to note however that when the Staffordshire bull terrier came to America in the late 1800s, a breeding split occurred that effectively gave us two different dogs. Those breeders who wanted to maintain the breed's fighting roots continued to selectively breed for aggression. Others, who merely fancied the breed, attempted to remove the aggressive traits and make the pit bull into a family pet. This is evident throughout the early 1900s when the pit bull terrier enjoyed a positive reputation. World War I support posters depicted the pit bull draped in an American flag. They appeared in advertisements to sell stereo equipment and shoes. And Stubby, a stray pit bull terrier from Connecticut, was brought to France to provide companionship for his owner while he fought in the war. Stubby was actually a decorated war hero and considered by many to be the world's first therapy dog. The most popular of all pit bulls, Petey (of the hit show *Our Gang, the Little Rascals*), was once viewed by many as America's dog. Despite this softer image, there were still many people who enjoyed watching dogs engage in bloody combat. As a result, pit bulls continue to be bred for fighting purposes today.

Fighting Classifications

There are generally three categories of fighting dog owners:

1. *The professional:* This person makes a substantial investment in purchasing, training, and conditioning the dogs. The professional might travel around the country to attend and participate in fights and is often knowledgeable about law enforcement investigation techniques. Fighting dogs owned by the professional are frequently on performance-enhancing steroids and/or chronic antibiotic therapy to treat infections. Additional payoffs come from stud fees and higher stakes matches.
2. *The hobbyist:* This person fancies the breed and enjoys the local fighting circuit. The hobbyist usually spends minimal time on training and may or may not engage in all the activities associated with conditioning. Fights are arranged, and gambling is the main focus as a means to win back the owner's investment.
3. *The street fighter:* The street fighter is usually associated with other forms of illegal activity, such as local street gangs and is utilized for more than fighting purposes. The street fighter's dog is aggressive toward humans and is more likely to cause a fatal attack than any other type of fighting dog. These dogs are frequently kept in substandard conditions and may show obvious signs of physical abuse. Because of this, the street fighter's dogs are the type more likely to be observed by veterinarians and shelter personnel.

Training and Conditioning

As shelter veterinarians, it is helpful to understand how fighting dogs have been trained and conditioned prior to coming into the shelter. The ideal fighting dog undergoes an extensive training regimen to build strength and endurance and to reinforce aggressive behaviors. A daily training routine starts at a very young age and continues on throughout a fighting dog's career. Puppies are exercised extensively and encouraged to engage in very rough play. Oftentimes a live small animal is used as a toy. The owner/trainer may hold the animal above a puppy's head enticing him to jump up, grab, and hold on. This is one of the first steps trainers take in making their dogs aggressive toward other animals.

As the pit bull puppy grows older, the animals used in training, commonly referred to as *bait* animals, are more likely to suffer fatal injuries. Cats, rabbits, and smaller, weaker dogs are used to build the dog's confidence and again reinforce the desirable aggressive behavior. It is not uncommon for fighters to steal neighborhood pets and use them as bait for their dogs. Bait animals who survive training sessions may later be found abandoned with injuries.

As the young dog in training becomes more confident in his fighting abilities, he will be put up against a fully trained and conditioned dog in a controlled fight. This practice is referred to as *rolling*. In addition to combat training, the dogs undergo strenuous endurance-building activities. Dogs may be forced to run on homemade treadmills for several hours a day, sometimes to exhaustion (see figure 30.2). A small animal is sometimes suspended at the end of the machine as bait to entice the dog, who may later receive the bait as a reward at the end of a training session.

As previously mentioned, the hold, shake, and tear bite style was specifically bred into the pit bull terrier in an effort to increase the dog's chances of winning in a fight. This characteristic is reinforced and strengthened in training by a device called a *spring pole*. A spring pole usually consists of a large spring suspended from a tree limb or rafter with rope or hide attached to the end; however, they sometimes simply consist of a rope or tire hanging from a tree without the spring.

The dog is trained to jump up and bite down on the rope, hide, or tire and remain suspended in mid-

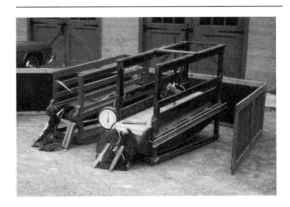

Figure 30.2. Treadmill.

air. While the dog hangs on, he will shake the target back and forth. Spring pole training provides muscle-building conditioning for the hind legs (jumping), making dogs better wrestlers, and strengthens the force of the dog's bite. Contrary to popular belief, pit bulls do not have locking jaws, nor are they born with any above-average bite power. Instead their genetically programmed style of bite along with this special training technique leads to an extremely powerful bite.

The nutritional programs provided to these dogs are also unique. Each meal is carefully calculated to ensure that the dogs are receiving the maximum levels of essential nutrients. Nutritional supplements like those used by today's bodybuilders are frequently added to diets. Supplements such as creatine monohydrate and other "muscle builder" products that can be purchased at local health food stores are added to the dogs' food along with various vitamin powders. Although dry kibble is a part of the dog's diet, the majority of the diet consists of meats such as boiled hamburger, eggs, and liver products. Homemade dietary programs are often sold by well-known fighters through various underground magazines.

Additional Uses for the Pit Bull Terrier

The street fighter in particular is more likely to utilize his dogs for other purposes in addition to fighting. Dog fighting is still very common with street fighters and gang members; however, it serves more as a source of entertainment or recognition of status. More often, however, an aggressive pit bull is essentially used much like a dangerous weapon, for protection and intimidation. Gang members use the dogs to successfully threaten and terrorize their neighborhoods, making it less likely that neighbors will report crimes. Reports of pit bulls acting as drug carriers are also not uncommon. Securing drugs inside the dog's collar or harness is one tactic used to hide drugs from police or others who might rob them of their drugs. This is an important detail to consider when examining dogs on intake at your facility. Be sure to remove and check all collars and harnesses for concealed drugs.

Pit bulls are also used as primary guard dogs, left standing guard over a criminal's home or illegal items. These dogs may be brought to a shelter or animal control facility by police or an animal control officer after execution of a search warrant against a suspected criminal. Pit bulls used as guard dogs for drug dealers or other persons carrying out illegal activities usually are receiving minimal care. They are often kept isolated, unsocialized, and underfed in unsanitary environments. Some may be debarked and declawed, allowing them to attack with minimal warning. Pit bulls raised for guard dog purposes can be some of the more dangerous ones to handle.

Medical Assessment

Dogs seized due to suspicion of fighting may need to be held as evidence for weeks to months, or even years, while owners await trial. It is most important to get a full physical assessment of the animal as soon as possible after arrival in the shelter or hospital. Upon entry to the facility, first evaluate whether it is safe to perform an exam on the dog. If handling would present a risk to staff or the dog, then medical assessment should be postponed until a later time. Staff safety should always be the first consideration. If the dog can be handled, then proceed with a thorough physical exam and document all of your findings. Bear in mind these dogs may come in heavily sedated or over tranquilized. If any ongoing treatments are to be administered, give careful consideration to the logistics of follow-up treatments in light of a more alert and potentially dangerous patient.

Throughout the intake and exam process remember that maintaining a chain of evidence is most critical to the successful outcome of the prosecution. Since the condition of the dog upon entry is likely to be used as evidence in the prosecution's case, thorough written and photographic documentation is invaluable. (See chapters 27 and 28 for more information on cruelty investigations.)

As it may be a while before the case goes to trial and the dog's condition will likely change while under your care, be careful to document initial conditions as well as improvements with time. In the physical exam, pay particular attention to all wounds, scratches, abscesses, and scars, cataloguing each in a detailed manner. The ears of pit bulls used in fighting are often cropped very close to the head so their opponents cannot grab and tear the pinna. In some cases, their ears are cropped by the owners themselves, resulting in abscesses and infection. See Figure 30.2. These dogs have a relatively high threshold of pain; therefore, lack of painful responses on exam does not rule out the possibility of serious injury (for example, gunshot wounds). Make an initial assessment of body condition scoring, document body weight, and continue to do so throughout the animal's stay. These dogs frequently have conditions related to substandard housing and care. For example, ringworm, staphylococcus pyoderma, external parasites (mange and flea infestations), heartworm disease, and intestinal parasite burdens are not uncommon. You may also want to consider taking several radiographs to document fractures in various states of healing if suspected. In an effort to maintain a chain of evidence, photographic evidence should be taken to supplement the written record. Take photographs of each animal. In each photo, hold a card in front of the dog that documents the date, animal identification number, and a brief description. Be sure that the animal is identified by a collar or microchip for follow-up exams. This is particularly important in a large-scale seizure. And, finally, be sure to date the written report and sign your name along with your assistant's name as a witness to that exam.

It is important to note that pit bulls are predisposed to several health problems unrelated to fighting. These include false pregnancy, hip dysplasia, anterior cruciate ligament rupture, demodectic mange, ringworm, allergic contact dermatitis, flea allergy dermatitis, acute moist dermatitis, acral lick granulomas, and pressure calluses (Clark 1994). The breed is also highly susceptible to parvovirus so precautions should be in place to minimize likelihood of infection at the shelter or other holding facility. Subclinical carriers of *Babesia gibsoni* have been reported at a very high frequency in American Pit Bull Terriers (Macintyre et al., 2002). (See chapter 16 for more information on Babesia.)

Routine medical care of dogs who will be held for extended periods of time should include appropriate vaccinations, deworming, heartworm testing, and prevention. While being held these dogs have a tendency to gain weight easily probably due to the less energetic lifestyle inherent in kennel housing, so weekly records of weight should be taken if feasible.

Owners of these dogs often inappropriately administer antibiotics for prolonged periods of time. Ask the investigator if antibiotics were found at the scene and document these for future reference. Should the dog need antibiotic therapy while in your care, you may find it unresponsive due to antibiotic resistance, and a different course of antibiotics will need to be selected.

Identifying Dogs Used in Fighting Activities

Identifying dogs used in fighting activities should be done carefully as the presence of scars may not always be an indication of fighting. Many nonfighting dogs are kept in fenced pens or debris cluttered yards, and it is not unusual for these dogs to have scars consistent with injuries sustained in this type of living environment. Scars primarily covering the top of the head and shoulders are more likely indicative of lacerations resulting from an attempted escape. Scars associated with fighting are usually located on the chest, face, and forelegs as seen in Figure 30.3. It is important to carefully study any scars thought to have resulted from bites. Always look for corresponding wounds or scars that would indicate upper and lower dental arcades. For example, the wounds shown in Figure 30.4 are

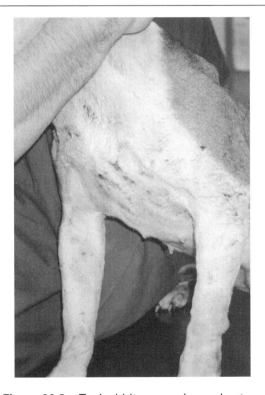

Figure 30.3. Typical bite wounds on chest, neck, and legs of pit bull. Photo credit Scott Giacoppo.

located on the inside of the leg and are matched by wounds on the opposite side as seen in Figure 30.5. A distinct upper and lower arcade scar pattern is seen on the chest of a dog in Figure 30.6.

Other injuries frequently seen in fighting or bait dogs include infections, abscesses, and healed or partially healed fractures of the legs and jaw (see Figures 30.7 and 30.8). Owners often have attempted treatment at home using suture kits, bandages, and over-the-counter medical supplies and ointments.

Sheltering Fighting Dogs

There are many special needs and precautions to consider when housing a fighting dog at a shelter. First, these dogs are often very valuable. As a result, it is not uncommon for dogs to be stolen from a shelter or

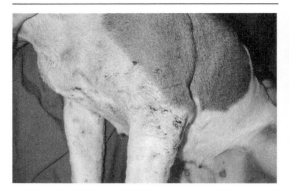

Figure 30.5. Bite wounds on lateral side of same leg in Figure 30.4. Photo credit Scott Giacoppo.

holding facility. Effective building security should be maintained at all times, during both public hours and after hours. Dogs should always be kept away from the public view and in an area restricted to staff

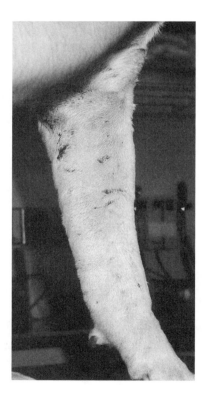

Figure 30.4. Bite wounds on medial left foreleg of pit bull. Photo credit Scott Giacoppo.

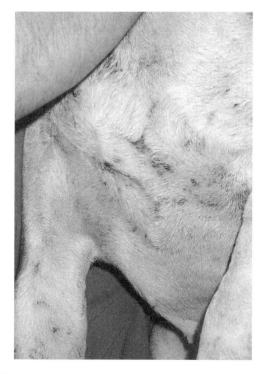

Figure 30.6. Upper and lower arcade bite wound pattern on chest of pit bull. Photo credit Scott Giacoppo.

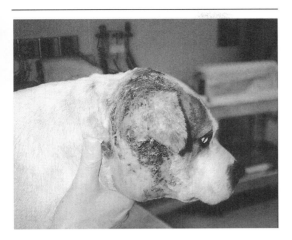

Figure 30.7. Bite wounds and abscess on head of pit bull. Photo credit Scott Giacoppo.

members only. Volunteers or service workers should not be allowed access to these dogs.

Pit bulls have a tendency to bond more closely to a handler, so it is advisable to assign as few people as possible to their care in order to maintain consistency. All staff members must be made aware of these dogs' potential for aggression and unpredictable behavior. Remind staff to remain alert to the dog's behavior at all times, even if a staff member may feel comfortable with the dog's temperament. There are many reports of handlers being attacked by sheltered fighting dogs, who had seemed even-tempered throughout their stay. Because of this, two people should always be present when handling and/or exercising these dogs.

In some instances, particularly with the professionally trained fighting dog, pit bulls show minimal signs of aggression toward people. They do, however have a strong drive to attack and kill other animals, making it important to exercise plenty of caution when walking or moving them. Walk the dogs individually and avoid any visual or physical contact with other dogs. Because they are often well conditioned and strong, be sure the staff member can physically manage the dog on leash, especially if he should become unruly. You may want to consider double leading, head halters (if it is safe to place on the dog), or a limited choke collar to improve control and safety. In certain cases, a dog may be so aggressive that daily handling will be limited. Be sure that the staff is well trained on the use of control poles, muzzles, and other safety equipment. It is also advisable to have a window in the door leading into the room where pit bulls are housed with the light switch outside in the hall. This allows the staff to safely ensure that no potentially dangerous dogs have escaped their enclosures before entering the room. It would also be advisable to install a panic button in rooms housing pit bulls, particularly if there will be occasions when only one staff member is in the room cleaning or working.

Safer kennel maintenance can be achieved by using kennels with guillotine doors. The minimal handling required by these types of kennel setups allows for the safer movement of dogs between runs in need of cleaning. Although it is important to provide bedding in order to prevent pressure sores, be sure to check the bedding frequently as these dogs can be destructive chewers and may readily ingest the bedding. Powerful jaws combined with a strong drive to chew and the boredom of kennel life may result in destruction of water and food dishes, kennel, crates, and even copper piping from automatic watering systems. (See Figure 8.1 in chapter 8.)

Because of the strong drive to attack and fight, housing can present a challenge. All dogs (even puppies from fighting lines) should be housed separately. If housed side by side, a solid partition needs to be in place, as dogs have been known to grab and harm one another through chain link or gaps in partitions. Dogs should be prevented from making direct eye contact while kenneled as this adds to their agitation and aggression. In addition, be sure that the kennel has a top on it or reaches to the ceiling, because these dogs are known climbers and can readily escape standard kennels. Kennel doors should ideally be double secured with latches and locks. It is not uncommon for dogs to escape by banging or biting on kennel doors, causing latches to open. Continue to pay attention to the importance of separation even when cleaning. If you move the dog to a holding pen while cleaning a run, be sure to maintain physical and visual separation from other dogs at all times.

Psychological Well-being of the Fighting Dog in Your Care

Being strong, high-energy, athletic animals and having a tendency to bond to their owners, the fighting dog often has a difficult time adjusting to life in the kennel. There is a tendency to go stir-crazy due to lack of physical activity and owner contact. Sheltered pit bulls often exhibit stereotypic behaviors such as repetitive leaping, spinning, pacing, or cage biting. In addition, due to the frustration, boredom, and lack of exercise these dogs experience in the shelter environment, they will frequently engage in destructive behaviors—chewing and destroying kennels, bowls, toys, and bedding. Because their powerful jaws can readily damage even the strongest chain link, be sure to check all kennels daily for damage that might cause harm to the dog or allow for escape. Because these dogs can be so destructive, some may think it best to limit their access to toys and bedding, but this will only lead to more behavioral problems. For dogs kept in their kennels, try to provide as much behavioral enrichment as possible. Toys that keep their minds busy are the best, such as a Kong toy stuffed with treats, or a Buster Cube that requires lots of activity in order to receive a food reward. It may be necessary, however, to provide even sturdier items for them to play with, such as bowling balls or old rubber tires. Because pit bulls are short-coated dogs, it is always important to provide a soft bed for their comfort.

Physical exercise, if it can be done safely, is very important to the dog's overall well-being while in your care. Because these animals are most often being held as evidence, exercise should be on leash only and preferably within a secured, fenced-in area to prevent escape. As stated earlier, safety is a priority while exercising. Have two staff members present at all times, and exercise the dogs separately. Extreme caution should be used when interacting with these dogs because they tend to be easily aroused and over-stimulated once removed from the cage. They will often grab hold of their leash and tug fiercely as they walk. While in this state of high arousal, they can easily be triggered to become aggressive. Staff should never use physical punishment or harsh leash corrections on these dogs as this can elicit an aggressive attack. Muzzle those dogs with questionable temperament if necessary to ensure staff safety.

Long-term housing presents many challenges. It is very difficult to provide for the behavioral needs of fighting dogs in a kennel over long periods of time. Watch for the development of behavioral side effects such as depression, boredom, self-mutilation, increasingly destructive or aggressive behav-

iors, appetite changes, and weight loss or gain. Taking daily notes with regard to the temperament and behavioral health of the dogs is important. In certain circumstances, the court may use this information to force the signing over of dogs for euthanasia if long-term housing is causing undue stress or risk to the dog or staff.

Rehoming Pit Bulls

It is never advisable to rehome a known or suspected fighting pit bull. Rehabilitation of a dog that has been genetically engineered and trained to fight other dogs to the death is not only unsafe but also virtually impossible. Pit bulls that enter your facility as strays or who have been surrendered by their owners, however, may be placable after an extensive behavioral evaluation. There are certain breed characteristics, however, that make the pit bull unsuitable for most homes. Because of their incredible strength, intelligence, and energy level, they are usually too much for the average dog owner. Pit bull terriers are very easily aroused dogs with an intense play style that can be overwhelming to owners and other dogs. They tend to enjoy the game of tug, regardless of any past spring-pole type training and can become quite aroused and dangerous when playing in this manner. This trait makes them unsuitable for placement into homes with small children. They also have a very high prey drive, which can make them dangerous around other pets such as cats, rabbits, and ferrets. Because of their high intelligence, pit bulls are easily trained, but this intelligence can lead to behavior problems if the dog is under-stimulated. For all these reasons, extreme care should be used when placing a pit bull into a home.

Behavioral Evaluation

It is critical to carefully and extensively evaluate any pit bull that is being considered for rehoming. Because of their genetic predisposition for dog aggression, they should be introduced to a number of other dogs to determine their propensity for fighting. Even dogs that have not been trained or used as fighting dogs can show aggression toward other dogs. The dog in question should be introduced to the other dogs on a very strong lead and collar that it cannot slip out of. Two people should be present during the evaluation to ensure the safety of the handler and the other dogs. Because pit bulls do not generally give warning signals before attacking, and because of their lightning fast reaction time, evaluators must be extra attentive and observant. Extreme caution should be used when bringing the dogs together, and the evaluators should be looking for signs of intense focus on the other dog. This may be the only warning signal given prior to an attack. After a pit bull has decided to attack, it will be virtually impossible to stop him, and the other dog will undoubtedly be harmed. Dogs that do not show signs of intense focus and whose body language remains loose and friendly should be allowed to approach and interact with the other dog. The dog in question should be introduced to a minimum of four other dogs, preferably of different size, gender, and breed. Only those dogs that show absolutely no aggression toward the other dogs should be considered for placement.

Another very crucial aspect of the pit bull temperament that needs to be evaluated is the dog's arousal level. The evaluator should engage the dog in play to determine how quickly he becomes aroused, how intense the arousal level is, and how long it takes for him to settle down once the play has ended. Because tug-of-war is a favored game of the pit bull, the evaluator should entice the dog with a rope toy held up high above his head. This will test the dog's propensity for jumping, grabbing, and tugging. A dog that shows intense focus on the rope toy, jumps off the ground to get a hold of it, and relentlessly tugs, is a dog that may be unsuitable for placement. This intense arousal level is difficult to manage and can be quite dangerous. It has also been suggested that a spring-pole type device be hung from a tree to test whether the dog has been trained using this method. The evaluation would include walking the dog past the pole and watching his reaction. A dog who has been spring-pole trained can be very dangerous if he was ever to bite someone, as he has been conditioned to bite, hang on, and shake.

These dogs may be docile and easy to handle and pass temperament tests if sick or in compromised physical condition upon entry to your facility. As they recover medically, however, they can become increasingly aggressive. Because of this, behavioral evaluations may need to be done on multiple occasions as the recovery process progresses.

The placement of pit bulls should be done with extreme care. Anyone interested in adopting a pit bull should be advised to socialize their dogs to people and other dogs, provide aerobic exercise every day, and to train them to a high degree of reliability. Potential adopters should also be made aware that some pit bulls do not exhibit their genetically predetermined tendency to be aggressive towards other dogs until they reach social maturity at the age of 2–3 years. This late onset dog aggression often occurs regardless of the amount of socialization the dog has received as a puppy.

COCKFIGHTING

Although cockfighting is legal in only two states (New Mexico and Louisiana and under legal challenge in Oklahoma), the sport continues to be carried on illegally throughout the United States. It is an ages old sport not unfamiliar to many varied cultures. This chapter will focus mostly upon examination, handling, and housing of gamecocks.

Recognizing a Gamecock

The American Poultry Association publishes the American Standard of Perfection, which outlines varieties of poultry including the gamecocks. There are two main fighting varieties, the Spanish gamecocks (such as the Malay, Cubalaya, Shamo, and Yokohama) and the Yankee gamecocks (which include the Modern Game and Old English). Most frequently, the fighters we see in law enforcement and shelters are hybrids of these birds and do not resemble their pure-bred ancestors. Fighters have learned that by cross breeding varieties, they can achieve a maximally aggressive bird. When questioned, owners of fighting birds may claim they are in fact show birds. It is generally easy to disprove this by simply referring to the show standards relating to size and color as outlined in the book. The build and coloring of fighting gamecocks today is greatly varied from the breed standards. In addition, show birds are required to be disease tested by the state and to wear leg bands at all times. Rarely if ever will fighting gamecocks have these leg bands. In fact, birds are frequently shipped live in crates without following any of the appropriate testing requirements.

In order to prevent injury during a fight, the combs and wattles of fighting cocks may have been trimmed. In addition, some fighters shave feathers around the legs and over the dorsal lumbar region. See Figure 30.8.

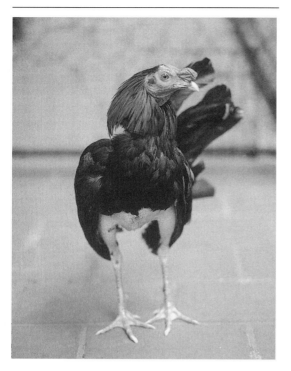

Figure 30.8. Typical fighting bird shaved by its owner to better detect "points" or injuries and to keep cool during the fight. Photo credit Mary Bloom.

Preparing for the Fight

All roosters will fight, and most fight with great vigor. Due to their breeding, the fighting gamecocks are even more territorial and aggressive than the standard rooster. In addition, they are forced into a ring where they have no choice but to fight and will fight until one or both are dead or too injured to continue. The purpose of this spectator sport is for entertainment and gambling. Because of this, fights must be intense, bloody, and relatively short to hold the audience's attention and allow for maximal gambling opportunities. In order to make the fight more gruesome, gamecocks often have their spurs filed down or cut off. The bird is then outfitted with razor-sharp steel blades or steel or plastic gaffs that are attached by boots to their legs. These artificial spurs ensure maximum injury during a strike on another bird.

Roosters do not undergo rigorous training programs like the pit bulls often do; nevertheless, rooster tread mills have been recovered from illegal operations. More frequently, the fighters use drugs to enhance the rooster's performance. Stimulants (strychnine is the most popular) are given to increase the rooster's aggression and agitation. Some receive hormones and even blood-clotting agents have been used to maximize their performance.

Housing and Handling Gamecocks

Seizure of gamecocks most frequently occurs on a large scale with numerous birds requiring housing in shelters and holding facilities. The birds may need to be held as evidence, sometimes for weeks or months, pending the owner's trial. Most shelters are not equipped to house large numbers of birds yet creative, safe, and secure shelter can be provided. It is important to remember that roosters will be stimulated to fight if they can see one another, so placement of visible barriers is equally as important as physical separation. Caging should be set such that minimal handling of birds (especially roosters) is necessary.

One housing technique that has worked well for temporary and long-term care is the use of standard dog show pens with a top that can be secured. Wood shavings are the preferred bedding. It is best to avoid using hay as it may present a risk of Aspergillosis to the birds. Wood shavings are spread on the floor (ideally a cement floor) where the birds will be housed. The pens are then set side by side in rows with at least a foot distance between each pen. It is important to separate the pens in this manner to prevent roosters from fighting and injuring one another through the pens. In addition, to minimize agitation and aggression, remember to provide visual barriers between each pen. Plywood or cardboard have been used successfully for this purpose. It is also important to secure the top of the pen with a clip or lock to prevent escape. The rows of pens should be set at least 4–5 feet apart, which creates a large walkway or aisle. This setup also allows for ease of cleaning. Simply spread clean shavings in the aisle, slide the pen with the bird inside over to the clean shavings, and then sweep and disinfect the floor where the pen once was.

Roosters should always be housed individually. If space is a problem, hens can be housed together, ideally in pairs, as they have less of a tendency to fight. This is because the fighting cock breeders do not select aggressive hens. Instead, they prefer to select hens who tend well to their clutch. Nevertheless, always be sure to monitor the behavior of paired up hens and be certain they will not fight before leaving them unattended. At the sign of any aggressive behavior, separate them immediately.

Medical Assessment and Common Injuries

Just like in the case of the seized fighting dog, it is imperative to maintain a chain of evidence. Careful and accurate documentation of the birds' condition upon entry and throughout their stay is very important. Both written and photographic documentation should be recorded, as this will all provide necessary evidence in a potential criminal trial.

Most wounds that result from fighting occur to the head. Birds that survive a fight will often have a great deal of swelling to their face and particularly around their eyes. Frequently the razors or gaffs will pierce eyes during a fight so it is important to look carefully past any facial or periocular swelling to assess the status of the globe and orbit. Noses can be encrusted with blood, making breathing difficult. In addition to facial injuries, birds may sustain punctured lungs and fractured wings and/or legs.

Some medications to have on hand that are useful in treating birds include topical ointments such as Furazone and triple antibiotic, and Terramycin powder that can be added to the water if needed.

If your facility houses other birds, be careful to appropriately quarantine the seized fighting birds and pay attention to avoiding any potential cross contamination. It is not uncommon for seized birds to develop laryngotracheitis secondary to stress. Be sure to consult with your state veterinarian or bureau of animal health/agriculture to learn which tests are required in your state. For example, in Massachusetts, all poultry must be tested for avian influenza and *Salmonella pullorum* when moved within state. It is thought that the illegal transport of fighting cocks may be contributing to the spread of poultry diseases in this country.

In 2002, an outbreak of exotic Newcastle Disease occurred in the southwestern states and is now considered an epidemic in that area of the country. It is suspected that this outbreak originated from fighting cocks smuggled in from Mexico. The nature of cockfighting further facilitates the spread of this disease as cockfighting inherently involves the congregation and subsequent dispersal of birds in a short period of time and after maximum exposure (housing and fighting at gaming events). Some state's animal health bureaus are concerned about

further spread of this disease within the United States and may now be requiring testing of these birds upon arrival to the shelter. Check with your local authorities for your responsibility in reporting arrivals of fighting birds to your facility.

Rehoming

Due to the highly aggressive nature of these birds, rehoming or placement into a sanctuary is not a realistic option. Fighting cocks cannot be housed with any other birds (even nonfighting varieties), as they are likely to kill them. Unfortunately, in most instances euthanasia will be the only option once a case is won and/or the fighting birds are legally turned over to you. Euthanasia should be performed using an intracoelomic injection of sodium pentobarbital.

CONCLUSION

Fighting animals add a unique dimension to shelter practice from a housing as well as medical standpoint. These animals often cannot be treated in the same manner as their "domesticated" or socialized counterparts, and safe handling is a major consideration. Indeed some of our greatest challenges lie in maintaining quality care and chain of evidence with animals that are frequently difficult and dangerous to handle.

REFERENCES

American Poultry Association. 2001. *The American Standard of Perfection*: The American Poultry Association.

Clark, R. D., and Stainer, J. (eds.). 1994. *Medical and Genetic Aspects of Purebred Dogs*, Fairway, KS: Forum Publications.

Colby, L. B. 1997. *Colby's Book of the American Pit Bull Terrier*: Neptune City, NJ: TFH Publications.

Dundes, A. 1994. *The Cockfight: A Casebook*. Madison, WI: University of Wisconsin Press.

Kirkwood, S. 1997. *Animal Sheltering*. Dogfighting: Sheltering the Victims. Washington, DC: The Humane Society of the United States.

Macintire, D. K., M. K. Boudreaux, et al. 2002. *Babesia gibsoni* infection among dogs in the southeastern United States. *Journal of the American Veterinary Medical Association* (220): 325–9.

Manley, F. 1998. *The Cockfighter*. Minneapolis, MN: Coffee House Press.

Stratton, R. F. 1991. *The Truth About the American Pit Bull Terrier*. Neptune City, NJ: TFH Publications.

Stratton, R. F. 1992 *World of the American Pit Bull Terrier*. Neptune City, NJ: TFH Publications.

Appendix 1
Animal Welfare Organizations and General Information

ORGANIZATIONS

These organizations provide advice, publications, training, and other support for the shelter animal care professional.

American Humane (AH)
63 Inverness Drive East
Englewood, CO 80112
303-792-9900 or 800-227-4645
www.americanhumane.org

American Society for the Prevention of Cruelty to Animals (ASPCA)
424 East 92nd Street
New York, NY 10128
212-876-7700
www.aspca.org

Doing Things for Animals (DTFA)
59 South Bayles Avenue
Port Washington, NY 11050
516-883-7767
Fax 516-944-5035
www.dtfa.org

Humane Society of the United States (HSUS)
2100 L Street, N.W.
Washington, D.C. 20037
202-452-1100
www.hsus.org

National Animal Control Association (NACA)
P.O. Box 480851
Kansas City, MO 64148
913-768-1319
Fax 913-768-0607
www.netplace.net/naca

World Society for the Protection of Animals (WSPA)
29 Perkins Street

P.O. Box 190
Boston, MA 02130
617-522-7000
www.wspa.org.uk

OTHER RESOURCES

American Red Cross
Offers an on-line booklet, *Pets in Natural Disasters*.
www.redcross.org/disaster/safety/pets.html

Animal Care and Equipment Services (ACES)
340 South Highway 138
Crestline, CA 93325
909-338-1791
800-338-ACES; fax 909-338-2799
www.animal-care.com

Petfinder.com
A national network that offers a state-by-state listing of animals available for adoption, lost and found, and shelters. Provides the largest searchable database of animals. Back page for members only offers advice from the ASPCA's National Shelter Outreach experts, including an on-line library, and provides a networking resource to shelters and rescues. Membership is free.
908-810-1976
www.petfinder.com

Pet Savers Foundation
Offers a shelter supplies discount program.
750 Port Washington Boulevard, Suite 2
Port Washington, NY 11050
516-944-5025
Fax 516-944-5035
www.petsavers.org

SPAY/USA
This organization provides nationwide service to shelters by providing referrals to local low-cost spay/neuter

programs and by helping to develop new programs and clinics.

750 Port Washington Blvd
Port Washington, NY 11050
800-248-SPAY
www.spayusa.org

VETERINARY ORGANIZATIONS

American Animal Hospital Association (AAHA)
12575 W. Bayaud Avenue
Lakewood, CO 80228
303-986-2800
www.aaha.net

American Association of Veterinary State Boards (AAVSB)
4106 Central
Kansas City, MO 64111
816-931-1504
www.aavsb.org

American Veterinary Medical Association (AVMA)
1931 North Meacham Road, Suite 100
Schaumburg, IL 60173
847-925-8070 or 800-248-AVMA
www.avma.org

Association of Shelter Veterinarians
Shelter veterinarian list service at sheltervet-subscribe@yahoogroups.com
www.sheltervet.org

University of California at Davis Veterinary College
Companion Animal Health Department
Maddie's Shelter Medicine Program
www.vetmed.ucdavis.edu/CCAH/Prog-ShelterMed.htm

ANIMAL BEHAVIOR RESOURCES

A trainer learns his or her craft through apprenticing, assisting in group classes, volunteering at animal shelters, attending seminars, and working with as many dogs as possible. Although thousands of people call themselves trainers, this is an unlicensed profession in most states, so quality and methodology vary tremendously.

Canine trainers offer group classes, private lessons, or board-and-train sessions. All manner of canine etiquette and dog sports are taught in group classes. Private lessons are best for solving in-home problems or for obedience instruction when owners have erratic schedules. Board-and-train allows someone else to train the dog without owner supervision. For this to be effective, the caretakers must be brought up to speed on what the dog was taught and how, as well as how to reinforce it.

Applied animal behaviorists have an advanced degree in animal behavior and may also be certified by the Animal Behavior Society. They work with the client's veterinarian to rule out any physical causes for behavior problems, and treatment can include drug therapy. The field is well suited for solving severe fears and phobias, obsessive/compulsive disorders, and aggression.

Veterinary behaviorists are the newest members of the problem-solving triad, as the specialty just became available for board certification by the American Veterinary Medical Association's Behavior College in 1995. These professionals may perform the diagnostic tests needed to rule out physical sources for a problem behavior (or, more likely, refer you to your own veterinarian) and then recommend appropriate behavior modification techniques, coupled with nutritional and drug therapies, if needed. For more information, contact the following organizations:

American Veterinary Society of Animal Behavior
avsabe@yahoo.com
www.avma.org/avsab

Animal Behavior Society
www.animalbehavior.org

Association of Pet Dog Trainers
P.O. Box 385
Davis, CA 95617
800-PET-DOGS
www.apdt.com

Index